# Making Senses of the Past

Visiting Scholar Conference Volumes

Processual and Postprocessual Archaeologies: Multiple Ways of Knowing the Past (Occasional Paper No. 10) *edited by Robert W. Preucel*

Paleonutrition: The Diet and Health of Prehistoric Americans (Occasional Paper No. 22) *edited by Kristin D. Sobolik*

Integrating Archaeological Demography: Multidisciplinary Approaches to Prehistoric Population (Occasional Paper No. 24) *edited by Richard R. Paine*

Material Symbols: Culture and Economy in Prehistory (Occasional Paper No. 26) *edited by John E. Robb*

Hierarchies in Action: *Cui Bono?* (Occasional Paper No. 27) *edited by Michael W. Diehl*

Fleeting Identities: Perishable Material Culture in Archaeological Research (Occasional Paper No. 28) *edited by Penelope Ballard Drooker*

The Dynamics of Power (Occasional Paper No. 30) *edited by Maria O'Donovan*

Hunters and Gatherers in Theory and Archaeology (Occasional Paper No. 31) *edited by George M. Crothers*

Biomolecular Archaeology: Genetic Approaches to the Past (Occasional Paper No. 32) *edited by David M. Reed*

Leadership and Polity in Mississippian Society (Occasional Paper No. 33) *edited by Brian M. Butler and Paul D. Welch*

The Archaeology of Food and Identity (Occasional Paper No. 34) *edited by Katheryn C. Twiss*

The Durable House: House Society Models in Archaeology (Occasional Paper No. 35) *edited by Robin A. Beck Jr.*

Religion, Archaeology, and the Material World (Occasional Paper No. 36) *edited by Lars Fogelin*

The Archaeology of Anthropogenic Environments (Occasional Paper No. 37) *edited by Rebecca M. Dean*

Human Variation in the Americas: The Integration of Archaeology and Biological Anthropology (Occasional Paper No. 38) *edited by Benjamin M. Auerbach*

# Making Senses of the Past

## Toward a Sensory Archaeology

*Edited by*
*Jo Day*

*Center for Archaeological Investigations*
Southern Illinois University Carbondale
Occasional Paper No. 40

*Southern Illinois University Press*
Carbondale and Edwardsville

Printed in the United States of America
16 15 14 13 4 3 2 1

**Library of Congress Cataloging-in-Publication Data**
Annual Visiting Scholar Conference (27th ; 2010 Carbondale, Illinois)
Making senses of the past : toward a sensory archaeology / edited by Jo Day.
p. cm. — (Occasional paper ; no. 40)
Includes bibliographical references and index.
ISBN-13: 978-0-8093-3287-8 (pbk. : alk. paper)
ISBN-10: 0-8093-3287-6 (pbk. : alk. paper)
ISBN-13: 978-0-8093-3313-4 (ebook)
ISBN-10: 0-8093-3313-9 (ebook)
1. Archaeology—Methodology—Congresses. 2. Senses and sensation—Congresses. 3. Archaeology—Social aspects—Congresses. 4: Archaeology—Psychological aspects—Congresses. 5. Material culture—Social aspects—Congresses. 6. Material culture—Psychological aspects—Congresses. I. Day, Jo (Jo Christine) II. Southern Illinois University at Carbondale. Center for Archaeological Investigations. III. Title.
CC75.7.A59 2013
930.1—dc23 2013006791

Copyedited by Mary Lou Wilshaw-Watts
Production supervised by Mary Lou Wilshaw-Watts
Designed and formatted by Linda Jorgensen Buhman, New Leaf Studio

Printed by authority of the State of Illinois.

For information, write to the Center for Archaeological Investigations, Faner 3479, Mail Code 4527, Southern Illinois University, 1000 Faner Drive, Carbondale, IL 62901; phone (618) 453-5031; or visit us online at www.cai.siu.edu.

The paper used in this publication meets the minimum requirements of American National Standard for Information Sciences—Permanence of Paper for Printed Library Materials, ANSI Z39.48-1992. ♾

# Contents


Figures vii

Tables xi

Acknowledgments xii

1. Introduction: Making Senses of the Past
*Jo Day* 1

2. *Dibéwagendamowin / Kārohirohi*: Reflections on Sacred Images on the Rocks
*William A. Allen, Gerard O'Regan, Perry Fletcher, and Roger Noganosh* 32

3. The Sound of Sulfur and Smell of Lightning: Sensing the Volcano
*Karen Holmberg* 49

4. Colored Monuments and Sensory Theater among the Mississippians
*Corin C. O. Pursell* 69

5. Maya Palaces as Experiences: Ancient Maya Royal Architecture and Its Influence on Sensory Perception
*Ryan Mongelluzzo* 90

6. Coming to Our Senses at Chavín de Huantar
*Mary Weismantel* 113

7. The Sensory Experience of Blood Sacrifice in the Roman Imperial Cult
*Candace Weddle* 137

8. Embodying the Divine: The Sensational Experience of the Sixth-Century Eucharist
*Heather Hunter-Crawley* 160

9. A Sense of Touch—the Full-Body Experience—in the Past and Present of Çatalhöyük, Turkey
*Ruth Tringham* 177

10. Musical Space and Quiet Space in Medieval Monastic Canterbury
*Joe Williams* 196

11. Sustenance, Taste, and the Practice of Community in Ancient Mesopotamia
*Marie Hopwood* 222

12. The Scent of Status: Prestige and Perfume at the Bronze Age Palace at Pylos, Greece
*Joanne M. A. Murphy* 243

13. A Whiff of Mortality: The Smells of Death in Roman and Byzantine Beth She'an-Scythopolis
*Emerson Avery* 266

14. Imagined Aromas and Artificial Flowers in Minoan Society
*Jo Day* 286

15. Craft and Sensory Play in Late Bronze Age Boeotia
*Anastasia Dakouri-Hild* 310

16. Scents and Sensibilities: The Phenomenology of Late Neolithic Iberian Slate Plaque Production
*Jonathan T. Thomas* 335

17. The Production Process as Sensory Experience: Making and Seeing Iron in Colonial New England
*Krysta Ryzewski* 351

18. Beyond the Display Case: Creating a Multisensory Museum Experience
*Catherine P. Foster* 371

19. Imagined Narratives: Sensory Lives in the Chacoan Southwest
*Ruth M. Van Dyke* 390

20. Afterword: Eleven Theses on the Archaeology of the Senses
*Yannis Hamilakis* 409

Contributors 421

Index 423

# Figures


| | | |
|---|---|---|
| 2-1. | Location of French River and Rock Lake, Ontario, Canada | 34 |
| 2-2. | The eastern rock painting panel visited at Rock Lake | 36 |
| 2-3. | William Allen at the eastern Rock Lake painted panel | 37 |
| 2-4. | Map of Lake Taupō, New Zealand | 38 |
| 2-5. | Kawakawa Bay bluffs | 39 |
| 2-6. | Perry Fletcher with *koru* rock painting | 40 |
| 3-1. | Olafur Eliasson, *The Body as Brain—Lava Floor* | 57 |
| 3-2. | Map of Volcán Barú | 58 |
| 3-3. | Volcanic bomb recovered during archaeological fieldwork and pestle from Yale University Peabody Museum | 61 |
| 4-1. | Map of Shiloh and Cahokia mounds in southeastern United States | 71 |
| 4-2. | Map of Shiloh showing mounds discussed in text | 71 |
| 4-3. | Thresholds of visibility | 75 |
| 4-4. | Types of presentational spaces | 76 |
| 4-5. | Mound A, approaching from the plaza: nonmonumental experience | 78 |
| 4-6. | Mound A, approaching from the river: experience of monumentality | 78 |
| 4-7. | Mound C, north approach: constrained monumental experience | 78 |
| 4-8. | Map of Shiloh representing the plaza as a ritual arena | 80 |
| 4-9. | Map of Shiloh representing the Mound A–plaza relationship as a ritual hall | 80 |
| 4-10. | Map of Shiloh representing the Mound C area as a restricted ritual hall | 81 |
| 4-11. | Map of Shiloh comparing two proposed ritual scenarios | 83 |
| 4-12. | Contrasting ideas as suggested by ethnohistoric data and tested at Shiloh | 85 |
| 5-1. | Map of Holmul site core | 92 |
| 5-2. | Map of Group III, Holmul | 93 |
| 5-3. | Three-dimensional reconstruction of Holmul palace | 93 |
| 5-4. | Plan view of Holmul palace | 98 |
| 5-5. | Map of Tikal site core | 99 |
| 5-6. | Cross section of the south profile of Holmul palace | 100 |
| 5-7. | Plan view of Tikal's Central Acropolis | 101 |
| 5-8. | Three-dimensional reconstruction of pronouncement stage, central inner courtyard, Holmul palace | 104 |

6-1. Map of Chavín de Huantar, Peru 115
6-2. Sketch plan of site of Chavín de Huantar 116
6-3. Underground gallery at Chavín de Huantar 119
6-4. Line drawing of "male cayman" on Obelisk Tello 121
6-5. Rubbing of Raimondi Stela 121
6-6. The Lanzón 123
6-7. The Black and White Portal 123
7-1. Relief showing a sacrifice on twentieth anniversary of Hadrian's reign 139
7-2. Detail of relief from honorary monument to Marcus Aurelius: sacrifice to Capitoline Jupiter 141
7-3. Refuse pit containing entrails, hooves, blood, and waste at Istanbul Kurban Bayram sacrificial area 144
7-4. A woman cleans entrails in front of blood-covered concrete wall at Kurban Bayram sacrificial area 145
7-5. Blood falling from Kurban Bayram trailer platform following slaughter of bull 146
7-6. Kurban Bayram refuse pit, filled with dirt and concrete, 50 days after sacrifices 147
8-1. Riha paten 164
8-2. Riha chalice 166
8-3. Riha fan 168
8-4. Bronze incense burner 170
8-5. Cross-shaped polycandelon 171
9-1. Map of location and excavation areas of Çatalhöyük, Turkey 179
9-2. Three different kinds of touch: global touch, reach touch, and extended touch 181
9-3. Contact traces that might survive archaeologically from different kinds of touch 182
10-1. Map showing location of Canterbury, United Kingdom 198
10-2. Justified access maps of St. Gregory's Priory and St. Augustine's Abbey 203
10-3. Format of graph used to obtain levels of presence availability for spaces in a system 205
10-4. Presence availability diagram of St. Augustine's Abbey, including exterior 206
10-5. Presence availability diagram of St. Gregory's Priory, including exterior 207
10-6. Quiet space presence availability genotypes of St. Gregory's Priory (SGP) and St. Augustine's Abbey (SAA) 211
10-7. Details of PA diagrams of St. Gregory's Priory and St. Augustine's Abbey, showing cloisters and neighboring spaces 213
11-1. Regional map of modern Turkey and Syria, showing location of Fıstıklı Höyük in southeastern Turkey 228
11-2. Fıstıklı Höyük settlement as it existed at height of occupation in Phase IIIa 228

11-3. Restricted vessel shapes from Fıstıklı Höyük 230
11-4. Unrestricted vessel shapes from Fıstıklı Höyük 230
11-5. Examples of painted pottery from Fıstıklı Höyük 236
12-1. Map of Mycenaean sites mentioned in text 245
12-2. Linear B tablet Un 718 245
12-3. Parts of the brain connected with smell and memory 247
12-4. Plan of the Palace of Nestor, Pylos, indicating areas of feasting, storage, production, and the lower town 250
12-5. Stirrup jar 252
13-1. Late Roman Palestine, with sites mentioned in text 267
13-2. Detail of Beth She'an Northern Cemetery, with tombs 269
13-3. Plan of Tomb 210 269
13-4. Plan of Tomb 201 270
13-5. Byzantine-period lamps from Tombs 206 and 224 271
13-6. Mirror plaque from Tomb 208 272
13-7. GC-MS chromatogram for silylated sample extracted from unguentarium 29-105-647 274
13-8. Entrance to Tomb 239 278
14-1. Maps of eastern Mediterranean and Crete, showing locations mentioned in text 288
14-2. Stone blossom bowl, Milatos 291
14-3. Egyptian lotiform chalice 291
14-4. Kamares-ware jug with painted rosette, Phaistos 294
14-5. Krater with floral relief, Phaistos 295
14-6. Bowl with "floating" flower, Sphoungaras 295
14-7. Pedestal with relief petals, Phaistos 297
14-8. Calyx cup, Knossos 297
15-1. Citadel of Thebes with surrounding cemeteries and distribution of workshops 314
15-2. House of Kadmos with distribution and absolute quantities of workshop-related finds and production stages and states represented by agate 315
15-3. Types of recognizable artifacts represented by agate assemblage 317
15-4. Failed artifacts among agate finds 318
15-5. Multiple lives of an agate object 318
15-6. Affordances of agate in action 321
15-7. Shiny things 324
15-8. Pattern and contrasts in agate finds 325
15-9. Free-style agate objects 327
16-1. Enigmatic engraved slate plaque from Valencina de la Concepción (Seville, Spain) featuring common cross-hatched triangle pattern underneath more rarely occurring ocular imagery 338
16-2. Only known plaque production site at Águas Frias (northern Portugal), where entire *chaîne opératoire* is evident 341
16-3. Experimental slate plaque preforms being ground into trapezoidal shapes on pavement 341

| | | |
|---|---|---|
| 16-4. | Engraved slate plaque from Pedra Branca used as template | 343 |
| 17-1. | Map of Rhode Island with Greene Farm, Potowomut, and Coventry—Greene family iron-production sites | 353 |
| 17-2. | Smith iron forging at Mystic Seaport Museum, Connecticut | 356 |
| 17-3. | Craftsperson judging iron's material and sensory properties | 358 |
| 17-4. | One of the last remaining outcrops of cumberlandite ore, Cumberland, Rhode Island | 358 |
| 17-5. | Anvil and anchor from eighteenth-century Greene family forge, Potowomut, Rhode Island | 361 |
| 17-6. | Electron microscope image of slag structures in wrought-iron tool from Greene Farm | 362 |
| 17-7. | Optical microscope image of nail sample from Greene Farm | 362 |
| 17-8. | Photomosaic of cross section of wrought nail from Greene Farm | 363 |
| 17-9. | Optical microscopy image of iron tool from Potowomut | 364 |
| 17-10. | The smith and his audience at Colonial Williamsburg | 366 |
| 18-1. | *Lived Experience in Ancient Judah*, Badè Museum of Biblical Archaeology, Berkeley, California | 376 |
| 18-2. | Archaeology as faith: *What Remains*, 2010, by Pamela Blotner | 379 |
| 18-3. | Quantification of senses: *Six Visions*, 2010, by Pamela Blotner | 380 |
| 18-4. | Musical rhythms of daily life: *Day by Day*, 2010, by Pamela Blotner | 381 |
| 18-5. | Social sense of community: *Gathering*, 2010, by Pamela Blotner | 383 |
| 19-1. | Map of San Juan basin showing Chaco Canyon, outlier great houses, and other landscape features circa 1020–1100 C.E. | 392 |
| 19-2. | Great house of Pueblo Bonito, looking south from the north rim of Chaco Canyon | 393 |
| 19-3. | Navajo archaeologist Davina Two Bears contemplates tenth-century enclosure at Willow Canyon complex south of the Chaco Wash, along the route described in the imagined narratives | 395 |
| 19-4. | Group of Colorado College students approaching Pueblo Bonito from east, along modern park-service trail | 396 |

# Tables


| | | |
|---|---|---|
| 10-1. | St. Augustine's Abbey: Access Analysis Data for Quiet Spaces | 204 |
| 10-2. | St. Gregory's Priory: Access Analysis Data for Quiet Spaces | 204 |
| 11-1. | Dates and Descriptions for Fıstıklı Höyük Occupational Phases | 229 |
| 11-2. | Percentages of Coarse Ware Sherds by Categories of Vessel Use across the Four Occupational Phases at Fıstıklı Höyük | 231 |
| 19-1. | How Narrative Decision Points Articulate with Existing Issues and Lead to New Research Questions | 400 |

# Acknowledgments

My initial words of thanks must go to all my colleagues at the Center for Archaeological Investigations and in the Department of Anthropology at Southern Illinois University Carbondale for deciding to take a gamble on a conference topic that, to some, may have seemed a little extraordinary. The support of them and their families throughout my year in Carbondale, and their kindness to a stranger in a strange land, made my experiences there enjoyable and memorable. To the many friends who guided me through the occasionally baffling intricacies of daily life in southern Illinois, I hope some day I will be able to repay the favor back in Ireland.

The conference could not have happened without the help of numerous people. At the CAI, the advice and assistance of Brian Butler, Kathy Lundeen, Heather Lapham, and Mark Wagner made my job ten times easier; in the Department of Anthropology, special thanks go to Paul Welch, Susan Ford, David Sutton, and Tony Webster. Thanks, too, to the CAI selection committee for their input into the lineup of speakers. I benefited greatly from the archive of previous visiting scholar conferences and am much obliged to my predecessors for their words of wisdom. Behind the scenes, the unfailing energy of Pat Eckert and Kim Goforth of the Division of Continuing Education, SIU Carbondale, ensured that everything was well organized.

That the event itself was a success is thanks to the wonderful multitasking student volunteers: Ayla Amadio, Samantha Hayes, Lea Hinchcliff, Craig Kitchen, Go Matsumoto, Kayeleigh Sharp, and Qiaoyun Zhang. The generosity of the many publishers who contributed to the conference book display was greatly appreciated, as was the technical support provided by the staff at Morris Library. I'm very grateful to Yannis Hamilakis for delivering the keynote address and to Robin Beck, who gamely accepted the challenge to be the conference discussant on somewhat short notice. Needless to say, the speakers and all the other attendees should be commended for creating an atmosphere that fostered discussion of many exciting ideas over the course of the weekend.

The process of turning conference papers into a coherent book is a lengthy and sometimes challenging one, and I'd like to express my gratitude to all the authors for their cooperation and patience during this metamorphosis. The feedback from the anonymous reviewers is much appreciated too. Thanks also to my graduate seminar class, who explored sensory methodologies in archaeology with me during my year at SIU Carbondale, often opening my eyes to new approaches, new critiques, and new material.

Finally, and most important in the context of this volume, a huge "thank you" to Mary Lou Wilshaw-Watts (CAI publications editor) for her guidance and advice, her editorial skills, her good humor, her emergency sweater, and her friendship.

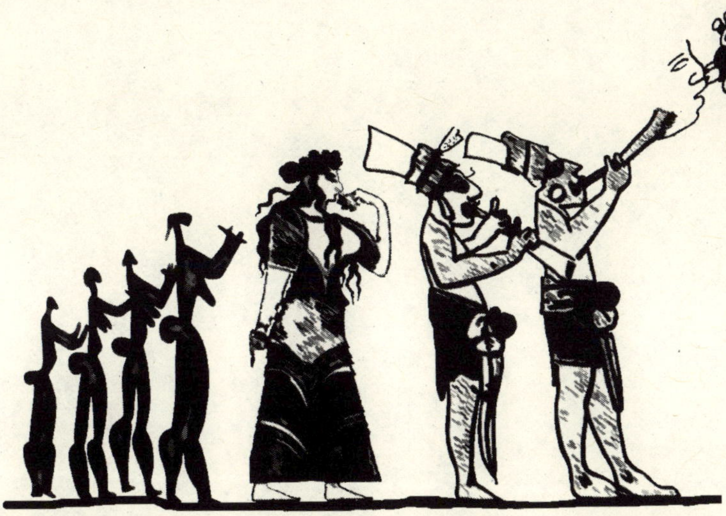

# 1. Introduction: Making Senses of the Past

*Jo Day*

*Correspondances*
La Nature est un temple où de vivants piliers
Laissent parfois sortir de confuses paroles;
L'homme y passe à travers des forêts de symboles
Qui l'observent avec des regards familiers.

Comme de longs échos qui de loin se confondent
Dans une ténébreuse et profonde unité,
Vaste comme la nuit et comme la clarté,
Les parfums, les couleurs et les sons se répondent.

Il est des parfums frais comme des chairs d'enfants,
Doux comme les hautbois, verts comme les prairies,
—Et d'autres, corrumpus, riches et triomphants,

Ayant l'expansion des choses infinies,
Comme l'ambre, le musc, le benjoin et l'encens,
Qui chantent les transports de l'esprit et des sens.
—Baudelaire (1972:10)

A euphonic song of ecstasy of body and soul, Charles Baudelaire's paean to a multisensory world evokes colors, sounds, and a rich array of scents. Perfumes as cool as infant skin, as soft as oboes, or as green as meadows perfectly capture the multisensory aspects of living and being. Indeed, such was the sensual nature of some of the poems in this collection of 1857, *Les fleurs du*

*Making Senses of the Past: Toward a Sensory Archaeology,* edited by Jo Day. Center for Archaeological Investigations, Occasional Paper No. 40.  ISBN 978-0-8093-3287-8.

*mal*, that both the publisher and the poet were prosecuted for offending public morality.[1] Baudelaire, of course, was not alone in understanding that the senses are the mediums through which humans experience their world, but while artists (in the broadest sense of the word) have generally been indulged with a certain amount of freedom for sensory explorations, such themes have only recently become accepted as legitimate subjects of academic investigations outside their more traditional home in the science laboratory. The proliferation in the last decade or so of journal articles and books concentrating on varying aspects of sensory studies in the humanities (e.g., Berg's Sensory Formations series), as well the emergence of a new journal dedicated to this topic (*The Senses and Society*), testifies to an interdisciplinary interest in the actual bodily experience of being human, of tasting, touching, smelling, hearing, and seeing. Much of the initial impetus for this came from the Concordia Sensoria Research Team (CONSERT), based at Concordia University, Montreal. CONSERT members David Howes and Constance Classen have consistently produced work that both shapes and redefines sensory studies (Classen 1990, 1993, 1997, 2005; Howes 1991, 2003, 2005, 2009), and their influence, as well as that of Paul Stoller (1984, 1989, 1997), is evident across an array of disciplines including history, sociology, ethnography, sociocultural anthropology, food studies, human geography, art and cinema, and archaeology.

It was the last of these, archaeology, and the senses that was the theme of the 27th Annual Visiting Scholar Conference at the Center for Archaeological Investigations, Southern Illinois University Carbondale, held in March 2010. The papers presented, many of them published in this volume, demonstrated the multiplicity of ways archaeologists are engaging with sensory studies.[2] This is not the first book to take sensory archaeology as its subject; previous publications have focused on exploring specific aspects of the sensorium: for example, acoustics (Scarre and Lawson 2006) or color (Jones and MacGregor 2002). In contrast, this volume covers a broad spectrum of sensory modalities, highlighting their interconnections, as well as their distinct roles in past societies. Neither does it claim to be a how-to manual for "doing" sensory archaeology, a historiography of the subject, nor a detailed discussion of the theoretical foundations of a sensory approach to archaeology.[3] It should be added that, in general, this volume does not venture into the realms of "science" (although see Chapter 12 for a summary of the workings of the human olfactory system). This is deliberate, and while archaeologists are indebted to the physiological and neurological discoveries that allow us to better understand the human sensory apparatus, this book is not the place for a detailed discussion of such things.[4] No apology should be necessary for the broad range of material and sites included here, from the Aegean Bronze Age to the American Southwest; rather, this diversity should be embraced as stimulating and challenging and as evidence that a more embodied approach to the past is possible regardless of archaeological specialization. In fact, this endeavor gives lie to the assertion that "'archaeology of the senses' remains focused upon a narrow range of prehistoric topics" (Borić and Robb 2008:1), and it is hoped that this volume will open minds to future multisensory investigations of the past.

It is important to mention that beyond academia there is a palpable interest in all things sensory, spurred in part by ever-changing technology. For example, the emergence of electronic books (e-books) and their accompanying readers, such as Amazon's Kindle, has led to debates about the experience of reading on-screen versus on a page. At the center of many of these discussions lies a heartfelt plea that such technology disposes of sensory interaction involving the feel of the pages, the sound of turning them, even the smell of new purchases or of old and familiar books (and bookshops). However, new sensory experiences are being formed simultaneously: for example, when using the touch-screen technology of an iPad or iPhone. Research into virtual reality and the computer-game industry, too, are pushing virtual sensory experiences into ever-closer approximations of real life. While the mid-twentieth-century movie experiments using Smell-O-Vision and AromaRama were not enduring commercial successes, products that promise to transmit aromas via the Internet and computer still seem to fascinate (e.g., DigiScents Scent Dome, Scratch-N-Sniff Pro, AromaJet IPsmell). A recent attempt to make practical use of the close link between smell and memory involved aiding student recall with "memory oils."[5] Food lovers, too, have been on the receiving end of a sensory revolution. Eating is always a deeply multisensory act, yet advocates of the style of cooking often termed "molecular gastronomy" have been striving to enhance consumption through creating richly layered sensory experiences. Heston Blumenthal, chef and owner of the Fat Duck restaurant in Bray, in the United Kingdom, has developed a dish called "Sound of the Sea" that explores sound's influence on the perception of flavor (see also Zampini and Spence 2010). It is eaten while listening to wave noises on an iPod, thus enhancing the experience of flavor of the seafood.[6] The Slow Food movement and the rising interest in *terroir*, or the taste of place (e.g., Trubek 2008), have also contributed to a broader awareness of both taste and overall sensory experiences.

## Sensory Revolutions

### *The Senses and Society*

One of the essential tenets of contemporary sensory research is that the senses, five of which are mentioned above, are as much culturally constituted as physically given. The contemporary Western sensorium happens to name and recognize five (taste, touch, olfaction, hearing, and vision), but this is neither the sole way nor the "right" way to order perception. Ethnographic studies have been invaluable in opening our eyes (to use a visual metaphor!) to other possibilities, where more or fewer than five senses are apparently conceptualized and accorded varying social importance (e.g., Classen 1990, 1993). Alongside this differential saliency, the senses are laden with symbolic meaning: Seeger's (1975) discussion of the Suya shows how they socially define themselves through hearing and speaking, while vision is associated with witches and smell with animals. Moreover, the significance in some cultures of interoceptive sensations—those that are perceived within the body rather than with external organs like the nose, skin, or ear—is only beginning to be recognized (Geurts 2002, 2003; Stroeken 2008). Irrespective of how the senses are culturally organized, the layers of meaning will permeate all aspects of society, from the language used to moral values to emic ideas of personhood (Geurts 2002:227). This variety of sensory experience suggests that projects such as the all-embracing "natural history of the senses" (Ackerman 1990) are well-nigh impossible.

As culture-specific sensory orders were noted, the accompanying realization of an apparent hegemony of vision pervading all aspects of modern Western life also emerged. Seeing has become synonymous with rationality and reason, with phrases such as "Do you see?" (as opposed to, say, "Do you smell?") equated with "Do you understand?" Explanations of this phenomenon have been detailed elsewhere (Classen 1997; Howes 2003; Smith 2007; Synnott 1991a), so a succinct summary follows below. Several intertwining threads have combined to produce this ocularcentrism attributed to the Euro-American world, one of which presents Aristotle as its originator. Writing in the fourth century B.C.E., he offered an analysis of the human sensory apparatus that defined the five canonical senses, among them privileging vision (e.g., *De Sensu* and *De Anima* II) (Jütte 2005:31–46, 54–71). Others have preferred to take the philosophy of Descartes as the starting point for a general downgrading of all things corporeal in contrast to the primacy of the mind (the famous Cartesian dualism), which he felt distinguished humans from animals. Descartes believed that the fallibility of the senses meant that only the mind could be trusted to reveal the truth (Synnott 1991a:70). However, it is important to remember that not all philosophers agreed with this position, and, for example, both David Hume and John Locke stressed the link between sensory perception and knowledge (Jütte 2005:127–128).

Nevertheless, an increasing intellectualization of vision did occur in the early modern era and was aided by the invention of various instruments that enhanced viewing, such as telescopes, microscopes, and cameras. With such instruments allowing glimpses of realms far away or tinier than could be seen with the naked eye, sight became a gateway to new worlds and associated with science, knowledge, measuring, and proof. Such supposedly inverse connections between intellect and the nonvisual senses were supported by the voyages of exploration that brought Europeans into contact with "primitive" peoples who were expected to show a natural predilection for the "lower" senses of taste, touch, and smell (Howes 2003:5). The most infamous example of such thinking is the hierarchical classification devised by natural historian Lorenz Oken combining sensory orders with racial types: The rational European eye-man was placed at the top; the Asian ear-man was just below and followed by the Native American nose-man and then the Australian tongue-man; until, on the lowest rung of the scale, was the tactile African skin-man (Classen 1997:405). Nineteenth-century scholarship became more interested in the measurement and comparison of human sensation, rather than in philosophical debate (Geurts 2002:8). Indeed, the association of sensory investigations with inherent racism probably contributed to academia's rejection of such studies in the first half of the twentieth century (Howes 2003:6). More recently, Marshall McLuhan and Walter Ong contributed to the marginalization of other sensory ways of knowing when they proposed a divide between visual and oral-aural societies based on technologies of communication (Smith 2007:8–13). Reading and writing were intimately linked to seeing, while tribal societies were thought to emphasize speaking and hearing. However, ethnographic work has now shown that there are no universalist sensory models of cultures such as those proposed by McLuhan and Ong, but rather a wide range of culture-specific sensory orders (Classen 1997:404; also see Goody [1987] on the concepts of written and oral cultures).

### *Archaeology and the Senses*

Where does all of this leave archaeology, a discipline completely ignored in a recent review of sensory research (Porcello et al. 2010)? During the first half of the twentieth century, as the influence of different theoretical approaches ebbed and flowed within the discipline, emphasis tended to be placed, at one end of the scale, on typologies and material classification, and at the other end, on large-scale processes such as social organization and state formation. Later, processual methodologies adhered to the "archaeology as science" mantra and focused on measurable results and testable hypotheses. The emergence of postprocessualism in the 1980s as a response to New Archaeology encouraged archaeologists to jump off Hawkes's "Ladder of Inference" (1954), an influential model that reified an approach in which understanding ideology and symbolism was believed beyond the capabilities of archaeology. All of these approaches form part of archaeology's own disciplinary biography and are certainly not being dismissed here. Yet, even as agency and the individual were stressed by postprocessualists, material culture was read as a text, and so the physicality of objects and corporeal human experiences were still missing from interpretation. Indeed, Howes (2005:1–4) sees the current sensory revolution as at least partly a reaction to this paradigm of discourse that was prevalent in much of social science and humanities research during the late twentieth century. Certainly by the 1990s, a realization that the past as re-created by archaeology was peopled by "faceless blobs" (a phrase first used by Ruth Tringham [1991:94]) became a call to arms. Influenced by research in the newly invigorated sensory studies and encouraged by a current scholarly climate that fostered debate, reflexivity, and multivocality, an archaeology that considers a more sensory, sensual, emotional, and experiential past began to emerge. Seminal works—such as those by Hosler (1994), Houston and Taube (2000), Tarlow (2000), and Hamilakis, Pluciennik, and Tarlow (2002)—laid the groundwork for later research in this field.

Concurrent with archaeology's discovery of sensory studies, modern philosophy offered new approaches to explorations of past humanity. Both Heidegger and Merleau-Ponty developed phenomenological approaches whereby the world becomes meaningful through human interaction with things. Merleau-Ponty (2002) proposed the sensing/perceiving human body as the primary avenue for creating meaning and understanding the human experience. His work has had a significant impact on landscape archaeology in particular, as further discussed below. Michel Serres (2008), through his reaction against the dominance of language and vision and his celebration of multisensory existence, has also inspired new lines of archaeological inquiry. Crucially, these involve reexamining many of the concepts that archaeologists had assumed immutable, such as color, time, or nature (Insoll 2007). Nevertheless, amid such sensory adventures, archaeology remains a very visual discipline, and no one would doubt the benefits or, indeed, the necessity of using maps, plans, section drawings, photographs, Munsell color charts, sketches, and reconstructions. Similarly, while archaeological fieldwork is a very physical activity and the process of survey or excavation is a multisensory one (as noted by both Tringham and Weismantel in this volume), no one would suggest dispensing with vision as a valued tool. A more sensory approach to archaeology and the past, therefore, does not call for the abandonment of visual analyses, or the privileging of any other sensory order, but is aware of maintaining a balance between contemporary best practice, the use of archaeologically grounded data, and the re-embodiment of the human pasts that we reconstruct.

Bridging the gap between past and present experiences has been a major challenge for archaeologists, and, famously, Binford's development of middle-range theory was seen as one way to surmount the problem. Acknowledgment of our shared human corporeality can be seen as another, and so the body becomes the starting point for sensory archaeology. This body is the physical, perceiving body, the body equipped with the sensory organs found in a fully functioning human being: nose, mouth, eyes, ears, skin, brain and nerves, as well limbs to allow movement. This body is common to humans across the world today and is shared with humans in the past from the moment anatomically modern *Homo sapiens* first emerged as a distinct species. This physical body or the body as a cultural artifact is itself a topic of increasing interest to archaeologists (e.g., Borić and Robb, eds. 2008; Joyce 2005). Numerous theoretical and methodological debates have surrounded "writing the body in archaeology," to borrow the title of Lynn Meskell's (2000) précis of the subject, but sensory archaeology aims to do more than read or write bodies, to go beyond the body's surface toward its multiple somatic experiences. It is crucial, of course, to recognize that all individuals exist in distinct historical and cultural contexts, the confines of which cannot be conveniently overlooked to reembody the past. However, through combining archaeologically informed contextual information with the opportunities provided by a shared sensing body, it is possible to formulate new ideas about past experiences of material culture and place. Or, as summed up by Christopher Tilley, sensory archaeology could be said to enable a focus on "culturally constructed individuals whose personhoods differ while possessing a universal body" (2010:487).

## Sensing Landscapes, Sensing Buildings, Sensing Power(s)

Tilley, of course, is one of the archaeologists who brought the issue of the sensing body to the foreground in archaeological work, commencing with his 1994 publication of *A Phenomenology of Landscape*. In particular, it was British prehistorians who adopted this so-called phenomenological approach, which draws on the philosophical works of Heidegger and Merleau-Ponty and emphasizes an "embodied engagement with the material world" (Brück 2005:46), without getting too involved in the ontological nuances that underpin the original philosophy. Landscape archaeology became the main forum for proponents of this methodology; the archaeologist "enters into the landscape and allows it to have its own effect on his or her perceptive understandings" (Tilley 2010:26). An awareness of the physicality of the landscape and monuments therein, as well as the interrelationship of these features, and a recognition of the agency they possess as more than just backdrops for human activity heralded new ways of thinking (and writing) about the past, all based on experiences in the present (e.g., Bender 1998; Cummings and Whittle 2004; Edmonds 1999; Scarre 2002). Such an approach is not without its critics (e.g., Barrett and Ko 2009; Fleming 2006), and the flaws in a phenomenological approach to landscape archaeology, at least in the earlier stages of its development, are evident. Most apposite for this volume is its reliance on vision, where what can or cannot be seen was granted primary importance (perhaps to be associated with the increased prominence of geographic information systems [GIS] in archaeology), while other sensory impressions were less emphasized or even ignored completely. Another criticism of the phenomenological approach is that it highlights the experience of the individual—frequently a white, Western academic, often male—and therefore omits many other potential interactions with the landscape, such as those of children, women, or groups. Closely connected to this is the question of the degree of familiarity of the researcher with the area. Long-term dwelling and regular habituation to place will produce experiences and memories that contrast with those of an infrequently visiting archaeologist. Many of the studies also tend to focus on ritual monuments in the landscape, at the expense of mundane experiences (Hamilton et al. 2006:33, 35). A final complaint has been the untestable nature of such research: How can a "subjective epistemology" (Barrett and Ko 2009:279) ever be replicated or verified? It should be noted, however, that Tilley himself has recently taken a more multisensory approach to his research and has responded in print to his critics (2010:471–481).

One of the ways archaeologists have been able to gain a culturally situated and sensorially aware understanding of past landscapes has been to cooperate with indigenous peoples where possible (Fowles 2010).[7] The work of William A. Allen and Perry Fletcher with their indigenous partners Gerard O'Regan and Roger Noganosh, which combines First Nations and Maori understandings of the landscape with more traditional archaeological techniques, is very much in this tradition. In Chapter 2, they explore a potential link between the locations of rock paintings and the ephemeral phenomenon of "shimmer," the visual effect noted when sunlight reflects off the surface of water and brings the painted rock face to life. The transience of such occurrences precludes a regular archaeological study; indeed, shimmer may not even be noticed unless the archaeologist is already attuned to looking beyond the image itself. However, an awareness of the indigenous beliefs relating to the surrounding landscape, where spirits and ancestors are understood to reside, means that interpretations of such numinous phenomena can move away from metaphor and toward recognition of actual powers in the land itself. The flickering light and dancing painting animate the rock as a nonhuman person, or a coactor, in rituals performed there. It should not be a surprise to find that something as apparently inanimate as rock can be perceived as alive, potent, and even a gateway to another world; indeed, other works have highlighted this issue in different cultures (e.g., Herva 2006; Lewis-Williams and Dowson 1990). Seeing beyond the static image is only one aspect of experiencing these rock-art sites, and sound, too, can play a key role (see also Boivin et. al 2007; Goldhahn 2002; Waller 2006). Spirituality of place may be further emphasized by the kinesthetic experiences required to create or interact with these Maori and First Nation sites: They are accessible only by water during favorable conditions, and thus the journey to the site also becomes incorporated into its meaning (Tilley 2008).

Karen Holmberg (Chapter 3) too stresses the link between a living landscape and its inhabitants, in this case, the supersensory experience of volcanic eruption. She uses analogies from her own life in New York City to draw attention to the mutability of landscapes, moving from benign to dangerous and back again to benign, replete with new (bodily) memories. Reconstructions of past perceptions must always be carried out in the distant present, but the experience of an erupting volcano is perhaps one of the few events during which it may be possible to at least approach past corporeal effects, whatever about their associated cultural meanings. Based on fieldwork in Panama, Holmberg demonstrates how these active landscapes make their way into myths and folktales, which through their retelling across generations help make sense of the violence of nature. In a similar fashion, the curation of material remnants of eruptions may also guide social memory and even offer a sense of regaining control over an unstable world. Her discussion of art exhibitions based on volcanic themes highlights that, while archaeology remains essentially text-bound, artists can produce the type of multisensory presentation that best encompasses something as intense as a volcano. This debate about presenting a sensory past in the present is returned to in greater detail later in the volume in Chapters 18 and 19.

Corin C. O. Pursell's work (Chapter 4) moves from thinking about the landscape to considering both the interaction between a settlement and its setting and the interaction of specific monuments within the settlement, in this instance Shiloh Mounds in Tennessee. Focusing on ritual action in public monumental settings, he explores control of space and the perception of mounds using a methodology that combines angles of visual perception with the actual form of public space. In discussing the different functions and audience experiences of Mound A and Mound C, he concludes that not only did each mound support varying social agendas within the community but that Mound A also functioned as a statement to the outside world. Furthermore, Pursell's research ties in to the important archaeological work on the symbolic roles of color (e.g., Cleland and Stears 2004; Hosler 1994; Houston et al. 2009; Jones and McGregor 2002), and his careful contextual examination of the use of red and white sediments in Mounds A and C suggests shifting control of symbolic media and potentially fluid meanings that changed over time.

The theme of elite-controlled experience of place as an expression of power is a concept Ryan Mongelluzzo also explores in Chapter 5 on Maya Classic palaces. Comparing Holmul and Tikal, Mongelluzzo discusses the interplay between architectural design and bodily effects. Unlike the situation with many other prehistoric societies, detailed iconographic and epigraphic evidence allows some insight into the Maya sensorium, and Mongelluzzo draws on these culture-specific understandings of seeing and hearing for his chapter. Indeed, when possible, sensory archaeologies should make use of contemporary texts to complement the physical remains, albeit with due caution. Movement within the Maya palace, as well as from inside to outside spaces and from public to private spaces, was accompanied by constantly changing sensory effects; smells, temperatures, light, colors, viewsheds, and sound filters all combined to reproduce and reinforce the social hierarchy in a spatial dimension. Mongelluzzo's chapter analyzes how this intricate palace design therefore affected and even controlled sensory perception. This work pushes a phenomenological approach toward new directions, focusing on a complex built environment rather than on the more usual landscape setting.

In a similar vein, Mary Weismantel presents a study of the sensory interfaces at the well-known site of Chavín de Huantar in Peru (Chapter 6). She notes that current archaeological interpretations of both the carved stone monuments and the site layout are heavily dependent on contemporary techniques of seeing, which use line drawings to offer instant totalizing narratives. However, when confronted with the physical reality of the monuments and architecture, a completely different way of viewing is required, necessitating bodily interaction and providing a far more fragmentary understanding of the whole. Whereas Mongelluzzo's chapter focuses on one entity—the palace—Weismantel considers the site as a whole to be moved through in processional fashion, with the elements of unpredictability and wonder essential to the experience of Chavín as a pilgrimage site. She also draws attention to the divergent experiences of place, based on the different social roles of the subject(s), reminding us that there is no one true past experience but rather a multiplicity of valid experiences.

## Embodied Rituals

The merging of more than one sense is a feature of many of the chapters in this volume, corresponding to the normal multisensory human experience. Although research has suggested culturally specific hierarchies of senses, whereby one particular mode of sensory perception becomes the dominant paradigm, it is accepted that all humans rely on the full sensorium in their daily lives. Chapters 7 through 9 emphasize this aspect of sensory archaeology, focusing on the interplay among the senses at specific ritual events or places. In Chapter 7, Candace Weddle explores the experience of sacrifice in Roman imperial cult through analogy with contemporary Islamic animal sacrifice in Turkey. Animal sacrifice was an important element in many of the rituals of ancient Rome and has long been the focus of academic inquiry. Perhaps unsurprisingly, study of the phenomenon has relied primarily on literary sources and iconographic evidence, leading to what Weddle terms "senseless" examinations of the ritual. In the tradition of autoethnographic research, she investigates the impact of large-scale animal sacrifice on both the worshipper and the location itself, although she is careful not to claim that her experiences replicate a precise historical moment. To see this chapter as merely aiming to shock via graphic descriptions and images of animal sacrifice is to miss one of the author's main points: Experiencing the full multisensory sacrificial process led her to formulate new research questions pertaining to activities before and after the fatal moments frozen in iconography or texts.

Ritual is also the focus of Heather Hunter-Crawley's research, but her Chapter 8 concentrates on a later period: the world of sixth-century Christianity. Complementing Weddle's emphasis on the bodily experience of being a worshipper, Hunter-Crawley considers the sensory affordances of the material culture used in Eucharistic ritual. Taking the Riha Hoard as her case study, she discusses the multisensory experiences associated with the chalice, paten, and fan, as well as related ecclesiastical objects such as censers and lamps, the use of which allowed worshippers to physically encounter the divine. Like Mongelluzzo, Hunter-Crawley is able to draw on texts describing early Christian attitudes toward the senses, such as the idea of the "tactile eye," itself derived from earlier Classical concepts of extramission. These support her suggestion of a more nuanced and interrelated notion of body and soul, in contrast to the Cartesian mind-body duality often imposed on the same material. To merely "read" artifacts is, as Hunter-Crawley states, to deny them their own materiality and presents an intellectual challenge to archaeologists grappling with the concept of material culture (e.g., Boivin 2008; Gosden 2005; Hurcombe 2007; Knappett 2005; Meskell 2005). Certainly objects become interesting as they reveal the "social and individual self-creation" associated with them (Olsen 2003:91; see Miller 2008 for a recent anthropological study of people and their things). However, objects are also interesting because of their "thingness," or materiality, which actively affects their creation and uses and which is perceived by humans through our senses. An approach to material culture informed by sensory archaeology, therefore, considers not just the associated symbolism and potential social meanings of things, but it also pays close attention to the bodily effects of things on people within a culturally specific context. This theme is returned to later in this volume in chapters by Day and Dakouri-Hild.

In contrast to the specific religious rituals discussed by Weddle and Hunter-Crawley, Ruth Tringham (Chapter 9) focuses on the rituals of daily life in a study of the senses of touch in the past and the present at Çatalhöyük. Previous archaeological studies on touch have concentrated on what Rodaway (1994:50) termed "reach touch," that is, active tactile encounters, usually with the hands. MacGregor's (1999) work on carved stone balls is the genesis of this genre and other researchers have followed in his footsteps, adding a haptic dimension to studies of stone (Tilley 2004), rock art (Ouzman 2001) and monuments (Cummings 2002). Ingold (2004) has also drawn attention to "pedestrian touch," focusing on feet instead of hands, which should certainly not be overlooked in studies of the past. In contrast to these studies, "global touch" (Rodaway 1994:48–50) lies at the heart of Tringham's chapter. Using Ingold's concept of the taskscape, Tringham explores the "full-body haptic-tactile-kinesthetic sensual experience," reminding us that since movements construct places, an awareness of our experiences in the here and now can be a guide to experiences of past peoples. Crucially, she grounds her theories in archaeological evidence from the site; hence, osteological results suggest habituation to squatting, and architectural remains demand certain movements—crouching, climbing, perhaps even falling. This exploration of the rhythms of activity that effectively help "places make sense" as "senses make place" (Feld 1996:91) demonstrates that a sensory archaeology is not restricted to elite or elaborate events and places but can also elucidate everyday experience (as demonstrated by King and Sánchez Santiago 2011).

## Exploring Sensory Modalities in the Past

Although Tringham's contribution is mainly about touch, it is clear that such a separation of the senses is an artificial one created to enable an academic presentation of a particular facet of human experience. The following chapters focus on other individual senses (hearing, taste, and smell) but by no means suggest that these senses are prioritized within the societies under discussion. Rather they are explorations of aspects of an interconnected human sensorium, separated here to allow an archaeological investigation of previously overlooked aspects of the material. In a similar way, the surge of publications focusing on individual senses sought to redress the apparent ocularcentrism of academia but were not intended to herald a new sensory hierarchy; select examples include acoustics (Bull and Back 2003), taste (Korsmeyer 2005), touch (Classen 2005), and smell (Classen, Howes and Synnott 1994; Drobnick 2006). It is also important to ensure that, when other senses are emphasized in academic studies or fieldwork, research with a visual basis is not forgotten or denigrated, as one visual anthropologist has warned against (Grimshaw 2001:6; see also Edwards and Bhaumik 2008). To that end, Pursell (Chapter 4) shows how to take visual research in new directions.

### *Archaeoacoustics*

The archaeology of sound is perhaps the most well developed of sensory studies that focus on the past, and research falls roughly into two categories. First, there is the study of ancient sound-making devices, often including experiments on how to play them or otherwise establish the range of notes that could be produced, although actual melodies and rhythms cannot generally be apprehended. Such work is often grouped under the heading "archaeomusicology," and includes such examples as Tutankhamun's trumpets (Kirby 1947) and Irish bronze horns (Coles 1967). Investigations into the earliest production of music by humans are related to this category (e.g., Dams 1985; Zhang, Xiao, and Lee 2004), but this topic spreads far beyond archaeology into evolutionary and neurobiological studies (Mithen 2006; Wallin, Merker, and Brown 2000).

The second category is a study of the behavior of sound—not just music—at archaeological sites; these can be either natural places featuring evidence of human activity and even modification, such as caves and rock-art locales (e.g., Boivin 2004; Goldhahn 2002; Loose 2008; Ouzman 2001; Reznikoff and Dauvois 1988), or man-made monuments, such as passage graves and stone circles (Devereux and Jahn 1996; Watson 2001; Watson and Keating 1999). All such studies emphasize that considering soundscapes is as important as considering visual effects and that a more integrated multisensory investigation may help in understanding the functions of the sites in question. In their earlier manifestations, these archaeoacoustical studies focused on measuring resonance and sound frequencies at the sites, thus providing quantifiable scientific data (e.g., Jahn, Devereux, and Ibison 1996). Indeed, the physiological and psychological results of certain sonic effects have been noted (Cook, Pajot, and Leuchter 2008; Watson and Keating 1999), fueling speculation about a link between monument design and the use of sound in ancient rituals, whether to attain an altered state of consciousness or to induce feelings of awe, fear, inclusion, or exclusion (see Needham [1967] and Tuzin [1984] for seminal articles on the power of sound).

As the archaeology of sound has become more established and has been influenced by wider sensory studies, measuring sound waves, while still providing intriguing food for thought (see the recent work on the prehistoric structures of Malta, for example, presented by Linda Eneix at this conference), is being complemented by a deeper engagement with the social meanings of the construction and use of sound and soundscapes (Boivin et al. 2007; King and Sánchez Santiago 2011). Feld's (1996) concept of "acoustemology" is useful here, drawing attention to acoustic knowing and sound's role in making sense of place. Ethnographic case studies provide opportunities to broaden our understanding of the myriad ways humans perceive and make sense of sound (e.g., Feld 1990; Porath 2008; Stoller 1984). The challenge for archaeologists, in acknowledging this diversity, is to tease out the deeper meanings of sounds and sound-making devices for past societies.

Chapter 10 by Joe Williams is a welcome addition to the archaeological corpus on sound and is unusual for focusing, not on prehistory, but on medieval England. Using the concepts of access analysis and copresence zones, he analyzes the musical space and the quiet space within two monastic structures, with the second of these categories perhaps inverting what is normally considered within the remit of archaeoacoustics. But quiet, silence, and the absence of noise can be culturally meaningful, too, yet are often overlooked in the clamor to focus on sound. At his chosen sites, aural experiences were structured by the architecture as well as by the different rules followed at each location according to the monastic order of the participants. Drawing on excavation reports, Williams is able to comment on the various types of noises that permeated the monastic walls—the human and background noises—as well as the temporal quality of the sounds. Moreover, as Weismantel also points out, there were many possible experiences of a (monastic) soundscape, varying according to the identity of the hearer—whether monk, visitor, tradesman, or even dog!

*Eating, Tasting, Remembering*

Moving from ears to mouths, Marie Hopwood's contribution (Chapter 11) turns to the sensuous world of food: of cooking, eating, and tasting as evidenced in archaeological material. Somewhat surprisingly, taste was the least well represented of the traditional five senses at the Carbondale conference. Within archaeology, focus on food has shifted over the last century from ignoring, or at best merely recording faunal and paleobotanical material, via a subsistence-driven outlook typical of processual approaches, toward studying the social meanings of eating and, in particular, feasting (Dietler and Hayden 2001; Wiessner and Schiefenhövel 1996). Until recently, therefore, the dominant approach within archaeology "focused mainly on procurement-production, rather than consumption" (Hamilakis 2000:56). The concept of feasting is one that archaeologists have embraced wholeheartedly, although attending to the sensory act of eating has been overwhelmed by using the feast to frame social and political issues, such as status negotiation, resource control, and the roles of commensality. There are signs though, at least in some branches of archaeology—for example, the Aegean Bronze Age—that the multisensory feast is gaining prominence (e.g., Day this volume; Fox 2008; Hamilakis 2008).

Despite this increasing interest in the archaeology of food, little has been done on actual taste. The term *taste* is, of course, an ambiguous one, entailing moral or ideological judgment ("to have good taste"), but here it is used to imply flavor preferences. Taste is one of the most intimate of the senses, as tasting only occurs once something has been incorporated into the body, via the mouth. As with exploring other senses from the past, a skeptical response is that it is impossible to say anything meaningful about something as personal and ephemeral as taste. After all, food preferences vary among people who share a culture, as well as within individuals as they move through different life stages (Macbeth and Lawry 2006:3). However, taste is also a cultural phenomenon, and even allowing for economic and ecological variables, it is closely linked to beliefs about what is "good to eat," often reinforced through taboo, dietary restrictions, or social hierarchies. This concept of social taste in turn is tied in to the material used in storing, preparing, and serving these substances. This, then, is how archaeology can approach taste: not on the individual level, but on that of the society and is the approach taken by Hopwood.[8] Through a study of the ceramic use alteration at the site of Fıstıklı Höyük in Turkey, diachronic changes in the shape and size of vessels point to fluctuations in cooking and storage needs within the community. Like Tringham, Hopwood's chapter considers quotidian performances (of food preparation here) rather than extraordinary events. By focusing on vessel changes as related to the foodstuffs within, rather than as isolated technological changes, she builds up a picture of a past cuisine that encompasses tastes and activities together (cf. Isaakidou 2007; Joyce and Henderson 2007). It is to be hoped that a future exploration of ancient tastes might combine Hopwood's ceramic-based approach with Isaakidou's focus on faunal remains and Valamoti's (2009) discussion of plant foods, approaching ever closer to the "gustemology" (Sutton 2010:215) of past societies.

Eating, tasting, and food are intimately tied in to memory, a theme that pervades many of the chapters in this volume. While Hopwood does not explicitly discuss this in relation to food at Fıstıklı Höyük, the powerful bodily memories created by the consumption of food and drink have been of considerable interest to anthropologists (Holtzman 2006; Seremetakis 1994; Sutton 2001). More broadly, Paul Connerton's (1989) work has been influential in archaeologies of memory, with his concept of "incorporating practice" in particular becoming pivotal for sensory studies. For it is not just tastes or recollections of food that are evocative, but smells, sounds, sights, and kinesthetic memories also recall similar moments in the past, what he calls "mnemonics of the body" (Connerton 1989:74). However, Connerton's traceless incorporating practices do not take into account the material culture—the cups, the food, the incense—that enables bodily memories to be created. As a result, Hamilakis has recently suggested abandoning the opposing categories of incorporating and inscribing mnemonic practices and instead focusing on the "shared mnemonic power of all material sensorial interaction" (2010:192).

Archaeological studies of memory also draw on Pierre Bourdieu's concept of *habitus*, where bodily practices both reflect and reproduce elements of society, as well as the idea that material culture can be seen as a means for "storing memory in extrabodily form" (Jones 2007:1). It is this characteristic of archaeological finds that facilitates the use of archaeology in nationalist agendas and imaginations. Material remains can be seen as providing emotional and tangible links to the past, in embodied support of present ideologies (e.g., Hamilakis 2007). It is obvious that memory is currently riding a wave of popularity within archaeology: The work of Van Dyke and Alcock (2003) was an early foray, while more recently, Mills and Walker (2008), Borić (2009), Georgiadis and Gallou (2009), and Lillios and Tsamis (2010) have all explored different aspects of the theme. Perhaps this is not surprising; after all, it can be said that "all archaeology is about memory" (Hamilakis 2010:188). As with all subjective experiences, however, there is never one true memory to be investigated but rather a concept operating on multiple levels simultaneously, whether individual, social, or even invented (Holtzman 2006:363). Archaeologists, while exploring the role of the senses in remembering the past in the past, must remain aware of whose memory they are presenting in the present.

### *Smelling the Past*

Smell is especially noted for its mnemonic powers, and the fame of the Proustian moment, combining smell, taste, and memory, is far-reaching. While the following three chapters (12, 13, and 14) on olfaction in the past do not take memory as their specific concern, the close link between remembering and scent is an integral element in each work. Archaeologies of smell are not common, although Insoll (2007:49–53) briefly discussed a material-based methodology for such explorations. Considering that an aroma cannot be excavated, this careful reliance on the archaeological material is essential and is a shared feature of these chapters. Joanne M. Murphy's contribution (Chapter 12) provides a summary of the physiology behind the human sense of smell, highlighting the particularly close connection between the olfactory system and the brain. While she stresses that all senses are used by humans in evaluating the world around them, scientific studies suggest that smell has a very immediate effect on the brain and, hence, on our emotions and memories. Murphy explores this idea through the lens of perfume manufacture and use at the Late Bronze Age palace of Pylos, in Greece. The decipherment of Linear B texts revealed a world of palatial administration, where perfumed oil was one of a number of goods closely controlled by the elite. While perfume manufacture contributed to the Pylian smellscape at large, the restricted use of the finished commodity helped create and maintain social hierarchies. As Synnott remarked, odor "is above all a statement of who one is" (1991b:438), and the links between smell and identity are strong. Furthermore, by thinking about the corporeal effects of the Pylian perfume industry, Murphy takes studies of Mycenaean wealth finance and elite gift exchange in new directions: A gift of perfume carries a reminder of social obligations with every inhalation, a truly embodied memory.

The scent of perfume wafts through Emerson Avery's Chapter 13 too, but here it mingles with the smells of death and decay. Focusing on the experience of visitors to Roman and Byzantine era tombs in the cemetery of Beth She'an-Scythopolis, Avery reminds us that not all smells are pleasant. In the close, lamplit environment of the chamber tomb, the proximate senses come to the fore, and the pungent mixture of perfumed oils, foodstuffs, and human remains would have created in the visitor a very specific bodily memory, made all the stronger by the use of many familiar items in this unfamiliar context (see also Hamilakis 1998). Unpleasant sensory experiences have been less well explored in archaeology and anthropology, with a few notable exceptions (Bartosiewicz 2003; Bubandt 1998; Corbin 1986; Holtzman 2010; Stoller and Olkes 1986; see also Miller 1997). Crucially, Avery emphasizes that olfactory likes and dislikes are culturally conditioned; indeed, olfaction has been described as "a moral construction of reality" (Synnott 1991b:438), enabling an "othering" of those who smell differently, in every meaning of the phrase (e.g., Almagor 1987). Thus, learning to smell correctly is an essential element in socialization, and laboratory tests have demonstrated the experience-dependent nature of odor perception (Ayabe-Kanamura et al. 1998). On a broader scale, this also reminds us that it is essential not to impose a contemporary Euro-American or Western construction of sensuousness onto other societies (Holtzman 2009:57–61) and, of particular importance for archaeology, onto those of the past.

Chapter 14, by Jo Day, returns to Bronze Age Greece, this time to the island of Crete and the Minoan civilization. The concept of synesthetic material culture is used here to investigate new ways of understanding stone and ceramic vessels with relief floral decoration. True synesthesia, where the subject automatically experiences cross-modal perception, such as attributing smells to colors or shapes to tastes (e.g., Cytowic and Eagleman 2009), is not the focus of this study. Rather, it discusses how the deliberate stimulation of one sensory modality can trigger other sensory responses. As with Hunter-Crawley's (Chapter 8) work, the emphasis is on the user's bodily interaction with the chosen objects, but links to olfaction in particular are explored, with the vessels' decoration suggesting a deliberate attempt to stimulate the sense of smell at communal events. On a larger scale, it is also suggested that in the light of a range of other archaeological evidence, olfactory stimuli were regularly manipulated in Minoan society to create emotional and mnemonic bonds and may have had ritual significance. This chapter also engages with the challenge of how to depict something as ephemeral as a smell or a sound, demonstrating that in fact this apparent difficulty resides within contemporary Western epistemology and need not be problematic in other societies.

## Sensory Production

There are many different archaeological approaches to understanding ancient technology and production, usefully summarized in Dobres (2010). The next three chapters in this volume (Chapters 15, 16, and 17) shift emphasis from consumption onto matters of production, in particular the idea of interplay between object and craftsperson. That objects or materials have "social lives" is not a new concept (Appadurai 1986), but it is the sensory aspects of this interdependence (e.g., Saunders 2001) that are brought to the fore here. Anastasia Dakouri-Hild considers the multiple material lives of agate objects in Late Bronze Age Thebes through the unusual approach of focusing on "unfinished, failed, and partially recycled" artifacts (Chapter 15). A key difference between her study and the more traditional *chaîne opératoire* approach to object biographies is that she allows for a dynamic relationship between the craftsperson and the material itself. Thus, the very materiality of agate may help direct the craftsperson's work—its stripes and bands suggesting forms to the experienced eye, its weight and cool smoothness perhaps pleasing in the hand—and failed artifacts offer opportunities for "sensory play." Relating these discarded objects to Theban society more broadly, Dakouri-Hild wonders whether a form of "sensory pruning" was carried out by the elite, where "workmanship of risk" (Pye 1995) was not appreciated and adherence to a certain aesthetic was preferred by those in authority.

The sensory experiences involved in manufacturing are also to the fore in Jonathan T. Thomas's contribution (Chapter 16), where he recounts experiments in crafting Late Neolithic Iberian slate plaques. Thomas writes of the specific sounds made when carving patterns into the stone, of the acrid smell and taste that accompanied the activity, and of the pain carvers experienced as their hands became raw. These are truly the embodied experiences of craftsmanship, and like Avery's (Chapter 13) aromas of decay, these unpleasant effects are as important as the pleasing tactile interaction with the smooth finished artifacts. Thomas reminds us, however, as Tringham (Chapter 9) and Murphy (Chapter 12) also note, that habituation changes the nature of the sensory experience. He proposes, therefore, that if those who made the plaques in Neolithic times were more experienced than his novice students, the acuteness of the perceived sound, smell, and pain would have lessened over time, perhaps to be replaced by other dominant reactions and mnemonics or perhaps even to be enjoyed rather than disliked (remembering that sensory likes and dislikes are culturally conditioned).

It is interesting, too, to situate Thomas's work within experimental archaeology more generally. Despite its aim of testing hypotheses about past practice using an experience-based approach, many archaeologists manage to ignore the actual experience in their results. As Thomas himself notes, publications focus on how many kilocalories it takes to chop down a tree with a stone ax or what precise temperature is needed to cook meat in a skin (Coles 1973:51). On the other hand, Mathieu (2002:4–5) has recently identified the emergence of a form of behavioral replication he calls "phenomenological," noting that if better controls were in place human perception could indeed be approached through experimental archaeology (for an example of this approach, see Molloy 2008). It is surely to be expected that future experimental archaeology will follow in this direction.

Krysta Ryzewski (Chapter 17) switches from an emphasis on the body of the craftsperson to the body of the actual artifact and examines the sensory experiences that lie embedded within metal at a microscopic level. Using the material from three family-run iron production sites in colonial period Rhode Island, she investigates the sensory cues that facilitated successful smelting and ironworking, as well as the transfer of this specialist knowledge. As Thomas wonders who the audience for plaque making was, in the preceding chapter, so Ryzewski also considers craft production as performance. Public display of the production process showcased the skills of the ironworkers while simultaneously creating a distinction between their specialized knowledge and the uninitiated audience (see also Carter 2007). This same audience, of course, were the ones who complained about what were, to them, the unpleasant smells and sounds that accompanied the process, yet again reminding us of the diverse sensory perceptions of the same activities.

## Telling a Multisensory Story

The final two chapters in the volume revolve around how to present the past and how best to communicate the results of sensory research. Catherine P. Foster (Chapter 18) discusses the dissemination of sensuous pasts and presents at the Badè Museum of Biblical Archaeology and Doug Adams Gallery. Her curation of an exhibition *Lived Experience in Ancient Judah* allowed Foster to create thematic multisensory experiences for the visitors, where contrary to the norm in most contemporary museums, they were encouraged to "Please Touch Gently." Interacting with the exhibits in such a tactile way harks back to practice in the earliest museums, where touching the artifacts was deemed an essential and expected part of the visit (Classen 2007). Only later in the nineteenth century did the past become secured in glass cases, to be appreciated solely with an educated eye.

Foster, like Tringham in Chapter 9, alludes to the developments in technology, in particular haptics and virtual touch, that allow ever more realistic encounters with artifacts without actually touching the real thing. This "digital touch" has been discussed in detail elsewhere (Paterson 2007) and was the subject of a paper by Linda Hurcombe at the Carbondale conference. Yet digital touch removes the opportunity to interact with the authentic and eliminates the personal engagement with the past engendered by handling objects from the lives of others or feeling "what others have felt" (Classen and Howes 2006:202). Such reproductions and non-artifacts (antifacts?) may therefore deliver a less satisfactory experience, an intangible sense of diluted "aura," to borrow Walter Benjamin's (1992) term. It should be asked whether the opportunity for experiences of the authentic will continue to be restricted to museum staff, archaeologists, and other such trained professionals, in the name of preserving and protecting artifacts. This was one of the issues that sparked debate at the conference, and although perhaps heretical, the idea of designating certain items as "sacrificial objects" to be handled, played with, and even broken by museum visitors should perhaps be considered. After all, why should we expect the public to be content with replicas and digital copies, while maintaining our own privilege of touching the genuine past?

The second exhibition that Foster discusses was a contemporary artist's exploration of "an archaeology of the senses." Whereas Foster strived to create holistic sensory experiences in her exhibition curation, Pamela Blotner focused on individual senses in each of her archaeologically inspired works to build up a layered effect of a full sensorium. Foster's comment that contemporary art can make archaeologists conceptualize material culture in new ways accords with Holmberg's (Chapter 3) comments on art's potential to convey experience. It is undeniable that archaeologists cannot avoid text and images as the current standard means to communicate research. But perhaps further cooperation with artists would allow more imaginative and emotional responses to the past to be explored beyond the self-imposed limits of a reproving academia.

To accompany her multisensory museum visit, Foster developed what she terms a *micro-narrative*, where the material was enhanced by textual explanations written from the point of view of a young girl in the ancient community, albeit mediated by the curatorial voice behind it. Ruth M. Van Dyke further develops this theme in Chapter 19, the book's final chapter, in which she tackles the potentially contentious issue of writing a more sensuous archaeology. While sociocultural anthropologists have been relatively proactive in considering the subjective nature of their writing (e.g., Clifford and Marcus 1986; Geertz 1988; Waterston and Vesperi 2009), archaeological writing generally has strived to maintain a patina of scientific objectivity, despite now recognizing the interpretive nature of even the most basic report (see Joyce 2002 for discussion on archaeological writing). So-called thick description, a descriptive and contextual style of ethnographic writing celebrated by Clifford Geertz (1973), is perhaps most closely approximated in archaeology by the writings of Tilley and other "landscape phenomenologists." Their accounts are bound by the researcher's first-person field observations (thus providing ammunition for those who critique the highly personal and subjective nature of such writing), a point Tilley sidesteps through exaggeration, stressing that he does not wish "to go around pretending to understand something from the point of view of a female Neolithic weaver with twins" (Tilley 2010:474). This protest against past voices masks lost opportunities, as Van Dyke explains, because imagined narratives offer the chance to present a multivocal past. The two accounts she presents here of a visit to Chaco Canyon, by a teenage girl and by the girl's grandmother, allow a freer exploration of different experiences of the same place and different understandings of the same material culture. Thus, side by side, they combine to present a fluid, dynamic, and more human interpretation of a past culture. Although the voices are fictions, all that her protagonists say and do is rooted in Van Dyke's own knowledge of the archaeology of Chaco and her own multisensory experience of the place.

Of course, Van Dyke is not the first to employ imagined narratives in archaeological writing. An issue of *Historical Archaeology* (32.1, 1998) was devoted to archaeological story-telling, and Mark Edmonds, for example, felt encouraged to experiment with intermingling story, material, and theory because "[t]he past contructed on the page was peopled either by dull archetypes who spent their lives chasing and producing food, or automata, blindly reproducing abstracted and simplistic symbolic codes" (Edmonds 1999:x). In contrast to Van Dyke's individual voices, Edmonds adopted the omniscient narrator perspective, a tactic that subtly underlines the sense of distance between past and present. Certainly, if we are to follow Stoller's exhortation to replace "bloodless language" with "sensuous scholarship" (1997:xv), a new way of writing the past must be utilized, at least in tandem with traditional scholarship.

It is often assumed that the target audience of these works must be the rather daunting "interested but nonspecialist member of the general public." With their vernacular language and lack of academic baggage (e.g., references, footnotes, and tentative framing of hypotheses), such works are undoubtedly more accessible to all, but that should not preclude these narratives from making other archaeologists rethink what they know and how they know it. Imaginative explorations of the past are carried out as much for the writer as for the reader (Gibb 2000:5) and can be valuable guides to future research, as Van Dyke herself points out. Her list of decision points encountered during the crafting of her Chacoan narrative provides an insight into her creative process. However, this "interpretive narrative archaeology" (McCarthy 2003) is not without its critics (e.g., Fleming 2006:275–276; Hummler 2008), and archaeologists must bear in mind the responsibility inherent in creating imagined or fictional pasts that may be understood elsewhere as definitive presentations. In the context of this volume, it is prudent to remember, too, that we must tread carefully to avoid projecting our own sensory values into these narratives, even if we can perceive sensory experiences in a similar fashion.

## Sensing the Past in the Future

The irony of presenting multisensory archaeological research in a standard edited volume is not lost on the contributors and editor. Papers at the conference were accompanied not just by the now-standard PowerPoint presentations, but also by videos, sound recordings, and replica artifacts for handling. To some degree, therefore, a written version can be seen as an "anticlimax" (Howes 2003:57). Indeed, during the social events that followed the day's papers, ideas were (only half-jokingly) bounced around about whether this book could have a tactile cover or scratch-and-sniff pages or colored and textured paper or pop-out images and sound effects. A supporting Web site to host the various multimedia materials was also investigated as a more feasible option (e.g., see King and Sánchez Santiago 2011 for online supporting aural material), but issues of intellectual property rights prevented its inception. But would such features have added anything to the scholarly value of the end product or just been attention-grabbing tricks? The answer depends on how such elements are used, much like sensory archaeology itself. Whether an approach to the past informed by sensory theories represents a paradigm shift, as debated more than once at the conference, or is just the latest sparkly new trick in the archaeologist's toolbox depends on what happens next. It is no longer enough for us to shout that the "faceless blobs" need to be given bodies and emotions. In line with Herzfeld's (2001:240–253) comments on an anthropology of the senses, an archaeology of the senses must avoid becoming a catalog of case studies and a marginalized branch of archaeology; rather, it needs to be seamlessly adopted into future interpretations of past cultures.

A number of themes emerge from this book that are pertinent for this incorporation of a sensory approach into mainstream archaeology. Many of the authors here are concerned with techniques of the body, unsurprising considering that the senses are ultimately corporeal in origin. Habituation, daily lived experience, movement through landscapes and around sites and buildings, apprenticeship, and performance are elements common to many of the chapters. While none of these themes are the prerogative of a sensory approach, the addition of sensory information enriches them further. The active manipulation of the senses is a second theme, whether that manipulation is by elites, authorities, craftspeople, or cooks and effected through landscapes, buildings, or material culture. We are also asked on more than one occasion to reflect on unpleasant sensory experiences—such as smelling foul odors (bearing in mind their cultural specificity), falling, or getting lost—as well as on the material results of sensory experiences—such as imperfectly crafted artifacts—all of which remind us that the past was far from a perfect world. Interestingly, only two chapters refer to altered states of consciousness (Weismantel; Day), although if the full gamut of past sensory experiences are to be recognized, these other ways of knowing and perceiving must be taken into account too (see Price 2001 and Hume 2007 for such an approach). It could even be suggested that the desire and capacity to experience other worlds or the feelings of awe when faced with natural phenomena such as sunlight shimmer or volcanic eruptions are candidates for recognition as other human senses. A caveat: The potential richness of sensory approaches must not lure archaeologists into "peopling the past with people like us," as discussant Robin Beck cautioned at the conference.

Perhaps most provocatively, the issue of presenting a multisensory past arises. Some museums are moving toward including greater interactivity with artifacts and/or replicas, and the developments in digital technologies will undoubtedly lead to ever more "real" virtual experiences. Whether these are as satisfying, both emotionally and intellectually, as touching the actual objects or visiting the sites remains to be seen (see Chatterjee 2008 for debate). Writing archaeology in a way that allows for greater scope to experiment with interpretation and multivocality (another theme common to several chapters) may well become a regular accompaniment to traditional texts. As Praetzellis (1998:1) noted, "The site contains many potential stories, but every one is a product of the archaeological imagination that pulls together historical and archaeological facts into an intepretation that is more than the sum of the parts of which it is made and more than its excavator can document in the usual way." We are all storytellers, and the reader of this volume may note the relatively high degree of subjectivity with which many of the authors write, unabashed in their use of *I* and the validity of drawing on their own embodied experiences to inform their archaeological interpretations. Simultaneously though, and of equal importance, some of them also voice their doubts and methodological concerns, reflecting the exploratory nature of their research and of the sensory field in general. Certainly, not every archaeologist will feel the need to write "imagined narratives," nor should they; scientific results need appropriate scientific presentation, and there is room for a whole spectrum of writing styles and techniques within the discipline. To paraphrase Frank (2000:482), it is important to ask, What can an archaeologist accomplish by using fiction and what is given up in the process?

It should also be asked to what extent sensory archaeology might affect archaeological practice, beyond the current phenomenological surveys. Research by Sarah Pink (2009) has focused on this very issue in ethnographic fieldwork. Excavation is a multisensory experience, and perhaps unconsciously, archaeologists already rely on touch and hearing (and smell to a lesser degree) as well as vision to guide their actions and interpretations. Is it possible to conceive of a future in which site-recording forms have spaces not just for soil color and texture, for example, but also for soil smell or sound? And what impact would this have on the resulting site interpretations, which are always guided by the questions one thinks to ask? However, it is not just field archaeology that may have to deal with "new" senses: The future promises developments in investigating the broader human sensorium. It is well known that training can enhance extant sensory perceptions (e.g., wine tasting), but research in neuroscience suggests that, with practice, it may be possible to acquire new senses such as magnetoreception (Nagel et al. 2005), and the ongoing fascination with sending aromas via computer may finally produce viable results. Moreover, who is to say whether Aldous Huxley's futuristic "feelies" will not become the norm for moviegoers everywhere? It is possible, of course, that among some circles this book may be seen as heretical as Baudelaire's sensual poems once did, but hopefully this will not lead to the prosecution of either the publisher or the editor and authors for crimes against archaeological morality. Rather, we should be confident that in this era of reflexivity and innovative thinking, it will be recognized that a sensory archaeology allows us to carefully explore previously inconceivable issues related to the very experience of being human in the past.

## Acknowledgments

For their helpful comments on various drafts of this introduction, thanks to Astrid Nyland, Conor Trainor, Corin Pursell, Bretton Giles, David Sutton, and Yannis Hamilakis.

## Notes

1. *Les fleurs du mal* can be read online at http://fleursdumal.org, in the original French and in various translations.

2. Papers by Kim Porter, Stacie King, Linda Eneix, Vasilis Tsamis, and Linda Hurcombe were not submitted for publication in this volume.

3. The forthcoming Cambridge University Press monograph *Archaeology of the Senses* (2013), by Yannis Hamilakis, will provide a more detailed examination of sensory archaeology. See also Skeates (2010) for an outlined methodology and archaeological application.

4. Those who wish to learn more about this aspect of sensory studies are directed to core texts such as Calvert, Spence, and Stein (2004) and the work of bodies such as the Crossmodal Research Laboratory at Oxford and the Multisensory Cognition Group at Trinity College Dublin.

5. Thanks to Joe Williams for passing on the link to the relevant Times Educational Supplement feature, available at www.tes.co.uk/article.aspx?storycode=6060248, accessed October 8, 2010.

6. See the restaurant's Web site (www.thefatduck.co.uk) for a more detailed exploration of Blumenthal's philosophy on food and sensory perception.

7. See also the forum on "Indigenous Archaeology" in *American Antiquity* (75:211–243).

8. In the case of societies with literary remains, it may be possible to reconstruct taste based on texts, albeit a taste filtered through the authors' own judgments. See, for example, Feldman (2005) on Roman taste.

## References

Ackerman, Diane
1990 *A Natural History of the Senses*. Random House, New York.

Almagor, Uri
1987 The Cycle and Stagnation of Smells: Pastoralists-Fisherman Relationships in an East African Society. *Res: Anthropology and Aesthetics* 13:106–121.

Appadurai, Arjun (editor)
1986 *The Social Life of Things: Commodities in Cultural Perspective.* Cambridge University Press, Cambridge.

Ayabe-Kanamura, Saho, Ina Schicker, Matthias Laska, Robyn Hudson, Hans Distel, Tatsu Kobayakawa, and Sachiko Saito
1998 Differences in Perception of Everyday Odors: A Japanese-German Cross-Cultural Study. *Chemical Senses* 23:31–38.

Barrett, John C., and Ilhong Ko
2009 A Phenomenology of Landscape: A Crisis in British Landscape Archaeology? *Journal of Social Archaeology* 9:275–294.
Bartosiewicz, László
2003 "There's Something Rotten in the State . . .": Bad Smells in Antiquity. *European Journal of Archaeology* 6:175–195.
Baudelaire, Charles
1972 [1857] *Les fleurs du mal*. Le Livre de Poche, Paris.
Bender, Barbara
1998 *Stonehenge: Making Space*. Berg, Oxford.
Benjamin, Walter
1992 [1936] The Work of Art in the Age of Mechanical Reproduction. In *Illuminations*, translated by Harry Zohn. Fontana, London.
Boivin, Nicole
2004 Rock Art and Rock Music: Petroglyphs of the South Indian Neolithic. *Antiquity* 78:38–53.
2008 *Material Cultures, Material Minds: The Impact of Things on Human Thought*. Cambridge University Press, Cambridge.
Boivin, Nicole, Adam Brumm, Helen Lewis, Dave Robinson, and Ravi Korisettar
2007 Sensual, Material and Technological Understanding: Exploring Prehistoric Soundscapes in South India. *Journal of the Royal Anthropological Institute* 13:267–294.
Borić, Dušan (editor)
2009 *Archaeology and Memory*. Oxbow, Oxford.
Borić, Dušan, and John Robb
2008 Body Theory in Archaeology. In *Past Bodies: Body-Centered Research in Archaeology*, edited by Dušan Borić and John Robb, pp. 1–7. Oxbow, Oxford.
Borić, Dušan, and John Robb (editors)
2008 *Past Bodies: Body-Centered Research in Archaeology*. Oxbow, Oxford.
Brück, Joanna
2005 Experiencing the Past? The Development of a Phenomenological Archaeology in British Prehistory. *Archaeological Dialogues* 12:45–72.
Bubandt, Nils
1998 The Odour of Things: Smell and the Cultural Elaboration of Disgust in Eastern Indonesia. *Ethnos* 63:48–80.
Bull, Michael, and Les Back (editors)
2003 *The Auditory Culture Reader*. Berg, Oxford.
Calvert, Gemma A., Charles Spence, and Barry E. Stein (editors)
2004 *The Handbook of Multisensory Processes*. MIT Press, Cambridge, Massachusetts.
Carter, Tristan
2007 The Theatrics of Technology: Consuming Obsidian in the Early Cycladic Burial Arena. *Archaeological Papers of the American Anthropological Association* 17:88–107.
Chatterjee, Helen J. (editor)
2008 *Touch in Museums: Policy and Practice in Object Handling*. Berg, London.
Classen, Constance
1990 Sweet Colors, Fragrant Songs: Sensory Models of the Andes and the Amazon. *American Ethnologist* 17:722–735.
1993 *Worlds of Sense: Exploring the Senses in History and across Cultures*. Routledge, London.
1997 Foundations for an Anthropology of the Senses. *International Social Science Journal* 153:401–412.

2007 Museum Manners: The Sensory Life of the Early Museum. *Journal of Social History* 40:895–914.

Classen, Constance (editor)
2005 *The Book of Touch*. Berg, Oxford.

Classen, Constance, and David Howes
2006 The Museum as Sensescape: Western Sensibilities and Indigenous Artifacts. In *Sensible Objects: Colonialism, Museums and Material Culture*, edited by Elizabeth Edwards, Chris Gosden, and Ruth B. Phillips, pp. 199–222. Berg, Oxford.

Classen, Constance, David Howes, and Anthony Synnott
1994 *Aroma: The Cultural History of Smell*. Routledge, London.

Cleland, Liza, and Karen Stears (editors)
2004 *Colour in the Ancient Mediterranean World*. BAR International Series 1267. Archaeopress, Oxford.

Clifford, James, and George E. Marcus (editors)
1986 *Writing Culture: The Poetics and Politics of Ethnography*. University of California Press, Berkeley.

Coles, John M.
1967 Some Irish Horns of the Late Bronze Age. *Journal of the Royal Society of Antiquaries of Ireland* 97:113–117.
1973 *Archaeology by Experiment*. Hutchinson, London.

Connerton, Paul
1989 *How Societies Remember*. Cambridge University Press, Cambridge.

Cook, Ian A., Sarah K. Pajot, and Andrew F. Leuchter
2008 Ancient Architectural Acoustic Resonance Patterns and Regional Brain Activity. *Time and Mind* 1:95–104.

Corbin, Alain
1986 *The Foul and the Fragrant: Odor and the French Social Imagination*. Harvard University Press, Cambridge, Massachusetts.

Cummings, Vicki
2002 Experiencing Texture and Transformation in the British Neolithic. *Oxford Journal of Archaeology* 21:249–261.

Cummings, Vicki, and Alasdair W. R. Whittle
2004 *Places of Special Virtue: Megaliths in the Neolithic Landscapes of Wales*. Oxbow, Oxford.

Cytowic, Richard E., and David M. Eagleman
2009 *Wednesday Is Indigo Blue: Discovering the Brain of Synesthesia*. MIT Press, Cambridge, Massachusetts.

Dams, Lya
1985 Palaeolithic Lithophones: Descriptions and Comparisons. *Oxford Journal of Archaeology* 4:31–46.

Devereux, Paul, and Robert G. Jahn
1996 Preliminary Investigations and Cognitive Considerations of the Acoustical Resonances of Selected Archaeological Sites. *Antiquity* 70:665–666.

Dietler, Michael, and Brian Hayden (editors)
2001 *Feasts. Archaeological and Ethnographic Perspectives on Food, Politics, and Power*. Smithsonian Institution Press, Washington, D.C.

Dobres, Marcia-Anne
2010 Archaeologies of Technology. *Cambridge Journal of Economics* 34:103–114.

Drobnick, Jim (editor)
2006 *The Smell Culture Reader*. Berg, Oxford.

Edmonds, Mark
1999 *Ancestral Geographies of the Neolithic*. Routledge, London.
Edwards, Elizabeth, and Kaushik Bhaumik (editors)
2008 *Visual Sense: A Cultural Reader.* Berg, Oxford.
Feld, Steven
1990 *Sound and Sentiment: Birds, Weeping, Poetics and Song in Kaluli Expression*. 2nd ed. University of Pennsylvania Press, Philadelphia.
1996 Waterfalls of Song: An Acoustemology of Place Resounding in Bosavi, Papua New Guinea. In *Senses of Place*, edited by Steven Feld and Keith H. Basso, pp. 91–135. School of American Research, Santa Fe, New Mexico.
Feldman, Charles
2005 Roman Taste. *Food, Culture and Society* 8:7–30.
Fleming, Andrew
2006 Post-Processual Landscape Archaeology: A Critique. *Cambridge Archaeological Journal* 16:267–280.
Fowles, Severin
2010 The Southwest School of Landscape Archaeology. *Annual Review of Anthropology* 39:453–468.
Fox, Rachel
2008 Tastes, Smells and Spaces: Sensory Perceptions and Mycenaean Palatial Feasting. In *DAIS. The Aegean Feast*, edited by Louise A. Hitchcock, Robert Laffineur, and Janice Crowley, pp. 133–141. Aegaeum 29. Université de Liège, Liège.
Frank, Katherine
2000 "The Management of Hunger": Using Fiction in Writing Anthropology. *Qualitative Inquiry* 6:474–488.
Geertz, Clifford
1973 Thick Description: Toward an Interpretive Theory of Culture. In *The Interpretation of Cultures: Selected Essays*, pp. 3–30. Basic Books, New York.
1988 *Works and Lives: The Anthropologist as Author.* Stanford University Press, Stanford.
Georgiadis, Mercourios, and Chrysanthi Gallou (editors)
2009 *Past in the Past: The Significance of Memory and Tradition in the Transmission of Culture.* BAR International Series 1925. Archaeopress, Oxford.
Geurts, Kathryn Linn
2002 *Culture and the Senses: Embodiment, Identity, and Well-Being in an African Community.* University of California Press, Berkeley.
2003 On Rocks, Walks, and Talks in West Africa: Cultural Categories and an Anthropology of the Senses. *Ethos* 30:178–198.
Gibb, James G.
2000 Imaginary, But by No Means Unimaginable: Storytelling, Science, and Historical Archaeology. *Historical Archaeology* 34(2):1–6.
Goldhahn, Joakim
2002 Roaring Rocks: An Audio-Visual Perspective on Hunter-Gatherer Engravings in Northern Sweden and Scandinavia. *Norwegian Archaeological Review* 35:29–61.
Goody, Jack
1987 *The Interface Between the Written and the Oral.* Cambridge University Press, Cambridge.
Gosden, Chris
2005 What Do Objects Want? *Journal of Archaeological Method and Theory* 12:193–211.

Grimshaw, Anna
2001 *The Ethnographer's Eye: Ways of Seeing in Anthropology.* Cambridge University Press, Cambridge.
Hamilakis, Yannis
1998 Eating the Dead: Mortuary Feasting and the Politics of Memory in the Aegean Bronze Age. In *Cemetery and Society in the Aegean Bronze Age,* edited by Keith Branigan, pp. 15–132. Sheffield Academic Press, Sheffield.
2000 The Anthropology of Food and Drink Consumption and Aegean Archaeology. In *Palaeodiet in the Aegean,* edited by Sarah J. Vaughan and William D. E. Coulson, pp. 55–63. Wiener Laboratory Monograph 1. Oxbow, Oxford.
2007 *The Nation and Its Ruins: Antiquity, Archaeology and the National Imagination.* Oxford University Press, Oxford.
2008 Time, Performance, and the Production of a Mnemonic Record: From Feasting to an Archaeology of Eating and Drinking. In *DAIS. The Aegean Feast,* edited by Louise A. Hitchcock, Robert Laffineur, and Janice Crowley, pp. 3–19. Aegaeum 29. Université de Liège, Liège.
2010 Re-collecting the Fragments: Archaeology as Mnemonic Practice. In *Material Mnemonics: Everyday Memory in Prehistoric Europe,* edited by Katina T. Lillios and Vasileios Tsamis, pp. 188–199. Oxbow, Oxford.
2013 *Archaeology of the Senses.* Cambridge University Press, Cambridge, in press.
Hamilakis, Yannis, Mark Pluciennik, and Sarah Tarlow (editors)
2002 *Thinking through the Body: Archaeologies of Corporeality.* Kluwer Academic/Plenum Publishers, London.
Hamilton, Sue, and Ruth Whitehouse, with Keri Brown, Pamela Combes, Edward Herring, and Mike Seager Thomas
2006 Phenomenology in Practice: Towards a Methodology for a 'Subjective' Approach. *European Journal of Archaeology* 9:31–71.
Hawkes, Christopher F.
1954 Archaeological Theory and Method: Some Suggestions from the Old World. *American Anthropologist* 56:155–168.
Herva, Vesa-Pekka
2006 Flower Lovers, After All? Rethinking Religion and Human-Environment Relationships in Minoan Crete. *World Archaeology* 38:586–598.
Herzfeld, Michael
2001 *Anthropology: Theoretical Practice in Culture and Society.* Blackwell, Oxford.
Holtzman, Jon D.
2006 Food and Memory. *Annual Review of Anthropology* 35:361–378.
2009 *Uncertain Tastes: Memory, Ambivalence, and the Politics of Eating in Samburu, Northern Kenya.* University of California Press, Berkeley.
2010 Remembering Bad Cooks: Sensuality, Memory, Personhood. *Senses and Society* 5:235–243.
Hosler, Dorothy
1994 *The Sounds and Colors of Power: The Sacred Metallurgical Technology of Ancient West Mexico.* MIT Press, Cambridge, Massachusetts.
Houston, Stephen D., Claudia Brittenham, Cassandra Mesick, Alexandre Tokovinine, and Christina Warinner
2009 *Veiled Brightness: A History of Ancient Maya Color.* University of Texas Press, Austin.

Houston, Stephen D., and Karl A. Taube

2000 An Archaeology of the Senses: Perception and Cultural Expression in Ancient Mesoamerica. *Cambridge Archaeological Journal* 10:261–294.

Howes, David

2003 *Sensual Relations: Engaging the Senses in Culture and Social Theory*. University of Michigan Press, Ann Arbor.

Howes, David (editor)

1991 *The Varieties of Sensory Experience*. University of Toronto Press, Toronto.

2005 *Empire of the Senses: The Sensual Culture Reader*. Berg, Oxford.

2009 *The Sixth Sense Reader*. Berg, Oxford.

Hume, Lynne

2007 *Portals: Opening Doorways to Other Realities Through the Senses*. Berg, Oxford.

Hummler, Madeleine

2008 Review of Stone Worlds: Narrative and Reflexivity in Landscape Archaeology. *Antiquity* 82:1156–1157.

Hurcombe, Linda

2007 A Sense of Materials and Sensory Perception in Concepts of Materiality. *World Archaeology* 39:532–545.

Ingold, Tim

2004 Culture on the Ground: The World Perceived Through the Feet. *Journal of Material Culture* 9:315–340.

Insoll, Timothy

2007 *Archaeology: The Conceptual Challenge*. Duckworth, London.

Isaakidou, Valasia

2007 Cooking in the Labyrinth: Exploring 'Cuisine' at Bronze Age Knossos. In *Cooking Up the Past: Food and Culinary Practices in the Neolithic and Bronze Age Aegean*, edited by Christopher Mee and Josette Renard, pp. 5–24. Oxbow, Oxford.

Jahn, Robert G., Paul Devereux, and Michael Ibison

1996 Acoustical Resonances of Assorted Ancient Structures. *Journal of the Acoustical Society of America* 99:649–658.

Jones, Andrew

2007 *Memory and Material Culture*. Cambridge University Press, Cambridge.

Jones, Andrew, and Gavin MacGregor (editors)

2002 *Colouring the Past: The Significance of Colour in Archaeological Research*. Berg, Oxford.

Joyce, Rosemary A.

2005 Archaeology of the Body. *Annual Review of Anthropology* 34:139–158.

Joyce, Rosemary A., with Robert W. Preucel

2002 *The Languages of Archaeology: Dialogue, Narrative and Writing*. Blackwell, Oxford.

Joyce, Rosemary A., and John S. Henderson

2007 From Feasting to Cuisine: Implications of Archaeological Research in an Early Honduran Village. *American Anthropologist* 109:642–653.

Jütte, Robert

2005 *A History of the Senses: From Antiquity to Cyberspace*. Translated by James Lynn. Polity Press, Cambridge.

King, Stacie M., and Gonzalo Sánchez Santiago

2011 Soundscapes of the Everyday in Ancient Oaxaca, Mexico. *Archaeologies: Journal of the World Archaeological Congress* 7:387–422.

Kirby, Percival R.
1947 The Trumpets of Tut-Ankh-Amen and Their Successors. *Journal of the Royal Anthropological Institute* 77:33–45.
Knappett, Carl
2005 *Thinking Through Material Culture: An Interdisciplinary Perspective.* University of Pennsylvania Press, Philadelphia.
Korsmeyer, Carolyn (editor)
2005 *The Taste Culture Reader: Experiencing Food and Drink.* Berg, Oxford.
Lewis-Williams, J. David, and Thomas A. Dowson
1990 Through the Veil: San Rock Paintings and the Rock Face. *South African Archaeological Bulletin* 45:5–16.
Lillios, Katina T., and Vasileios Tsamis (editors)
2010 *Material Mnemonics: Everyday Memory in Prehistoric Europe.* Oxbow, Oxford.
Loose, Richard W.
2008 Tse'Biinaholts'a Yałti (Curved Rock That Speaks). *Time and Mind* 1:31–50.
Macbeth, Helen, and Sue Lawry
2006 Food Preferences and Taste: An Introduction. In *Food Preferences and Taste: Continuity and Change.* 2nd ed. Edited by Helen Macbeth, pp. 1–13. Berghahn, Oxford.
McCarthy, John P.
2003 More than Just "Telling the Story": Interpretive Narrative Archaeology. In *Ancient Muses: Archaeology and the Arts,* edited by John H. Jameson Jr., John E. Ehrenhard, and Christine A. Finn, pp. 15–24. University of Alabama Press, Tuscaloosa.
MacGregor, Gavin
1999 Making Sense of the Past in the Present: A Sensory Analysis of Carved Stone Balls. *World Archaeology* 31:258–271.
Mathieu, James R.
2002 Introduction–Experimental Archaeology: Replicating Past Objects, Behaviors, and Processes. In *Experimental Archaeology: Replicating Past Objects, Behaviors, and Processes,* edited by James R. Mathieu, pp. 1–10. BAR International Series 1035. Archaeopress, Oxford.
Merleau-Ponty, Maurice
2002 [1945] *The Phenomenology of Perception.* Translated by Colin Smith. Routledge Classics, London.
Meskell, Lynn M.
2000 Writing the Body in Archaeology. In *Reading the Body: Representations and Remains in the Archaeological Record,* edited by Alison E. Rautman, pp. 13–21. University of Pennsylvania Press, Philadelphia.
Meskell, Lynn M. (editor)
2005 *Archaeologies of Materiality.* Blackwell, Oxford.
Miller, Daniel
2008 *The Comfort of Things.* Polity Press, Cambridge.
Miller, William I.
1997 *The Anatomy of Disgust.* Harvard University Press, Cambridge, Massachusetts.
Mills, Barbara J., and William H. Walker (editors)
2008 *Memory Work: Archaeologies of Material Practices.* School of Advanced Research Press, Santa Fe, New Mexico.
Mithen, Steven
2006 *The Singing Neanderthals: The Origins of Music, Language, Mind, and Body.* Harvard University Press, Cambridge, Massachusetts.

Molloy, Barry P. C.
2008 Martial Arts and Materiality: A Combat Archaeology Perspective on Aegean Swords of the Fifteenth and Fourteenth Centuries B.C. *World Archaeology* 40:116–134.
Nagel, Saskia K., Christine Carl, Tobias Kringe, Robert Märtin, and Peter König
2005 Beyond Sensory Substitution—Learning the Sixth Sense. *Journal of Neural Engineering* 2(4):R13–R26.
Needham, Rodney
1967 Percussion and Transition. *Man*, n.s. 2:606–614.
Olsen, Bjørnar
2003 Material Culture after Text: Re-Membering Things. *Norwegian Archaeological Review* 36:87–104.
Ouzman, Sven
2001 Seeing Is Deceiving: Rock Art and the Non-Visual. *World Archaeology* 33: 237–256.
Paterson, Mark
2007 *The Senses of Touch: Haptics, Affects and Technologies*. Berg, Oxford.
Pink, Sarah
2009 *Doing Sensory Ethnography*. Sage, London.
Porath, Nathan
2008 Seeing Sound: Consciousness and Therapeutic Acoustics in the Inter-Sensory Shamanic Epistemology of the Orang Sakai of Riau (Sumatra). *Journal of the Royal Anthropological Institute*, n.s. 14:647–663.
Porcello, Thomas, Louise Meintjes, Ana Maria Ochoa, and David W. Samuels
2010 The Reorganization of the Sensory World. *Annual Review of Anthropology* 39:51–66.
Praetzellis, Adrian
1998 Introduction: Why Every Archaeologist Should Tell Stories Once in a While. *Historical Archaeology* 32(1):1–3.
Price, Neil S.
2001 An Archaeology of Altered States: Shamanism and Material Culture Studies. In *The Archaeology of Shamanism*, edited by Neil S. Price, pp. 3–16. Routledge, London.
Pye, David
1995 *The Nature and Art of Workmanship*. Herbert Press, London.
Reznikoff, Iegor, and Michel Dauvois
1988 La dimension sonore des grottes ornées. *Bulletin de la Société Préhistorique Française* 85:238–246.
Rodaway, Paul
1994 *Sensuous Geographies: Body, Sense and Place*. Routledge, London.
Saunders, Nicholas J.
2001 A Dark Light: Reflections on Obsidian in Mesoamerica. *World Archaeology* 33:220–236.
Scarre, Chris (editor)
2002 *Monuments and Landscape in Atlantic Europe*. Routledge, London.
Scarre, Chris, and Graeme Lawson (editors)
2006 *Archaeoacoustics*. MacDonald Institute for Archaeological Research, Cambridge.
Seeger, Anthony
1975 The Meaning of Body Ornaments: A Suya Example. *Ethnology* 14:211–224.

Seremetakis, C. Nadia (editor)

1994 *The Senses Still: Perception and Memory as Material Culture in Modernity.* Westview, Boulder, Colorado.

Serres, Michel

2008 [1985] *The Five Senses: A Philosophy of Mingled Bodies.* Translated by Margaret Sankey and Peter Cowley. Contiuum, London.

Skeates, Robin

2010 *An Archaeology of the Senses: Prehistoric Malta.* Oxford University Press, Oxford.

Smith, Mark

2007 *Sensing the Past: Seeing, Hearing, Smelling, Tasting, and Touching in History.* University of California Press, Berkeley.

Stoller, Paul

1984 Sound in Songhay Cultural Experience. *American Ethnologist* 11:559–570.

1989 *The Taste of Ethnographic Things: The Senses in Anthropology.* University of Pennsylvania Press, Philadelphia.

1997 *Sensuous Scholarship.* University of Pennsylvania Press, Philadelphia.

Stoller, Paul, and Cheryl Olkes

1986 Bad Sauce, Good Ethnography. *Cultural Anthropology* 1:336–352.

Stroeken, Koen

2008 Sensory Shifts and 'Synaesthetics' in Sukuma Healing. *Ethnos* 73:466–484.

Sutton, David E.

2001 *Remembrance of Repasts: An Anthropology of Food and Memory.* Berg, Oxford.

2010 Food and the Senses. *Annual Review of Anthropology* 39:209–223.

Synnott, Anthony

1991a Puzzling over the Senses: From Plato to Marx. In *The Varieties of Sensory Experience,* edited by David Howes, pp. 61–76. University of Toronto Press, Toronto.

1991b A Sociology of Smell. *Canadian Review of Sociology and Anthropology* 28:437–459.

Tarlow, Sarah

2000 Emotion in Archaeology. *Current Anthropology* 41:713–730.

Tilley, Christopher Y.

1994 *Phenomenology of Landscape: Places, Paths and Monuments.* Berg, Oxford.

2004 *The Materiality of Stone: Explorations in Landscape Phenomenology* 1. Berg, Oxford.

2008 *Body and Image: Explorations in Landscape Phenomenology* 2. Left Coast Press, Walnut Creek, California.

2010 *Interpreting Landscapes: Geologies, Topographies, Identities. Explorations in Landscape Phenomenology* 3. Left Coast Press, Walnut Creek, California.

Tringham, Ruth E.

1991 Households with Faces: The Challenge of Gender in Prehistoric Architectural Remains. In *Engendering Archaeology: Women and Prehistory,* edited by Joan M. Gero and Margaret W. Conkey, pp. 93–131. Blackwell, Oxford.

Trubek, Amy B.

2008 *The Taste of Place: A Cultural Journey into Terroir.* University of California Press, Berkeley.

Tuzin, Donald

1984 Miraculous Voices: The Auditory Experience of Numinous Objects. *Current Anthropology* 25:579–596.

Valamoti, Soultana Maria

2009 Plant Food Ingredients and 'Recipes' from Prehistoric Greece: The Archaeobotanical Evidence. In *Plants and Culture: Seeds of the Cultural Heritage of Europe,* edited by Jean-Paul Morel and Anna Maria Mercuri, pp. 25–38. Edipuglia, Bari.

Van Dyke, Ruth M., and Susan E. Alcock (editors)
2003 *Archaeologies of Memory*. Blackwell, Oxford.
Waller, Steven J.
2006 Intentionality of Rock-Art Placement Deduced from Acoustical Measurements and Echo Myths. In *Archaeoacoustics*, edited by Chris Scarre and Graeme Lawson, pp. 31–39. Macdonald Institute for Archaeological Research, Cambridge.
Wallin, Nils L., Björn Merker, and Steven Brown (editors)
2000 *The Origins of Music*. MIT Press, Cambridge, Massachusetts.
Waterston, Alisse, and Maria D. Vesperi (editors)
2009 *Anthropology Off the Shelf: Anthropologists on Writing*. Wiley-Blackwell, Oxford.
Watson, Aaron
2001 The Sounds of Transformation: Acoustics, Monuments and Ritual in the British Neolithic. In *The Archaeology of Shamanism*, edited by Neil Price, pp. 178–192. Routledge, London.
Watson, Aaron, and David Keating
1999 Architecture and Sound: An Acoustic Analysis of Megalithic Monuments in Prehistoric Britain. *Antiquity* 73:325–336.
Wiessner, Polly, and Wulf Schiefenhövel (editors)
1996 *Food and the Status Quest: An Interdisciplinary Perspective*. Berghahn, London.
Zampini, Massimiliano, and Charles Spence
2010 Assessing the Role of Sound in the Perception of Food and Drink. *Chemosensory Perception* 3:57–67.
Zhang, Juzhong, Xinghua Xiao, and Yun Kuen Lee
2004 The Early Development of Music: Analysis of the Jiahu Bone Flutes. *Antiquity* 78:769–778.

# 2. *Dibéwagendamowin / Kārohirohi*: Reflections on Sacred Images on the Rocks

*William A. Allen, Gerard O'Regan, Perry Fletcher, and Roger Noganosh*

*Abstract:* Observations of reflected sunlight shimmering on ancient rock art have previously been reported with the implication that the visual effect adds to the significance of the images or locality (Arsenault 2004a:305; Hyder 2004:89). This paper provides an account of the landscape features at a number of water's edge rock faces in northern Ontario in Canada and Lake Taupō in New Zealand where the phenomenon appears on or about painted images. It explores factors to be considered in determining whether there is an actual correlation between the reflected light and the placement of the rock paintings and, if so, how such reflections may have been interpreted within the traditional worldviews of the Anishinaabeg in Canada and the Māori in New Zealand.

Northern Ontario's French River was the main route of access from eastern Canada to Lake Huron and its connecting long-distance routes to the upper Mississippi River and to Canada's great Northwest. In October 2008, Ontario archaeologist William Allen, accompanied by local elders, introduced Gerard O'Regan, a rock art researcher from Ngāi Tahu, a Māori tribe of New Zealand, to the sites of some French River rock paintings. The localities could only be visited by boat, from which in the calm, sunny, autumn conditions we observed shimmering sunlight reflected from the water onto the red ochre rock paintings. We pondered. Would the creators of the paintings have seen such shimmering light, and might it have influenced where they chose to paint? Would subsequent

*Making Senses of the Past: Toward a Sensory Archaeology*, edited by Jo Day. Center for Archaeological Investigations, Occasional Paper No. 40.  ISBN 978-0-8093-3287-8.

visitors to the rock paintings have seen the shimmer and could it have contributed to the experience of the paintings and the place? Moreover, to what extent can such modern observations reasonably be related to past activities?

In a review of archaeological approaches to landscape, Arsenault (2004b:80) calls for archaeologists to enhance their interpretations of sacred landscapes by better incorporating the traditional knowledge of indigenous worldviews and further developing tools for investigating what might be described as sensory factors such as sound, touch, and light effects (Arsenault 2004a:303–306). Such an approach would allow for broader perspectives than can be achieved through strict examinations of static, visual perspectives and would better reflect the range of phenomena that Indigenous Peoples are understood to appreciate at sacred places. We have found this approach to be valuable when considering specific heritage sites of two unrelated cultures on either side of the globe. In this regard, we discuss our observations of shimmering reflected sunlight on rock paintings in Ontario, Canada, and in New Zealand.

## Ontario Observations

In calm conditions slight movement in the water surface from currents or ripples caused by a gentle breeze can create unevenness in the concentration of reflected sunlight on neighboring surfaces. This can result in an observable shimmering effect on those surfaces if they are sufficiently broad, angled appropriately to the source of the light reflections, and partially reflective themselves, as is the case, for example, with the hull of a boat or a clear rock surface. Rock paintings in Ontario are almost always positioned on vertical rock faces at the water's edge. During two days of field visits to rock painting sites on French River and Rock Lake (Figure 2-1), the shimmering light effect was noticeable at four different localities. All four sites were visited by boat in calm, sunny conditions. After initially observing the shimmering reflections, we recorded the effects from the boat using a handheld Canon Si5 camera in 640 × 480, 30 fps video mode. Care was taken to ensure that there was no disturbance of the water surface or light source by the boat or its wake; this sometimes required filming from a distance, using high zoom settings on the camera. Given these factors, the resulting video recordings contain considerable shaking and jitter, but there is sufficient stable footage to clearly document the natural shimmering light effect on the painted rock surfaces.

The first recording was made at a rock bluff on the northern side of French River about 1 km west of the Trans-Canada Highway bridge. There, a sheer bluff drops vertically into deep water. Near the center of the bluff, a human figure is painted in red ochre about 1.5 m above river level. This places it at about eye level for people standing in a small open boat, such as did the elders on our trip who led the placement of tobacco offerings—a documented traditional practice at sacred sites (Arsenault 2004a:299)—which reflects the sacred regard that these places and paintings are held in today. With the vessel sitting midriver—some 30 m from the bluff—so that the wider landscape settings could also be viewed,

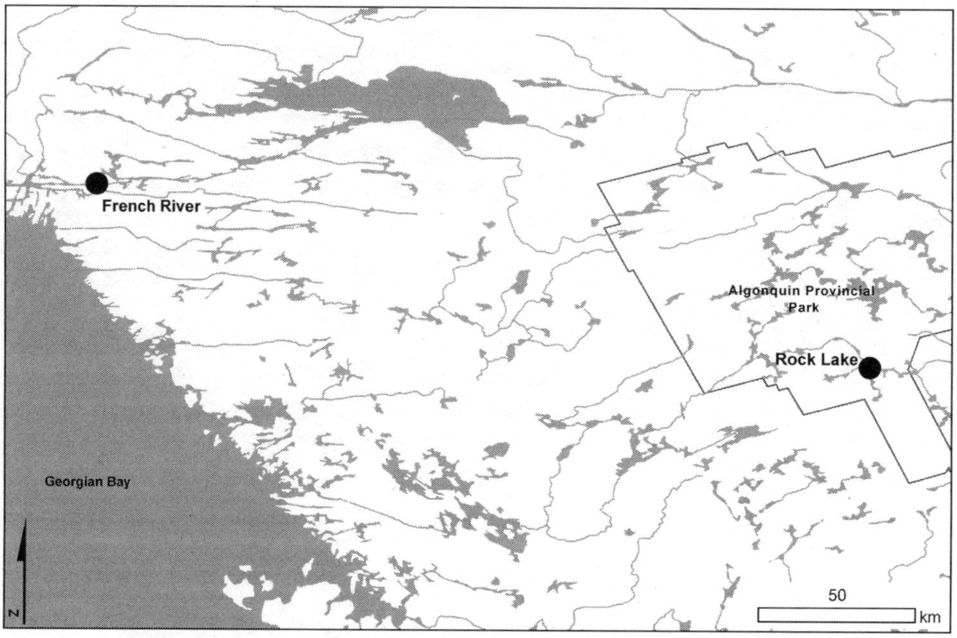


**Figure 2-1.** *Location of French River and Rock Lake, Ontario, Canada. (Map by Gerard O'Regan.)*

the shimmering effect of reflected sunlight was first noticed where it was most vivid—about a shadowed crevice just above water level at the eastern end of the bluff—and then recognized as extending over the lower level of the bluff toward the rock paintings.

Another site visited a short time later is also on the north bank of the river, just east of the Trans-Canada Highway bridge. Documented in 1793 in the journal of John MacDonell (Gates 1965:85), it is at the base of a precipitous cliff. The paintings are positioned about 2 m above river level on a smooth panel that overhangs deep water. The figures include an upright anthropomorph with one arm raised, an apparent animal at the feet of the upright figure, and two curved lines. During the midafternoon visit, the shimmering reflected sunlight was especially intense over these rock paintings and surrounding panels.

Having been advised by First Nation elders about the cultural interpretation of forms in natural features at sacred places, Allen had observed during a previous visit to the site that in certain light conditions the particular panel has the appearance of a face with two eyes formed by shadows in shallow depressions in the rock (Allen 2009). Also of possible cultural interest, local participants on the present visit noted that a small, river-level rock ledge that protrudes over deep water just to the west of the painted panel would have been a particularly good spot for spearing fish.

Later that same day, the site was viewed from the top of the high banks on the opposite side of the river. The shimmering light was still very pronounced on both the painted panel and adjacent rock but not elsewhere along the cliff face.

Also from that vantage point, a break in the vertical bluffs can be seen immediately above the painted panel. It has not been determined whether or not the cliff face there is actually scalable; if so, it would be a very steep and dangerous climb, even for an agile person, and especially so in wet or icy conditions. As the locality is most readily accessible by river and given the distance and orientation of the panel from the protruding rock ledge, the rock paintings were most likely produced by someone on the river.

Allen and O'Regan also made an afternoon visit to two sets of rock paintings along the base of another waterside bluff at Rock Lake, near the East Gate in the south of Algonquin Provincial Park. Again, with flat water and sunny conditions, reflected light shimmer was a notable visual feature over the rock paintings in both localities.

Accessible only from the lake, a sheer rock face that drops vertically into deep water forms the panel for the easternmost set of paintings (Figures 2-2 and 2-3). Three vertical and parallel red ochre strikes about 30 cm long are painted near the center of the panel at about 1.5 m above the lake's surface, the approximate head height of a standing adult. About 2 m to the north and lower on the panel, a little less than 1 m above the lake's surface, is a red painted figure about 30 cm high with splayed limbs, large pointed ears, and a tail. The figure may represent Nanabush, a significant ancestor in Algonquin traditions who sometimes took the form of a hare and is featured in rock paintings elsewhere in Ontario (Devereux 2008:21). At the time of the visit, the reflected light shimmered particularly along the bottom of the panel covering this figure, but shimmer was also discernible over the higher three strikes and especially in a small horizontal crevice in the rock adjacent to them.

The second group of rock paintings is situated near the western end of the same bluff. A group of six weathered red ochre lines about 30 cm in length accompanied by two smaller dashes fan out over a small vertical panel just above current lake level and just before the cliff face breaks to a landing of fallen rocks. A further eight red strikes are located on a panel adjacent to and about 1.5 m above the first. Reflected light shimmer was noted over all the markings but was particularly bright along the rock at the water's edge and over the lower panel.

These two sets of markings are the only rock paintings recorded on Rock Lake and are only accessible by boat. It is possible to land on fallen rocks next to the second group of rock paintings, but the lower of these is just beyond the dry landing. Shimmer was not observed anywhere else along the cliff face.

These French River and Rock Lake examples are not the first Canadian rock painting sites at which observations of sunlight related phenomena have occurred. Arsenault (2004a:305) discusses nine finger-painted sites in Quebec, of which he considers seven oriented so as to receive maximum sunlight. Strong reflections of sunlight off the smooth rock surface and silica film at Nisula site, Upper North Shore, can make the red ochre paintings there momentarily difficult to discern (Arsenault 2004a:305–306). Allen previously saw shimmering reflections immediately beside a rock painting in the Barron Canyon, Ontario. This site is a good example of the challenge of "transience of evidence" for archaeologists (Corbin 2005:131), as it displays both transient shimmering light and transient

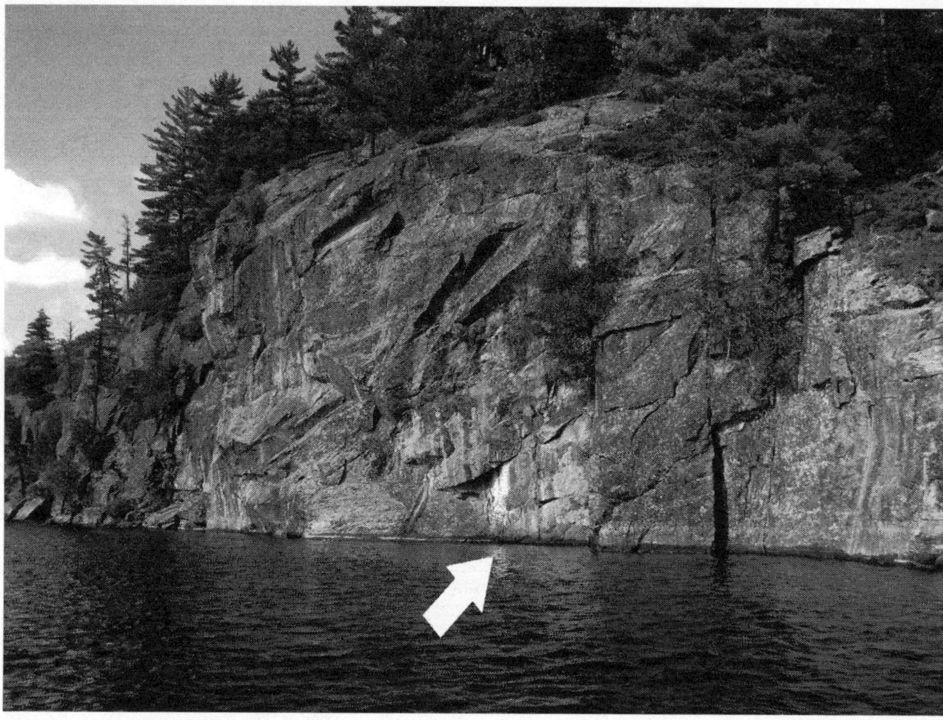

**Figure 2-2.** *The eastern rock painting panel visited at Rock Lake. (Photograph © Gerard O'Regan.)*

auditory experience. In certain wind conditions, waves lap against a flat-roofed cave at the waterline, intermittently closing and opening the cave's entrance and causing a deep gurgling sound that resembles a mumbling voice coming from the rock. Similarly, the sound of water flowing through a deep fissure in the large carved Kinomagewapkong ("Teaching Rocks") at Petroglyphs Provincial Park has also been suggested as possibly related to the voices of manitous, or spiritual beings (Devereux 2008:27–28).

## New Zealand Observations

Situated between latitudes 38° and 39° south on the other side of the globe, *Taupō Moana*, the 30 km wide Lake Taupō, sits in a large volcanic crater in the center of the North Island of New Zealand (Figure 2-4). Perry Fletcher has spent 30 years recording pre-European Māori sites around this region, including rock paintings on a peninsula on the northern edge of the lake. During a site tour in November 2009, the start of New Zealand's summer, Fletcher and O'Regan noted shimmering light on and about the rock paintings' localities, similar to that which O'Regan had recorded with Allen in Canada.

Four groups of markings, collectively registered as T18/102 in the New Zealand Archaeological Association site record system, are located along 120 m of

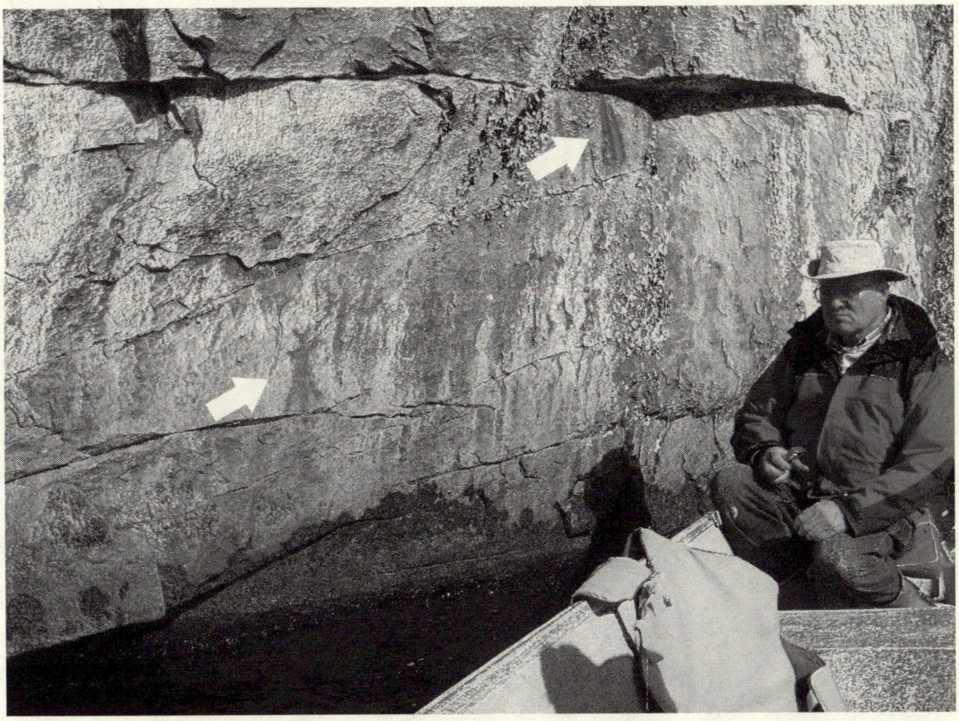

**Figure 2-3.** *William Allen at the eastern Rock Lake painted panel. White arrows indicate the paintings (enhanced). (Photograph © Gerard O'Regan.)*

a stone bluff on a peninsula that forms the eastern edge of Kawakawa Bay and separates it from neighboring Whangamata Bay (Figure 2-5). The paintings are most readily accessible by water, with steep, dangerous cliff-face climbs required to visit the localities otherwise. Therefore, all the markings can only be viewed with ease from the lake.

The southernmost set is visually dominated by a vertical rectangular panel about 1 m wide that has been completely covered in thick red ochre, red being a color associated with *tapu,* or sacredness, in traditional Māori culture. Nine small red strikes up to 30 cm in length are on immediately adjacent panels, but unlike the large red patch that can be seen in clear conditions from over 100 m away on the lake, the smaller red strikes are visible only when close to the cliff. At the time of the site visit, early afternoon sunlight reflected off the lake and shimmered over the lower cliff face in the vicinity of the paintings, including over the red strikes and the overhang immediately above the markings.

From a vantage on the lake, even some distance from the shore, another set of markings is also visible on the north end of the bluffs. Local Māori tradition has it that the remains of the war canoe *Te Reporepo* lie at this location. Three vertical red strikes, each about 75 cm long, are painted about 3 m above present lake level. Shimmering reflected sunlight was observed in a small dark overhang above and faintly at the top of the rock panel with the markings. The marked panel is oriented slightly to the south, and during the midafternoon visit, the

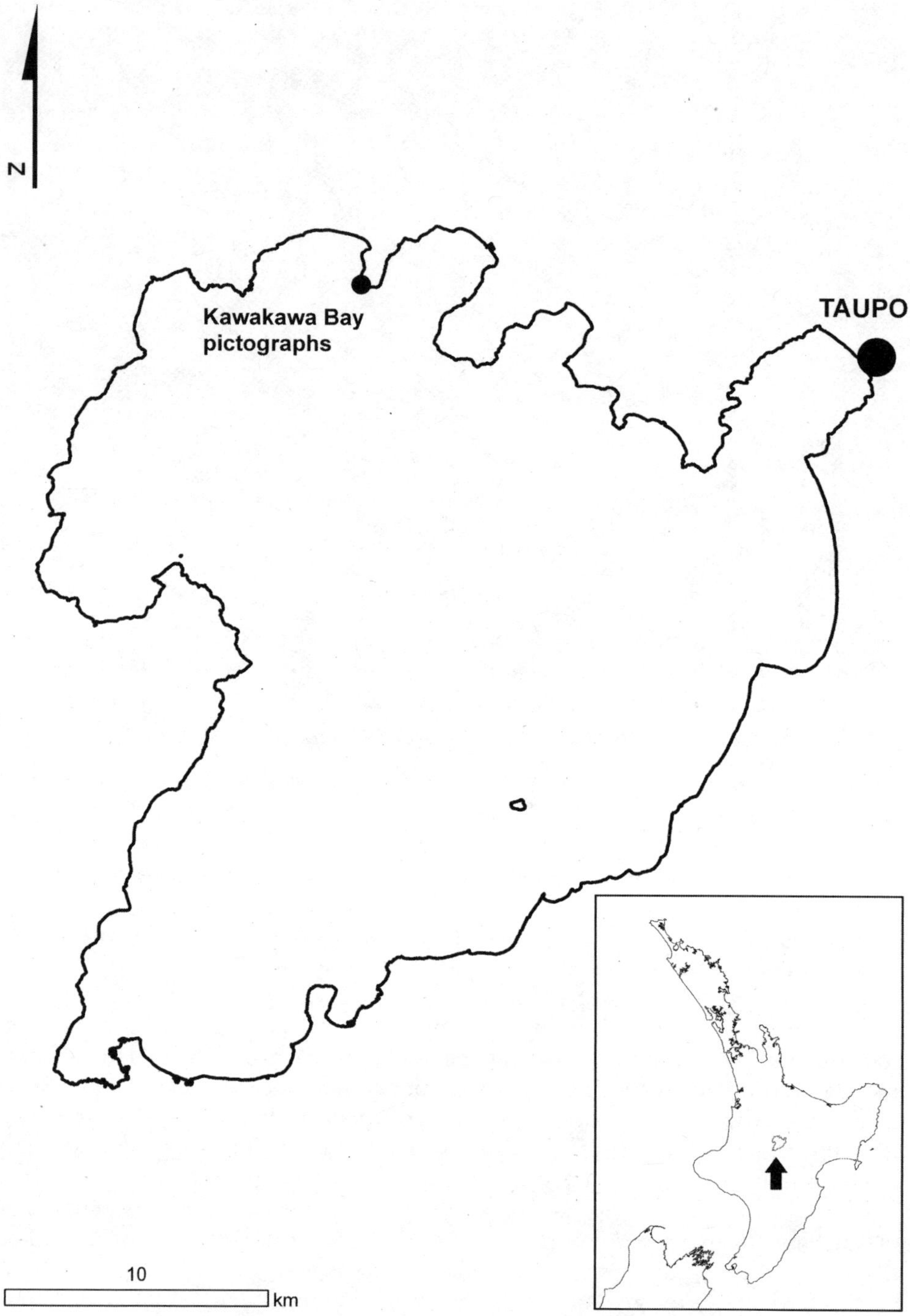


**Figure 2-4.** *Lake Taupō, New Zealand. (Map by Gerard O'Regan.)*

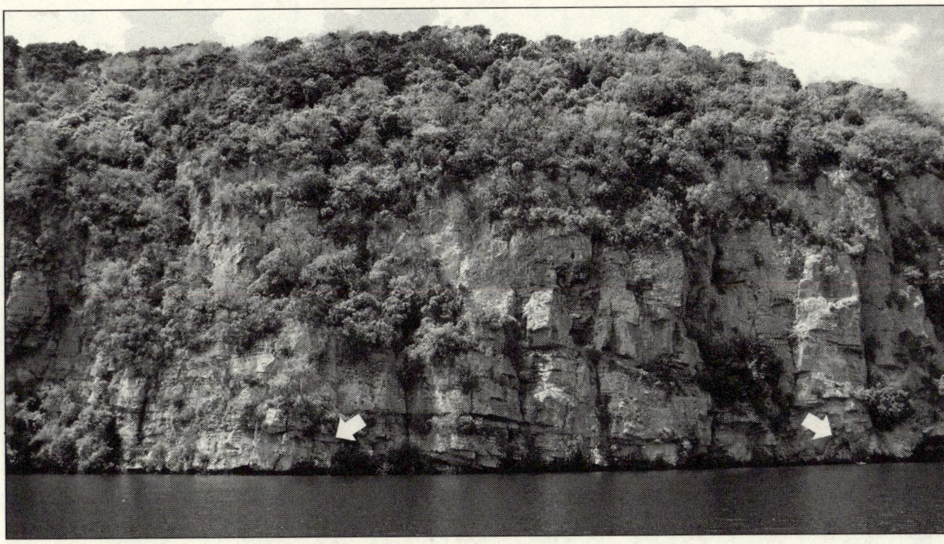

**Figure 2-5.** *Kawakawa Bay bluffs. Arrows indicate the three red strikes (left) and about 80 m to the right, the grotto with the koru (spiral) painting. (Photograph © Gerard O'Regan.)*

shimmering reflections were particularly vivid under overhangs on the adjacent more westerly oriented face.

About 20 m from these and only about 1 m above current lake level, is a 25 $cm^2$ composition of two vivid red curving rock paintings that flank a central red dot. These have been interpreted as bird motifs, with one local from nearby Kinloch describing them to O'Regan as depicting the moa, an extinct large flightless bird pictured in rock art in the South Island, but the images do not have sufficient form for the subject matter to be confidently identified. No light reflections were observed in association with these rock paintings, which were visited en route to the northern end of the peninsula but which were not revisited later in the afternoon, at the time other recordings of reflections were made. Sixty meters south, and about 40 m north of the large red rectangle, an overhanging panel at head height outside a small grotto also has a red ochre design. The single 50 cm long rock painting is a *koru*, or spiral design, typical of late pre-European Māori wood carving and tattooing (Figure 2-6). A small area of vivid shimmering light was recorded on the painted panel, although the boat partially blocked the reflections that otherwise would have covered the whole panel. It is worth noting that had the reflection come from the boat itself, then the light would have been static and no shimmer indicative of movement in the water's surface would have been visible. From a slight distance offshore, the most spectacular shimmer observed at any of the sites discussed was recorded around the immediate cliff face, including the painted panel and grotto. No cultural material was evident in this particular grotto, although artifacts and human remains have been found carefully positioned in similar places in the surrounding area.

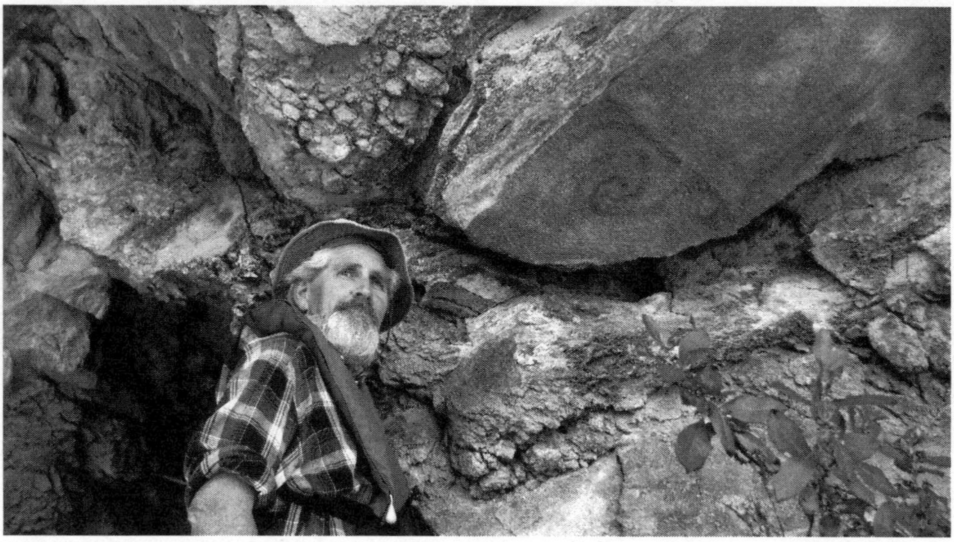

**Figure 2-6.** *Perry Fletcher with the koru rock painting. (Photograph © Gerard O'Regan.)*

## Past Conditions

Having described the rock paintings, their physical settings, and the phenomena observed in relation to these, there remains the question of whether the shimmer that we see today was also visible when the paintings were created or viewed in the past. Fundamental to this are the circumstances of the people at the locations, the climatic conditions likely to have been experienced at the time, and any changes to the natural settings likely to have occurred since then.

A key factor is that none of the locations discussed are occupation sites. Due to their situation at the base of bluffs, some are entirely inaccessible from land without abseiling, and all are most practicably and safely visited by boat. Landings can be made at only two of the Taupō sites, the red rectangle and the *koru* sites, but even these are small, barren, rocky spaces inhospitable for extended stays or encampment. None of the Canadian images discussed could have been readily accessed by land. Although it is conceivable that they were painted during times of firm winter ice, this is thought to be unlikely for a variety of reasons: flowing rivers can be free of winter ice, rocks are often ice covered, paint may not adhere to frozen rock, it is uncomfortable or even hypothermic to mix and apply paint in winter weather, and the sturgeon cerebrospinal fluid used for binding the paint is not readily available in winter. Given these factors, engagement with both the Ontario and Lake Taupō sites would most likely have been for visits (1) of a short duration and (2) made by canoe.

Both Māori in New Zealand and First Nations people in Canada traditionally showed spiritual and practical respect for the bodies of water over which they traveled. As noted above, the networks of rivers and lakes were traditional travel routes in Ontario and were navigated by canoe (using vessels that gave rise to the traditional Canadian canoe that remains popular today). Offerings are known to have been proffered to engender spiritual protection during travel, such as those at the Great Sacred Turtle, a natural bedrock formation on Georgian Bay, Ontario (Allen 2006:65; Jameson 1990:530; Melnick 2008). The descendants of Polynesian voyagers of the Pacific, pre-European Māori used canoes extensively to travel on rivers, on lakes, around the coast, and across the notoriously rough straits between the islands. Their various forms of canoes were their only means of transport other than by foot. Although Lake Taupō does not freeze over, it is a deep lake that draws melted snow from nearby mountains and remains a cold body of water. The caution with which Māori set out on it is described by the European explorer Ernest Dieffenbach, who recorded in his 1843 journal that "[t]he natives are afraid of trusting themselves on the lake whenever there is the slightest indication of bad weather" (Dieffenbach 1843:335) and so delayed his impatient European traveling party by two days. Subsequently, in a large but laden canoe, he "perceived that the natives had been right, as the waves of the lake still rose high even from the moderate winds. . . . If we had been upset we should not have had much chance of saving ourselves by swimming, as the western shore consists of high cliffs of a trachytic rock, which are washed by deep water" (Dieffenbach 1843:336). The *Journal of Ensign Best 1837–1843* similarly records cautious reluctance by Māori guides to voyage on Lake Taupō during anything other than prime conditions.

> $12^{th}$ A fine morning: blowing a little fresh. This was made an excuse for more Mauri [Māori] delay. First we were to start directly then long stories were told of all who had ever been drowned in the Lake. Poof said I, I am a soldier I am not afraid of being drowned. Ah said several if you were drowned there are plenty to replace you but we are few. [Taylor 1966:308]

Given such practical regard, the most likely occasions people would have been visiting the rock painting localities would have been in safe conditions of calm weather and when the general area was warmed by direct sunlight. These conditions are also those that give rise to the shimmer effect of reflected sunlight.

As with climatic conditions, the natural features of the rock painting settings would have had a major bearing on the past visibility of any reflected light shimmer. Despite seasonal variability and, in the case of Lake Taupō, a slightly raised water level due to the construction of a hydroelectric dam, most of the paintings discussed are well above the water. Even allowing for lower water levels in former times, the area of light reflections would be similar to those seen today and would encompass the positions of the rock paintings.

Sheer rock cliffs over deep water provide little opportunity either now or in the past for vegetation cover substantial enough to influence the light characteristics or sense of space at most of the sites. Even on Lake Taupō, where the water level was 1 m lower in the past, there would have been (at best) only minimal footholds for plants on small rock ledges subject to wave action and only in front of two of the sites. The paintings there are above the height of low scrub. All the paintings discussed are also on stable surfaces that have changed little since the rock paintings were created. Some surrounding markings may have been lost due to differential weathering, but if so, such loss does not negate recognition of the shimmering light on those paintings that do survive today. It is likely then that the main features of the physical environment in the past would have been very similar to those that exist today. Given this and the weather conditions during which these places were likely to have been visited, it is certainly conceivable that shimmering light reflections were visible at the time the rock paintings were painted and very probable that they were evident during a high proportion of subsequent visits to the sites and observations of the markings.

## What Might They Have Seen?

If the artists and subsequent indigenous observers saw the reflected light shimmering on the rocks and paintings, it must then be considered whether they would have attributed any cultural significance to this phenomenon. The presence of rock art can be used to assess something of the significance that past people attached to what are otherwise unaltered features of the natural landscape (Bradley 2000), perhaps sometimes even indicating the spiritual dimensions in "inner worlds" of rock (Taçon and Ouzman 2004). It is well known that past generations of Indigenous People in both New Zealand and Canada saw their worlds as alive with spirits on a variety of scales. In 1897, George B. Hayes hired Native guides to take him on the long canoe trip to Kitchi Mikinak Assin, a 30-ton turtle-shaped rock perched facing southwest in Ontario's Algonquin Provincial Park. It is of historically documented sacred significance (Laidlaw 1922:83) and Hayes's (1897) photo shows the series of small stone cairns in front of the Turtle. According to Whitley (2008:558), the religious or sacred origin of rock art is widely acknowledged in North America. In western Canada, the Stoney people of the Kootenays traditionally viewed the ochre used in rock paintings as red clay spirit, a powerful symbol made by *Waheambah*, the Sun. The pigment was believed to hold the power to yield the life strength of blood (Lakustra 2007:85). Mazinaw Rock, in Bon Echo Provincial Park, Ontario, is painted with over 200 Algonquian red ochre rock paintings and "fits exactly what is known about the believed dwelling places of rock *manitous*, especially the meeting of tall, broad rock faces with water" (Devereux 2008:21). Added to this is what Saunders describes as a "pan-Amerindian philosophy of light" (1998:226) where dazzling colors and light effects were indicative of spiritual attributes (Saunders 1999:245).

In New Zealand, Māori traditionally view the world as ordered through descent relationships from the gods to all living things, including ancestors and other spiritual elements embedded in the land. The elements are personified: Ārohirohi or Pareārohi being the female embodiment of heat shimmer and in one account, the wife of Rehua—himself the incarnation of the star Antares and whose name is associated with the heat of summer (Best 2005:310). Another example of this spiritually imbued landscape is provided by Grace (1970:496), who outlines traditions of supernatural guardians said to have haunted the volcanic peaks (Mounts Tongariro, Ruapehu, and Ngāuruhoe) of the sacred mountain immediately to the south of Lake Taupō. These guardians would visit and bring grief upon those who infringed the stringent laws associated with the mountain. In crossing the barren volcanic Rangipo Desert to the east of the mountain, past Māori would avoid looking at the volcanoes, asking questions of the stunted vegetation, using charred timber found about the desert for cooking, or preparing food until clear of the desert. Infringement would result in the offender perishing in sweeping snow and sleet, with it being said that "the bones of those who offended the spirits of the mountain in earlier days can be found uncovered even today, bleaching on the dark and ever-shifting sands of Rangipo" (Grace 1970:496).

O'Regan's (2007:18–23) review of Māori concepts of the spirituality of place draws on ethnohistorical accounts as well as contemporary observations by authorities in Māori studies (a recognized scholastic discipline in New Zealand). He notes that for Māori people the mountains are not just representations of ancestors, but actually are ancestors. Rocks and places may have indwelling spirits put in place by the gods, guardian spirits put in place by religious leaders, or the residual "sacredness" that draws from an important individual's connection to a place. O'Regan's (2007:172) spatial analysis of rock painting placement in two South Island Māori rock shelters has demonstrated that in at least some sites Māori did have regard for the spiritual attributes of places when deciding where to position their rock paintings.

Given such worldviews, it is suggested here that, if the ancestors saw shimmering light reflections on the rocks and rock paintings, they are likely to have interpreted the shimmer as indicative of a life force or spirit in that place and image. Of course, drawing a connection between rock art and moving light effects is not a novel suggestion. Lewis-Williams (2001) outlines the neuropsychological approach to rock art research that relates some otherwise abstract rock paintings to entoptic patterns. These light percepts are generated internally by the neural system and appear during altered states of consciousness. In shamanistic societies, they may accompany the shaman's transition into spiritual dimensions. Moving light need not necessarily be limited to interpretation as "spirit" in itself, and it may be the effect of variable light in animating the rock paintings that has significance. Hyder (2004:89) describes the rock art images of the Cave of the Whales on San Nicholas Island, California, appearing to be alive in the play of reflected sunlight and among the noise of fauna and pounding waves. Noganosh observes that from his indigenous perspective, it is not a case of the light shimmering on the Canadian rock paintings but rather of the rock paintings dancing through the light. Similarly, talking of the renowned Opihi *taniwha*, reptilian creatures painted on the ceiling of a South Island rock shelter, contemporary Māori artist Manos Nathan (personal communication 2010) considers that the painter would have been conscious of apparent movement in the figures caused by shifting shadows as the angle of sunlight changed over the textured surface during the course of producing such large images. Interestingly, a Māori traditional regard for the visual effect of light is evident in the widespread use of iridescent abalone (*Haliotis iris)* shell in the eyes of ornaments and wood carvings to enliven the ancestral figures represented.

## Discussion

This paper is the result of a study of the sometimes-dramatic visual phenomena observed at several different waterside rock painting localities. Above we outline why we believe this same phenomena would have been witnessed by Indigenous People in the past and consider its relationship to spiritual aspects of the images or places. Indeed, as Arsenault (2004a:305) suggests regarding the reflective quality of rocks for Algonkian motifs, it may be reasonable to speculate that shimmering reflected light could have influenced the choice of rock painting placement. However, until further systematic data collection and analyses have been carried out, the anecdotal nature of the observations must be acknowledged. Whitley (2005:125) notes with regard to many archaeoastronomical associations drawn with rock art, that regardless of how visually dramatic the association with an observed phenomena appears, there must be some reasonable basis for believing that it is the result of intentional behavior if it is to have inferential value. Therefore, it must be considered whether or not the apparent association between reflected shimmering light and rock paintings is simply a random or coincidental occurrence.

Further investigation of these issues would involve documenting a much larger sample, taking measurements of the frequency of times when a rock painting site can be accessed, and quantifying the frequency of reflected light occurrences at sites. Such research would need to determine whether the episodes and locales of shimmer are more statistically significant in the vicinity of rock paintings than elsewhere and also whether shimmer, when not associated with rock paintings, is associated with other kinds of cultural sites or natural places that traditional knowledge would suggest have similar spiritual attributes. Such quantification is necessary for a meaningful exploration of whether the shimmering light phenomenon is a plausible determinant of rock painting location, as has been argued for acoustic properties at certain rock art sites in southern India (Boivin 2003; Boivin et al. 2007), Scandinavia (Goldhahn 2002), and Micronesia (Rainbird 2008:266) (see also Whitley 2005:128). Only when such research has been undertaken will we be able to say for certain that the link between shimmer and rock art is more than simply a widespread characteristic of the steep waterside bluffs on which the paintings occur.

Beyond our current observations, the shimmering reflections may turn out to be ubiquitous at water's edge rock faces given particular weather conditions and different times of day. Alternatively, there may be other water's edge rock painting sites where shimmering light does not occur, possibly negating any sensible "inference about art placed on an unaltered earth feature . . . , especially when there are potentially many more examples of similar art at other nearby locations that may not exhibit the same phenomenon or effect" (Whitley 2005:126). Indeed, no shimmering reflections were noted at a more easterly French River rock painting site visited earlier than those discussed here. Nor were any seen at other rock painting sites on Lake Taupō visited by Fletcher and O'Regan, although this can plausibly be explained by the sites being in shadow at the time of the visit. An absence of shimmer at other rock painting sites need not, however, necessarily dismiss consideration of shimmer at sites where it has been observed. A variety of characteristics, perhaps individually or sometimes in combination, may have been at play in the choice of places for rock paintings or the behavior involved in marking such places. Acoustic properties have already been noted. By way of another example, O'Regan has also noticed that red colored natural features are prominent about several North Island Māori rock art sites he has visited. Rock paintings elsewhere may have been animated by other sources of flickering light, such as by fires in rock shelters or by torch light during traditional canoe-based fishing expeditions in Canada, which could have caused a shimmer effect on water's edge paintings also.

Even if such light effects were not evident when the paintings were produced, and so not a factor in their positioning, at least with regard to the specific rock paintings discussed here, we can expect that many subsequent visitors saw these places with the light reflections shimmering on the rock and that the shimmer may have been seen as animating the rock painting and evoking the spirituality within the image or the place.

## Conclusion

For people whose worldview included seamless connections to the natural environment, a meditative, reflective process would have been a continual and integral part of daily interaction with their environment, a process that allowed connection to the "Seen" and the "Unseen" within the landscape. Whitley notes that "we will only understand prehistoric religions when we adequately apprehend traditional non-Western religions, and use our knowledge of them to aid in our understanding of the prehistoric past" (2008:559). Our observations have been made in relation to two unrelated cultures in quite different parts of the world. Yet in both cases, we have found value in considering the sensory experience in combination with the particular cultural worldview and in reflecting on the situational and physical contexts related to the different sets of rock paintings. Given what is known of the traditional worldviews of Indigenous Peoples in Canada and New Zealand and the context in which the images have been created, it is reasonable to view an attribution of animation or spiritual significance to shimmering light on the rock paintings of the particular cultures. Such attributions may be an appropriate starting point for further archaeological investigations at places where shimmering light continues to be evident.

It has been noted elsewhere that observations that draw on both traditional indigenous and archaeological perspectives will have richer insights (Allen 2008:18–24; Allen, Brady, and Decontie 2008:283; Marshall and Bartlett 2009). It is our current experience that having a regard for the traditional worldviews and engaging multiple senses to recognize spiritual aspects of place facilitate recognizing and recording the subtle and changing nuances at rock painting sites. Combining this with appropriate analytical consideration can broaden and enrich archaeological interpretations of these places.

Having made the observations and considered the climatic, environmental, and cultural circumstances surrounding the rock paintings, we believe there are sufficient grounds to entertain further detailed exploration of the phenomena observed in relation to the paintings. The primary purpose of this chapter has been to draw attention to the apparent association between the shimmering light reflections and the rock paintings we visited. We hope it serves as encouragement for further recording and analyzing of such observations. These observations will be further strengthened by examining any relevant comments on sunlight reflections encountered in the ethnographic records and by continuing to gather and take on board perspectives informed by indigenous worldviews. In this work, we concur with the aims Arsenault (2004b:80) outlines as appropriate for the study of sacred landscapes, particularly the integration of traditional knowledge and the development of standardized field methods for recording observations that would allow models to be scientifically critiqued. Furthermore, we hope that in the future a sufficient body of information will permit the consideration of light reflections in association with rock paintings to move beyond the anecdotal and toward forming a substantiated contribution to the continuing and broadening exploration of sensory factors at these sacred painted places.

## Acknowledgments

Parks Canada, particularly through Sheryl Smith and Jim Molnar, generously supported Allen and O'Regan's fieldwork during which the Canadian observations were made. The observations on French River were made under the guidance of First Nations and Métis leaders of the Cultural Advisory Committee of the French River Visitor Centre. We thank Ngāti Tūwharetoa for their support in our discussion of their heritage at Lake Taupō. Daniel Parker kindly helped produce the maps, and we are thankful for the comments of all those who have reviewed this paper. Kia ora ra. Ginawaydaganuc.

## References

Allen, William Arthur

2006 Summary of 2001 Research. In *13th Annual Archaeological Report Ontario 2002*, edited by Dena Doroszenko, pp. 58–79. Ontario Heritage Trust, Toronto.

2008 Dbaajmoowin: Dialogue with the Elders. In *Rethinking Protected Areas in a Changing World: Proceedings of the 2007 George Wright Society Biennial Conference on Parks, Protected Areas, and Cultural Sites*, edited by Samantha Weber and David Harmon, pp. 18–24. George Wright Society, Hancock, Michigan.

2009 Archaeologists Come to Their Senses, Looking Beyond Visual Archaeological Evidence. *Ontario Archaeological Society Arch Notes* 14(6):10–11.

Allen, William A., Liam M. Brady, and Peter Decontie

2008 Manaadjiyindj iyaa manidoo nayaagadjitoodj kije-asin mazinaakobiihiganan Honouring the Spirits of Sacred Pictographs. In *Preserving Aboriginal Heritage: Technical and Traditional Approaches, Proceedings of Symposium 2007*, edited by Carole

Dignard, Kate Helwig, Janet Mason, Kathy Nanowin, and Thomas Stone, pp. 277–289. Canadian Conservation Institute, Ottawa, Canada.

Arsenault, Daniel

2004a From Natural Settings to Spiritual Places in the Algonkian Sacred Landscape: An Archaeological, Ethnohistorical, and Ethnographic Analysis of Canadian Shield Rock-Art Sites. In *The Figured Landscapes of Rock-Art: Looking at Pictures in Place*, edited by Christopher Chippindale and George Nash, pp. 289–317. Cambridge University Press, Cambridge.

2004b Rock-Art, Landscape, Sacred Places: Attitudes in Contemporary Archaeological Theory. In *The Figured Landscapes of Rock-Art: Looking at Pictures in Place*, edited by Christopher Chippindale and George Nash, pp. 69–84. Cambridge University Press, Cambridge.

Best, Elsdon

2005 [1924] *Maori Religion and Mythology*, Pt. 2. Dominion Museum Bulletin No. 11, Te Papa, Wellington.

Boivin, Nicole

2003 Rock Art and Rock Music: Petroglyphs of the South Indian Neolithic. *Antiquity* 78:38–53.

Boivin, Nicole, Adam Brumm, Helen Lewis, Dave Robinson, and Ravi Korisettar

2007 Sensual, Material, and Technological Understanding: Exploring Prehistoric Soundscapes in South India. *Journal of the Royal Anthropological Institute*, n.s. 13:267–294

Bradley, Richard

2000 *An Archaeology of Natural Places.* Routledge, London.

Corbin, Alain

2005 Charting the Cultural History of the Senses. In *Empire of the Senses—The Sensual Culture Reader*, edited by David Howes, pp.128–139. Berg, Oxford.

Devereux, Paul

2008 The Association of Prehistoric Rock-Art and Rock Selection with Acoustically Significant Landscape Locations. In *The Archaeology of Semiotics and the Social Order of Things*, edited by George Nash and George Children, pp. 19–29. Archaeopress, Oxford.

Dieffenbach, Ernest

1843 *Travels in New Zealand; With Contributions to the Geography, Geology, Botany and Natural History of That Country.* John Murray, Albemarle Street, London.

Gates, Charles M. (editor)

1965 The Diary of John MacDonell. In *Five Fur Traders of the Northwest*. pp. 63–119. Minnesota Historical Society, St. Paul.

Goldhahn, Joakim

2002 Roaring Rocks: An Audio-Visual Perspective on Hunter-Gather Engravings in Northern Sweden and Scandinavia. *Norwegian Archaeological Review* 35:29–61.

Grace, John Te H.

1970 *Tuwharetoa: The History of the Maori People of the Taupo District.* A. H. and A. W. Reed, Wellington.

Hayes, George B.

1897 From South River to Rainy Lake via Cedar Lake and White Trout Lake 1897. Private photograph album on file, Algonquin Park Archives, Whitney, Ontario.

Hyder, William D.

2004 Locational Analysis in Rock-Art Studies. In *The Figured Landscapes of Rock-Art: Looking at Pictures in Place*, edited by Christopher Chippindale and George Nash, pp. 85–101. Cambridge University Press, Cambridge.

Jameson, Anna
1990 [1838] *Winter Studies and Summer Rambles in Canada*. McClelland and Stewart, Toronto.

Laidlaw, George
1922 Ojibway Myths and Tales. In *33rd Annual Archaeological Report 1921–22 Being Part of Appendix to the Report of the Minister of Education Ontario*, edited by R. B. Orr, pp. 83–99. Legislative Assembly of Ontario, Toronto.

Lakustra, Ernie
2007 *The Intrepid Explorer: James Hector's Explorations in the Canadian Rockies*. Fifth House, Calgary, Alberta, Canada.

Lewis-Williams, J. David
2001 Brainstorming Images: Neuropsychology and Rock Art Research. In *The Handbook of Rock Art Research*, edited by David S. Whitley, pp. 332–357. AltaMira, Walnut Creek, California.

Marshall, Albert, and Cheryl Bartlett
2009 Co-Learning re: "Talking and Walking Together" of Indigenous and Mainstream Sciences. Eskasoni Mi'kmaq First Nation and Cape Breton University. Electronic document, http://www.integrativescience.ca/uploads/articles/2009February-Bartlett-Marshall-Integrative-Science-Two-Eyed-Seeing-Aboriginal-CEPI-Indigenous-knowledge-environmental-planning.pdf, accessed April 25, 2012.

Melnick, Zachary (director)
2008 *Rooted in Stone—Reflections on West Parry Sound's Past*. Produced by Yvonne Drebert. 2 hr. 10 min. DVD. The Shield—Ontario Visual Heritage Project. Lock 3 Media.

O'Regan, Gerard
2007 Wahi Tapu and Rock Art: An Intra-site Analysis of Two Southern Maori Rock Art Shelters. Unpublished Master's thesis, Anthropology Department, University of Auckland.

Rainbird, Paul
2008 The Body and the Senses: Implications for Landscape Archaeology. In *Handbook of Landscape Archaeology*, edited by Bruno David and Julian Thomas, pp. 263–270. Left Coast, Walnut Creek, California.

Saunders, Nicholas J.
1998 Stealers of Light, Traders in Brilliance: Amerindian Metaphysics in the Mirror of Conquest. *RES* 33:225–252.
1999 Biographies of Brilliance: Pearls, Transformations of Matter and Being, c. A.D. 1492. *World Archaeology* 31:243–257.

Taçon, Paul S. C., and Sven Ouzman
2004 Worlds Within Stone: The Inner and Outer Rock-Art Landscapes of Northern Australia and Southern Africa. In *The Figured Landscapes of Rock-Art: Looking at Pictures in Place*, edited by Christopher Chippindale and George Nash, pp. 39–68. Cambridge University Press, Cambridge.

Taylor, Nancy M. (editor)
1966 *The Journal of Ensign Best, 1837–1843*, R. E. Owen, Government Printer, Wellington.

Whitley, David S.
2005 *Introduction to Rock Art Research*. Left Coast, Walnut Creek, California.
2008 Religion. In *Handbook of Archaeological Theories*, edited by R. Alexander Bentley, Herbert D. G. Maschner, and Christopher Chippindale, pp. 547–566. AltaMira, Lanham, Maryland.

# 3. The Sound of Sulfur and Smell of Lightning: Sensing the Volcano

*Karen Holmberg*

*Abstract:* In this chapter I use Michel Serres's *The Five Senses* and *The Natural Contract* as conduits through which to enter a discussion of the role of bodily experience in scientific interpretation and the framing of natural phenomena as a form of "violence." I consider bodily perception and its relation to the phenomena of radically changing environments, for which I use the volcano in eruption as an exemplar. In so doing, I purposefully conflate the categories of "cultural" and "natural" forms of violence. Nature and culture are messily combined and not viewable as easily separated entities; through perception, a humanized or cultured nature exists. Drawing on Hegel's views of the roles of art and science and Kant's framing of the volcano as a perceptual object, I propose that violently changing environments are in many ways *supersensible*: They lie beyond what we are able to mentally grasp through our senses and reason. We can only attempt to understand them based on our prior experience and knowledge. How we interpret the material and immaterial correlates of others' human experience is entirely dependent on our own sensoria, or sum of perceptions, which provide a map of the objective world. It is, I propose, incumbent on archaeologists to attempt to evaluate sensory correlates of human experience, despite the difficulty of the endeavor, in order to provide more complete and more accurate conceptions of the past.

> The five senses, still on the verge of departure toward another adventure, a ghost of the real timidly described in a ghost of language, this is my essay.
>
> —Serres [2008:345]

The socially and politically confronting novel *Senselessness* (Castellanos Moya 2008) utilizes the titular lack of "sense" as an evocation of the violence inflicted on indigenous peoples in Central America. The book's title refers to an

*Making Senses of the Past: Toward a Sensory Archaeology,* edited by Jo Day. Center for Archaeological Investigations, Occasional Paper No. 40.  ISBN 978-0-8093-3287-8.

absence of sense both in terms of logic and in bodily capability when attempting to create an account of violence in the past in the context of the present. Without a sensory component, only a shadow of human life exists. This sentiment is echoed by French theoretician Michel Serres (2008), who proposes that scientific studies or any other systems of knowledge cannot be divorced from bodily experience without losing a vast amount of comprehensiveness or meaning. In prior work, Serres (1995) argued that environmental change forces us as humans to reconsider our relationship to nature and what he terms the "violence" with which it can act. In this chapter, I combine these threads of Serres's body of work in order to consider bodily perception and its relation to the phenomena of radically changing environments, for which I use the volcano in eruption as an exemplar. In so doing, I purposefully conflate the categories of "cultural" and "natural" forms of violence. Nature and culture are messily combined and not viewable as easily separated entities (Haraway 1991; Latour 1991, 2009; Skúlason 2005; Strathern 1992; Žižek 2008a). The ineffectiveness of Cartesian dualism in the nature and culture construct is not a product of the late modern era but an enduring component of human life.

The cover of *The Natural Contract* by Serres (1995) portrays a volcano in eruption as emblematic of a turbulent and potentially violent Earth. In doing so, Serres parallels Icelandic philosopher Páll Skúlason, who holds that the volcano "symbolizes the earth itself" and is "independent of human existence" (Skúlason 2005:21). The volcano, as a highly mutable entity, can by no means be seen as "timeless" despite its monumentality (Massey 2005:133). I propose that volcanic eruption can be seen as an example of a highly contextual changing environment that humans have experienced over the extreme *longue durée*. In past work, I have urged a focus on the interstices of volcanic eruptions as being crucial to understanding the lived experience of volcanic landscapes over the long term (Holmberg 2005, 2007). In general, the focus on an "event" of eruption with a "before" and "after" is one that I find highly problematic and unhelpful in examining the role of past environmental changes and how they should be interpreted as lessons for the present or augurs for the future (Holmberg 2013). In this chapter, however, I would like to change tack and focus very specifically on volcanic eruption. In doing so, I frame it as an experience with intensely rich phenomenological resonance that can become embedded in social memory. In this chapter, I query the archaeological ability to encompass this in our analyses.

## Metasense and Making Sense

In drawing on *The Five Senses* by Serres (2008), I am implicitly working from a cultural norm that assumes that sight, hearing, touch, smell, and taste govern how we collect information about our world. This division draws on Aristotle's distinction of senses, though Aristotle suggested that there were only four senses, as it permitted each to be correlated to one of the four elements (vision = water; hearing = air; smell = fire; touch = earth); taste was considered a modified form of touch (Sankey and Cowley 2008:2). The lack of integration of these senses, however, led Aristotle to suggest an additional quasi sense, the *sensus communis,* which mediated the others and served as a metasense. This metasense is something that is fed by sensory perception and is a concept that I will return to later in this chapter. In so doing, however, I do not imply that the concept of five primary senses is entirely portable either culturally or temporally.

A vast amount of cultural variation exists in the way that the senses are accessed and ordered so as to provide information (e.g., Howes 2003, 2004). While there are physiological bases for perception, the way that sensory data are translated is dependent on cultural norms: One culture may not have a word for a particular color; another may not smell a particular odor (Marks 2000:203). Additional senses, such as balance, sentiment, or intuition are also noted in some cultures (Gibson 1966), while others may designate fewer senses. The Hausa group of Nigeria are most commonly cited to illustrate this variability, as they linguistically refer to only two senses, sight and experiencing (Keating and Hadder 2010:118; Ritchie 1991). Senses can promiscuously merge in the way they are perceived: Music can produce tastes (Beeli et al. 2005) or colors can be sensed as smells (Keating and Hadder 2010:120). The impairment of senses is also an important cultural marker (Keating and Hadder 2010).

## Sensing What We Know

As individuals, we can only work from what we know, both intellectually and personally; to follow a line of reasoning begun by Kant in *Critique of the Power of Judgment* (1987 [1790]), we only know that which we can gain knowledge of through our senses. Building on Kant, Burke (2008:x [1757]) added that "the senses are the great originals of all of our ideas," while Schiller then expounded on the human desire to put our "sensuous nature" at ease (Schiller 1993:31 [1801]). Working from the more bodily vantages of Burke and Schiller that built on Kant's definition of the *sublime,* I'd like to propose that the volcano—certainly sublime in many terms—is effectively *supersensible*: It lies beyond what we are able to mentally grasp through our senses and reason, particularly in times of eruption. We can only attempt to understand it based on our prior experience and knowledge.

How we interpret the material correlates of others' human experience is entirely dependent on our own sensoria, or sum of perceptions, which provide a map of the objective world (Marks 2000:203; Varela et al. 1991). As a New Yorker for a decade prior to and now a decade after 2001, I find that I tend to mentally reference the destruction of the World Trade Center towers as synecdochic for the transformation of familiar environments—particularly monumental landscapes that seem solid—when they suddenly, radically, and threateningly change. I'd spent considerable time in the towers. I could see them from the rooftop of my apartment building, took multiple photos of them over the years, and unfailingly used them as a reference point for lost tourists to help them determine uptown from downtown. They were a very lived part of my landscape.

Throughout the autumn of 2001, my downtown apartment was filled with a metallic-tasting dust that burned my lungs and nose and made it seem as though I was peering through fog in my living room. The sound of sirens or of fighter planes overhead made me jump; the sight of tanks in the streets and parks made my skin feel cold. For months, when the wind blew from the south, the unmistakable smell of burning bodies filled the air and my nose. My dreams were hyper-vivid and apocalyptic. It was a heavily sensory-based experience with a substantial emotional load; I assumed that the city would never return to normal or ever be the same. With the passage of time, however, the feelings have faded from a raw bruise to something that is simply a part of personal narrative and cultural memory. I experienced the violence and its aftermath, in sum, but was not catastrophically affected by it.

Objects can provide a material prompt for memory (Bergson 1991). Recently, I jogged past the stone benches in front of the Winter Harbor boat basin in front of what is now called Ground Zero. People taped paper notes to the benches by the waterfront in the months following the collapse of the World Trade Center towers seeking the strangers they had met that day. The notes detailed conversations people had had and stories they had told about their lives before they jumped into the Hudson River or caught the last ferry to leave that day. People left contact information so that they could meet again. The stone benches, like less friendly versions of Proust's madeleine, elicit the involuntary memory of those stories for me.

Not long ago, jogging by these same benches, I noticed a large clump of worried-looking firemen and police personnel scanning the waterfront beside them. Emergency workers had cordoned the bench area with police tape. Several dozen more firemen were slightly farther down, looking toward the water. There were two fireboats hovering along the same stretch of waterfront with full decks of officials, who were also peering at the water, and as I rounded the corner of shops, I saw the lights of nearly a dozen fire trucks parked at the scene. Something was clearly wrong. It was only later that I realized what I had felt as I watched this: I had felt nothing, really, other than mild curiosity. It did not occur to me to be concerned or to connect that spot, so extremely close to a location where thousands of people died traumatically and unexpectedly, to any sense of unreasonable risk or discomfort. The residue of a very large-scale event was now a component of memory. The monumental landscape, in which the World Trade Center towers still exist in many ways—through the lights used as noumenal annual prosthetics for them, by the fact that the subway station is still named for them, and by the numerous photos of them for sale by street vendors—was no longer one of fresh trauma and had somehow again become one that was very lived and nonthreatening.

The Manhattan landscape is clearly culturally, temporally, and contextually separated from the pre-Columbian landscapes that I study archaeologically. The way in which I understand how human life has experienced volcanic landscapes in the past, however, is very much colored by my own phenomenological experience—my sense—of a landscape that was benign, then threatening, and then benign again, yet filled with new stories and memories. This frames the way I understand archaeological contexts that have long, repeated intersections with volcanism. Catastrophic volcanic eruptions rarely lead to sustained abandonment of occupied regions or prompt large-scale culture change (Grattan and Torrence 2007); they are, however, highly experiential and remain lodged in cultural memory for sometimes exceptionally long periods.

## Sensing the Environment

A recent journal article by Meltzer and Holliday (2010) queries whether or not Paleoindians living in North America would have sensed the climatic changes occurring around them during the Younger Dryas Chrozone (11,000–10,000 $^{14}$C years B.P.), when widespread cooling beset much of the globe and returned it to near-glacial conditions. The authors determine that the event probably escaped perception and center their argument on their interpretation of the lack of severe, rapid changes or evidence for large-scale cultural change or collapse. While I appreciate the authors' assessment that Paleoindians were highly mobile and did not expect stable or unchanging environments, I also assume that there was a strong chance that they were perceptually aware of the changes in their environment. In both past and present, climate is "relatively invariant in its variations: quick and slow, catastrophic and mild, regular and chaotic," hence rare phenomena may not be surprising but will still be perceptually striking (Serres 1995:3). The lack of any material correlates for the Paleoindians' senses of their environment reduces their past perceptions to something even more spectral than the "ghost of the real" that Serres (2008:345) claims is provided by the senses. While the research frameworks utilized in the Paleoindian study potentially did not permit collection of data that would provide material correlates for climate change perception, it is also quite possible that no such correlates exist. Perception in the archaeological record is not easy to excavate.

Unlike gradual environmental changes like those considered by Meltzer and Holliday (2010), I propose that the concentrated natural violence of volcanic eruptions makes the perception of them less debatable for anyone within their vicinity. This does not imply, however, that all people will perceive the eruption in the same way. Perception of volcanic eruption can be extremely varied even within very local populations and is crosscut by issues such as gender, status, and age (Cronin et al. 2004). Further, the way in which the senses are utilized is highly culturally contextual (e.g., Classen 1993; Howes 2004). It is my opinion, however, that volcanic eruption rarely escapes the perception of those close to it.

While Pompeii provides the most commonly known and materially rich volcanic context explored by archaeologists, myriad other studies use artifactual evidence to provide evocative discussions of volcanism and its impact on people in the Holocene (e.g., Grattan and Torrence 2007; Plunket and Uruñuela 2008; Sheets 2008). The ability to make plausible social-scientific interpretations regarding how people perceived eruption in the past becomes more challenging and conjectural with greater time lapse and lesser material evidence.

The pitfalls that exist when trying to address experiential or sensory elements in the deep past are clearly evident in the context of Laetoli in Tanzania.

Discovered in 1976, the footprints left by three early humans as they walked away from the Sadiman volcano over 3.5 million years ago continue to provide important data regarding hominid morphology and bipedalism (e.g., Raichlen et al. 2010). While a general search on the Internet for *Laetoli* produces many in situ photographs or casts of the footprints, at the time of this writing roughly half of the images retrieved were artists' renditions of the early humans walking through volcanic ash during the eruption. The images provide strikingly contrasting visions of the living context in which the footprints formed. Six images, in particular, can be found repeatedly recycled on Web sites. In one representation, two frail adults of indeterminate gender walk across a barren, blackened landscape in single file: The adult walking behind carries an infant and the three cast long, ominous shadows as several large birds stand nearby and a giraffe browses a treetop. In a second image, a muscular adult male and female walk through powdery white ash under blue skies as more ash spews from the close-by slope of the volcano; some large birds, but no other animals or juvenile individuals, are represented. The male puts his arm, perhaps protectively, around the shoulders of the female, and both appear either apprehensive or curious. A third image shows three extremely slender, upright, and alien-looking adults; one, seemingly female, walks resolutely through a brown and dusty landscape while dust clouds billow overhead and a zebra or similar animal stands under a tree.

A fourth image portrays three small, dark, ape-like creatures; their heavy black fur contrasts with the thick layer of white ash that covers the ground like snow. Unlike the other images, this one shows a nighttime scene. The three hominids are being hunted by a large cat that looms over them on an ash-covered rock, and they crouch fearfully as the cat snarls. The crater of the volcano is visible at the top of the illustration, spewing black soot. In a fifth image, two hirsute, barrel-chested adults walk with purpose, but without apparent concern, through a hazy dusk; no animals or third individual is visible. The individual in front looks either to the back or to the side, and it is unclear if he or she is are viewing the volcano, which is not imaged, or seeking a companion from the corner of his or her eye. A final image shows a cartoonish, extremely erect-postured woman with graceful, slender legs and a ponderous skull. She holds the hand of an adolescent as they walk with purpose and determination through mud, while a blue sky and the slopes of the volcano are visible to the side of the illustration.

The illustrations were all originally produced for use in museums or textbooks but are also used and reused by educators, bloggers, and religious organizations both to support and repudiate human evolution. None of the representations indicate that the footprints of hundreds of other animals—including hyenas, wildcats, baboons, wild boars, giraffes, gazelles, rhinos, antelope, buffalo, elephants, and birds—also are recorded in the ash. A light rain, also not shown in the illustrations, cemented the ash and preserved the prints. As the tracks were not obscured by or superimposed by the prints of other animals, it is evident that the ash fell thick and quickly. Each of the artists' renderings is evocative and seeks to add an experiential component to the preserved footprints, yet the images impose on past individuals unsupported assumptions of nuclear family composition, emotion, and close interpersonal interaction. Avoiding such conjecture or projection is the challenge for archaeologists interested in providing a more sensory-rich investigation of the past.

One of the primary weaknesses of the artists' varied Laetoli renditions is their sole reliance on visuality in conveying interpretations of the past experience of the eruption. A firmly established postprocessual critique in archaeology notes the inapplicability of post-Enlightenment, Western emphases on visual perception to many past contexts and strongly questions the dualism it creates between subject and object (e.g., Ashmore 2007:261; Barrett 1994; Bender 1993; Edmonds 1999; Gosden 1994; Shanks and Hodder 1995; Thomas 2001; 2004:178–180; Tilley 2008:33). This critique, in part, stems from phenomenological discussions of the corporeal and social context of visuality (Merleau-Ponty 1962:226).

Heavily visual fields, like film studies, have recently placed more focus on the multisensory component of human experience (e.g., Barker 2009), and recent social-science projects similarly highlighted additional senses, such as hearing (e.g., Loose 2008). Senses other than that of sight are invoked in the perception of the environment by Ruiz-Ballesteros et al. (2009:163), who hold that sound or its absence, strong smells, and sensations of heat or dryness are exceptionally important conduits of information and memory. Our perceptions create a "particular sense of nature" in which sensory aspects are inseparable from one another and from their affective or cognitive aspects (Ruiz-Ballesteros et al. 2009:163). Through perception, a humanized or cultured nature exists.

Using purely visual representation, the artists' renditions of Laetoli could not incorporate the fact that the heavy ash fall would have made visibility low without entirely obscuring the image. As recent accounts of the Eyjafjallajökull eruption in Iceland highlight, the lack of visibility possible from ash clouds can be extreme (e.g., Knowlton 2010). I assume that this low visibility could provide one explanation for why the Laetoli hominids' footprints indicate that they were moving slowly, despite the extraordinary circumstance of the eruption and the large number of other potentially unfriendly animals. Their sense of sight was largely obscured. We could plausibly assume that the early humans' mouths likely felt dry and acute discomfort would have begun once the moisture of their bodies combined with any fine ash particles that entered their lungs (International Volcanic Health Hazard Network [IVHHN] 2010). Their eyes and noses likely felt as though they were burning and irritated (IVHHN 2010). Other components are entirely outside of responsible supposition and can only be left as question marks. Was there an unruly chorus of animal noises or an eerie quiet? Did the ash smell acrid or feel warm as it fell around them? Did the Laetoli hominids see lightning flashing from the charged particles of the ash clouds, and if so, what did they think of it? There is no material basis on which to gauge an answer to these questions, and hence they are archaeologically inaccessible.

The desire to base social-science interpretations on robust data implicitly concedes a greater flexibility to artistic representations than is allowed in archaeological assessments. The contrast between what the sciences and the arts are able to address regarding sensory experience is touched on by Hegel (1975:1), who states that art is the "science of sensation, of feeling." Art, for Hegel, serves as a "mediator between reason and sense" and something that "presents itself to *sense*, feeling, intuition, imagination; it has a different sphere from thought" and "demands an organ other than scientific thinking" (Hegel 1975:4–5).

Two recent art exhibitions reflect some of what Hegel is expressing with regard to volcanic landscapes. The first, an exhibit held in New York City (Nov. 13, 2009–Jan. 2, 2010) entitled *Volcano Lovers*, combined the work of artists from Iceland and Japan because of their shared commonality of volcanic landscapes (ISE Cultural Foundation 2009–2010). *Dark Lamp*, an installation by Icelandic artist Haraldur Jónsson, required "viewers" to sit in a small closet in complete darkness while a recording of an unknown woman's voice read out the names of 200 colors. The artist stated that the experience of the piece "takes place between the senses" (Jónsson 2009). Danish-born artist Olafur Eliasson's project, *The Body as Brain–Lava Floor* (Figure 3-1), filled a gallery in Switzerland with lava from Iceland (Eliasson 2007). The intended purpose of this was to provide the sensory-rich experience of being in a volcanic landscape. Visitors were forced to walk over the material; it was uneven and caused one to stumble, it smelled of primal earth, it crunched beneath one's feet.

As Hegel (1975:7–8) states, art displays reality "sensuously, bringing it thereby nearer to the senses, to feeling, and to nature's mode of appearance. What is thus displayed is the depth of a suprasensuous world" that is freed from overly intellectual reflection and "rescues itself from the here and now, called sensuous reality and finitude." Eliasson touches on this in his work by shifting the bodily senses to the forefront, over the brain or intellect, in his lava-floor piece. Art provides a more salient way to plumb the sensory experience of a volcanic landscape than archaeology can offer; Hegel's point that science is bound by logical, intellectual reasoning is valid. The negation of sensory components in archaeological practice, however, leaves a vacuum in which Laetoli-like caricatures or sterile, dehumanized views of the past can be created. Archaeologists should not overreach what the data can reasonably provide regarding sensory experience in the past, but we can expand how we query experience in the past.

## The Little Frog and the Big Volcano

Over the past decade I have conducted research in western Panamá in a 240-km$^2$ area to the east of the Volcán Barú summit (Figure 3-2). The sites I have excavated range from 7 to 20 km from the volcano. As the majority of physical impact from Barú eruptions occurs to the west of the volcano, I was able to study a population that was experientially but not catastrophically affected by eruptions. My accelerator mass spectrometry dates and ceramic chronologies show a continuous occupation from 200 C.E. to 1400 C.E.; people farmed, made stone tools and pottery, and buried their dead without obvious interruption. At least three, and perhaps as many as four, eruptions occurred during the time span of this uninterrupted occupation, with eruptions spaced fairly regularly every several hundred years (Anchukaitis and Horn 2005; Behling 2000; Sherrod et al. 2007); these eruptions did not catastrophically affect people living in the research area (Holmberg 2009). A lack of abandonment or culture change, however, does

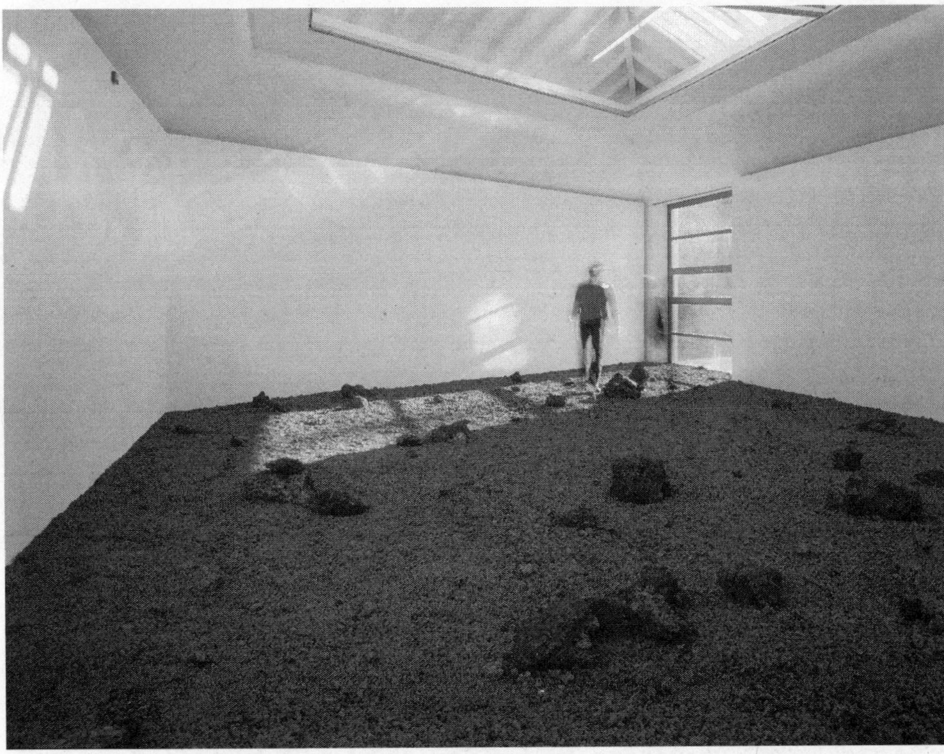

**Figure 3-1.** *Olafur Eliasson,* The Body as Brain—Lava floor: Projekt Sammlung (5), *2007. Installation view at Kunsthaus Zug, Switzerland, courtesy of the artist; Neugerriemschneider, Berlin and Tanya Bonakdar Gallery, New York. (Photograph © Florian Holzherr. © 2007 Olafur Eliasson.)*

not indicate that people did not perceive changes in their environment (cf. Meltzer and Holliday 2010).

I collected stories from local people about the volcanic landscape during fieldwork. The stories people told about large snakes slithering down the mountain, boulders exploding into the sky with fire, and caves speaking with one another and with the volcano all indicate to me a residue of long-term cultural memory linked to eruption. In this discussion, I will focus on one story from the indigenous Bribí group that was recorded by Costa Rican anthropologist María Bozzoli (1979). The story describes Kchabuckè, a little frog made of *achiote,* the seed used to make a red dye for body paint and a flavoring for cooking.

> The sea was a pregnant woman, and she was bitten by a snake and died. When it came time to bury her, two consecutive claps of thunder were heard, but it wasn't actually thunder as the sound came from the corpse. It sounded four more times. Then God called the tiny frog made of *achiote* and told her to sit on the woman/sea's body and by the mouth of her stomach, which is on her liver. They were about to bury the body when the corpse began making more

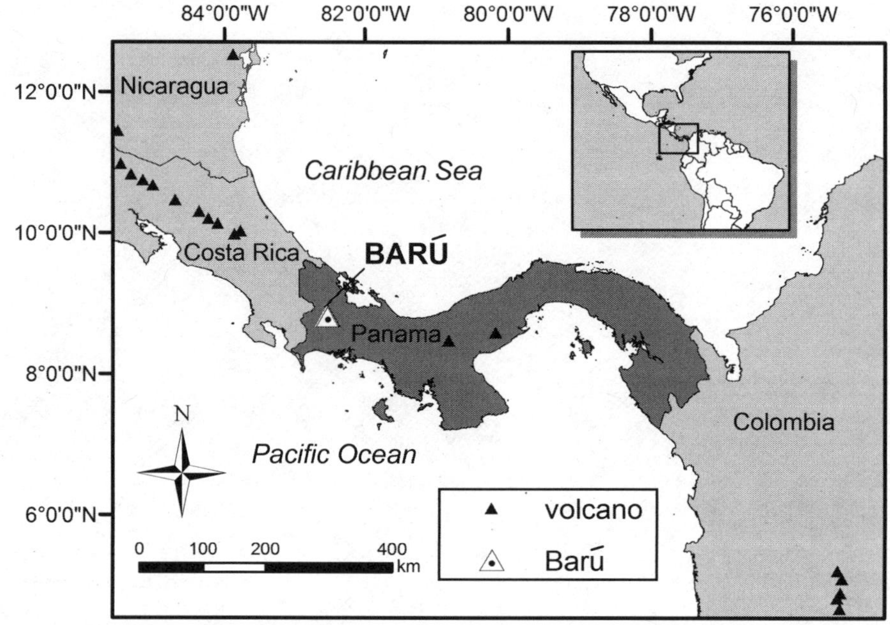


**Figure 3-2.** *Map indicating the location of the Volcán Barú in western Panamá in relation to other active Holocene volcanoes in Central America and the isthmus. Data are from the Smithsonian Global Volcanism Project.*

> loud sounds and the ground began to shake. God told the little frog not to move, and it was trapped there and hungry as it had not eaten anything. They buried the body under a mound of earth, but it began to make an incredible amount of noise. God told the little frog to stay on the burial mound over the stomach, but even still the noises continued. At noon on the fourth day the little frog still had not eaten, but then she saw a worm and decided to eat it. She had to move slightly off of the mound to catch the worm and was not able, no matter what she did, to jump on top of the body again. Because of this, the body swelled and burst and a tall tree grew exploded from it through the earth and continued to grow continually toward the sun [Peraldo and Montero 1994:49].

The story is ripe with information about how the frog experienced an unusual and violent event. Hearing, not sight, is the first and longest sensory description. As Edmund Burke (2008:123 [1757]) wrote, "excessive loudness alone is sufficient to overpower the soul, to suspend its action, and to fill it with terror," and this seems indicated by the primacy of the strange and terrifying noises in the story. The frog next felt the shaking of the ground below her. She experienced what must have been great hunger after days without sustenance. She saw food and longed for it though she was under explicit orders to keep at her post. She felt frustration as she tried repeatedly to return to her duty but was physically unable to do so. She watched as something exploded from the ground and grew to extraordinary heights. It is only after all of these descriptions that sight is highlighted when she watches as a tree grows high into the sky. This sequencing of the senses is an inversion or shuffling of the sensory hierarchy we are most used to, one that preferences sight, in ways that mirror examples from other non-Western contexts (e.g., Howes 2003:35).

For Costa Rican volcanologists Peraldo and Montero (1994:50), the story of the frog plausibly encapsulates a very accurate record of a particular eruption of the Volcán Barú. The tremors felt by the frog parallel what is felt when an underground magmatic mass opens new passages to the surface due to an obstruction in the main crater. The swelling of the ground is a reasonable description of the buildup of magma. Earthquakes accompany the explosive release of the magma. The description of the tree's rapid and excessive growth forms an easily grasped metaphor to describe the column of gases and ash that rose rapidly from the crater during Barú eruptions.

The "sense" that something unusual was occurring must have struck the pre-Columbian residents of the Barú area during eruptions. Ash plumes from eruptions extended at least 10 km into the sky (Sherrod et al. 2007:6). Earthquakes, loud noises from seismic shifts, glowing pyroclastic flows at nighttime, and ash-generated lightning very commonly accompany ash plumes at stratovolcanoes like Barú. People most certainly remembered and told stories about the eruptions for many generations following each one. While I do not dispute the possibility that Peraldo and Montero (1994) are correct and that the story of the frog describes one concise eruption of Barú, I propose that another plausible interpretation is that the narrative for each new eruption was likely folded into the stories of prior ones and the blended tale was used as a way to understand or convey the eruption experience.

Rather than only recording what individuals experienced during a Barú eruption, I suggest that there is additionally the concept of a "metasense" implied by the direct communication from God to the little frog regarding her duties. While informed by the bodily senses, the metasense mediates and "makes sense" of the available information. I find it noteworthy that the frog does not perish in the story nor does the story make reference to punishment from God for her neglecting her duty by seeking food. The story describes, in essence, the experiences of volcanic eruption as witnessed from a close distance but devoid of catastrophic impact for the narrator or main character. In such a case, a radical transformation occurs in the way that the landscape is perceived; it goes from silent to violent and then returns to a normal that is slightly modified.

## Experiential Bombs

The "strangeness and untranslatability" of experience is incredibly difficult to convey to others who have not had the same experience, yet sense memory comprises an important part of social memory (Marks 2000:199). This, per Serres (2008:345), is the limitation of the "ghost of a language" with which we are forced to convey sensory information. In examining the role of objects and bodily perception in cinematography, Laura Marks draws on the work of Nadia Seremetakis (1994) when she states that "sense memory and material artifacts work in the same way; both are emissaries of cultural experience" (Marks 2000:201). While memory of the senses can itself be a cultural artifact according to Marks (2000) and Seremetakis (1994), the challenge for archaeologists is the determination of what the representations of social memory could be. Immaterial ideas and ideals are often expressed in material form (Miller 2005). While archaeological investigation is intimately linked to material culture, a great deal of what survives from the past—even if it is collected—is not easily incorporated into analyses (Buchli 2007:183).

In addition to the stories that I collected about the volcanic landscape, I also recovered a number of objects during my fieldwork that were not easily classified. One highly unusual object I recovered at a site 14 km from the Volcán Barú seems to indicate some past importance assigned to it that can no longer be definitively interpreted (Figure 3-3). The object appears to be a volcanic bomb, which is defined as any volcanic material ejected during an eruption that is larger than 64 mm in diameter. Volcanic bombs are found at Ceren in El Salvador in a structure interpreted from its unusual artifact assemblage to be a divining site associated with a female shaman (Simmons and Sheets 2002). Those bombs, however, were part of the heavy inundation of tephra that destroyed and preserved the Maya farming village (see Miller 2002:Figures 2.7 and 2.8). The low level of impact from volcanic materials on the eastern flanks of Barú, the lack of an impact crater, and the distance of the site from the volcanic crater all speak against the possibility that the bomb was ejected to the location by eruption. A bomb of this size could fall only within several hundred meters of the vent (David Sherrod, personal communication 2008). The bomb fell somewhere near the volcano's summit and was carried to the site.

That casts of corn cobs made of lava from the Sunset Crater volcano in the U.S. Southwest were carried four kilometers and then broken attests to the transport of volcanic materials devoid of tradition functional purpose in the prehistoric past (Elson et al. 2002, 2007). The "corn rocks" at Sunset Crater, however, were purposefully made for what Elson et al. (2002, 2007) assume was ritual usage. The bomb from Barú is clearly "natural" and shows no evidence of modification. It very strongly resembles, however, the form of a stone pestle from the Barú area (MacCurdy 1911:34, Figure 32). The bomb was found in association with both chipped and ground stone tools that show obvious utilitarian use, as well as a stone obelisk that was clearly modified and has a smoothed base but shows no evidence of use as a grinding or pounding tool. The bomb has no perceptible functional use. It is definitively linked to volcanic eruption in its formation; what provides a tantalizing and frustratingly opaque question for me, however, is whether the bomb had immaterial or sensory links to the volcano for the people who seemingly transported it a considerable distance from its original location.

If we feel a reversal of our sense of mastery when the earth acts on us (per Serres 1995:33), then perhaps the curation of the bomb, intimately linked to eruption, provided a material way to resume mastery once the exceptional transformation of the usually placid volcano was over. Alternately, sociologist Maurice Halbwachs (1980 [1950]) proposed that memories and stories survive when they accrue to material objects to which they are linked. Perhaps, then, the transplanted bomb

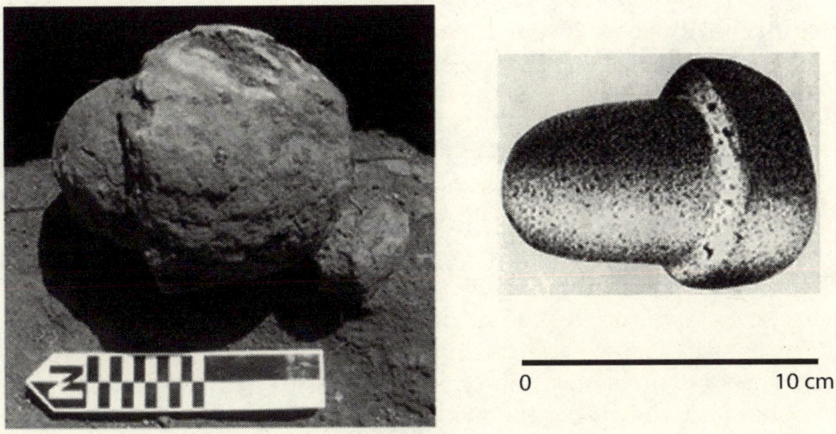


**Figure 3-3.** *A volcanic bomb recovered during archaeological fieldwork (left) and a pestle held in the collections of Yale University Peabody Museum from the study area (right). (Photograph © Karen Holmberg. Illustration from MacCurdy [1911:Figure 32].)*

served the same purpose as the story of the little frog. That is to say, it potentially provided a way to remember the experience of viewing a volcanic eruption and convey it to others. Many additional alternative hypotheses might be formed, and it is unlikely that a definitive consensus of which is most valid could exist. Perhaps such a consensus is not desirable due to the inability to truly understand the perceptions of the past in the present: The way that we perceive objects from the past can sway widely from the way they were perceived in the past (Serres 1995).

## Science with Sense

Violence is generally considered to be a product of human action that is inflicted on other people (e.g., Arendt 1970); violence can be more broadly defined, however, as a "reduction in being" (Schinkel 2010). With such an inclusive definition, the tendency in the social sciences toward a deprivation of sensory or experiential components when considering past people can in itself be viewed as an act of violence, in that it reduces the embodied experience that comprises human life. In such a case, of course, the injury or disservice is not to the people of the past but to ourselves and to our understanding of past life and how it relates to the present. Sensory experience can be highly collective and integral to cultural practice; ignoring the senses provides academic writing that is divorced from the corporeality of human life (Howes 2003:xi–xiii).

In this chapter, I have explored the concept of "natural" violence, which is inextricably connected with human life, per the conception of Serres (1995), with a focus on volcanic eruption as a radical example of environmental change. In looking at an extreme, obvious, and spectacular form of violence, I have neglected the vast phenomenological range of violence that exists in human life (per Schinkel 2010; Žižek 2008b). In so doing, however, I seek to avoid questions of whether past people were perceptually aware of their changing environment (per Meltzer and Holliday 2010) and examine instead how they might have perceived those changes.

The examination of changing environments in the past is a topic of growing archaeological interest. I feel that what we are largely seeking archaeologically in looking at changing environments is a metasense through which to understand our own present through the past. We are, however, only able to do so through what we know via our own senses and experiences. I perceive landscapes as capable of changing from benign to violent to benign again for those inhabitants not catastrophically affected. In so doing, I merge my own perception of a site of "cultural" violence in contemporary New York City with the "natural" violence of pre-Columbian volcanic eruptions.

By no means do I intend to essentialize experiences of the past. I do, however, propose that pre-Columbian people who lived near the Barú volcano during its fairly regular eruptions registered its monumental presence in the landscape prior to eruptions. I further propose that they would have noted its dramatic changes. For those who lived a safe distance from the volcano and were not catastrophically affected, the perception of the landscape would gradually return to one that was moderately benign. Violence is, perhaps, best defined by the bystanders who witness it, not by its victims (Žižek 2008b). Witnesses of large-scale violent events who are not disastrously affected perceive the event and then continue their lives while folding the experience into their sensoria.

Our perception of the world around us is always multisensory and merges and interlinks our senses to understand and translate our bodily experience (Beeli et al. 2005; Keating and Hadder 2010:120; Tilley 2008:33). In volcanic landscapes, components of nature and culture and sensory experience would be highly merged during the unusual occurrence of eruption. How people in the past perceived such phenomena is, of course, contextual to their own sensoria, though I propose that defined categorizations—such as smell, taste, hearing, and sight—would coalesce into one experiential package. The stench of live burning material, the feel of warm ash, the sound of massive telluric movements, the feel of charged ions in the air, and those charged ions visible as lightning in the volcanic ash clouds would all provide overlapping stimuli that were likely not experienced in the same way by everyone. To return to Aristotle's delineation of four senses that are linked to four elements; all eight would be very messily combined in an eruption of a volcano such as Barú. For those who experience such an unusual circumstance without catastrophic impact, the memory would remain even if the landscape returned to its prior normalcy.

The farther back in time we stretch our analyses, and the fewer material correlates available to analyze, the more difficult it is for us as social scientists to responsibly assess past sensory perception. The artists' renditions of the early human experience at Laetoli are iconic nearly to the point of cliché; I have used them as an example of what we do not want to replicate in archaeological assessments of the past in terms of projection of cultural norms and conjecture. While art may provide a more fluid way to explore sensory experience, archaeological research provides the only way to create plausible and data-derived interpretations of human experience in the past.

Archaeologically, we are accustomed to dealing with material culture, yet a great deal of our current material culture is highly immaterial; the archaeology of ourselves is of value (Harrison 2010). I have highlighted an ethnohistoric story of a frog that experiences a probable volcanic eruption as one way to consider how past people made "sense" of the phenomena in immaterial ways. In so doing, I accept that oral history forms one way to try to translate social memory, though it can only be interpreted through the lens of the present (Connerton 1989).

The presence of interpretively difficult objects, like the volcanic bomb, and the absence of clear material indications of their meaning or significance prevent easy assessments of their importance. Such materials, however, indicate that there are categories of data and elements that elude us and that we do not regularly consider but should. Drawing on Hannah Arendt's statement that "the things of the world have the function of stabilizing human life" (1958:137), Bill Brown (2010:191) states that "our sense of ourselves and what we call identity stabilize foremost in relation to concrete objects." My own sense is that the bomb could have signified a material remnant of the eruption—the epitome of instability—which then led to a sense of control or ownership.

As Kant (1987:120 [1790]) writes, the sublime violence of a volcano when viewed from a safe distance creates a sensation or "the courage [to believe] that we could be a match for nature's seeming omnipotence." Sublime objects like the volcano relocate human objects "within unhuman history—the history, not of the world, but of the earth . . . or, one might say, some new history of the *earth* as *world*" (Brown 2010:199). While large-scale geophysical events can be catastrophic for some, they provide a highly varied and highly sensory experience for others; as Serres (1995:124) states, "I tasted joy during the earthquake that terrified so many people around me." While acknowledging the archaeological limitations on what we can plausibly say about the bodily experience of the past, I hold per Serres (2008:345) that the senses form an important ghost of adventure to explore in a ghost of language.

## References


Anchukaitis, Kevin, and Sally Hor

2005 A 2000-Year Reconstruction of Forest Disturbance from Southern Pacific Costa Rica. *Palaeogeography, Palaeoclimatology, Palaeoecology* 221:35–54.

Arendt, Hannah

1958 *The Human Condition*. University of Chicago Press, Chicago.

1970 *On Violence*. Harcourt, Brace and World, New York.

Ashmore, Wendy

2007 Archaeologies of Landscape. In *A Companion to Social Archaeology*, edited by Lynn Meskell and Robert Preucel, pp. 255–271. Blackwell, Malden, Massachusetts.

Barker, Jennifer

2009 *The Tactile Eye: Touch and the Cinematic Experience*. University of California Press, Berkeley.

Barrett, John
1994 *Fragments from Antiquity*. Blackwell, Oxford.
Beeli, Gian, Michaela Esslen, and Lutz Jäncke
2005 Synaesthesia: When Colored Sounds Taste Sweet. *Nature* 434:38.
Behling, Hermann
2000 A 2860-Year High-Resolution Pollen and Charcoal Record from the Cordillera de Talamanca in Panama: A History of Human and Volcanic Forest Disturbance. *The Holocene* 10:387–393.
Bender, Barbara
1993 Introduction. In *Landscape: Politics and Perspectives*, edited by Barbara Bender, pp. 1–7. Berg, Oxford.
Bergson, Henri
1991 *Matter and Memory*. Translated by Nancy Margaret Paul and W. Scott Palmer. Zone Books, New York.
Bozzoli, María
1979 *El Nacimiento y la Muerte entre los Bribris*. Editorial Universidad de Costa Rica, San José.
Brown, Bill
2010 Objects, Others, and Us (the Refabrication of Things). *Critical Inquiry* 36:183–207.
Buchli, Victor
2007 Material Culture: Current Problems. In *A Companion to Social Archaeology*, edited by Lynn Meskell and Robert Preucel, pp. 179–194. Blackwell, Malden, Massachusetts.
Burke, Edmund
2008 [1757] *A Philosophical Enquiry into the Origin of Our Ideas of the Sublime and Beautiful: And Other Pre-Revolutionary Writings*. Oxford University Press, Oxford.
Castellanos Moya, Horacio
2008 *Senselessness*. Translated by Katherine Silver. New Directions, New York.
Classen, Constance (editor)
1993 *Worlds of Sense: Exploring the Senses in History and across Cultures*. Routledge, London.
Connerton, Paul
1989 *How Societies Remember*. Cambridge University Press, Cambridge.
Cronin, Shane, David Gaylord, Douglas Charley, Brent Alloway, Sandrine Wallez, and Job Esau
2004 Participatory Methods of Incorporating Scientific with Traditional Knowledge for Volcanic Hazard Management on Ambae Island, Vanuatu. *Bulletin of Volcanology* 66:652–668.
Edmonds, Mark
1999 *Ancestral Geographies of the Neolithic*. Routledge, London.
Eliasson, Olafur
2007 *The Body as Brain—Lava Floor: Projekt Sammlung* (5). Kunsthaus Zug, Switzerland.
Elson, Mark, Michael Ort, Kirk Anderson, and James Heidke
2007 Living with the Volcano: The 11th Century A.D. Eruption of Sunset Crater. In *Living under the Shadow: Cultural Impacts of Volcanic Eruptions*, edited by John Grattan and Robin Torrence, pp. 107–132. One World Archaeology Series. Left Coast, Walnut Creek, California.

Elson, Mark, Michael Ort, Jerome Hesse, and Wendell Duffield
2002 Lava, Corn, and Ritual in the Northern Southwest. *American Antiquity* 67:119–135.
Gibson, James J.
1966 *The Senses Considered as Perceptual Systems*. Houghton Mifflin, Boston.
Gosden, Christopher
1994 *Social Being and Time*. Blackwell, Oxford.
Grattan, John, and Robin Torrence (editors)
2007 *Living under the Shadow: Cultural Impacts of Volcanic Eruptions*. Left Coast, Walnut Creek, California.
Halbwachs, Maurice
1980 [1950] *The Collective Memory (Le Memoire Collective)*. Harper & Row Colophon, New York.
Haraway, Donna
1991 *Simians, Cyborgs, and Women: The Re-Invention of Nature*. Free Association, London.
Harrison, Rodney
2010 Exorcising the 'Plague of Fantasies': Mass Media and Archaeology's Role in the Present; or, Why We Need an Archaeology of 'Now'. *World Archaeology* 42:328–340.
Hegel, Friedrich
1975 *Aesthetics: Lectures on Fine Art*, Vol. 1. Translated by T. M. Knox. Clarendon, Oxford.
Holmberg, Karen
2005 The Voices of Stones: Unthinkable Materiality in the Volcanic Context of Western Panamá. In *Archaeologies of Materiality*, edited by Lynn Meskell, pp. 190–211. Blackwell, Malden, Massachusetts.
2007 Beyond the Catastrophe: The Volcanic Landscape of Barú, Western Panamá. In *Living under the Shadow: Cultural Impacts of Volcanic Eruptions*, edited by John Grattan and Robin Torrence, pp. 274–297. Left Coast, Walnut Creek, California.
2009 Nature, Culture, and the Volcano: The Archaeological Significance of the Volcán Barú in the Chiriquí Province of Panamá. Ph.D. dissertation, Department of Anthropology, Columbia University, New York.
2013 An Inheritance of Loss: Archaeology's Imagination of Disaster. In *Humans and the Environment: New Archaeological Perspectives for the 21st Century*, edited by Matthew Davis and Freda Nkirote. Oxford University Press, Oxford, in press.
Howes, David
2003 *Sensual Relations: Engaging the Senses in Culture and Social Theory*. University of Michigan Press, Ann Arbor.
2004 *Empires of the Senses: The Sensual Culture Reader*. Berg, Oxford.
ISE Cultural Foundation
2009–2010 *Volcano Lovers from Iceland and Japan*. Curated by Birta Gudjonsdottir and Shinya Watanabe. November 13, 2009–January 2, 2010. New York.
IVHHN (International Volcanic Health Hazard Network)
2010 The Health Hazards of Volcanic Ash. Electronic document, http://www.ivhhn.org/images/pamphlets/Health_Guidelines_English_WEB.pdf, accessed September 17, 2010.
Jónsson, Haraldur
2009 Artist's Talk on *Dark Lamp*, November 14. ISE Cultural Foundation, New York.

Kant, Immanuel

1987 [1790] *Critique of the Power of Judgment*. Translated by Werner S. Pluhar. Hackett, Indianapolis.

Keating, Elizabeth, and R. Neill Hadder

2010 Sensory Impairment. *Annual Review of Anthropology* 39:115–129.

Knowlton, Brian

2010 Icelandic Volcano Began Rumbling in March. *New York Times*. New York. Electronic document, http://www.nytimes.com/2010/04/16/world/europe/16iht-scene.html?scp=1&sq=Icelandic%20volcano%20began%20rumbling%20in%20March&st=cse, accessed April 15, 2010.

Latour, Bruno

1991 *We Have Never Been Modern*. Translated by Catherine Porter. Harvard University Press, Cambridge.

2009 Will Non-Humans Be Saved? An Argument in Ecotheology. *Journal of the Royal Anthropological Institute* 15:459–475.

Loose, Richard

2008 Tse'Biinaholts'a Yalti (Curved Rock That Speaks). *Time and Mind: The Journal of Archaeology, Consciousness and Culture* 1:31–50.

MacCurdy, George

1911 *A Study of Chiriquian Antiquities*. Memoirs of the Connecticut Academy of Arts and Sciences, Vol. 3. Yale University Press, New Haven.

Marks, Laura

2000 *The Skin of the Film: Intercultural Cinema, Embodiment, and the Senses*. Duke University Press, Durham.

Massey, Doreen

2005 *For Space*. Sage, London.

Meltzer, David J., and Vance T. Holliday

2010 Would North American Paleoindians Have Noticed Younger Dryas Age Climate Changes? *Journal of World Prehistory* 23:1–41.

Merleau-Ponty, Maurice

1962 *Phenomenology of Perception*. Translated by Colin Smith. Routledge, London.

Miller, C. Dan

2002 Volcanology, Stratigraphy, and Effects on Structures. In *Before the Volcano Erupted: The Ancient Cerén Village in Central America*, edited by Payson D. Sheets, pp. 10–23. University of Texas Press, Austin.

Miller, Daniel (editor)

2005 *Materiality*. Duke University Press, Durham.

Peraldo, Giovanni, and Walter Montero

1994 *Temblores del Período Colonial de Costa Rica*. Editorial Tecnológica de Costa Rica, Cartago.

Plunket, Patricia, and Gabriela Uruñuela

2008 Mountain of Sustenance, Mountain of Destruction: The Prehispanic Experience with Popocatépetl Volcano. *Journal of Volcanology and Geothermal Research* 170:111–120.

Raichlen, David, Adam Gordon, William Harcourt-Smith, Adam Foster, and William Randall Haas

2010 Laetoli Footprints Preserve Earliest Direct Evidence of Human-like Bipedal Biomechanics. PLoS ONE 5(3):e9769. doi:9710.1371/journal.pone.0009769.

Ritchie, Ian

1991 Fusion of the Faculties: A Study of the Language of the Senses in Hausaland. In

*The Varieties of Sensory Experience*, edited by David Howes, pp. 192–202. University of Toronto Press, Toronto.

Ruiz-Ballesteros, Esteban, José Valcuende, Victoria Quintero, José Cortes, and Elena Rubio

2009 Naturalizing the Environment. *Journal of Material Culture* 14:147–167.

Sankey, Margaret, and Peter Cowley (translators)

2008 Sense and Sensibility: Translating the Bodily Experience. In *The Five Senses: A Philosophy of Mingled Bodies*, by Michel Serres, pp. vii–xii. Continuum, London.

Schiller, Friedrich

1993 [1801] On the Sublime (Toward the Further Development of Some Kantian Ideas). In *Essays*, edited by Walter Hinderer and Daniel Dahlstrom, pp. 22–44. Continuum, New York.

Schinkel, Willem

2010 *Aspects of Violence: A Critical Theory*. Palgrave Macmillan, New York.

Seremetakis, Nadia

1994 *The Senses Still: Memory and Perception as Material Culture in Modernity*. Westview, Boulder.

Serres, Michel

1995 *The Natural Contract*. Translated by Elizabeth MacArthur and William Paulson. University of Michigan Press, Ann Arbor.

2008 *The Five Senses: A Philosophy of Mingled Bodies*. Translated by Margaret Sankey and Peter Cowley. Continuum, London.

Shanks, Michael, and Ian Hodder

1995 Processual, Postprocessual, and Interpretive Archaeologies. In *Interpreting Archaeology: Finding Meaning in the Past*, edited by Ian Hodder, Michael Shanks, and Alexandra Alexandri, Victor Buchli, John Carman, Jonathan Last, and Gavin Lucas, pp. 3–29. Routledge, London.

Sheets, Payson

2008 Armageddon to the Garden of Eden: Explosive Volcanic Eruptions and Societal Resilience in Ancient Middle America. In *El Niño, Catastrophism, and Culture Change in Ancient America*, edited by Daniel H. Sandweiss and Jeffrey Quilter, pp. 167–186. Dumbarton Oaks, Washington, D.C.

Sherrod, David, James Vallance, Arkin Tapia Espinosa, and John McGeehin

2007 *Volcán Barú: Eruptive History and Volcano-Hazards Assessment*. Open-File Report 2007-1401. United States Geological Survey.

Simmons, Scott, and Payson Sheets

2002 Divination at Cerén: The Evidence from Structure 12. In *Before the Volcano Erupted: The Ancient Cerén Village in Central America*, edited by Payson D. Sheets, pp. 104–113. University of Texas Press, Austin.

Skúlason, Páll

2005 *Reflections at the Edge of Askja*. University of Iceland Press, Reykjavik.

Strathern, Marilyn

1992 *After Nature: English Kinship in the Late Twentieth Century*. Cambridge University Press, Cambridge.

Thomas, Julian

2001 Archaeologies of Place and Landscape. In *Archaeological Theory Today*, edited by Ian Hodder, pp. 165–186. Polity Press, Cambridge.

2004 Mind, Perception and Knowledge. In *Archaeology and Modernity*, pp. 171–201. Routledge, London.

Tilley, Christopher
2008 *Body and Image: Explorations in Landscape Phenomenology* 2. Left Coast, Walnut Creek, California.
Varela, Francisco, J. Evan Thompson, and Eleanor Rosch
1991 *The Embodied Mind: Cognitive Science and Human Experience*. MIT Press, Cambridge, Massachusetts.
Žižek , Slavoj
2008a Unbehagen in der natur. In *In Defense of Lost Causes*, by Slavoj Žižek, pp. 420–461. Verso, London.
2008b *Violence*. Picador, New York.

# 4. Colored Monuments and Sensory Theater among the Mississippians

*Corin C. O. Pursell*

*Abstract:* Recent research has demonstrated that colorful sediments were frequently used to surface Mississippian earthworks. This paper interprets one such colorful monumental space, Shiloh Mounds in southwestern Tennessee. Engagement with the sensuous past of Shiloh changes our understanding of the site, inverting assumptions about the power dynamics in the construction of two of the main mounds. Shiloh was constructed using red and white sediments, which were deposited in discrete areas of the site and distinctly cap the two mounds in question. Many southeastern Native Americans characteristically split both their ideological and social realities into the dichotomous categories of Red or White, which were key symbols for a suite of related concepts—including clan, directional, and animal symbolism—tied to various personal or social attributes. This paper shows that broad ethnographic generalizations about power do violence to the locally contextual, historically contingent metaphors of Shiloh, in which monumental Red and White, in quotidian and ritual experience, were used to accomplish surprising social goals. The manipulation of color and perspective create the powerful impact of a small white burial mound and modify that of a large red "chief's" mound.

Traditionally, most Mississippian monuments have been portrayed as being either brown or grass-covered, as we living archaeologists project backward from our present experience into the prehistoric past. The typical experience today is that of a broad, grass- or tree-covered swath of open plaza and low mounds. Despite that, we are aware that the lived experience of the mound towns of southern Tennessee would have included the smell of roasting deer and

*Making Senses of the Past: Toward a Sensory Archaeology,* edited by Jo Day. Center for Archaeological Investigations, Occasional Paper No. 40.  ISBN 978-0-8093-3287-8.

corn, the sound of an early dialect of Chickasaw, and the feel of a surrounding crowd and houses. Similarly, we now realize that many Mississippian mounds were quite brightly colored, darkly colored, or sharply contrasting (Anderson and Cornelison 2002; Pursell 2004; Sherwood and Kidder 2011). Mounds were the central sacred architecture of the Mississippian peoples, a physical feature that literally served as either a backdrop or platform for the majority of the important political and religious events of a person's life (Knight 1981, 1986). With that in mind, it is difficult to think that this color play was not done with purpose. This paper will particularly focus on the visual and meaning-laden experience of place created by the construction and use of two major earthworks using colored earths in the thirteenth century C.E. at an important Mississippian political center along the Tennessee River (Figure 4-1).

Shiloh has been under erosional threat for decades and has been the subject of intense archaeological scrutiny since 1998. Recent reexamination of old work has been combined with new excavations to create a more complete whole (Anderson and Cornelison 2002; Sherwood and Kidder 2011; Welch 2006). An important result of this research was the discovery of the complex use of colored sediments in large primary Mound A, particularly distinct red sediment caps. Excavations in the 1930s showed that Mound C, a smaller burial mound, also had colored sediments—in this instance, layers of white (Figure 4-2). These colored sediments have been interpreted previously in terms of ethnographic analogy to Charles Hudson's description of the Red and White structural dichotomy in historic Native American groups of the southeastern United States (Anderson and Cornelison 2002; Hudson 1976:234–239; Welch 2006:408–409). Red and White were shown to act as extended metaphors for kin divisions and for War and Peace respectively, with a variety of associated symbolic concepts. As stated by Hudson, European observers had an incomplete understanding of how this system operated and may have reported misleading information about practices related to dual organization in the Southeast (1976:234). Only a limited grasp of the historic practices tied to this color dichotomy and the related suite of concepts is available. Another study inspired by the Shiloh work has recently addressed the subject from a geoarchaeological perspective with some useful reflections on social importance (Sherwood and Kidder 2011), and a study on color meaning in the Mississippian ceramics known as head pots presents a possible relationship of color meaning to time or temporality (Cobb and Drake 2008). The actual ways these colors were used, experienced, and manipulated within prehistoric communities have not been addressed.

In order to study color symbolism at the site, the specific archaeological contexts of the use and experience of color are the best archaeological correlates to examine. The study of the experience of space and the control of spatial perception are major avenues for understanding ritual activity in public monumental environments (Ashmore and Knapp 1999; Fogelin 2003; Giddens 1986; Moore 1996). Two approaches may be usefully applied to Shiloh, one drawn from archaeological work in Peru and the other from such work on the Indian subcontinent. Jerry Moore (1996) proposed that Peruvian monumental structures can be studied through examination of the angles of visual incidence and the distance

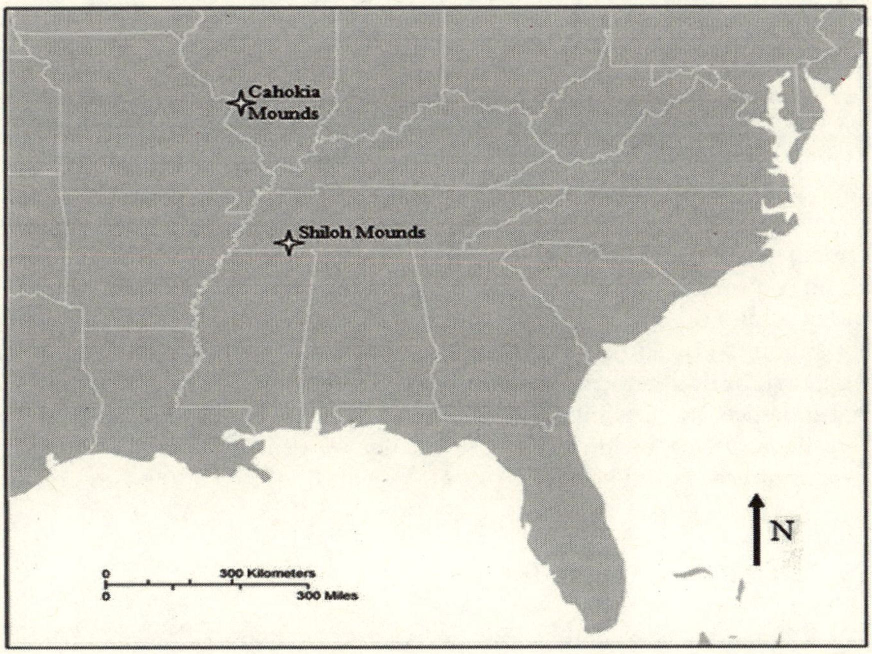


**Figure 4-1.** *Location of Shiloh and Cahokia mounds in the southeastern United States.*

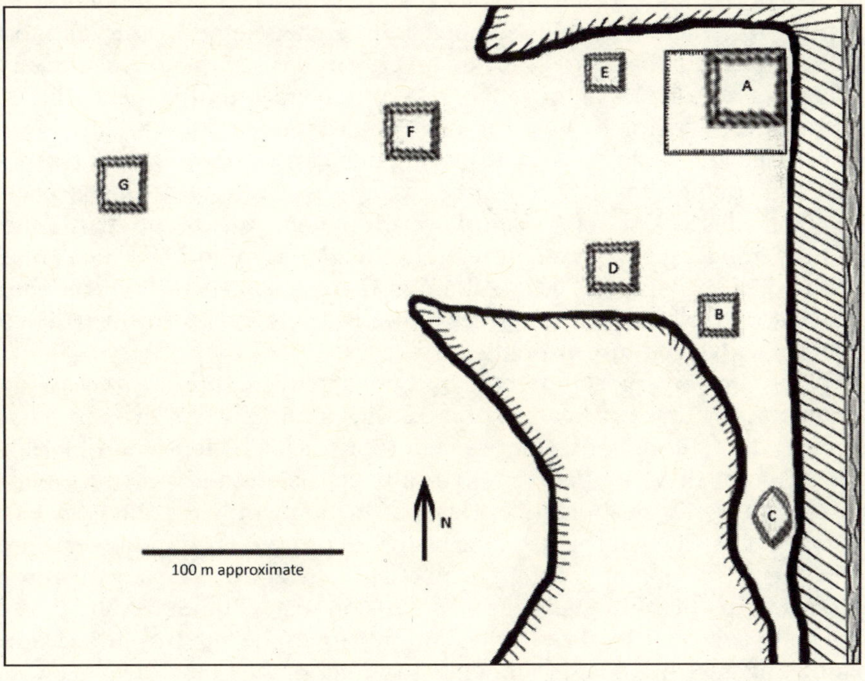


**Figure 4-2.** *Map of Shiloh showing mounds discussed in the text.*

of the observer from the activities related to the structure. Lars Fogelin (2003:135) proposed that the goals of construction and use can be identified from the form of a ritual space. As Mississippian mound centers are both monumental and make up a ritual space, Mississippian sites are amenable to both techniques. A similar study was successfully accomplished in Crete at the same time this research was originally proposed, demonstrating its utility in stone architecture (Letesson and Vansteenhuyse 2006). This study will instead use these ideas in the study of Mississippian earthen architecture.

The combination of the two approaches reveals different functions of and intended audiences for Mounds A and C at Shiloh. Mound A, the presumptive "chief's mound," is shown to be a public locale able to act as a predominantly Red symbol for both a local community audience in the plaza and an extracommunal audience approaching from outside, with markedly distinct effects depending on the audience. Mound C is shown to be a restricted ceremonial locale for the performance of elite-controlled White burial ritual to a limited audience.

## Color in Archaeology

This research follows up on Warren DeBoer's (2005) exhortation to archaeology to stop "playing second fiddle" in studies of color symbolism and instead to directly engage with the ancient use of color in practice. Color symbolism and the independent cognitive study of cross-cultural color perception have two different histories in anthropology, each of which bears on this study. When attempting to understand color symbolism in archaeological contexts, most archaeologists have either turned to some version of direct-historical analogy (as per Charles Hudson [1976]) or to the idea of universal, multivocal bodily referents proposed by Victor Turner (Turner 1967; Erdogu and Ulubey 2011). Despite the advantage archaeology has in exploring deep time depth, color is rarely held to possess its own history. By contrast, the cognitive anthropology approach has given color a history, but a specifically evolutionary one, emphasizing the development of basic color terms in sequence (e.g., Berlin and Kay 1969; Hays et al. 1972; but see Chapman 2002). Although there is some flexibility, neither the cognitive nor the symbolic approaches typically study long-term change in color referents in a given culture or polity.

My research diverges from these traditions in this important way, following those who assert that genealogies of meanings are important even in the three basic red/white/black body-color system (Borić 2002:39; Jones and MacGregor 2002:7–9). Color does not have a universally consistent meaning even within a single culture at a single moment but is given meaning only in context and in use. Cobb and Drake (2008) recognized the historical process of color meaning, claiming that the prehistoric use of color symbolism may at times be a deliberate allusion to a sort of "monumental time," an allusion to a distant past and a broadly shared belief system. Ritualized behavior often gives the feel and surface appearance of being ancient and eternal, while itself being the home of constant social renegotiation beneath this immortal veneer (Bell 1992:138–169). The creation of a new set of color uses at Mississippian sites drew on this ancient color history to give power and legitimacy to the colors' new social meanings.

Colored mounds can be seen from the Middle Woodland period (ca. 2500–1500 B.P., varying in chronological range by region), including red, white, and yellow Kolomoki, yellow Pinson, light and dark Mound House, and ubiquitous red, black, white, and yellow at the major Hopewell sites such as Tremper Great House, Turner, and the Hopewell site (Buikstra et al. 1998:84–88; DeBoer 1997; Mainfort 1986, 1988; Pluckhahn 2003; see also Hall 1997:17–23, 27). Research has done well looking at real associations of color, material, and location within archaeological sites, seeking patterning that is both locally unique and referential to broader color schemes. Results from the Ohio Hopewell and Illinois Hopewell appear distinct, as does the completely different color use at Kolomoki, suggesting that regional and local traditions of color use may predate the Mississippian.

Mississippian use of colored sediments should not surprise archaeologists, therefore, as Mississippians are heirs to these varied traditions and surely equally able to manipulate color in public architecture for their novel symbolic needs. Shiloh itself represents a new material transformation of color meaning: an aesthetic, a religious, and a political reinterpretation of color's long-held meanings in large-scale public rituals of construction, creating a newly materialized symbolic order that surrounded and structured the lives of the inhabitants of Shiloh. The roles of materialization, public performance, aesthetic objects and agency, and memorialization are thus all relevant to this new set of negotiated color meanings at Shiloh (for further discussion of these topics see Gell 1998; Giddens 1986; Gosden 2001; Inomata and Coben 2006; Jones 2007; Miller 2005; Robb 1998; Stewart and Strathern 2003; Van Dyke and Alcock 2003).

## Concepts—Visual Restriction and Presentational Formats

Moore and Fogelin confronted differing research questions related to monumentality. Moore's Peruvian structures were characterized by being vertically imposing but restricted in the avenues of approach and visual appreciation. Fogelin's Indian Buddhist structures were characterized by distinctive ways of manipulating and controlling the attention and movement of an audience in an enclosed space. Mississippian mound centers can be seen in both senses. As with nearly all studies of architecture and practice, this research operates with the assumption stated by Giddens (among others) that architecture both shapes daily practices and is shaped by them (Giddens 1984:110–161). The analyses by Moore, Fogelin, and me are also united by the precepts laid out by Moore: that public ritual serves as communication, that human perception limits that communication, that different rituals for different audiences involve distinct perceptions, and that ceremonial architecture reflects those rituals and the related body of perception (1996:135–136).

Moore examined the variability in *huacas* in the Andes by examining a number of variables of monumental structures. He showed that many variables of ritual architecture can be used by archaeologists to illuminate the associated social contexts and ceremonial patterns of an archaeological culture. Although he described a variety of useful variables, only Moore's concept of *visibility* is operationalized here. In this context, visibility includes the ability to see (or otherwise perceive) a structure or an architectural element.

The vertical angle of view and the distance from the observer to the performance are the two primary factors of visibility that can be put into operation (Figure 4-3). In the most basic conception, elevation above the rest of the community is a simple way to mark social difference (Lewis et al. 1998), but the experiential impact of a mound's height and scale is a step beyond this interpretation. Monuments perceived as taller, or larger, are more visible and thus more salient in the experience of a monumental site, which has an effect on the inhabitants. This argument is buttressed strongly by studies done on the biological and physical limits of human perception, in which certain limitations of angle perception may be noted. At differing thresholds above or below the horizon and the level gaze of the human eye, the viewer becomes more or less able to perceive such features as color and physical scale. These thresholds of human perception are relevant to this analysis. When confronted by a small object or distant large object that takes up less than 18° of the vertical field of perception, viewers do not have a monumental experience; such distant objects appear as background in the visual field, not as imposing monuments. At a vertical angle greater than 18°, a massive structure is experienced by the observer as monumental. The monument fills enough of the visual range of the viewer so as to appear to be a large object. At an angle of 27°, the structure fills the observer's visual range (Moore 1996:160). Partially because the human upper limit for visual perception is only around 50–55° above the horizon, an object filling more than 45° of the vertical visual field will be perceived as a vertical surface rather than as a monument. These points were originally argued by Märtens (1890) and are thus known as Märtens's rule (Letesson and Vansteenhuyse 2006). An important subsidiary point is that rises or depressions between the observer and the subject can serve to respectively decrease or increase the experience of vertical scale.

By contrast, Lars Fogelin (2003) examined the variability in ritual presentation in Buddhist *stupa* complexes using concepts derived from theater studies. The ritual contexts examined essentially varied along a continuum from an arena to a hall format (Figure 4-4). Following Fogelin's analysis, arena formats are presentational spaces in which the performance occurs in the center of a surrounding audience. Such a performance context encourages participatory behavior, reduces the ability of any one performer to manipulate the entire audience, de-emphasizes the social distance between audience and performers, and is associated with communal ritual. The faces of other audience members are serve as a continuous visual backdrop to performances in such an arena, and any performers must face at most half the audience at one time. Observing the reactions of other participants and audience members provides continuous feedback on appropriate group behavior and further unifies the experience. At the opposite end of the spectrum is the hall format, a presentational space in which the performance occurs at one

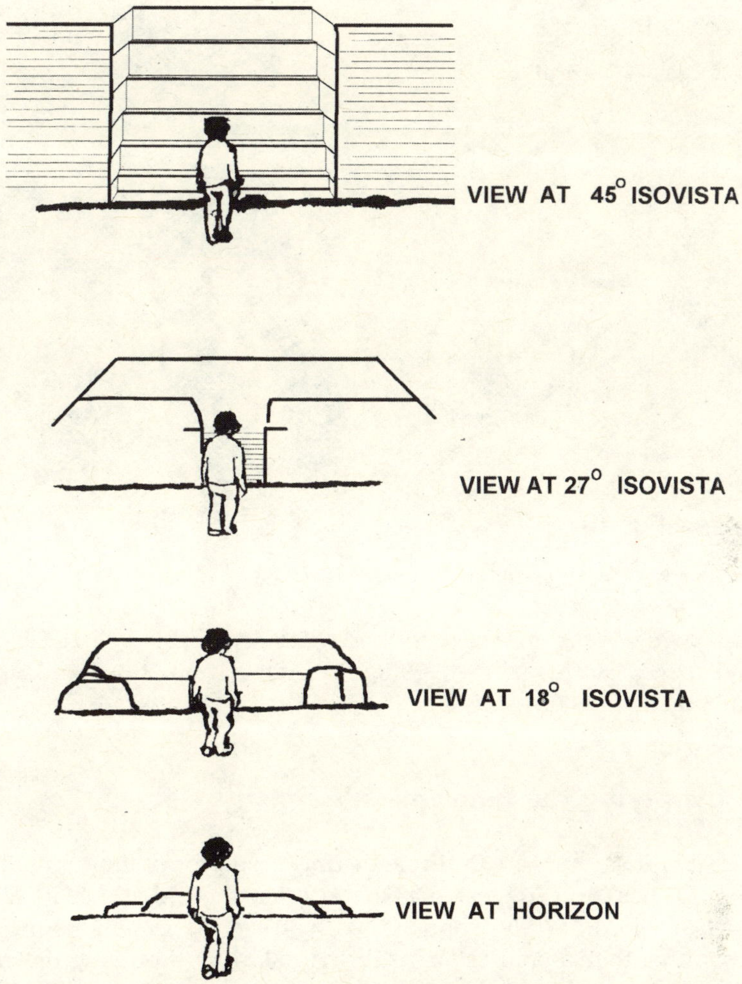


**Figure 4-3.** *Thresholds of visibility (Moore 1996:Figure 3.4).*

end, with the audience oriented toward that locale. Such a context discourages participation, constrains communal ritual, emphasizes social distance between the performer and the audience, permits the manipulation of the entire audience by a single individual, and is associated with ritual led by a practitioner in a leadership role and is also known as corporate ritual. The entire audience is oriented toward the performers, with their attention directed toward a single point. Fogelin does not argue that these two are exclusive categories that should be contrasted but rather that they are extreme ends of a continuum on which most presentational spaces may be placed. Most architectural spaces used for ritual fall somewhere between these extremes. In no case does the form of the ritual space strictly determine the ceremonial practices performed therein; they simply lend themselves more effectively to one or the other.

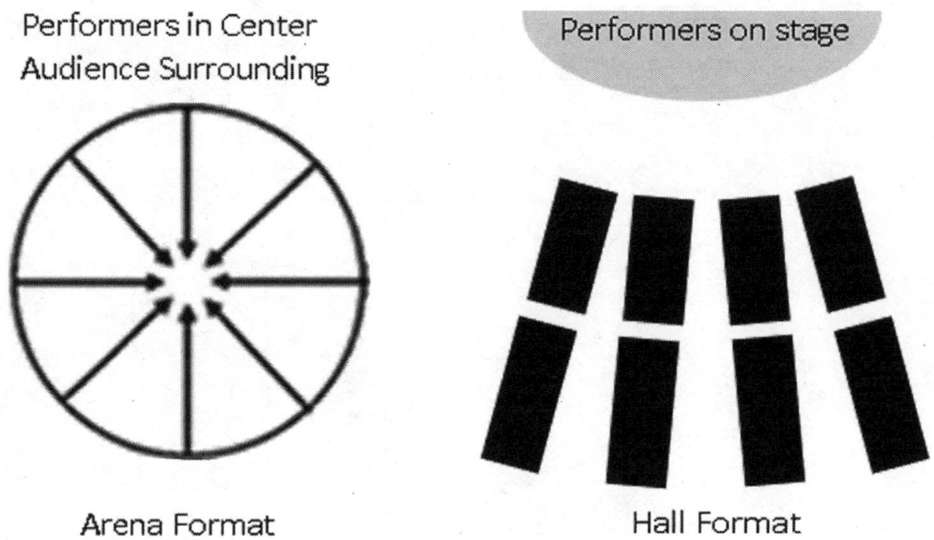


**Figure 4-4.** *Types of presentational spaces.*

Both Moore's ideas of verticality and visibility and Fogelin's ideas of presentational spaces can reveal archaeological information about the deployment of monumental architecture.

## Applying the Concepts—Visibility

At Shiloh, there are multiple distinct scenarios of monumental experience. Mound A has been suggested as the primary mound at the site (Anderson and Cornelison 2002:6), while Mound C has been seen as a small mound fulfilling a religious, rather than a political, role (Welch 2006:408). Applying the methodology described above, Mound C is seen to be potentially a more politically powerful tool of the elite within the community than is Mound A, in which more than one social agenda is expressed. However, due to its size and bluff-top placement, Mound A also acts powerfully as a community statement to the outside world.

Mound A is not currently the same height it would have been during its use. At least one historic structure has been constructed and removed from atop the mound, perhaps reducing the overall height, and a bit of superficial erosion may have occurred over time. On the other hand, Shiloh has experienced relatively little surface erosion compared to many other Mississippian sites, as can be seen from the many low house mounds surrounding the plaza, whose collapsed wattle-and-daub structures have never been plowed. The present-day height of Mound A is thus a reasonable proxy of the height of the final use layer of the mound before its abandonment, and any height loss does not significantly affect the final analysis. The first red layer found during excavation was quite near the surface, indicating that the final red-capping episode was within a meter or two of the height used in the following estimates. It should be noted that the following analysis applies only to the final stage of the mound and that earlier construction episodes would have appeared significantly less monumental both to the community and to outsiders. Mound C, by contrast, was built in only one or two episodes and would have been experienced in basically only three ways: the prepared ground before construction, the ritual of construction, and the final product, examined below.

Mound A, as seen from most of the plaza, is not experienced as monumental in the sense that Jerry Moore (1996) describes (Figure 4-5). An observer does not cross the critical threshold of 18° of visual elevation until closer than about 22 m to the mound. As noted earlier, at a visual angle of less than 18° a structure is experienced more as background than as monument. The plaza itself extends approximately 120 m east–west and 70 m north–south, so most of a potential community audience in the plaza would not experience the mound as monumental. In order for the mound to fill one's visual field, an approach of closer than 14 m from the mound is needed. Further decreasing the experience of monumentality is the existence of a deliberately constructed apron surrounding Mound A. Moore (1996) has shown that an intervening rise reduces the effect of the visual experience of monumentality. Thus, the apron acts as a deliberate artificial reduction in the perceived social distance between the mound top and the plaza. The eroded west apron would have been almost as broad as the area in which monumental perception would have been possible, greatly decreasing the number of audience members who could potentially experience the mound as monumental. The apron had two construction episodes, and during each there were some structures atop the apron (Welch 2006:208–222). The apron itself may have been constructed after the main body of Mound A (Welch 2006:216). These structures are poorly dated but obscure the mound only partially when viewed from within the plaza. Because of the lack of data on the structures, it is not clear whether they would enhance or decrease the vertical experience of the mound, but certainly they would reduce the visual impact of the red surface when viewed from within the community.

Mound A when seen from the river to the east is a different story (Figure 4-6). Because of the steep descent of the bluff face, Mound A presents a greatly enhanced sense of vertical distance when seen from outside the community. The mound–bluff face would be experienced as monumental for almost 100 m, affecting many people passing the site and anyone approaching from the riverside. While Mound A's apron and apron structures serve to de-emphasize elite power within the community, Mound A's bluff-edge locale serves to greatly emphasize elite power to outsiders. The Tennessee River is likely to have been a major thoroughfare of travel and exchange for the entire region, indicating that almost any passing outsider would have experienced Shiloh's primary mound as monumental.

Mound C is barely visible from the river in the same way, but perhaps more important, it lacks any intervening apron when approached from the north (Figure 4-7). When approaching from the north, only those persons within 10 m of the mound would experience it as monumental. This would not be significant if it were possible to approach the mound from any other direction, but the surrounding environmental hazards mean that the only approach from within the

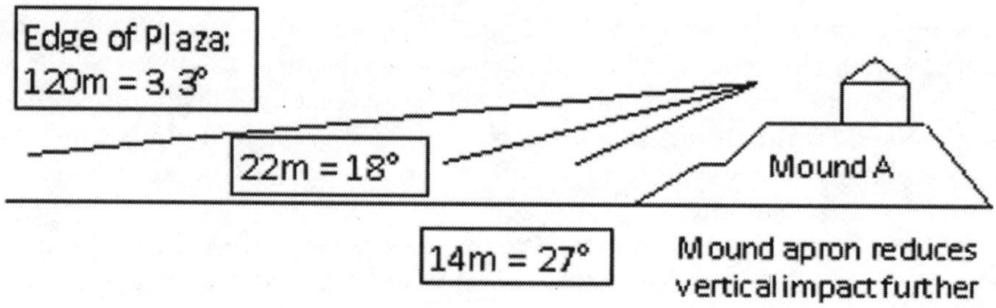


**Figure 4-5.** *Mound A, approaching from the plaza: nonmonumental experience.*

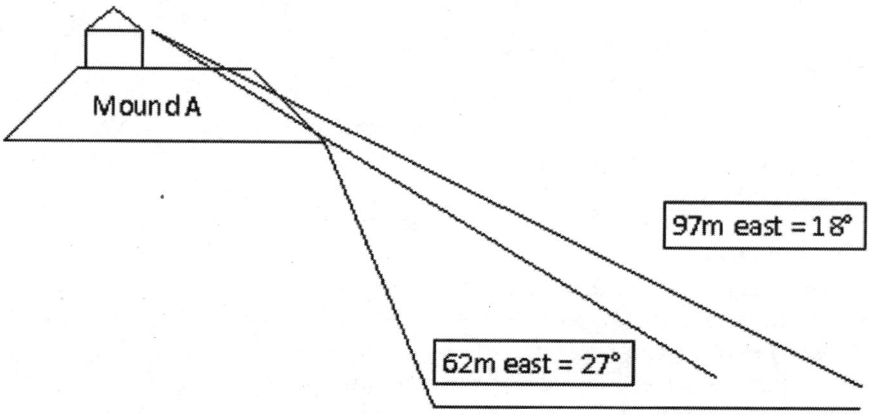


**Figure 4-6.** *Mound A, approaching from the river: experience of monumentality.*

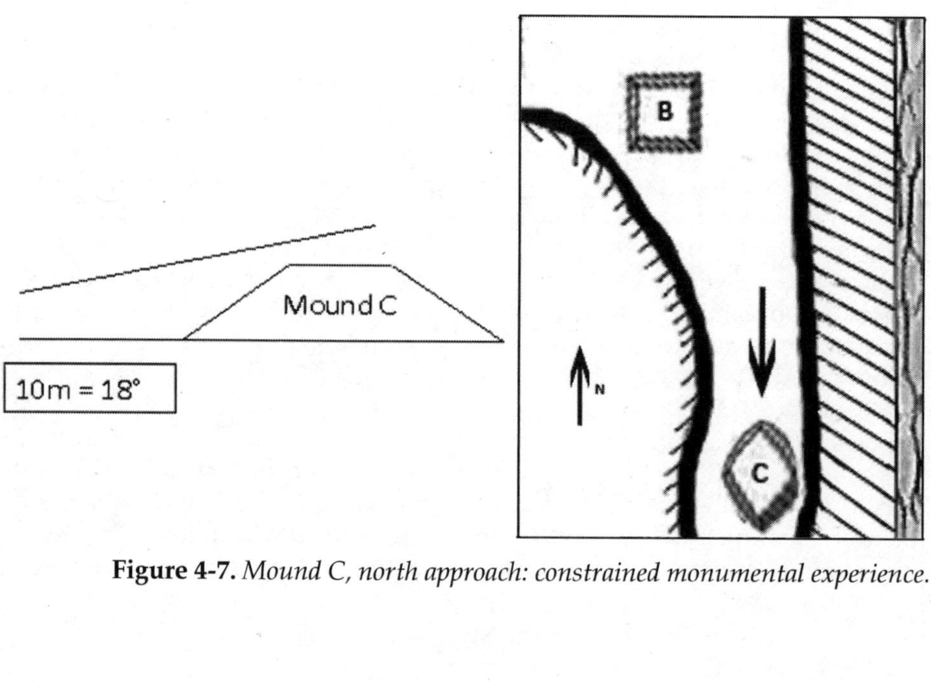


**Figure 4-7.** *Mound C, north approach: constrained monumental experience.*

community is from the north. The reduced audience space and surrounding ravines and river bluff thus control and restrict the audience's vantage point to emphasize the height of the mound. Furthermore, the lack of an apron means that the distance of monumental perception for Mound C is almost the same as for the much larger Mound A. The verticality and monumentality of Mound C are emphasized in this space just as they are de-emphasized within the plaza for Mound A.

## Applying the Concepts—Halls and Arenas

Turning to the subject of audience control, multiple different audience scenarios are evident. Ritual or symbolic gestures involved in the construction or use of mounds may have had many intended audiences; four have relevance in this analysis. A ritual may have occurred in the plaza with the audience in the plaza experiencing the mounds as background. Mound A may have been viewed by an audience in the plaza. Mound A may have been viewed by an audience on or across the river to the east, below the bluff face. Finally, Mound C may have been viewed by an audience in the restricted area between the river and the ravine.

In the first scenario, ritual acts related to the Shiloh plaza would clearly fit into the arena end of the continuum, with an open space lacking any elevation or differentiation of performers (Figure 4-8). Such use implies probable communal ritual with less significant elite mediation and matches well with historic data on acts in common areas and plazas of the Southeast, which include ritualized cleaning and dancing activities (Hudson 1976:78, 113, 212–213; see also Knight 1981). In this case, mounds serve only to delimit activity and are experienced as landscape background, not as monumental architecture. Note that this does not preclude elite mediation; plaza spaces simply lend themselves best to communally organized ritual behavior that is less directly supportive of elite control.

While the plaza could clearly act as an arena, it could also serve as a hall if a performance were observed atop one of the mounds, during the mound construction, or atop a mound apron (Figure 4-9). The surrounding mounds and structures could serve to contain and orient the audience. The elevated position of the mound tops or aprons at the end of the plaza could act as a stage for the performance of corporate ritual by an elite mediator-performer. Such behavior has some support in the historic record (e.g., Hudson 1976:78; Knight 1981:45). Whether the southwest portion of Mound A might have served this function is not known because this portion of the mound has not been excavated. In this case, the broad plaza space would allow a large audience for potentially powerful elite performer(s), but this ritual space evidently could be open to participation by the entire community.

Mound C presents the most hall-like ritual format (Figure 4-10). The mound rests upon a narrow spit of flattened land between the bluff and river to the east and a ravine to the west. Access to the spit is further controlled by the placement of Mounds D and B, which partially block access from all directions but due north. Due north of Mound C is an open flat area some 80 m long and 20

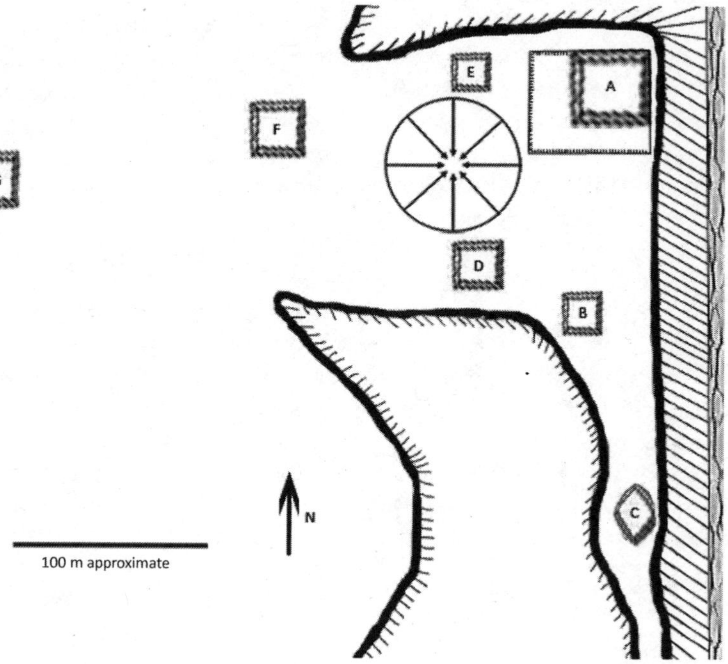


**Figure 4-8.** *Map of Shiloh representing the plaza as a ritual arena.*

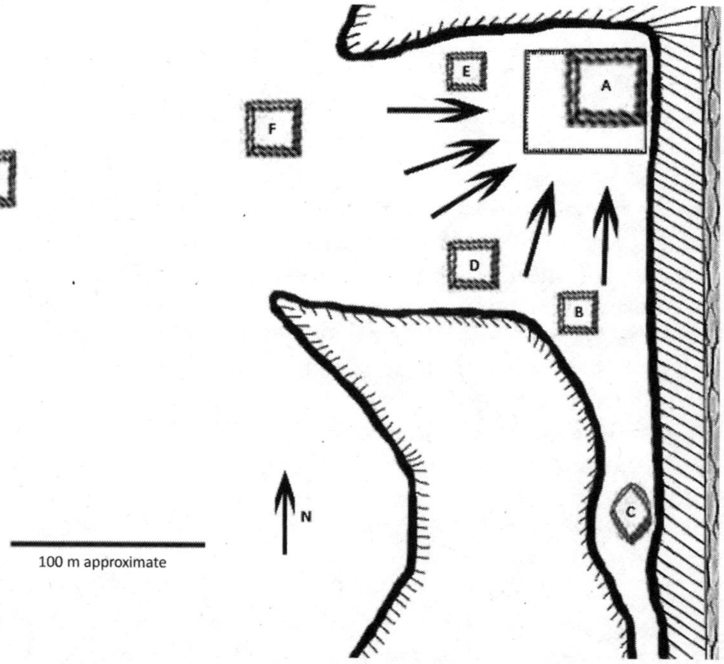


**Figure 4-9.** *Map of Shiloh representing the Mound A–plaza relationship as a ritual hall.*

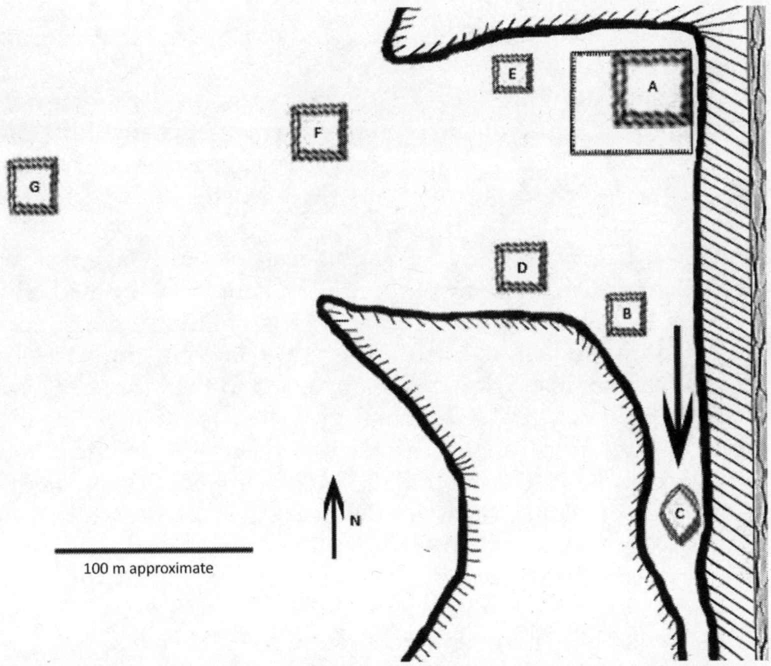


**Figure 4-10.** *Map of Shiloh representing the Mound C area as a restricted ritual hall.*

m wide. The partially restricted approach and the constrained audience area would create a ritual environment strongly constraining to communal or participatory ritual and would act to spatially control the crowd. Such control, combined with the vertical elevation provided by Mound C, would serve to emphasize the power and authority of the performers during mound-related ritual events. The presence of a structure almost immediately north of Mound C, known as House Mound K (Welch 2006:237), would potentially act as a further restriction, maintaining the audience within the zone of monumental perception of the mound. Unfortunately, there is no date for this house, so its relationship to the mound is unknown.

## The Experience of Red and White

This case study of the deployment of color meaning in Mississippian architecture indicates some of the ways Mississippian peoples negotiated meaning in the public sphere. Such an interpretation turns on their heads some of the assumptions about the relationship of mound building to elite power. To reiterate the scenario, Mound A is the largest mound at the site, positioned at the east edge of the plaza (see Figures 4-9 and 4-10). The combination of its large size and central location would traditionally be interpreted to indicate it as the primary locus of elite power at the site. Although it would customarily still be seen as an elite-dominated venue, Mound C is smaller and more peripherally located, leading to the assumption that it is of lesser importance.

Mounds A and C (Figure 4-11) are the best examples of the use of colored sediments at Shiloh. The use of such sediments represents an additional investment of labor and meaning in these mounds. However, each mound represents a distinct use of color, which seems comprehensible when seen as part of the overall design of the site.

Mound C has been shown to be a burial locale at which layers of white clay were used and, thus, carries a body of symbolic meanings associated with White. Mound C is the location of the manipulation and control of burial contexts by elites, supported by the hall-like spatial format, relatively emphasized vertical experience, and spatial restriction of the approach to the mound. This strongly indicates elite control of white sediment and related White meanings, which in turn seems to correspond strongly with the demonstrated historic-ethnographic relation of chiefs and White (Hudson 1976:223, 235). In partial agreement with the historic symbolism of White, the archaeological evidence suggests white is tied to burial, chiefs, elite power, and ancestors and that access to power related to the color white is private or restricted. The evidence presented here indicates that all ceremonies in this locale, both the rituals of use and the rituals of construction, involved elite mediation. This overall relationship of meaning appears to be supported by the inclusion in Mound C of the Shiloh Pipe, a flint-clay figurine probably originating at Cahokia and indicating a claim to alliance or affiliation with elites at Cahokia (Welch 2006:410–411). This pipe and one other object, also found with a burial in Mound C, are the only pieces of highly valued Mississippian display goods recovered from Shiloh, indirectly suggesting that most individuals did not have access to such materials and that only a small number of social elites were able to acquire such items. The pipe may also bear "peace" connotations and White symbolism itself, as per historic peace pipes, although accounts of the Southeast also refer to similar red stone "war pipes" (Swanton 1918:67). Welch's previous tentative interpretation of Shiloh as a symbolically White community is not necessarily contradicted by the interpretation presented here, as our presumptive chiefly burial and elite contexts are all symbolically White (Welch 2006:408–409). However, it is clear that that would be an insufficiently complex examination of the ways color is used at the site.

Mound C is not simply an earthwork. A log chamber tomb with five to six individuals was contained within the center of the mound. This chamber tomb was excavated in antiquity into a low mound of yellowish clay built previous to all other construction but as part of this one major event. Three bodies were discovered during the initial phase of excavation. In addition to the Shiloh Pipe, copper-inlaid shell ornaments, shell beads, and small ornaments of coal and lead were placed with the three bodies (Welch 2006:11–24). Interestingly, although these three bodies appear simply to be flexed burials, one of the original excavators described them as sitting facing the pipe, as if at a social event. The bundled long bones of two or three other individuals were found at one end of the same tomb by later excavators. At least 19 other bodies were identified throughout the mound; they lacked grave goods, were buried at a variety of depths, and were

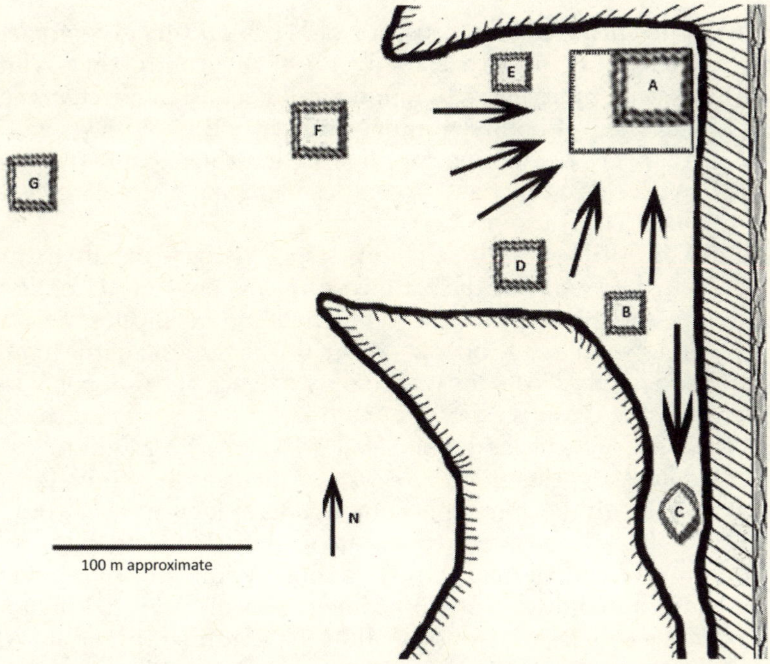


**Figure 4-11.** *Map of Shiloh comparing the two proposed ritual scenarios.*

deposited either during the construction or as intrusive additions later (Welch 2006:32–35). The initial deposit of the log tomb was immediately covered by a white clay cap approximately 1 m high; collectively, this deposit has been previously suggested to represent a single important event to the Shiloh community (Welch 2006:274). The final mound was 3 m tall, but the entire mound appears to have been one episode; in other words, the yellowish surface, the excavation of the low chamber tomb and its construction, the deposit of the five or six individuals and their esoteric goods, the capping with white clay, and the covering of the entire display with 2 m of earth were conducted as one extended event. Other than the presumably communal construction—itself a performative, ritual event—performance or ritual related to this event was evidently conducted for a relatively small audience constrained within the area to the north of Mound C. While the meter-tall white burial mound would have been the powerful focus of audience attention, the final 3-m tall mound memorializing the event would have created the lasting vertical visual effect for the rest of the duration of the Shiloh community.

Turning to Mound A, there appears to have been a greater negotiation of meaning among social groups. While Mound A still seems to have involved the sort of labor commitment and scale that is generally held to have supported elite power, the community was intimately involved in the meanings created. The involvement of Mound A in the arena-like plaza complex also suggests communal involvement in the rituals of use and construction, rather than strictly elite-controlled, elite-mediated ritual behavior. The mound is predominantly red in terms of the sediments used in its construction. These factors in combination suggest that Red meanings involve a lesser degree of elite control than White meanings do. At the same time, the red mound would act as an effective message to outsiders, a statement of both community power and elite power indicating a threat to outsiders. The archaeological evidence indicates that Red symbolism at Shiloh is tied to the community and to conflict, matching historic understandings of Red symbolism (Hudson 1976:234).

Mound A is still poorly understood despite being partially excavated by Frank Roberts in the 1930s and the Southeastern Archaeological Center in recent years. Recent research has allowed for a detailed understanding of the mound's stratigraphy (Sherwood and Kidder 2011), but only a fraction of the mound's surface is understood. Roberts demonstrated the existence of a number of structures on and beneath the apron west of the main body of the mound, but the relationship of these structures and associated artifacts with Mound A is unclear. Available evidence suggests that there were structures atop both construction episodes that make up the apron, but some of this evidence is very fragmentary (Welch 2006:221–222). Excavation records are vague and the methods used in recovery do not meet contemporary expectations. A single burial, lacking grave goods and laid in a shallow pit, also predated the apron's construction. An atypical layer of mussel shells was found within the apron stratigraphy. While this evidence makes for intriguing fodder for speculation, the lack of detailed records and context precludes the information from being incorporated into this discussion in any greater detail.

In the interpretation proposed herein, Shiloh both matches and elucidates our understanding of Southeastern color meaning (Figure 4-12). Charles Hudson and others have noted the many salient structural relationships construed through Red and White symbolism in the historic Southeast (Hudson 1976:234–235; Knight 1986:678; Swanton 1928:197–248; Waring 1968:54). Shiloh provides a possible test for such ideas. While White meanings may very well have had all the meanings recognized historically, at Shiloh, we recognize a limited number of controllable variables. White is associated with the south, burials, and elite power, as shown by the characteristics of visibility and presentation discussed above. This does indicate a potential match, identifying historic chiefs with prehistoric elites and burials of respected ancestors associated with ancient, pure, White wisdom. In a possibly related vein, the Creek and Chickasaw placed symbolically White structures in the south of their communal square ground, and Mound C is in the south of the site. By the same token, both the clear threat to outsiders projected by and the association with foreigners at Mound A could be indications of continuity or renegotiation of shared meanings. The Creek and Chickasaw tended to place the house of the warriors or the house of the foreigners (both symbolically Red) in the east side of the square ground, and Mound A is in the east of the plaza. My argument is not that Shiloh should be interpreted by use of Creek analogy but rather that the archaeological data from Shiloh illustrate a unique architectural interpretation of structural relationships that may have been shared by many groups of the Southeast. Shiloh should ideally be interpreted by reference to itself: This is the way that the people of Shiloh negotiated

| Concepts Associated with Historic Red Symbolism: | Concepts Associated with Historic White Symbolism: |
|---|---|
| War | Peace |
| Disunity | Unity |
| Impurity | Purity |
| Warriors | Chiefs |
| Foreigners | Councils |
| Dangerous | Venerable |
| **Archaeological Associations of Mound A:** | **Archaeological Associations of Mound C:** |
| East Direction | South Direction |
| Outsiders | Venerable Burials |
| Communal | Social Elite |
| Public Ritual | Restricted Ritual |
| Community Center | Community Margin |

**Figure 4-12.** *Contrasting ideas as suggested by ethnohistoric data and tested at Shiloh.*

and experienced public meaning through architectural deployment for their own social and ritual needs.

Although a clear-cut dichotomy of color and ritual has been described here, the actual deployment of color meaning was more complicated. Despite the fact that Mound A is predominantly red colored, and that the final and largest capping episode (relevant to this analysis) was red, for at least one episode during its construction history, Mound A was yellow, gray, or whitish colored, as well as perhaps other colors at times (Sherwood and Kidder 2011). The color of the mound changed through time, perhaps as social conditions merited. Other mounds at the site appear to have been colored as well, including red layers in Mounds E and F and the limited use of white sediments in Mound F (Welch 2006:253, 261–266). This suggests that the control of symbolic media was not consistently in the hands of any one social group or individual and that the meanings intended for expression varied in content in different situations.

As a final aside, our understanding of color is unlikely to match that of the people of Shiloh, who in addition to having potentially radically different color terminology from our norms (Conklin 1955) may have emphasized or experienced marked synesthesia with brightness or shimmer (Saunders 1999) or other sensory phenomena (Houston and Taube 2000). This study is not designed to address a variety of other possible sensory phenomena associated with the mounds, such as the feel of the earth, the scent of the burials or of the tobacco smoked with the Shiloh Pipe, the taste of feasting associated with mound construction, the unique echoes and other acoustic effects created by the architectural form of the site through time, or myriad other research questions. While the salient nature of the color of the mounds begs for interpretation, these other phenomena may have been of great importance as well.

## Conclusion—The Idiosyncrasy of Red and White

Previous research indicated that the use of architectural color symbolism among the Mississippians is a localized phenomenon that cannot be interpreted as simply representing a general trend or matching exactly the historic structural relationships of color among native peoples. Archaeological data nevertheless indicate a long-standing tension between the colors Red and White in much of the Southeast. At Shiloh Mounds, two distinctly colored ritual areas exist, involving idiosyncratic deployment of these two colors. Through a study of the manipulation of space and visual understanding, archaeologists can comprehend the intended meanings contained within the functional structures. At Shiloh, this leads to the conclusion that White and Red color symbolism match some of the known historic meanings among Muskogean groups, while also involving situational and contextual reinterpretation during creation and use. In this, archaeological data must be privileged over ethnographic analogy.

Shiloh is particularly well suited to this sort of analysis. However, I contend that each Mississippian mound center might be similarly examined in order to understand the ways local communities negotiated these broader bodies of shared meaning, such as the tension between Red and White and the mound symbol itself, for their own use.

## Acknowledgments

Many thanks to Jo Day, Paul Welch, Lars Fogelin, John Kelly, T. R. Kidder, Tim Pauketat, Susan Alt, Meghan Buchanan, Anne DiCosola, Robin Beck, Tamira Brennan, and three anonymous reviewers for various forms of guidance, assistance, and comments on versions of this work. Special thanks to David Anderson, John Cornelison, and the Southeast Archaeological Center for the opportunity to work at Shiloh.

## References

Anderson, David G., and John E. Cornelison Jr.
2002 Excavations at Mound A, Shiloh: The 2002 Season. Manuscript on file, Southeast Archaeological Center, Tallahassee, Florida.
Ashmore, Wendy, and A. Bernard Knapp
1999 *Archaeologies of Landscape: Contemporary Perspectives*. Blackwell, Malden, Massachusetts.

Bell, Catherine
1992 *Ritual Theory, Ritual Practice*. Oxford University Press, Oxford.
Berlin, Brent, and Paul Kay
1969 *Basic Color Terms: Their Universality and Evolution*. University of California Press, Berkeley.
Borić, Dušan
2002 Apotropaism and the Temporality of Colours: Colourful Mesolithic-Neolithic Seasons in the Danube Gorges. In *Colouring the Past: The Significance of Colour in Archaeological Research*, edited by Andrew Jones and Gavin MacGregor, pp. 23–44. Berg, New York.
Buikstra, Jane E., Douglas K. Charles, and Gordon F. M. Rakita
1998 *Staging Ritual: Hopewell Ceremonialism at the Mound House Site, Greene County, Illinois*. Kampsville Studies in Archaeology and History, No. 1. Center for American Archaeology, Kampsville, Illinois.
Chapman, John
2002 Colourful Prehistories: The Problem with the Berlin and Kay Colour Paradigm. In *Colouring the Past: The Significance of Colour in Archaeological Research*, edited by Andrew Jones and Gavin MacGregor, pp. 45–72. Berg, New York.
Cobb, Charles R., and Eric Drake
2008 The Colour of Time: Head Pots and Temporal Convergences. *Cambridge Archaeological Journal* 18:85–93.
Conklin, Harold C.
1955 Hanunóo Color Categories. *Southwestern Journal of Anthropology* 11:339–344.
DeBoer, Warren R.
1997 Ceremonial Centres from the Cayapas (Esmeraldas, Ecuador) to Chillicothe (Ohio, USA). *Cambridge Archaeological Journal* 7(2):225–253.
2005 Colors for a North American Past. *World Archaeology* 37:66–91.
Erdogu, Burcin, and Aydin Ulubey
2011 Colour Symbolism in the Prehistoric Architecture of Central Anatolia and Raman Spectroscopic Investigation of Red Ochre in Chalcolithic Çatalhöyük. *Oxford Journal of Archaeology* 30:1–11.
Fogelin, Lars
2003 Ritual and Presentation in Early Buddhist Religious Architecture. *Asian Perspectives* 42:129–154.
Gell, Alfred
1998 *Art and Agency: An Anthropological Theory*. Oxford University Press, Oxford.
Giddens, Anthony
1986 *The Constitution of Society: Outline of the Theory of Structuration*. Polity, Cambridge.
Gosden, Chris
2001 Making Sense: Archaeology and Aesthetics. *World Archaeology* 33:163–167.
Hall, Robert L.
1997 *An Archaeology of the Soul: North American Indian Belief and Ritual*. University of Illinois Press, Urbana.
Hays, David G., Enid Margolis, Raoul Naroll, and Dale Revere Perkins
1972 Color Term Salience. *American Anthropologist* 74:1107–1121.
Houston, Stephen, and Karl Taube
2000 An Archaeology of the Senses: Perception and Cultural Expression in Ancient Mesoamerica. *Cambridge Archaeological Journal* 10:261–294.
Hudson, Charles
1976 *The Southeastern Indians*. University of Tennessee Press, Knoxville.

Inomata, Takeshi, and Lawrence S. Coben (editors)
2006 *Archaeology of Performance: Theaters of Power, Community, and Politics*. Archaeology in Society Series, Altamira, Lanham, Maryland.

Jones, Andrew
2007 *Memory and Material Culture*. Topics in Contemporary Archaeology, Cambridge University Press, New York.

Jones, Andrew, and Gavin MacGregor (editors)
2002 *Colouring the Past: The Significance of Colour in Archaeological Research*. Berg, New York.

Knight, Vernon James, Jr.
1981 Mississippian Ritual. Ph.D. dissertation, Department of Anthropology, University of Florida, Tallahassee.
1986 The Institutional Organization of Mississippian Religion. *American Antiquity* 51:675–687.

Letesson, Quentin, and Klaas Vansteenhuyse
2006 Towards an Archaeology of Perception: 'Looking' at the Minoan Palaces. *Journal of Mediterranean Archaeology* 19:91–119.

Lewis, Barry R., Charles Stout, and Cameron B. Wesson
1998 The Design of Mississippian Towns. In *Mississippian Towns and Sacred Spaces: Searching for an Architectural Grammar*, edited by R. Barry Lewis and Charles Stout, pp. 1–21. University of Alabama Press, Tuscaloosa.

Mainfort, Robert C.
1986 *Pinson Mounds: A Middle Woodland Ceremonial Center*. Research Series No. 7. Division of Archaeology, Tennessee Department of Conservation, Nashville.
1988 Middle Woodland Ceremonialism at Pinson Mounds, Tennessee. *American Antiquity* 53:158–173.

Märtens, Hermann E.
1890 *Optisches Mass für den Städtębau*. Max Cohen und Sohn, Bonn, Germany.

Miller, Daniel (editor)
2005 *Materiality (Politics, History, and Culture)*. Duke University Press, Durham, North Carolina.

Moore, Clarence B.
1915 Aboriginal Sites on Tennessee River. *Journal of the Academy of Natural Sciences of Philadelphia* 16:171–428.

Moore, Jerry D.
1996 *Architecture and Power in the Ancient Andes*. Cambridge University Press, Cambridge.

Morgan, William N.
1999 *Precolumbian Architecture in Eastern North America.* University Press of Florida, Tallahassee.

Pluckhahn, Thomas J.
2003 *Kolomoki: Settlement, Ceremony, and Status in the Deep South, A.D. 350 to 750.* University of Alabama Press, Tuscaloosa.

Pursell, Corin C.
2004 Geographic Distribution and Symbolism of Colored Mound Architecture in the Mississippian Southeast. Master's thesis, Department of Anthropology, Southern Illinois University Carbondale.

Robb, John E.
1998 The Archaeology of Symbols. *Annual Review of Anthropology* 27:329–346.

Saunders, Nicholas

1999 Biographies of Brilliance: Pearls, Transformations of Matter and Being, c. A.D. 1492. *World Archaeology* 31:243–257.

Sherwood, Sarah C., and Tristram R. Kidder

2011 The DaVincis of Dirt: Geoarchaeological Perspectives on Native American Mound Building in the Mississippi River Basin. *Journal of Anthropological Archaeology* 30:69–87.

Stewart, Pamela J., and Andrew Strathern (editors)

2003 *Landscape, Memory, and History: Anthropological Perspectives*. Anthropology, Culture and Society, Pluto, London.

Swanton, John R.

1918 *An Early Account of the Choctaw Indians*. Memoirs of the American Anthropological Association 5:51–72.

1928 *Social Organization and Social Usages of the Indians of the Creek Confederacy*. Forty-second Annual Report for the Years 1924–1925, pp. 279–325. Bureau of American Ethnology, Government Printing Office, Washington, D.C.

Turner, Victor

1967 The Forest of Symbols: Aspects of Ndembu Ritual. Cornell University Press, Ithaca, New York.

Van Dyke, Ruth, and Susan E. Alcock (editors)

2003 *Archaeologies of Memory*. Blackwell, Malden, Massachusetts.

Waring, Antonio J., Jr.

1968 The Southern Cult and Muskhogean Ceremonial. *The Waring Papers: The Collected Papers of Antonio J. Waring, Jr.*, edited by Stephen Williams, pp. 30–69. Papers of the Peabody Museum of American Archaeology and Ethnology, No. 58, Harvard University, Cambridge.

Welch, Paul D.

2006 *Archaeology at Shiloh Indian Mounds, 1899–1999*. University of Alabama Press, Tuscaloosa.

# 5. Maya Palaces as Experiences: Ancient Maya Royal Architecture and Its Influence on Sensory Perception

*Ryan Mongelluzzo*

*Abstract:* This work examines ancient Maya Classic (250–900 C.E.) palaces, with a focus on new evidence recovered from the royal court at Holmul, Guatemala. Ancient Maya palaces were designed and modified as expressions of authority and through nonverbal communication maintained the power and position of the rulers who were anchored inside them. I take a phenomenological approach using a series of spatial analyses and intersite comparisons with the main palace at the site of Tikal, the largest power near Holmul, to deduce how palace morphology affected sensory perception and movement. Uncovering ancient palace spatial systems is an integral part of understanding ancient Maya rulership, Maya tenets of architectural design, and how we as humans experience our built landscapes.

## Architecture, Power, and the Senses

Palaces were the architectural embodiment of royal power. These buildings were not only a potent symbol but they also actively communicated that power in a dialectic with the people within and around their bounds. This communication was enacted through the use of behavioral, conceptual, and emotional cues built into the morphology of the architecture. A palace must give every entrant the realization that they are a member, guest, or trespasser and that they should behave, think, and feel accordingly. This was accomplished by controlling sensory

*Making Senses of the Past: Toward a Sensory Archaeology,* edited by Jo Day. Center for Archaeological Investigations, Occasional Paper No. 40.  ISBN 978-0-8093-3287-8.

perception. The palace would communicate messages like "Look" or "Listen" or "Do not see or hear." Efforts to control sensory perception are *strategies* in the sense advanced by de Certeau (1984:36). In the case of Maya palaces, this strategy would involve the communication and maintenance of power as delimited by place. All the design decisions by ancient Maya rulers that went into the construction of a palace would have comprised a "means of control, and hence of domination, of power," part of LeFebvre's (1991:26) theory of the social production of space.

Individuals are granted differential access in the ability to perceive a space, and Sanders (1990) has shown that concepts from environmental psychology, such as privacy and territoriality, are integral to exploring this phenomenon. Privacy can be defined as the control of unwanted personal interaction and communication (Sanders 1990:50). Key to this is information control. Territoriality is the definition of spaces, each marked for specific uses (Sanders 1990:49). Both privacy and territoriality were fluid in time—depending on occasion, day, and year—and this is at odds with the relatively static nature of architecture. However, at the design level, both of these factors are considered and subsequent uses of the spaces are constrained or facilitated by these design decisions.

## The Classic Maya and Holmul

Holmul is an ancient Maya site in the northeastern Petén of Guatemala. The site possesses features (Figure 5-1) that mark it as a major center, including large temple complexes, a ball court, and numerous stelae (Estrada-Belli 2002; Merwin and Vailliant 1932). Artifacts dating to the Late Preclassic period (250 B.C.E. to 250 C.E.) have been recovered from the lower strata of the site, with evidence for continued occupation through the Terminal Classic (800–900 C.E.) period. Group III at Holmul consists of two adjoining courts, each sitting on its own platform (Figure 5-2). The southeastern court (Court A) has a temple as its central focus, while the northwestern one (Court B), considered to be the palace proper, is centered around a multiroom building that possesses thrones (Figure 5-3). Each of the platforms is ringed by ancillary structures. It appears that Group III was the royal palace at least as early as the Early Classic (400–600 C.E.) period and was so up to and including the Terminal Classic (800–1000 C.E.) (Estrada-Belli and Mongelluzzo 2002; Mongelluzzo and Valle 2006a). The following analyses of the Holmul palace were completed after clearing excavations exposed large portions of the palace morphology, which was then planned and modeled in three dimensions using computer software. Subsequent comparisons to the Central Acropolis of Tikal are drawn solely using plans of that palace.

## Palaces Primer

Of primary importance is the very nature of Classic Maya palaces because their layout dictates a complex and dynamic array of sensory stimuli. I believe three chief concerns shaped the morphology of these palaces. First,

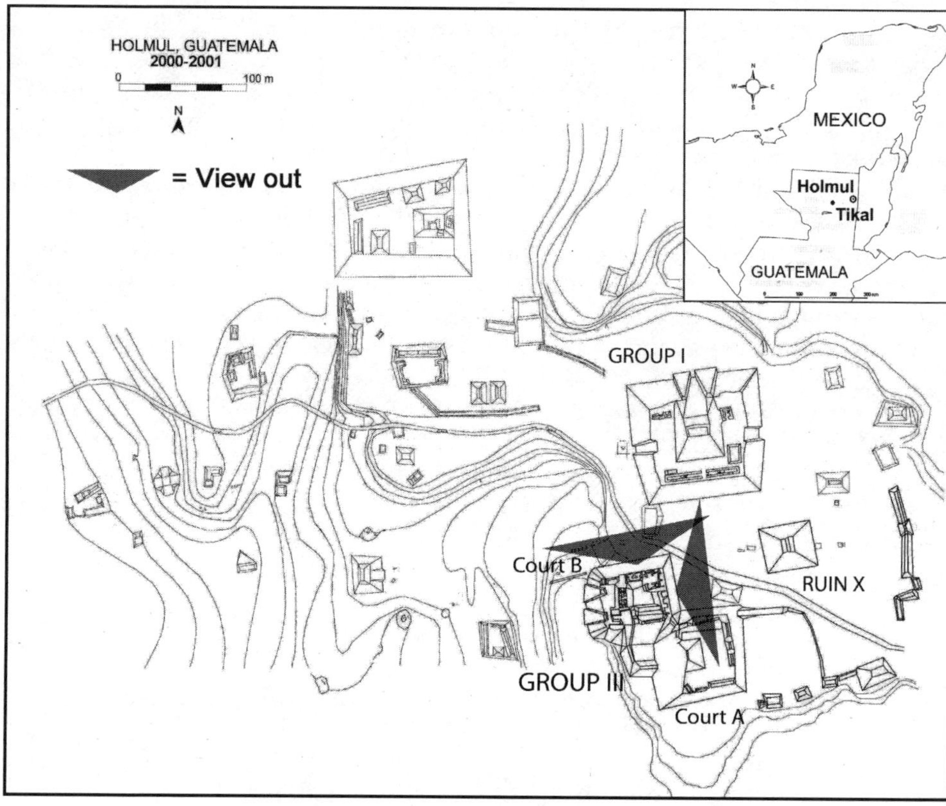


**Figure 5-1.** *Map of the Holmul site core. Views out are noted. Inset is map of the Maya area and indicates the two sites that are the focus of the analysis. Map courtesy of Holmul Archaeological Project.*

as residences, they were larger, more complicated versions of mounded house groups, which are a traditional form to this day. This meant that Maya palaces consisted of multiple structures arranged around open-air courtyards. Second, limits in the knowledge of architectural engineering led to the use of corbeling as the predominant method of raising a stone roof. Because corbel vaults can solidly span only limited distances, rooms were small and narrow. Finally, palaces were often occupied over multiple generations and for hundreds of years, which resulted in morphologically complex palimpsests.

The designers of ancient Maya palaces are unknown today. Unlike written works, which were sometimes signed by the scribe, royal buildings bear no such mark by their designers. While architects as a type of craft specialist were thought to have existed (Houston 1998:530; Karl Taube, personal communication 2010), evidence—other than the circumstantial type, such as the quality and complexity of a design—is scant. The buildings often do bear statements of dedication and patronage, which contain the names of the rulers who commissioned them. Palaces were viewed as materializations of royal power, legitimacy, and authority. Architects were the ones with the artistic, technical, and perhaps religious knowledge to

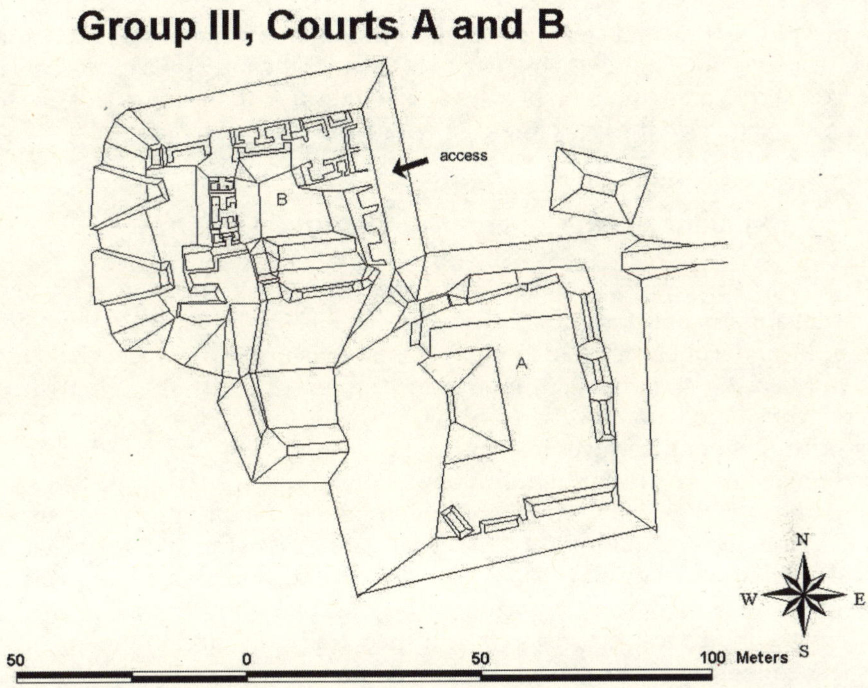


**Figure 5-2.** *Map of Group III, Holmul. Map courtesy of Holmul Archaeological Project.*

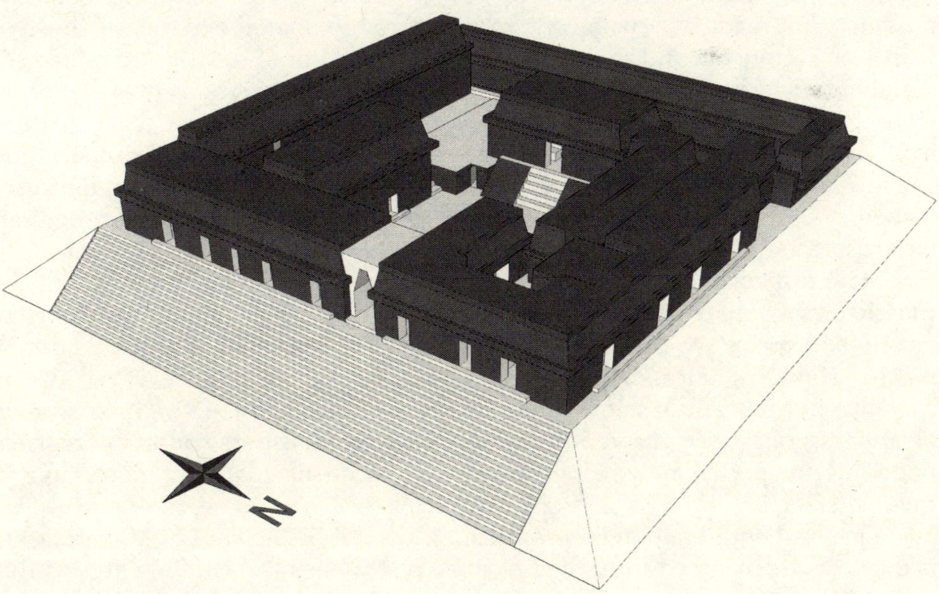


**Figure 5-3.** *Three-dimensional reconstruction of the Holmul palace. Base platform of the palace measures approximately 55 m wide and 5 m high.*

take this philosophy and create buildings, but this was done in conjunction with rulers as it was done under their auspices. Consider the use of the term *designer(s)* here to be a concomitant union of ruler and architect, with the knowledge that the relationship between the two obviously would have been hierarchical.

## Ancient Maya Concepts of Vision and Sound

Most of our understanding of emic concepts of the senses for the ancient Maya, particularly sight and hearing, have been drawn from the fields of epigraphy and iconography. In terms of sight, or vision, two concepts held by the ancient Maya are of particular importance for this work. The first is that viewing was not considered a passive sensory act. "What is crucial here is that the eye is *procreative*. It not only receives images from the outer world, but positively affects and changes that world through the power of sight—in short, it behaves as an 'emanating eye' that establishes communion between internal will and external result" (Houston and Taube 2000:281). That seeing something changed the very nature of what was viewed is a very powerful belief, and architecture was used to facilitate the gaze of some and control the gaze of others.

The second concept of vision is one specifically denoted in the textual records as relating to Maya rulers and is called *–ichnal*. This concept is defined as a perceptual field held by the ruler or deity that extends out in front of him or her and serves to witness and validate what perceived. Interestingly, *–ichnal* was constituted not only by the presence of the ruler but also by the objects and people in view, in particular the other perceivers present, and "served almost as a notarial presence that made actions more concrete through shared experience and participation" (Houston and Taube 2000:289). The concept of *–ichnal* also reified the social hierarchy by granting the ruler privileged spatial positions in the environment. Furthermore, "broad fields, issuing from the view bodies accorded *–ichnal* in Classic Maya rhetoric, impart meanings to architectonic spaces" (Houston and Taube 2000:289). When *–ichnal* was brought to bear in a palace setting, the space gained in significance, but what I demonstrate further here is that these settings were designed to express a sense of *–ichnal* to those present in the spaces.

With respect to hearing and sound, much evidence suggests that among the Classic Maya "there was a strong distinction between mere sound and songs of beauty and praise" (Houston and Taube 2000:276). Preferential consideration of types of sound is indicative of a larger system that categorized everything within a sound environment. While it is impossible to know if the cries of a macaw ever or always grated, the theoretical framework here considers sound as information: This perspective may help us understand acoustic goals and perceptions in royal architecture.

One sequence of sounds of particular interest in the case of Maya palaces is that which emanated from the lips of rulers. It has been credibly argued that rulers may have not always deigned to speak (Houston et al. 2006:229), but when they did, it "consisted not just of empty words but potent emanations, sometimes of an especially fiery nature" (Houston et al. 2006:228). Do not mistake the preceding description as one referring to simple oratorical skill because the "ancient Maya believed that vitalizing forces resided in the breath and other exhalations" (Houston et al. 2006:228). Vocalizations were materialized as speech scrolls on ceramic vessels and tied to the concepts of wind, gas, heat, and fire.

## Sensory Analysis: On the Landscape

Maya palaces were not isolated architectural features existing in a vacuum. In a very real sense, they helped comprise a landscape of social order (Knapp and Ashmore 1999:16). Maya royal palaces were located in civic centers along with public plazas and tall temple pyramids. While not attaining the heights of temples, palaces were quite large in footprint and were of comparable or greater heights than other monumental structures, including ceremonial ball courts. Palaces were linked visually with all other civic-ceremonial architecture and public space in site centers, given their size and proximity to said architecture. All of these structures and spaces had dynamic and real purposes but also were the backdrop for all activities that occurred in and around the city center, serving as a composite reminder to all of the social order.

### *Vision: Nonverbal Communication*

The stucco and plaster facades of ancient Maya monumental architecture were often painted predominantly red (Houston et al. 2009). This color would have contrasted strongly with the natural landscape (see Miller in Houston et al. [2009:72]), while also reducing glare from the formerly white plaster (Schele 1985:37). The color red was sometimes achieved using specular hematite, especially for floors, which resulted in a subtle sparkling effect when viewed. Citing David Stuart, Schele (1985) linked the use of this red exterior paint to a complex of hieroglyphic symbols that represent blood and, by extension, lineage and dynasty. More recently, Houston and colleagues (2009:30) pointed out that the Mayan word for red (*chak*) relates to such concepts as big and great. Obviously, these are symbolic ties that would relate directly to the rhetoric of divine kingship and would have been dominant in the views of palatial architecture. The inside of palaces are depicted using a much wider spectrum and "provided richly colored backdrops for the dazzling colors of personal adornment" (Houston et al. 2009:84) of rulers and courtiers.

Commonly, the facades of Maya palace buildings were covered in stucco sculptural elements (Schele 1998). Most of these were on the roofs or roof combs of palace buildings (roof combs being relatively lightweight vertical additions that made buildings appear taller without adding corresponding mass). These elements would have primarily depicted religious themes of rulers, deities, supernatural creatures, and elements corresponding to the political-religious tales of which they were a part. It is important to note that, in such adornments, rulers invariably linked themselves to these sacred themes in efforts to validate their power.

Portraits of rulers were also common visual elements of palace contexts, a phenomenon linking them to lineage and dynasty as portrayals of past rulers remained on display for generations. Sometimes, these representations were even moved to palace contexts later in their use histories. At Uaxactun, stelae were reerected at the primary entrance of the palace after being removed from other locations. Relating the image of the ruler, and images of past rulers, directly to the palatial architecture had multiple impacts, including reinforcing a justification of authority based on lineage history. It also tied the ruler to the building even when the ruler was not physically present or visible.

### *Sound: Signaling*

Before discussing sound, I caution that I have not discovered direct evidence that the ancient Maya engaged in an advanced science of acoustics. While the effects described in this work are present, they may have been side effects of controlling vision and movement, in a coincidental conjunction of goals. Of course, it is not a great leap to infer that the Maya designed architecture with concepts like privacy and quiet in mind, but there are more complex acoustic phenomena in place and, though unintended, these may have had the power to produce psychological or emotional responses. Nevertheless, this potential lack of intention should not undermine recognition of the presence of these effects and their power.

Ancient Maya palaces were very likely the origin point for sounds signaling where the ruler and palace residents were and what they were doing. Sounds emanating from the palace may have let the immediate population know that the ruler was entering or leaving the palace or, similarly, that the palace was the starting location of a royal procession. Rulers were often depicted with accompanying musicians (K1210, K1453, K1563, K3009, K4120, K5233, K6313, K6984),[1] who could have indicated changes in the ruler's status by playing their instruments. Rulers may have also signaled their own movement in an intriguing way. Taube (2005:32) has demonstrated how wearing jade celts would have augmented rulers' ritual performances as highly polished jadeite "emits high and sharp clinking sounds." There are also examples of these jade celts hanging nearby rulers seated on thrones (K530, K2784, K5456) and affixed to the thrones themselves (Taube 2005:28), suggesting that these celts were worn within the palace walls and that their distinctive clinking would have signaled a ruler on the move (Karl Taube, personal communication 2010).

## Sensory Analysis: Inside/Outside

The small room size of Maya palaces created an intricate and shifting set of stimuli to the senses as an individual moved through the various spaces. While direct room-to-room movement occurred, an exploration of the plans of the Holmul and Tikal palaces shows it almost never occurred through suites of more than three rooms. Therefore, there was constant movement between inside and outside spaces in order to interact with and within palace architecture.

A consistent shift between inside and outside spaces would have resulted in effects on vision, hearing, smell, and cutaneous sensations. During the day, palace rooms would have been lit only by ambient light from doorways and an occasional window. Movement to the outside by an individual would have resulted in his or her physical response to a much brighter environment and the consequent restriction in pupil dilation. In terms of hearing, this movement would have resulted in shifting between closed and open sound environments. Smells would have been more acute indoors and less so outside, although this is dependent, to a degree, on the origin of the odor. Because rooms tended to be darker, they were also cooler than outside. Upon a shift to the outside, an individual's skin would sense heat, both of the type held by the high humidity of the region and from direct contact with sunlight. Occasional breezes would have produced heightened sensation as the skin would be wet with sweat after little time outside. Though the multisensorial effects of movement through palaces are a fascinating set of phenomena, the analysis below focuses primarily on vision and hearing and how these senses were controlled utilizing the inside/outside boundary concept.

### *Vision: Views Out*

Analysis of the viewshed from a palace out across the rest of the city, or "views out," concentrates on spaces where views out from the palace were given wide or significant sightlines, what de Certeau (1984:36) called *panoptic practice*. Palace inhabitants were seemingly granted special purviews that were particularly large and wide in scope. I suggest that these perspectives emanating from the palace were *–ichnal* writ large across the urban landscape.

The north and east sides of the Holmul palace possess rooms that face out and away and, therefore, represent initiating points for a viewshed from the palace (Merwin and Vaillant 1932; Mongelluzzo 2005). The east side, on which sits the main entrance, possesses seven rooms that face out, yielding multiple opportunities to observe potential entrants to the palace from different observation posts (see Figure 5-1). The entrance stairway is capped by a platform that would have also provided a view out. The north side also had at least four outward-facing rooms. Additionally, there is a stair in the northwest corner, adjacent and to the east of Room 25 that led to a platform whose sole purpose may have been to provide a lookout to the north for the suite of rooms tucked away there (Figure 5-4). Views to the north would have looked out onto Group I and the path that led to the site's ball court and eventually Group II, all major civic components of Holmul.

By comparison, the Central Acropolis of Tikal, the palace for this great center, possesses outward-facing buildings on all but its western side. These buildings are predominantly structures with multiple doorways that are parallel to each other and face the same direction. The potential views out are numerous and redundant, creating an almost panoptic scenario (Figure 5-5). The North Acropolis and the adjacent Maler Causeway to the north, the Mendez Causeway to the east, and Temple V and the Palace Reservoir to the south were all clearly observable from the Central Acropolis.

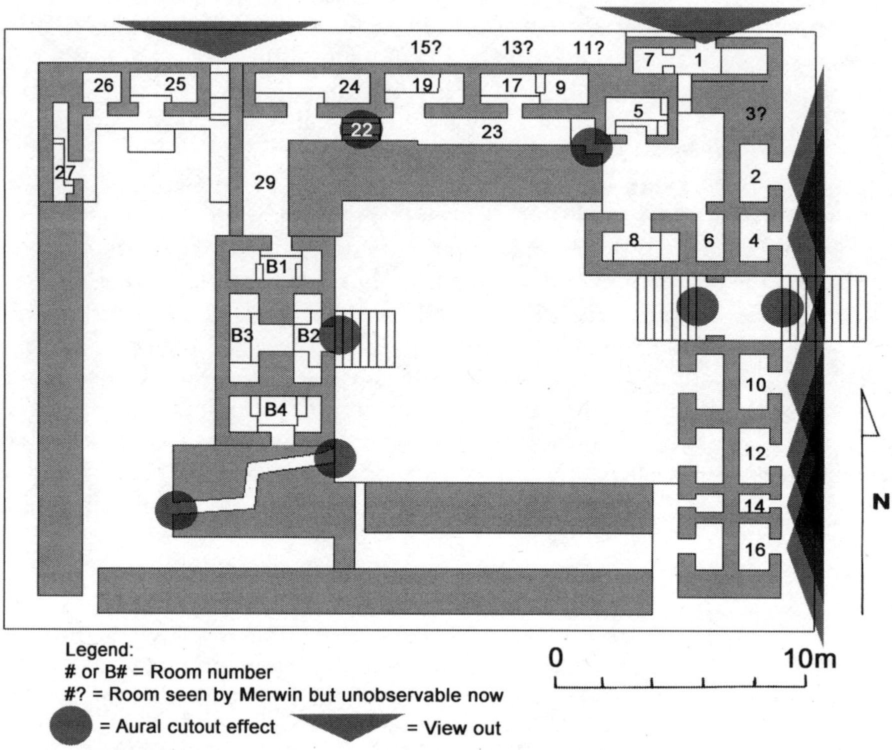


**Figure 5-4.** *Plan view of the Holmul palace. Views out and aural cut out effects are noted.*

### *Vision: Monitoring Outsiders*

Also important is how vision was controlled along major paths of movement in the vicinity of and within the palace. Actors within palace contexts would not have been motionless, and designers would have had to do more than control a single vantage point. The Holmul palace has a steep slope on its western side due to natural topography, which is augmented further by the height of the palace's base platform (over 4.5 m) and subsequent constructions. This slope would have impeded movement to the palace, and potential entrants would have had to approach instead from the east or northwest. The most likely entrance to the palace proper was from the east, and this was also the most direct route. This path would have taken a person by the pyramidal Ruin X and Court A of Group III with its central temple, with the massive Group I looming all the while in the arriver's peripheral vision (see Figure 5-1).

Approaches from the northwest would have brought one by the site's ball court and up to a curious building. During the Classic period, a structure blocked passage between the southwest corner of Group I and the northeast corner of Group III, Court B. It is obscured on the current map because it was effectively cut in half by a modern logging road. When the structure was whole, it may have

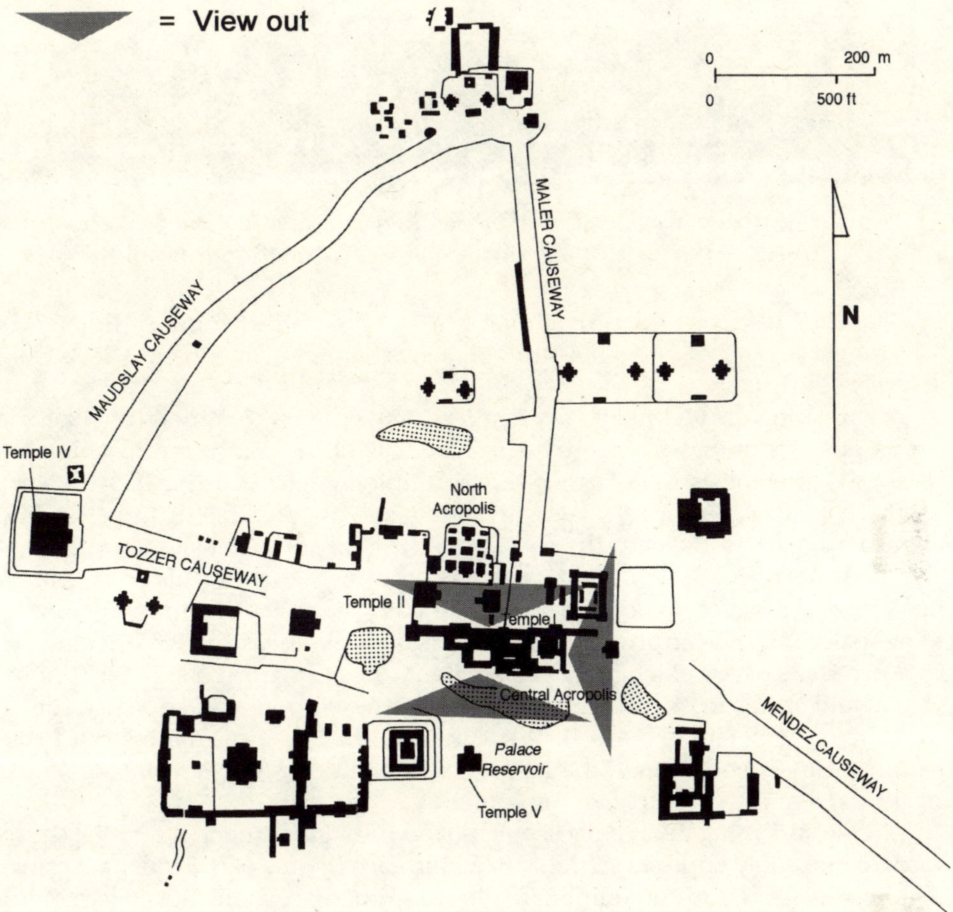


**Figure 5-5.** *Map of the Tikal site core. Views out are noted. Redrawn by Ryan Mongelluzzo after Harrison (1999:Figure 5).*

acted as a cue marking a transition in space and in expectations of appropriate behavior with passage into the site's main plaza. Both approaches are replete with messages that help describe the power of the palace's residents.

Within the Holmul palace, there were few options for movement, all of which were highly restricted and controlled. Entering the palace involved climbing a stair (flanked by outward-facing rooms), crossing westward through an archway, and descending into the main palace courtyard (Figure 5-6). From there, there were at least two choices. Climbing a stair on the opposite side of the courtyard would have led to the palace's throne room. Combined with the previously described architectural features, this stair created a very formal, almost processional, entrance to the palace's throne room from the outside. The pattern just described has been identified by Runggaldier (2009:307) as occurring in other Maya palaces as a formal entrance sequence. Veering to the left at the base of this stair would have led instead to the opening of a Z-shaped tunnel that went back

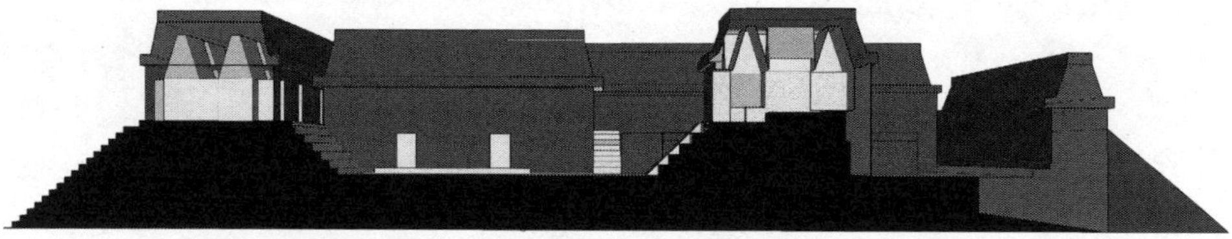

**Figure 5-6.** *Cross section of the south profile of the Holmul palace. Note the east-west path consisting of stairs and floors, demonstrated here in black.*

to what may have been the royal quarters (see Figure 5-4, south of Room B4). This tunnel was narrow and not straight, hence both movement and vision were severely restricted.

Comparing the Holmul palace again with the Central Acropolis of Tikal, the earlier analysis of views out provides some insight into paths approaching the palace. As previously stated, there are multiple views out from the northern, southern, and eastern sides, providing wide vistas of potential visitors. The only approach not viewable is to the west from the Tozzer Causeway originating at Temple IV (see Figure 5-5). Rather than a confusing anomaly, this arrangement may instead indicate something about the path of movement from Temple IV to the palace. The Central Acropolis possesses no obvious western oriented entrance; instead of approaching directly, potential visitors using the Tozzer Causeway would have had to swing up to the Northern Acropolis and approach southward between Temples I and II. What we see, then, is a formal entrance that required movement through the religious and political statements made by the stelae and temples of the North Acropolis.

In the sprawling Tikal palace, one moved through sequences of royal courtyards, conceivably under watchful eyes within each (Figure 5-7). Sequential courts within a palace context are reminiscent of the Ninomaru Goten, or Palace of the Second Compound, in Nijō Castle, Japan, which was built early in the Tokugawa era (1600–1868 C.E.), though this example concerns sequential buildings, not courts. As one progressed from one building to the next, access became more and more restricted in terms of who was allowed entry, finally culminating with the shogun's chamber (Coaldrake 1996:155).

However, Tikal's rulers did not sit within its historically most important and potentially most restricted court, Court 5D-6, the one that contained the "clan house" (Harrison 1999:76) of ruler Toh-Chak-Ich'ak I, who ruled in the fourth century C.E. We know that this ruler's throne structure was preserved almost unchanged for over five hundred years (Schele and Mathews 1998:94) and that new courts and throne structures were constructed for later rulers. When analyzing a plan of the palace, it is evident that there were multiple entrances to this hallowed court. A formal, almost processional, path through the later courts, likely under heavy observation, would be analogous to the Japanese example. Using a less formal, but more direct, path from the east or south would have been physically possible but perhaps only allowed at certain times or for certain personages. As for the later courts, Harrison (2001:91) has identified baffles in the palace that he believes were in place to restrict movement between them.

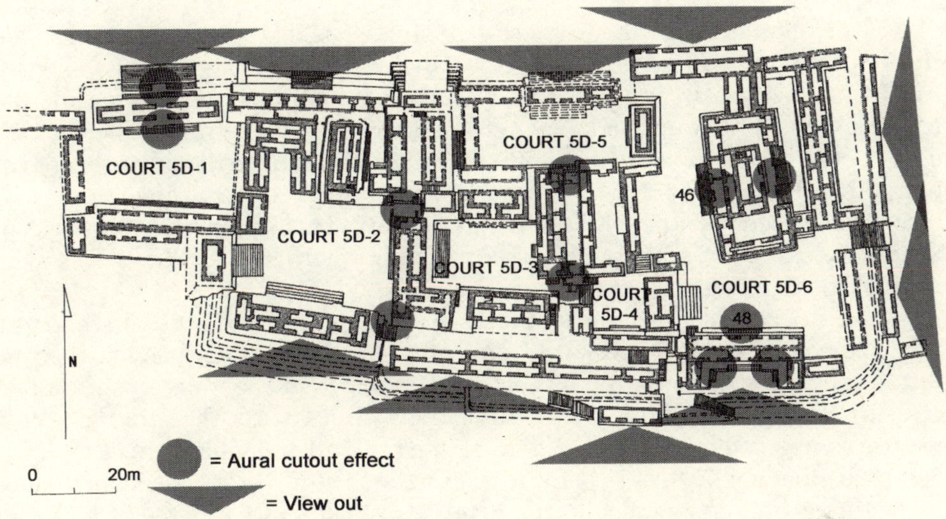


**Figure 5-7.** *Plan view of Tikal's Central Acropolis. Views out and aural cut out effects are noted. Redrawn by Ryan Mongelluzzo after Harrison (1999:Figure 118).*

### *Sound: Cut Outs*

This constant movement from inside to outside spaces caused an acoustical effect known as the *cut out*. This effect is a sudden drop in intensity of sound associated with an abrupt change in the spectral envelope of the sound or a modification of reverberation (Augoyard and Torgue 2006:29). This effect occurs because either the sound or the listener is in motion or because the sound environment is changed. Because of the change in space, the acoustics change, bringing a sound suddenly to the fore or ending it suddenly. Opening a window would produce this effect, as would passing by the open door of a busy nightclub. Cut out effects can mark transitions between spaces; for example, they can occur upon entering a room or crossing a courtyard (Augoyard and Torgue 2006:32). Our bodies are sensitive to the change in sound produced by a cut out. Augoyard and Torgue (2006:35) also argue that it is possible to emphasize the events initially following a cut out. In other words, at that initial change in the sound environment, a person is more aware as he or she tries to understand it.

Because of the nature of ancient Maya elite architectural morphology, a high number of cutouts are present. Outdoor courtyards are as common as, if not more common than, indoor hallways are at linking rooms together. Of course, crossing any indoor/outdoor threshold produces a cut out effect. But the only doorway cut outs noted in this initial study were those that acted as the main entrance to a palace or as entrances to main throne buildings. However, it is of interest to consider what effects people would experience when crossing from inside to outside to inside spaces. Given their locations, cut outs in the Maya palaces studied here served to help communicate differences between adjacent spaces. These differences may have been either functional or symbolic in nature.

The Holmul palace cut outs mostly distinguish what I have termed *transition zones* (Mongelluzzo and Valle 2006b) marking the function or meaning of spaces (see Figure 5-4). An arch creates a pair of cut outs for an individual entering the palace. As the individual proceeds, a turned corner and another arch create cut outs at each end of the northern hallway, Room 23. Perhaps the most severe cut outs, at least in terms of the amount of change produced in the sound environment, are located on either end of the tunnel that leads to the western precinct of the palace. There is another cut out along the northern side, one created by the lookout in the western precinct.

At Tikal, cut out effects are similarly in place at transition zones. In this case, they helped differentiate one court from another and communicate whatever the differences were between them. The main entrance to the palace necessitated crossing through a building, while transitions from Courts 5D-2 through 5D-5 were accompanied by cut outs created by the buildup of architecture (see Figure 5-7). The other cut outs were all produced in or around Court 5D-6: One relates to the throne building, while the others relate to an entrance into the palace from the south.

## Sensory Analysis: Power in Spatial Distances

Many artistic representations of ancient Maya rulers provide insight into how the Maya considered socially hierarchical relationships in a spatial sense. As they do in our society, high, up, and above in a spatial sense signaled authority and power to the Maya. Houston (1998:343) describes this ancient concept of verticality representing social hierarchy by citing the Kimbell Panel, which originally hung on a wall, and its depiction of overlord, lord, and captives at three different levels of height. Two other examples depicted on architecture can be seen in Palenque. One is the Oval Palace Tablet on which the ruler Janaab' Pakal is seen in a dominant position over his mother, who is handing him a crown. Also within the palace, on the western side of House C, six lords captured in 659 C.E. (Martin and Grube 2000:164) are depicted. The key to their representation is that they are at the base of the structure, where they simultaneously act as a symbolic base for power and as literal submissive underlings, depicted offering upward gestures of supplication. There are also many ceramic cylinder vases on which the ruler is depicted in various activities with those lower in the social hierarchy in subordinate spatial positions (Reents-Budet 2001:213).

### *Vision: Dominance*

Having tied power to a vertical spatial hierarchy, it is subsequently possible to see how this spatial dominance was employed in Maya palaces. To someone on the ground outside a Maya palace, the building loomed above, in the dominant position. Entry into every Maya palace required climbing at least a few stairs. The Holmul palace has over 5 m of stairs to climb. Reaching the throne room required climbing an additional stairway, repeating the spatial relationship of vertical dominance, this time between an individual and the locus of the ruler. Visitors to throne rooms, after their initial entry, often took a deferential position, such as sitting or kneeling and, therefore, were spatially lower than the ruler. Again, the *–ichnal* of the ruler comes into play here as "among the Classic Maya, this perceptual field is preferably 'down,' especially as it encompasses lower-ranking persons" (Houston et al. 2006:174).

### *Sound: Stages (Reverse Proxemics)*

Within the Holmul palace, the ruler could have communicated from three seemingly obvious places, which fall into two categories: pronouncement stages and throne rooms. Two of them are what I term *pronouncement stages*: places where the ruler would have spoken to a group of people, perhaps approximating the royal court. This concept echoes recent work by Inomata (2006), who focuses on royal performances that were mass spectacles that both integrated the community and reaffirmed a contested social hierarchy. However, Inomata (2006:203) also acknowledges royal performances on smaller scales, tied to palace architecture and, hence, for smaller audiences. Both of the Holmul pronouncement stages occur at the top of stairs, one looking down into the central inner courtyard of the palace (Figure 5-8) and the other looking down on the area just outside the main entrance of the palace (see Figure 5-3). In the former space, the ruler would have been framed by his throne building and, in the latter, by a stone arch spanning overhead. The third communication stage is the main throne room of the palace. The main throne is flanked by two *L*-shaped benches, which leave a limited amount of floor space and thus allow for fewer visitors and create a more intimate venue.

Inomata and Coben (2006:30) state that "it is essential in the analysis of theatrical space to place the human body as the point of action and sensory perception. We need to see such spaces not only from the position of 'God's eyes' (plan views) but also from those of performers and spectators." Hall (1990) coined the term *proxemics* for distinguishing social interactions that occurred at different spatial distances and he separates these interactions into four separate spatial distances: intimate, personal, social, and public, with each further subdivided into a close and a far phase. The bases of his research include the range of sensory effects and how they change from very close spatial distances to very distant ones. What is of interest here is that with these two types of sound environments, pronouncement stages and throne rooms, the architecture dictates spatial distance. Instead of social interaction regulating spatial distance as Hall observed, in Maya palaces architecture bounds social interaction and determines spatial distance. The pronouncement stages were at the Public Distance–Close Phase of interaction, in which Hall (1990:123) observed that the speaker's voice is loud, word choices are careful, and grammatical and syntactic shifts occur. The audience's visual focus would have been on the speaker's face, while 60° scanning would have filled their visual field with the speaker's whole body (Hall 1990:124).

Maya throne rooms would have caused interactions at the Personal Distance–Far Phase of interaction. These interactions would have been very intense. This distance occurs at about arm's reach, which Hall (1990:120) describes as the limit

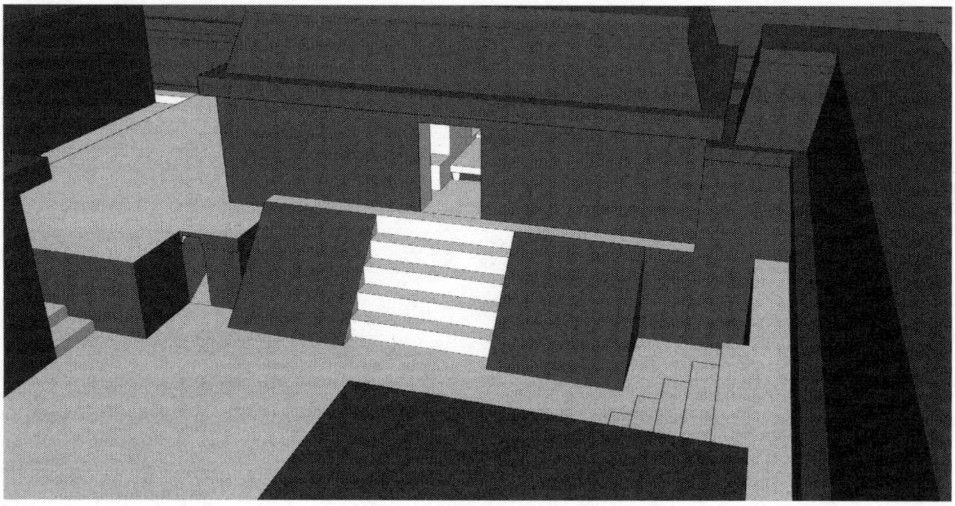

**Figure 5-8.** *Three-dimensional reconstruction of the pronouncement stage at the central inner courtyard of the Holmul palace. Doorway width is 1.6 m and faces out to the east.*

of literal physical domination. In terms of viewing the ruler, fine details—such as dental decoration and small jewelry like labrets—would have been visible. The typical 15° scope of clear vision would have allowed the viewer to concentrate on only the upper or lower face at one time (Hall 1990:120). Through a study of the depiction of gaze between ancient Maya courtly personages on pictorial ceramic vessels, Jackson (2009:74) recognizes the power of these interactions stating, "The privilege of direct or connective gaze not only suggests one element of a codified set of performed behaviors that defines elite identities, and differentiates among ranked elite identities, but also signals the ways in which ordinary actions and nonmaterialized patterns (not directly recoverable through the archaeological record) structured social interaction and marked difference in a lived context." Interestingly, vocalizations that Hall (1990:120) observed at this range were often cross-culturally below what he termed a normal speaking voice. History tells us that on August 5, 695 C.E., the ruler of Tikal, Jasaw Chan K'awil I, led a defeat over the rival city of Calakmul (Martin and Grube 2000:44). The decision to go to war may have been communicated with not much more than a whisper.

## Sensory Analysis: Efforts at Privacy

Sanders (1990:50) argues that physical and psychological opportunities for privacy increase with social complexity. As part of the effort to maintain power, it follows that royals must distinguish themselves from the rest of the community. It is clear that ancient Maya royals accomplished this in many ways: through dress, possessions, depictions in art, and sheer size of their homes, just to name a few. Granting or limiting access to the royals for individuals who were dependent on them was another way to differentiate and maintain social distance; therefore, some activities were private. It is important to note that complete privacy was not the goal. Complete privacy is isolationist and carries with it a bevy of psychological issues, and of course, palaces have public functions as well. Altman and colleagues (1981:115) studied privacy from a dialectical approach, treating it as desirable at some times and not at others. Spatially, this would lead to either spaces oscillating in function or multiple spaces, some private and others not. As will be shown, ancient Maya palaces at least exhibit evidence of the second possibility.

Creating privacy requires two realms of effort. The first is to create spaces of privacy. Obviously, the way these spaces become private is to limit sensory perception of them. Within architecture, this is accomplished by walling in spaces and by putting those spaces "deep" within the architecture. Walling in a space and restricting doorway size are ways to limit perception of subsequent activities within that space. By mandating a long path to a space, and navigation through multiple doorways, the designer ensures that perception is similarly limited.

The second realm of effort occurs after the private spaces are created, as the privacy therein is under constant threat of disruption (Sanders 1990:50). These invasions are not necessarily malicious; something as simple as curiosity can be at the root. In an effort to prevent such incursions, behavioral conventions are developed and then communicated in multiple ways. They become norms in society and are learned in the same fashion. But because of the importance of these conventions, they are also often communicated nonverbally using behavioral cues built into the architecture. Through rules governing access, social knowledge and physical-spatial representation work hand in hand to maintain privacy.

Territoriality is important because it ties activities to physical spaces. Specific private activities are attached to a space by being enacted in that space, and that territory is subsequently demarcated in some way from the space that surrounds it. This separation can serve to emphasize privacy but also to allow opportunities for behavioral cues and other nonverbal communication strategies to express that the space is particularly different. When considering territoriality, it is only in the most general sense that "possession" of space is the main point. Instead, the meaning is expanded and more nuanced so that it covers the associated functions of the spaces as well. In this sense then, a bedroom is a different territory than a hallway is, even though they may adjoin, because they serve different functions. It is from this point that space and privacy quickly become intertwined.

These territorial definitions carry markers for use of the space and for behavior within that space. These markers can be conceptual or physical, verbal or nonverbal. One must be enculturated to identify and understand the markers, though some are the same cross-culturally. Since the spaces under study are palaces, it is important to note that the more public the territory, the more necessary behavioral markers are (Sanders 1990:49). Palaces straddle the line between public and private space, having functions in both realms. It seems that behavioral markers would be even more important owing to the hybrid nature of the building type.

### *Vision: Views In*

Vision must be controlled for privacy to exist. This can be done with fixed features such as walls or semi-fixed ones such as doors and curtains. In this section I look at how much of a palace interior was visible from the outside and how much of a palace it would have been possible to navigate only by prior experience in the space. In other words, I will consider how many spaces within a palace were hidden and how a mental pathway through them was only possible to develop by direct interaction. To qualify, a space needed to be invisible from any entrances on the outside and be a transition zone away from its corresponding courtyard. These parameters ensure that the spaces were not seen from the outside or during cursory visits to outlying areas of the palace.

Also important is how much of a room was visible from outside its doorway. A constricted doorway would hide much of a room from an outside view, with the opposite being true for an open doorway. Instead of trying to figure out what the ancient Maya would have considered a restricted doorway, I look at the amount of the room hidden from view.

Many of the Holmul palace rooms and courtyards were not visible from outside. Aside from out-facing rooms, rooms and spaces not adjacent to the main courtyard were known of only by those people who had regular access to all areas of the palace. More complete excavations might reveal that even for an individual who had been granted access to the main courtyard, more than 50% of the Holmul palace would still have remained unknown and, in this sense, private.

Similarly, Tikal's palace has many rooms that are not visible from outside or from one of the entrances to the palace. The outside rooms on the south side of the palace would have been visible only from Temple V, and even then, it is not clear how visible they would have been given the distance. As the courts are nested, it is not surprising that the innermost ones, Courts 5D-2 and 5D-3, contain the most hidden rooms (see Figure 5-7). What is noteworthy is that visual access to the throne building with the oldest dynastic significance, Structure 5D-46 in the aforementioned Court 5D-6, was not more restricted, with subsequent building programs adding construction west of Structure 5D-46 instead of enveloping it completely from outside view. As later rulers had their thrones within subsequent courtyards to the west, this early structure and its courtyard held great symbolic value in communicating the origins of royal power and justifying its authority. Through time, the ancient Maya rulers of Tikal recognized this and allowed Structure 5D-46 to continue to resonate visually.

### *Sound: Filters*

When considering the relationship of sound to power, it is easiest to think of it in terms of the control of information. Maya royals would want some sounds to go unheard by all but a few, and in terms of privacy, there were some sounds they would not have wanted to hear. Obviously, there were other sounds (e.g., music, song, pronouncements, royal decrees) that the rulers would have wanted to be communicated clearly.

The first element to consider is preventing unwanted sounds outside the palace from being heard inside. Palaces are often in close proximity to the rest of the civic center and therefore would be exposed to two types of elements. One, termed *drone*, is a constant layer of stable pitch with no noticeable variation in intensity (Augoyard and Torgue 2006:40). This sound would be created by the constant activity in any city center, whether ancient or modern. Markets, religious ceremonies, celebrations, construction and repair, and conversations of hundreds or thousands of people at once would have combined for a drone effect.

Far more difficult sound effects to deal with are called *incursions*. These are effects that refer to unexpected sound events that modify the climate of a moment (Augoyard and Torgue 2006:65). Anything occurring unexpectedly in the sound environment would create an incursion. In contemporary Western culture, the ringing of a phone would be the epitome of incursion. In ancient Maya cities, examples of incursions might be the calls of kept birds or the crash after a tumpline broke. The Bonampak murals tell us that music and the cries of tortured captives were also an occasional issue.

Incursions can lead to an effect known as *decontextualization*. Augoyard and Torgue (2006:37) define this term as an incongruous intervention of sounds into an environment of different or unknown expectations. Essentially, these are sounds heard in an environment that do not belong to that environment. Private sounds in a public space or vice versa would both be examples. In terms of privacy, Maya royals would have wanted some sounds they produced not to be heard and would likewise not have wanted some outside sounds to enter the palace. The competing desires arise in conjunction with attempting to communicate power from a space and the architecture constructed there. How palace designers worked to lessen these aversive sound effects will be discussed below.

To ease discussion, I distinguish two types of sound filters: a closed filter attempts to block sound substantially or completely; an obscuring filter has the same goal, but concessions are made to allow some movement of sound through the space. Two almost ubiquitous filters used in Maya palaces are foundational platforms and curtains. The platforms serve to lift the buildings up and create some distance from the plaza level below. Curtains in doorways could have been closed, and depending on the material from which they were made, some degree of sound would have been kept out. Evidence for curtains is the presence of cordholders, which are widespread in Maya palace architecture but not always noted on plans. While neither of these elements is studied in more detail here, their importance in terms of controlling sound should not be underestimated.

There are two clear examples of closed filters in the Holmul palace. The first is a sealed hallway that connects Room 1 to the courtyard of Rooms 5, 6, and 8 (see Figure 5-4). When the hallway was open there would have been no filter from outside the palace into the courtyard because Room 1 possesses doorways on its north and south sides. What is interesting is that the closure is much thicker than is seen with any other door closures observed in the site core of Holmul. The other closed filter separates Room 29, which was actually a courtyard, from the western precinct (see Figure 5-4). In fact, that is the only purpose of the wall, as it is non-load bearing. The preserved height of the wall was well above head height, reaching almost 3 m.

Obscuring filters occur at both the main entrance of the Holmul palace (see Figure 5-4, just south of Room 6) and the entrance to the supposed royal quarters (the aforementioned Z-shaped tunnel). Obscuring filters are coupled with transition zones presumably to help keep the sounds of each place within that space. The transition zone in the main entrance is created by an archway and would have aided in keeping sounds outside the palace from getting in. The last two obscuring filters are walls within rooms that were added well after initial construction. One created Rooms 9 and 17 from a single room, and the other created a small space in Room B1 of the main throne building. This second example was originally the arm of a throne that was subsequently built upward.

The Central Acropolis at Tikal also contains many closed filters. Interestingly, they predominantly comprise the rear or medial walls of a structure. Therefore, these filters would have kept sound out of the central areas of the palace, but rooms near the outer limits probably would have been exposed to outside sound as the filters would not have been entirely effective in their immediate vicinity. Because the primary function of these walls is to be part of buildings, it is hard to know how important their filtering qualities were. The only closed filter that is not a load-bearing wall is located in the southeast corner of the palace in Structure 5D-48 (see Figure 5-7). It was created by sealing an inner doorway that originally had allowed an unimpeded path from outside the palace into Court 5D-6. However, its effects must have been minimal as it is flanked on each side by similar doorways that were not sealed.

Four obscuring sound filters are known in the Central Acropolis at Tikal. Each was created owing to a restriction of space by the construction of walls. An example of this would be a narrow hallway. The aforementioned baffles identified by Harrison (2001:91) as restricting people's movement may also have restricted sound travel, though it is not clear how high the baffles were built. Three of the four obscuring filters are located around Court 5D-3, the innermost and most private of the palace courtyards. Again, these examples demonstrate how access and sound restriction are intertwined for they are created by the same architectural features.

## Conclusions

Ancient Maya palaces must first be considered as part of the greater built urban landscape, within which they were a focal point. Spatial relationships to other buildings were quite meaningful. The symbolism carried on their decorated facades helped convey these meanings as well as communicate information about who resided within the palaces. More direct communications were also likely, as sounds emanating from or occurring within the palaces conveyed information too.

These palaces are marked by outward-facing buildings and rooms, though their functions are not entirely clear. Perhaps they held those who controlled access. What is apparent is that these outward-facing structures created opportunities for surveillance of the surrounding area, especially near palace entrances. All who approached the palaces or interacted near it could have been watched. Another morphological distinction of palaces is that they were broken into precincts, which were separated by transition zones marked by cut out auditory effects. The precincts were likely functionally different and the transition zones signaled these differences.

The most frequent location for interacting with the ruler was designed in a very specific way, which had strong sociospatial implications. Throne rooms were set up so that rulers were seated above their audience but almost within arm's reach. This combination of sensory dominance and intimacy was interwoven into interactions with the ruler. Another possible interaction space, the pronouncement stage would have caused the ruler to shift into an oratorical performance for his audience. Both of these stages offered the ruler a vantage point of visual dominance.

Privacy measures were also present in palaces, although it is difficult to assess the degree of intention behind some of them. Inward-facing courtyards and rooms with spaces not exposed to view by their doorways create controlled visual access to the palaces. Closed and obscuring sound filters occur, the latter more frequently than the former. While it is not evident if they were built specifically to affect sound travel, they were clearly present and had filtering effects.

Palaces were certainly part of the strategy of maintaining royal authority. What is now clear is that palaces accomplished this in much more complex and subtle ways than previously considered. By affecting, influencing, and at times, controlling sensory perception and the production of space, palace architecture served to reinforce the power of the ruler and that ruler's position in the social hierarchy. The visual and aural senses were exposed to behavioral and symbolic cues on multiple fronts. As a palace stood in the city landscape, it was a communicative beacon of royalty and of important information for the ruled social group. The morphological design within palaces necessitated multiple shifts from inside to outside as one moved through them. This phenomenon was orchestrated in multiple social aspects to reaffirm royal authority. Spatial distances, especially vertical ones, between people also became imbued with meaning. Finally, the concept of privacy was used in myriad ways to separate ruler from follower.

## Acknowledgments

I extend my sincerest gratitude to Jo Day for creating such an intriguing conference topic and to those at Southern Illinois University Carbondale, both students and staff, who helped her. I wish to thank IDAEH and the people of Guatemala for the opportunity of and assistance in excavating Holmul. None of the work would have been possible without Francisco Estrada-Belli and the Holmul Archaeological Project. Funding for research and conference travel was provided by the University of California, Riverside. For their tireless eyes and generous feedback with various versions of this manuscript, I would like to thank my advisor, Wendy Ashmore; Karl Taube; Laura Kosakowsky; and Michelle Butler. Last, but not least, I would like to thank Christina Halperin for her help with the various figures presented here.

## Note

1. K numbers refer to the catalog system of rollout photographs of ceramic vessels by Justin Kerr; see www.famsi.org.

## References

Altman, Irwin, Anne Vinsel, and Barbara B. Brown
1981 Dialectic Conceptions in Social Psychology: An Application to Social Penetration and Privacy Regulation. *Advances in Experimental Social Psychology* 14:107–160.
Augoyard, Jean-Francois, and Henry Torgue
2006 *Sonic Experience: A Guide to Everyday Experience*. McGill-Queen's University Press, Montreal.
Coaldrake, William H.
1996 *Architecture and Authority in Japan*. Routledge, New York.
de Certeau, Michel
1984 *The Practice of Everyday Life*. University of California Press, Los Angeles.
Estrada-Belli, Francisco
2002 *Archaeological Investigations at Holmul, Guatemala. Preliminary Report of the 2001 Season.* Submitted to Instituto de Antropología e Historia of Guatemala and the National Geographic Society. Available at http://www.bu.edu/homul/reports/HOLMUL_01_report.pdf.
Estrada-Belli, Francisco, and Ryan Mongelluzzo
2002 Holmul's Royal Seats: Excavations in Structure 43, Group III. Paper presented at the 67th Annual Meeting of the Society for American Archaeology, Denver.
Hall, Edward T.
1990 *The Hidden Dimension*. Anchor, New York.
Harrison, Peter D.
1999 *The Lords of Tikal: Rulers of an Ancient Maya City*. Thames and Hudson, London.
2001 Thrones and Throne Structures in the Central Acropolis at Tikal as an Expression of the Royal Court. In *Data and Case Studies*, edited by Takeshi Inomata and Stephen D. Houston, pp. 74–101. Royal Courts of the Ancient Maya, Vol. 2. Westview, Boulder.
Houston, Stephen D.
1998 Classic Maya Depictions of the Built Environment. In *Function and Meaning in Classic Maya Architecture*, edited by Stephen D. Houston, pp. 333–372. Dumbarton Oaks, Washington D.C.
Houston, Stephen D., Claudia Brittenham, Cassandra Mesick, Alexandre Tokovinine, and Christina Warinner
2009 *Veiled Brightness: A History of Ancient Maya Color*. University of Texas Press, Austin.
Houston, Stephen D., David Stuart, and Karl Taube
2006 *The Memory of Bones: Body, Being, and Experience among the Classic Maya*. University of Texas Press, Austin.

Houston, Stephen D., and Karl Taube
2000 An Archaeology of the Senses: Perception and Cultural Expression in Ancient Mesoamerica. *Cambridge Archaeological Journal* 10:261–294.
Inomata, Takeshi
2006 Politics and Theatricality in Mayan Society. In *Archaeology of Performance: Theaters of Power, Community, and Politics*, edited by Takeshi Inomata and Lawrence S. Coben, pp. 187–222. Alta Mira, New York.
Inomata, Takeshi, and Lawrence S. Coben
2006 Overture: An Invitation to the Archaeological Theater. In *Archaeology of Performance: Theaters of Power, Community, and Politics*, edited by Takeshi Inomata and Lawrence S. Coben, pp. 11–46. Alta Mira, New York.
Jackson, Sarah E.
2009 Imagining Courtly Communities: An Exploration of Classic Maya Experiences of Status and Identity through Painted Ceramic Vessels. *Ancient Mesoamerica* 20:71–85.
Knapp, A. Bernard, and Wendy Ashmore
1999 Archaeological Landscapes: Constructed, Conceptualized, Ideational. In *Archaeologies of Landscape: Contemporary Perspectives*, edited by Wendy Ashmore and A. Bernard Knapp, pp. 1–32. Blackwell, Malden, Massachusetts.
Lefebvre, Henri
1991 *The Production of Space*. Blackwell, Malden, Massachusetts.
Martin, Simon, and Nikolai Grube
2000 *Chronicles of the Maya Kings and Queens: Deciphering the Dynasties of the Ancient Maya*. Thames and Hudson, New York.
Merwin, Raymond Edwin, and George C. Vaillant
1932 *The Ruins of Holmul, Guatemala*. Memoirs of the Peabody Museum of American Archaeology and Ethnology Vol. 3, No. 2. Harvard University Press, Cambridge.
Mongelluzzo, Ryan
2005 Excavaciones en el Grupo III. In *Investigaciones Arquelógicas en la Región de Holmul, Petén, Guatemala. Informe Preliminar de la Temporada 2005*, edited by Francisco Estrada-Belli, pp. 28–43. Department of Anthropology, Vanderbilt University, Nashville.
Mongelluzzo, Ryan, and Judith Valle
2006a Espacio y Función del Palacio, Grupo III-B, Holmul, Petén. In *XIX Simposio de Investigaciones Arqueológicas en Guatemala, 2005*, edited by Juan Pedro Laporte, Barbara Arroyo and Hector E. Mejía, pp. 317–324. Asociación Tikal, Guatemala City.
2006b Ancient Traffic Signals of Holmul? Architectural Markers That Prompt Behavioral Changes. Paper presented at the 71st Annual Meeting of the Society for American Archaeology, San Juan, Puerto Rico.
Reents-Budet, Dorie
2001 Classic Maya Concepts of the Royal Court: An Analysis of Renderings on Pictoral Ceramics. In *Theory, Comparison, and Synthesis*, edited by Takeshi Inomata and Stephen D. Houston, pp. 195–236. Royal Courts of the Ancient Maya, Vol. 1. Westview, Boulder.
Runggaldier, Astrid
2009 Memory and Materiality in Monumental Architecture: Construction and Reuse of a Late Preclassic Maya Palace at San Bartolo, Guatemala. Ph.D. dissertation, Department of Archaeology, Boston University, Boston.
Sanders, Donald
1990 Behavioral Conventions and Archaeology: Methods for the Analysis of Ancient Architecture. In *Domestic Architecture and the Use of Space: An Interdisciplinary Cross-*

*Cultural Study,* edited by Susan Kent, pp. 43–72. Cambridge University Press, New York.

Schele, Linda

1985 Color on Classic Maya Architecture and Monumental Sculpture of the Southern Maya Lowlands. In *Painted Architecture and Polychrome Monumental Sculpture in Mesoamerica,* edited by Elizabeth Hill Boone, pp. 31–50. Dumbarton Oaks, Washington, D.C.

1998 The Iconography of Maya Architectural Facades during the Late Classic Period. In *Function and Meaning in Classic Maya Architecture,* edited by Stephen D. Houston, pp. 479–518. Dumbarton Oaks, Washington, D.C.

Schele, Linda, and Peter Mathews

1998 *The Code of Kings: The Language of Seven Sacred Maya Temples and Tombs.* Simon and Schuster, New York.

Taube, Karl

2005 The Symbolism of Jade in Classic Maya Religion. *Ancient Mesoamerica* 16:23–50.

# 6. Coming to Our Senses at Chavín de Huantar

*Mary Weismantel*

*Abstract:* Study of the sensory interface between bodies, artifacts, and archaeological sites produces new kinds of information that may more closely approximate the lived experience of past actors. This approach may be especially useful in the study of non-Western, precapitalist societies, whose perceptual practices differed from our own. Study of sensory interfaces at the Formative Peruvian site of Chavín de Huantar allows us to recognize the idiosyncratic site plan and "poor visibility" of designs carved on monumental stones as intentional practices on the part of their makers. Parallels between these interfaces point to recursive, intentional practices on the part of the site's builders and to differences between actors at the site.

As an empirical science, archaeology has always relied on the senses. I have seen bioarchaeologists close their eyes while probing a bone with their fingers; an expert on ceramics hold a sherd to her ear to listen to its distinctive "ping"; even a geomorphologist use his taste buds to analyze dirt samples. But few archaeologists consider sensory experience itself to be a valid topic for research, primarily because of concerns about objectivity. This is both a misplaced fear and a missed opportunity.

Asking questions about how humans used their perceptual capacities in the past can open our eyes to new forms of data that have been there all along but have escaped our attention. The scientific method requires researchers to reduce the complexities of the material world to a few measurable data points selected along a single narrow parameter. Unavoidably, this process strips away characteristics that were intrinsic to the object in its original material context and

*Making Senses of the Past: Toward a Sensory Archaeology,* edited by Jo Day. Center for Archaeological Investigations, Occasional Paper No. 40.  ISBN 978-0-8093-3287-8.

meaningful in its original cultural context. Among the information that gets lost in the process, and that might merit investigation, is the perceptual interface between the human body and archaeological sites and artifacts.

Some archaeological studies that espouse a phenomenological approach (e.g., Tilley 1994) have been criticized for ethnocentric and ahistorical assumptions (see, for example, Hall 2000:48–52; Smith 2003:62–63), but careful analysis of the body-artifact interface can be the opposite: a means to partially escape the inherent biases imposed on us by our formal and informal training as modern Western observers (Weismantel 2011). This is especially valuable when the object of study is a premodern, non-Western society, such as can be found in Formative South America.

Empirical science teaches us to think of perception as a series of invariant physiological responses to stimuli; in contrast, phenomenologist Merleau-Ponty explored the complex and multifaceted process that underlies the simple act of "seeing" (1964, 2002), and anthropologists have shown that looking and seeing are learned and culturally variable processes (Berger 1980; Howes 2005; Smith 2007). Human actors intentionally construct objects and buildings to engage our bodily and perceptual capacities in culturally sanctioned ways. These choices are built in to the material record in the way that artifacts and built environments constrain, prevent, or enable specific forms of interaction and perception. Analyzing these aspects of artifacts and site plans can provide valuable information about how members of past societies viewed their social and material worlds and how they acted to change them.

The site of Chavín de Huantar is an especially apt case for an archaeology of the senses. Theatrical elements that play with visitors' sensory perceptions can be found throughout the site (Burger 1992; Lumbreras et al. 1976; Rick 2004) and are a major factor in its continued fame and success as a pilgrimage site since at least 1000 B.C.E.

In this chapter, I confine my analysis to visual information, although I will review some evidence for soundscapes at the site. Analysis is focused on two specific aspects of the site: its carved stone monuments and its architectural plan. Each of these has been the subject of extensive study, but the primary tools of analysis—the line drawing and the map, respectively—direct our attention away from the phenomenology of seeing. A focus on the body-site and body-monument interfaces at Chavín can return our attention to neglected aspects of the physical evidence and integrate disparate lines of research. It can also provide information about the divergent experiences of different groups of actors at the site, a topic that is very briefly discussed at the end of this chapter. Each of these topics merits full-length consideration on its own; here, I provide only an outline in order to demonstrate what a sensory archaeology can accomplish.

## Archaeology at Chavín de Huantar

The site of Chavín de Huantar is located in the north-central Andes of Peru, at an altitude of 3,150 m asl (Figure 6-1). The chronology of the site is currently the topic of debate (Burger and Salazar 2008; Rick 2008; Rodriguez Kembel

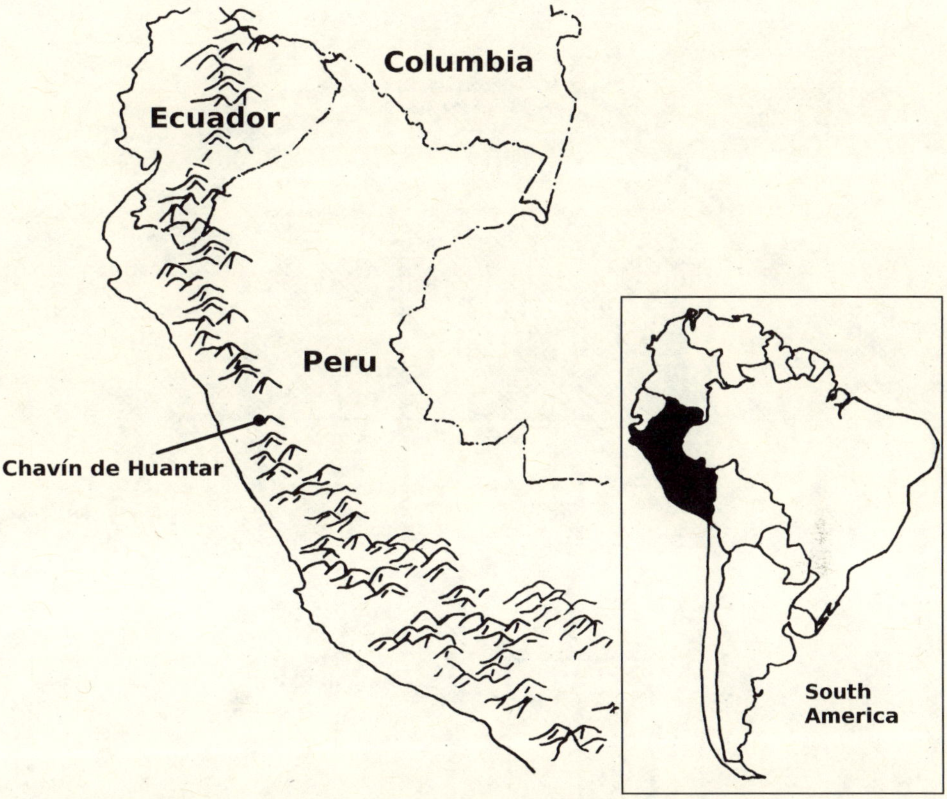


**Figure 6-1.** *Location of the site of Chavín de Huantar, Peru.*

2008), but Chavín was unquestionably thriving between 1000 B.C.E. and 500 B.C.E. Its major occupation is several centuries longer than that and falls primarily within the Early Horizon (900–200 B.C.E.), with significant occupation reaching back into the preceding Initial period (1800–900 B.C.E.).

The temple complex sits at the junction of two rivers and comprises stone-faced buildings, plazas, terraces, and staircases grouped into two contiguous *U*-shaped clusters: a smaller northern cluster surrounding a sunken circular courtyard and a larger area to the south that includes two rectangular plazas, one larger and one smaller (Figure 6-2). The entire complex is approximately .5 h in size (Rick 2008:17); the smaller cluster, which has received the most archaeological attention, is 123 m × 73 m, with a total construction volume of roughly 100,000 $m^3$ (Lumbreras 1977:2–3; Moore 1996:52). This complex is large for the highlands but quite small compared to earlier and contemporaneous sites on Peru's northern and central coasts. The site of Sechín Alto (2100–1000 B.C.E.) on Peru's north-central coast, for example, is so big that the entire temple complex at Chavín would fit easily inside any of its multiple plazas. The principal mound there has a base of 300 m × 250 m, rises 44 m above the ground, and is estimated to contain some 2,000,000 $m^2$ of building material (Pozorski and Pozorski 2002). At the time of its construction, it was the largest structure in the New World.

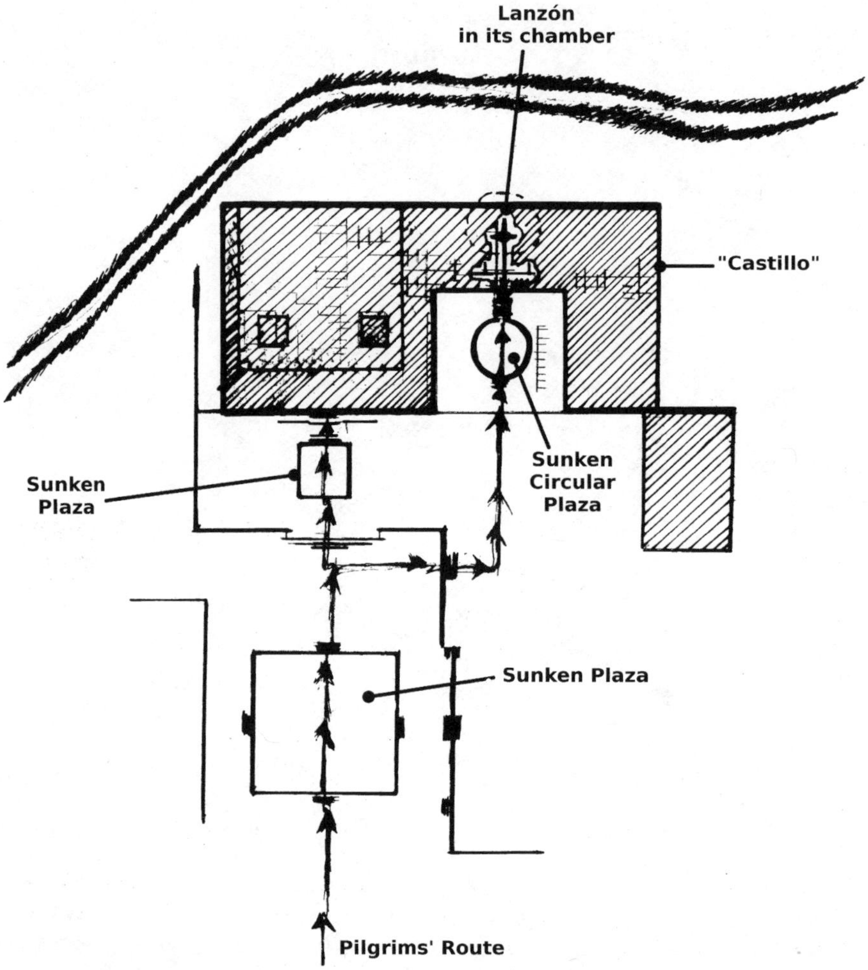


**Figure 6-2.** *Sketch plan of the site of Chavín de Huantar. (Drawing by Mary Weismantel after Burger [1992:Figure 120] and Rodriguez Kembel [2008:Figure 2.8].)*

Nevertheless, Chavín is the most famous Formative period site in Peru and has been since colonial times. One source of renown is its monumental stone carvings, executed in a distinctive style and bearing extraordinarily complex designs. A few of these remain in situ, but many were removed from their original settings long ago. Chavín is also known popularly in Peru for a network of passageways and chambers, referred to as galleries or *galerías,* that undergird parts of the complex (Silverman 1999). The walls of the largest building reach 12–14 m above ground, but the underground features extend vertically another 2–6 m below ground and extend horizontally in places beyond the limits of the aboveground architecture (Contreras and Keefer 2009; Lumbreras 1977:2–3, cited in Moore 1996:51; Rick 2008:17).

Excavations have recovered very little in the way of ordinary debris dating to the main periods of occupation, a fact that testifies to the sacred nature of the temple complex. During the site's apogee, the residential quarters were located across the river, away from the sacred temple area. The few artifacts from this period found in the temple precinct are noteworthy. Luis Lumbreras excavated an underground chamber full of fine ceramics, which he interpreted as offerings brought by pilgrims (Burger 1992:138–139; Lumbreras 1977); a second chamber excavated by John Rick in 2001 revealed a cache of incised conch (*Strombus*) shell trumpets with wear marks indicating many years of use as musical instruments (Rick 2004).

Archaeological evidence suggests that the temple fell into disrepair in the last few centuries of the first millennium B.C.E., but by the seventeenth century C.E., it had once again become a major religious pilgrimage site, described by Antonio Vasquez de Espinoza in 1616 as "one of the most famous of the heathen sanctuaries, like Rome or Jerusalem with us," a place that drew pilgrims "from all over the kingdom" of Peru (1968:491 [1620]; cited in Moore 1996:126). In the five centuries since then, Chavín has attracted a different kind of pilgrim. Throughout the colonial and national periods, artists, writers, explorers, and scientists made the difficult trek to the site and wrote glowing reports about the monumental stone art. The early republic of Peru celebrated Chavín as evidence that Peruvian civilization predated Spanish imperialism, and the site and its monuments continue to be important national icons for modern Peru (Cummins 2008), as well as attracting a small but steady flow of international tourists despite its rather inaccessible location.

### *Previous Research*

Chavín de Huantar was first excavated in 1919 by Julio C. Tello, a foundational figure in Peruvian archaeology. Intensive study of the site continued throughout the twentieth century, and many important figures in Andean studies have either worked at or written about it, including Tello, Wendell C. Bennett, Luis Lumbreras, Donald Lathrap, John Rowe, and Richard Burger. (For a brief overview of archaeological work at Chavín, see Contreras 2010:1–3. The best introduction to the site, and to Formative South America in general, remains Burger 1992; for an excellent recent edited volume on the site, see Conklin and Quilter 2008.) Since 1995, Stanford archaeologist John Rick and his students and colleagues have conducted annual excavations at the site, which is now a UNESCO World Heritage Site.

Two topics have been of long-standing interest in Chavín studies. One is the site plan, which is oddly asymmetrical and incorporates elements that appear to be borrowed from the monumental architecture of other regions, notably the north and north-central coasts of Peru. A second topic of intensive study is the massive stone carvings associated with the site, which feature complex iconography involving hybrid human-animal figures and costumed humans holding ritual paraphernalia. In the study of both architecture and art, much attention has been given to questions of chronology, which I will not address here. The phenomenological aspects of the site have often been commented on but have not been the topic of systematic theoretical discussion.

Evidence for Sensory Phenomena

As mentioned above, Chavín is known for its capacity to cause unusual sensory experiences. The windowless galleries, with their dead ends, right-angle turns, and sudden changes in floor height, seem designed to disorient and mystify (Figure 6-3). When the temple was fully functional, this dramatic spatial context must have intensified the effect of visual and auditory experiences, such as the sight of a costumed figure or the sound of a chanting voice. The small size of these chambers indicates that entrance was highly restricted; reminiscence, rumor, and reputation may have been important means for extending the impact of these sensory effects beyond those who directly experienced them.

Rick (2008) has made extensive efforts to recover the original soundscapes within the galleries and elsewhere on the site; his re-creations of the effect of the conch shell trumpets played within the galleries demonstrate that the volume and intensity of the sound echoing off the stone walls and reverberating down the corridors are truly awe inspiring. Even outdoors, they produce a high-volume cacophony.[1] A plausible explanation for the trumpets' findspot is that they were stored in the underground chamber where they were discovered; ritual practitioners could retrieve them and begin playing in procession through the galleries before emerging above ground; a possible ethnographic analogy is twentieth-century Pueblo ceremonies that began with chanting and drumming in the kiva (Ferguson 1931; Parsons 1923). Or, like the sacred musical instruments played within an Amazonian men's house, they might never have been seen by noninitiates but only heard (Gregor and Tuzin 2001; Hugh-Jones 1988; Murphy and Murphy 2004 [1985]).

Even without the help of human actors playing instruments, internal features built in to the galleries produce unexpected sensory impressions. An elaborate system of ducts, shafts, and apertures introduces fresh air into the galleries and channels humidity out of them; however, they are overengineered for this purpose, suggesting that they were constructed to serve other ends as well (Rick 2004). The ducts convey sounds produced in one chamber into other chambers, producing an unnerving impression of voices and whispers in an empty room. Luis Lumbreras suggested that some hidden channels might be responsible for the extraordinary roaring sounds still audible within the underground galleries when rain falls on the ground outside (Burger 1992:143; Lumbreras et al. 1976). Rick (2008) postulates that polished hematite mirrors found at the site may have been used to refract light into the galleries through the shafts. This would have produced an extremely eerie, seemingly inexplicable visual effect not unlike the character of the auditory effects.

One other intriguing piece of information about sensory perception at the site is evidence for the ingestion of psychotropic drugs (Roe 2008:181–182; Torres 2008). Carved ashlar blocks show costumed figures in procession carrying enormous San Pedro cacti; artifact inventories include paraphernalia for grinding and ingesting snuff (Burger 1992:157–159; Torres 2008:245–255.). Ethnographic,

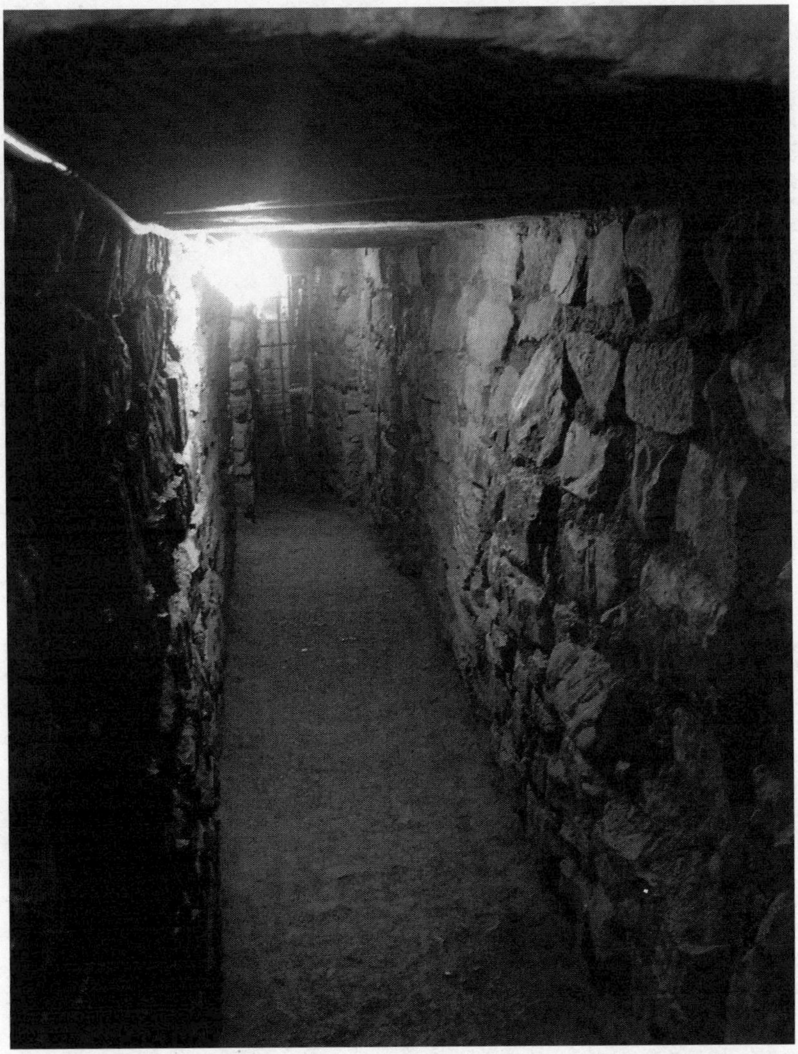

**Figure 6-3.** *Underground gallery at Chavín de Huantar. (Photograph © Mary Weismantel.)*

historic, and archaeological evidence establish these as part of a well-established South American cultural complex of psychotropic drug taking in religious contexts (Cordy-Collins 1977, 1980; Sharon 2000). Abundant imagery of jaguars and of hybrid figures incorporating human, feline, avian, and crocodilian ("cayman") features has been interpreted as depicting the transformations undergone by shamans under the influence of hallucinogens (Burger 1992:157–159; Cordy-Collins 1980:86–87; Torres 2008:245). Producing the desired human-artifact interface, then, was a two-sided project: It involved the engineering of galleries but also the temporary chemical manipulation of the human body in order to alter and intensify sensory perception.

While evidence for these sensory effects is fragmentary, some aspects are amenable to analysis. In the sections below, I will (1) describe specific aspects of the sensory interfaces with the human body created by Chavín's carved stone monuments and built environment; (2) argue that these two kinds of sensory interfaces create parallel kinds of experience, which relate to the site's function as a pilgrimage destination; and (3) suggest that studying the differing sensory interactions of various actors with these artifacts and buildings at the site would be a fruitful direction for further research.

## The Sensory Interface: Rematerializing Chavín

Standard archaeological practice makes use of a variety of technologies that enhance our ability to view an object in the way we want: in its totality, in one glimpse, with every detail clearly visible. For us, this kind of looking is "natural." We do not pause to reflect on the cultural history that produced our epistemological devotion to sensory perception that is impersonal and replicable (Howes 2005) and that led to the development of supporting technologies: microscopes, telescopes, and cameras, as well as specific kinds of drawing and drafting practices, including those that produce maps, plans, scale models, and scientific illustrations.

In other cultural contexts, such as the non-Western, premodern sacred space of Chavín, other kinds of perceptual practices may have been valued. If so, key artifacts should manifest physical characteristics that produce the desired forms of looking, just as our scientific implements and practices do. However, the tools used in archaeological research may unintentionally render the original perceptual interface invisible. This has often been the case with the monumental carvings and architectural site plan at Chavín.

### *Carved Stone Monuments*

The line drawing is an indispensable tool for iconographic analysis—precisely because it produces a very different viewing experience than actually looking at a monolith (Figure 6-4). Modern viewers confronted with one of Chavín's great stones, such as the Obelisk Tello, Black and White or Falcon Portal, Lanzón, or Raimondi Stela, struggle to see the carved designs. From Ayre's 1961 article in *American Antiquity* to John Rick in 2008, researchers have complained of "poor visibility," and have worked to overcome the problem through a variety of techniques, including artificial lighting, rollouts, rubbings, and other means (Figure 6-5).

These strategies enable technicians to produce accurate line drawings and to reproduce these drawings at a scale that is inexpensive to manufacture and comfortable for a human being to examine from a seated position (the size of a standard academic journal or book). They also allow researchers, students, and interested amateurs who cannot travel to Peru access to these works of art and their enigmatic designs. But now that we have solved the problem, we can pause to consider why it exists.

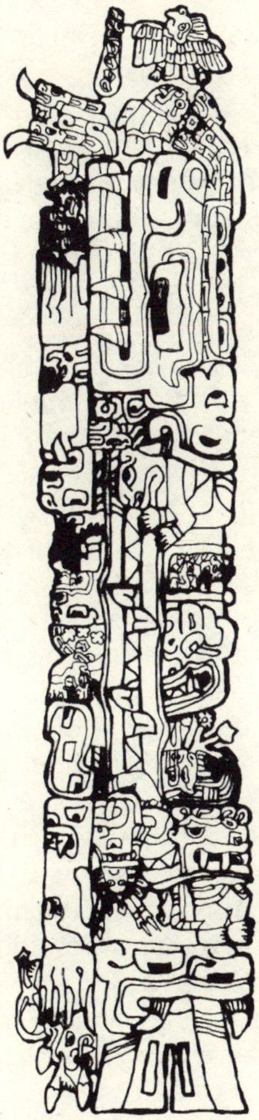

**Figure 6-4.** *Line drawing of the "male cayman" on the Obelisk Tello. (Drawing by Mary Weismantel after Roe [2008:Figure 7.1(b)].)*

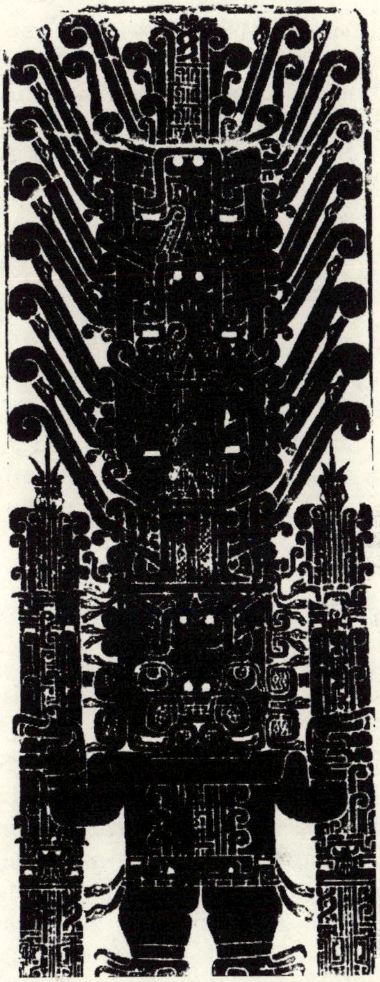

**Figure 6-5.** *Rubbing of the Raimondi Stela (Ayres 1961:Figure 16).*

The phrase *poor visibility* describes the physical experience of looking at these monuments with the naked eye. This experience does not result from any modern damage or deterioration; it is part of the original human-artifact interaction. This makes it a meaningful physical characteristic of the artifact that can be analyzed to recover information about how prehistoric viewers interacted with the carved stones (Weismantel 2011).

Among the key physical characteristics of the original three-dimensional object that are not reproduced in a two-dimensional line drawing are the following: scale, style of execution, material, shape, and placement. These characteristics work in concert to produce the particular kind of visibility that is so markedly typical of Chavín carved stone. Specifically, Chavín stones have a large scale (typically between 2 and 2.5 m in height); a style of carving that involves shallow, uniform incisions without modeling; very hard surfaces that are highly polished; two-sided symmetrical designs that wrap around three- or four-sided stelae or cylindrical columns; and placement that prevents immediate, full visibility.

If we consider the interaction of these characteristics with the human body, the following facts are evident: Many of the stones are taller than the human body by as much as 50%, so a significant amount of the carved design cannot be seen by a person standing in front of the stone; the shallow, uniform incisions and hard, highly reflective surfaces of the stone render the images almost invisible to the naked eye, no matter how well lit the stone is[2]; a two-sided image wrapped around a four-sided stone cannot be seen in its entirety by a stationary individual and is difficult to piece together even when walking around the stone to look at it from all sides. These limitations are recursive: If the style and material were different, the images would be visible despite their large size; if the scale were small and intimate, the images would be visible in their entirety despite the style of execution and material.

The two monuments that are still in situ offer further viewing challenges. Because of its placement within an extremely small chamber, seeing the design on the Lanzón requires some effort and cannot be accomplished all at once (Figure 6-6). What is possible is a series of partial glimpses from different angles, obtained by moving physically around the stone with some difficulty within the tight space (Cummins 2008). The twin pillars of the Black and White Portal, which are on the exterior of the temple, are more accessible—but because they are placed immediately adjacent to a framing wall, portions of the designs carved on them are completely inaccessible (Figure 6-7). Finally, the designs carved on ashlar blocks originally mounted on the building's exterior would have been 2–8 m above ground, a height that would have rendered their designs completely illegible, although it would have been possible to see that *something* was carved on them.

In sum, the designs carved onto worked stones at Chavín were not visible to their original audiences without considerable effort and, even then, only incompletely. The recursive, mutually reinforcing decisions made in executing these designs suggest that, rather than a failed or "poor" attempt at visibility, this was an intentional strategy on the part of their makers.[3] Instead of the immediate, synchronic, totalizing vision that is the goal of Western scientific illustration, the artists or artisans who carved and placed these stones manufactured a partial and fragmentary kind of vision and a slower viewing process, in which a partial or total image is gradually pieced together through a series of discoveries. Possible reasons for this viewing process are discussed below.

### *Site Plan*

The primary tool for analyzing the built environment at Chavín is the map or plan. This, too, is a familiar, indispensable tool for examining spatial data—yet it is an abstraction that differs from the actual site in every physical characteristic. A map may be "accurate," but it still produces a kind of "looking

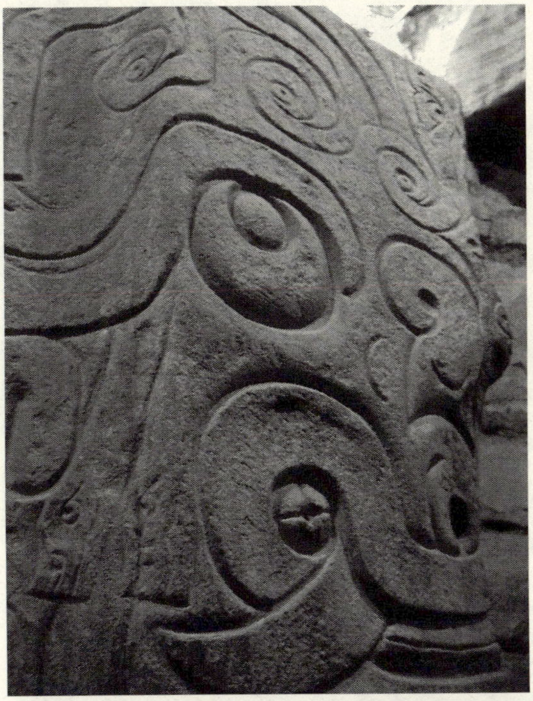

**Figure 6-6.** *The Lanzón. (Photograph © Mary Weismantel.)*

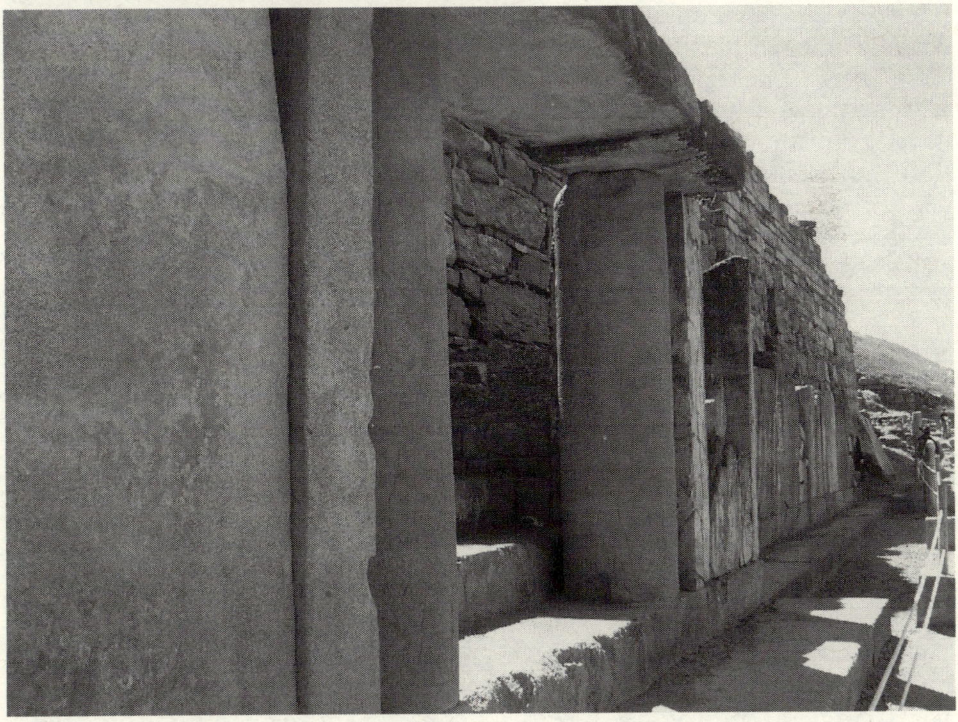

**Figure 6-7.** *The Black and White Portal. (Photograph © Mary Weismantel.)*

at Chavín" that differs greatly from any visual experience that could actually be had at the site.

One obvious difference is in perspective. The plan takes a bird's-eye view, which is ideal for allowing a researcher to see the entire site at a glance. Ancient people, too, often "looked" at site plans in this way: They thought of sacred space in abstract terms and built their temples, monuments, and other places of worship in cosmographic shapes or other ideal forms. However, even after construction they only "saw" these designs in recognizable perspective in their mind's eye.

Conventional maps and plans cannot reproduce the experience of the body on the ground moving toward and within a built environment (although innovations in visualization techniques are changing these limitations). Thinking about this kind of perceptual interface may contribute to two discussions about Chavín: debates about the influence of site designs from other regions and attempts to interpret its curiously asymmetrical plan. The builders of Chavín copied elements from elsewhere to create a novel, composite plan (Burger 1992; Burger and Salazar 2008); as they did so, they also constructed a particular visual interface. Analysis of this interface allows us to get a better sense, not only of how the site looked, but also of how it worked; in addition, this may allow us to better see the builders of the highland site as intentional actors working to create a particular kind of built environment to suit specific social and ideological needs.

In this call to consider the phenomenological effect of a site on the human body, I am of course following a common thread in recent archaeological studies of landscape (e.g., Ashmore and Knapp 1999; Hall 2000; Rodning 2009; Smith 2003; Tilley 1994). Developments in fields such as geographic information system (GIS) technology and a burst of new work by cultural geographers have introduced a human-scaled perspective into studies of built environments and introduced archaeologists to concepts such as the isovist and the vision field (Llobera 2007). Archaeologist Jerry D. Moore has applied some of these approaches to South American sites (1996, 2005); I rely on his insights here.

## Chavín as Processional

Chavín is located in the highlands, but its architecture makes formal reference to the western littoral zone, while the art makes iconographic reference to the eastern tropical lowlands. This obvious evidence of influence from elsewhere raises temporal and political issues far outside the scope of this chapter. Here, I only want to suggest that, in addition to formal elements, it may be worthwhile to consider the experiential aspects of the built environment when comparing sites. This might help us think about not only *what* was borrowed, and *when*, but also *why*.

Moore observes that some sites, such as the coastal sister sites of Sechín Alto and Las Haldas, have a "processional" structure.[4] He points out that the most impressive aspect of Sechín Alto from the ground is not the enormous pyramid[5] but rather the 1,400-m long succession of four plazas flanked by long, low mounds, which creates a long axis that draws visitors along it in a slow, processional movement toward the pyramid at the end (1996:110–111).

The concept of a processional site plan is extremely useful for thinking about a religious site like Chavín, and so too is the comparison to Sechín Alto. Both sites feature sunken circular plazas, a diagnostic feature of sites on the north-central coast that was apparently copied at Chavín (Lumbreras 1977). The southern axis of Chavín's ceremonial center is somewhat reminiscent of Sechín Alto, although on a vastly smaller scale. Phenomenologically, both sites have a processional structure, but the differences between them are also significant.

At Sechín Alto, the long central axis produces a human interaction with the built environment that is fragmentary and slow. Worshippers are led through courtyards of different levels connected by staircases, which require them to move up and down into different kinds of spaces as they approach the central pyramid. This vertical movement breaks up the journey into intermediary stages and fosters a focus on the process as well as on the end point. At Las Haldas, the central pyramid is literally invisible at many points along the journey toward it; at other points, it looks far more insignificant than it actually is (Moore 1996:110).

The kinesthetic experience of Chavín de Huantar is very similar. The dual northern and southern axes draw visitors from the periphery toward the interior in a steady north-south progression, but this horizontal progress is broken by alternating vertical surfaces (stairways, sunken plazas, platforms, and finally the gallery floors) that slow movement, change the spatial experience, and restrict visual access to parts of the site.

The visual experience of the highland temple, however, is strikingly different from that of massive sites on the coast, like Sechín Alto. Coastal sites demand that you stand in front of an enormous edifice and be overwhelmed with its magnificence and might. Chavín, in contrast, hides its wonders. The ultimate goal, the small chamber enclosing the Lanzón, is invisible even from a short distance away. The path to it is hidden from the main southern axis, which leads toward the temple; getting to it requires leaving this axis by a side staircase that provides access to the smaller northern axis. This less visible pathway takes visitors on an even more extreme kinesthetic journey down into, and then up out of, the sunken circular courtyard and into the buried galleries.

Another key difference between the two sites concerns symmetry: Unlike the rigid symmetry of the coastal processional, Chavín's asymmetrical plan draws pilgrims into a series of enclosing, interrupted visual experiences that are orderly, but unpredictable.

### Asymmetry and Unpredictability

The asymmetry of Chavín's site plan, with its two contiguous, dissimilar *U*-shaped clusters of buildings, plazas, platforms, and staircases, has been the topic of scholarly discussion at least since John Rowe's (1977) influential essay on the subject in 1962. Unlike typical New World monumental architecture, in which earlier phases are covered over by later enlargements, the temple complex at Chavín expanded through lateral growth.[6] The resulting plan involves two adjacent clusters that are different in shape and size, although parallel in orientation. It is a curious plan to look at: It appears oddly lopsided and lacks any apparent center. However, this asymmetry is most visible from the bird's-eye perspective available to the modern investigator. When a person walks through the site, the vistas that appear on either side are almost uniformly symmetrical.[7] The asymmetry of the site is present but invisible.

Experientially, this invisible asymmetry contributes a sense of unpredictability. Walking through the site, one encounters visual experiences that are clearly planned, but the sequence is not readily apparent: You cannot predict what's around the next corner. As in a haunted house, this unpredictability is unsettling and introduces elements of anticipation and surprise that greatly enhance the effect of any sight, sound, or other sensory stimulus that is introduced.

In sum, these brief analyses of the body-carved stone and body-site plan interfaces at Chavín demonstrate that attention to perceptual interfaces provides information that can be lost when using standard techniques for recording and analyzing visual data, such as the line drawing and the site map. In the next section, I point to parallels between the site plan and the carved stone monuments and suggest possible reasons Chavín's builders decided to create these particular kinds of perceptual interfaces.

## The Manufacture of Wonder

Research on Chavín to date has called on two very different kinds of expertise and produced a bifurcated scholarly literature. On the one hand, the site has attracted a series of highly skilled excavators who have grappled with questions including the site's difficult stratigraphy and its baffling location in a highland area devoid of large population or intensive agriculture. On the other hand, the complex iconography on the carved stone monuments offers a different kind of challenge. Many luminaries of Andean studies have tried their hands at deciphering the intertwined human, animal, and avian figures that cover the surfaces of Chavín stone, among them John Rowe (1977 [1962]), Donald Lathrap (1973), Peter Roe (2008), Tom Cummins (2008), and Gary Urton (2008).

For the most part, there is little overlap between these two lines of inquiry, despite the fact that the carved stones were originally integral to the architecture at the site (Urton 2008). (An exception is Cummins 2008.) This chapter demonstrates the potential value of looking at art and architecture together: Even a very preliminary analysis of the perceptual interface between the human body, the carved stones, and the site plan produces some surprising parallels.

As described above, Chavín's built environment includes the following characteristics: an asymmetrical plan that creates unpredictability; a processional pathway through the site in which vertical movement up and down creates an impeded, slowed-down progress enacted in stages; and an end point that is hidden from view underground, rather than openly displayed. In contrast, other pre-Columbian site plans typically include some or all of the following features: The central precinct is symmetrical and easily comprehended, allowing visitors to anticipate the bodily and visual experiences ahead; the pathway to and through this central precinct is straight and open, leading toward a central monumental space that is clearly marked as the goal; and major monuments are placed and designed for maximal visual impact. Parts of the central precincts of well-known Mesoamerican sites, such as Teotihuacán or La Venta, demonstrate these features, and many early Peruvian coastal sites conform to this model to varying degrees.

It could be said, therefore, that the site plan of Chavín is typical in some respects: It is satisfyingly monumental, is clearly planned, has a processional structure, and contains elements of symmetry and repetition. But it is the unique combination of these features at Chavín that creates a very particular kind of perceptual experience of unpredictability, interruption, and limited visibility.

Interestingly, the carved stone monuments do something similar. The designs use elements of symmetry and repetition, and the stones themselves are unquestionably monumental. But instead of an immediate, synchronic, total picture, the Chavín stones create a slow and impeded viewing process, in which a partial or total image is gradually pieced together through a series of discoveries. Consider how different this sensory interface is from that provided modern visitors to a museum. Instead of a well-lit, open space and a painting hung at just the right height with an informative label, visitors to Chavín were confronted with a series of frustrating partial glimpses of complex designs that are difficult to comprehend even when visible in their entirety. In both art and architecture, the effect at Chavín is to withhold the total picture from view.

This curious pattern is more comprehensible if we remember the site's function as a sacred pilgrimage center—and perhaps as an oracle, as it was in the seventeenth century (Vásquez de Espinosa 1968:491 [1620]; cited in Moore 1996:126). In contrast to the laboratory context of analyzing objects or the museum context of studying art, a sacred context may require perceptual interfaces that create an experience of wonder, awe, or the ineffable. Specific material objects and spatial arrangements that create the requisite kind of seeing may include (1) restricted access to enhance the visual impact of sacred images; (2) required actions within the sacred space that are constructed as journeys toward the sacred; and (3) a perceptual interface that structures the physiological and cognitive process of seeing so as to impart or reinforce an ideology, a philosophy, or a set of beliefs.

### Restricted Access

Around the world, the construction of sacred architecture entails provision for structures that hide certain objects or experiences from view. Sometimes this involves making such objects or experiences completely inaccessible to everyone, so that they are known only through memory or myth; restricting access to all but religious specialists, whose job it is to transmit to and interpret for nonspecialists the experience of being in the sacred presence; or allowing access only at particular times or after having undergone special preparations, as documented in Van Gennep's classic study of rites of passage (2004 [1960]). Modern religious ceremonies often combine these techniques, as for example in Jewish or Catholic rites in which a specialist (rabbi or priest) opens a sacred enclosure to reveal an object that only the specialist is allowed to touch but that the assembled congregation is invited to behold. In a native South American example of this practice, royal mummies were kept in palaces and attended by retainers in the Inca city of Cuzco. According to ethnohistoric sources, the incumbent Inca king and queen would regularly enter these palaces to pray to their ancestors; ordinary residents of Cuzco saw the mummies more rarely, when they were brought out and paraded around the city during specific calendrical rituals (Isbell 1997:38–68; Zuidema 1983).

Restricted access changes the experience of seeing. For example, a very short viewing period can heighten the emotional charge associated with the object, searing its image in the viewer's memory. This kind of viewing is often used for religious purposes: for example, when sacred icons are introduced to African initiates in coming-of-age rituals (Richards 1982; Turner 1967) or when funerary sculpture is used in Oceania (Kuechler 2002). A well-known example from the indigenous Americas is the use of sacred kachinas in Pueblo society (Kennard 2002 [1938]).

### The Sacred Journey

Chavín was a pilgrimage site: People traveled to it to have a transformative religious experience. The art and architecture at the site was constructed to fulfill this goal: Working together, they turned a visit to Chavín into a satisfying encounter with mysteries and marvels. The structure of the site itself makes reference to the pilgrim's journey—and not just metaphorically. The gradual process of crossing the space toward the sacred icons, and deciphering the images carved on those icons, creates the bodily experience of moving toward the goal of seeing something hidden—a goal that may never be fully achieved. (The sacred inner sanctum may not be accessible to all pilgrims; the entire image may never be fully decoded or even seen.)

Countless ethnographic and historic pilgrimages require the performance of a series of activities in prescribed stages (Morinis 1992; Turner and Turner 1978). The largest pilgrimage in the world today is the *hajj*, the journey to Mecca required of all Muslims (Peters 1995). This pilgrimage comprises two journeys: travel to Mecca and then the much more sacred journey from place to place within the site and its immediate environs, each of which demands a specific action: circling a cube-shaped building known as the Ka'bah; running between the hills of Al-Safa and Al-Marwah; drinking from the Zamzam Well; going to the plains of Mount Arafat to stand in vigil; and throwing stones in a ritual "Stoning of the Devil." After these structured movements toward and away from sacred places, pilgrims shave their heads, perform sacrifices, and finally celebrate the festival of Eid al-Adha.

In the Andean context, ethnohistoric accounts of pilgrims at the site of Pachacamac describe a series of approaches to various sacred precincts within the site, each of which required a specific regimen of fasting and ritual. According to Pedro Pizarro, the sacred precinct included a first court, which could only be entered after twenty days' fast; an upper court, which required a year's fast to enter; and the shrine itself, which was not entered by lay people at all until Pizarro forced the unwilling local political leaders to violate the inner sanctum (Pizarro 1970:123 [1533]; cited in Moore 1996).

### Imparting a Philosophy

The preceding discussion may make it sound as though Chavín, in particular, or religious rituals, in general, depend on a set of theatrical special effects designed to trick gullible viewers. Resolute empiricists and skeptical atheists will find this interpretation satisfying, but the entire cross-cultural, archaeological, and historical record attests to a widespread, ever-present human need for sacred places and things. We do not want to end where we began—by dismissing as a kind of "poor" or failed visibility the perceptual interface created at Chavín.

Instead, we can ask what the objective might be in instituting this kind of perceptual process. Like the trained scrutiny of the scientist, a kind of seeing that is specific to sacred places must serve highly specialized ends. What does it accomplish to construct a site and a series of sacred artifacts that are only allowed to be seen through a gradual process that begins with fragments and slowly moves toward a grasp of the whole? Is this simply a metaphorical way of making the pilgrim's journey an experiential reality or could there also be a larger philosophical statement expressed through this perceptual interface?

One place to look for answers is in the South American ethnographic record, especially that of indigenous Amazonians who still practice religious vision quests involving the use of hallucinogens, like the people of Chavín once did.[8] According to ethnographers, the vision of the world that underlies these practices teaches that ordinary perception is incomplete. When we perceive humans, animals, plants, minerals, and bodies of water as separate from one another, we fail to see the world as it really is. The purpose of shamanic ritual involving psychotropic drugs is to escape this limited, fragmented vision and to be able to see a hidden reality: an animate world in which all things are interconnected (Brown 1987; Harner 1984; Vivieros de Castro 1992).

No matter how strong the historical links or how apparent the similarities between a modern and a prehistoric society, twenty-first-century ethnography can only suggest hypotheses to be tested against the archaeological evidence. The Amazonian evidence is persuasive for several reasons: The Obelisk Tello from Chavín, which famously depicts Amazonian flora and fauna (Lathrap 1973); the abundant iconographic references to hallucinogenic drugs at the site, which parallel the documented use of hallucinogens in the Amazon; and the striking similarities between Amazonian animist beliefs and the strange hybrid creatures in Chavín iconography, which I hope to draw out in a future publication. However, I employ this ethnographic analogy here to serve a limited end, which does not depend on direct historic connection between the two regions. Amazonian religiosity holds that the mundane vision of the world is inherently fragmentary and incoherent and that it is only through ritual practices specifically aimed at changing one's perception that one may gain access to a more holistic and complete vision of the world. This notion of using religious learning in order to achieve a holistic vision is common to many religions and suggests a reason for the partial, fragmentary vision imposed on pilgrims at Chavín. A perceptual process that initially provides confusing, fragmentary glimpses that must be slowly put together into a whole may have been a means to teach a religious philosophy about the nature of reality—and of seeing itself.

Visitors to the site experienced a kaleidoscope of visual, spatial, auditory, and other sensory impressions and left with a lifetime of memories to contemplate and reflect on. Piecing these together into a coherent vision could well have been the means to achieving genuine philosophical insights, making the visit to Chavín a worthwhile intellectual exercise as well as an exciting, and unforgettable, sensory experience. Certainly this is the latent promise in Amazonian shamanic ritual and in pilgrimage practices such as the *hajj*.

In sum, the interrupted, fragmentary, partial form of sight constructed by both monumental art and architecture at Chavín and the emphasis on a process of attaining or movement toward a goal may be intentional aspects of the perceptual interface at the site. The repetition of this experience at different levels—from the pathways through the built environment to the surfaces of the carved stones—suggests recursiveness and intentionality. Furthermore, cross-cultural and South American ethnographic, historic, and archaeological examples of sacred sites and religious rituals suggest plausible interpretations for these choices on the part of Chavín's builders. Restricting access to the sacred; creating the experience of a journey; and imparting a philosophy, cosmology, and ideology are all goals that may have been achieved by constructing these kinds of perceptual interfaces.

However, we should also keep in mind that these interfaces were not the same for diverse actors. At least since Richard Burger's excavations of the residential area across the river from the temple complex (1984), archaeologists have thought about the presence of multiple actors at Chavín and their interpretations have taken into consideration the differences between leaders and ordinary people. The highly restricted access to the site's northern axis, where the small circular plaza and even smaller *galerías* are located, has been interpreted as a means of control over valued information, spaces, and objects (see, for example, Rick 2005). The difficult-to-grasp iconography of the carved stone monuments, similarly, may be seen as restricting access to sacred knowledge to an educated, specialist, priestly class.

There is also another related difference between actors at Chavín. A pilgrimage site by definition attracts pilgrims; it also requires a resident population, presumably both specialist and nonspecialist, to maintain the site and manage the experiences of those who come there. The fragmentary, surprising, nonreplicable viewing experience of the visitor is quite unlike the everyday access of the resident—a difference that has not been lost on archaeologists, who see the power differential between these forms of access.[9] A still greater difference in perceptual interface existed between the builders and artists[10] who erected and carved the great stone temple and those persons who only saw it. Both of these perceptual processes might be experienced as a journey toward an end, and both may have begun with a partial and fragmentary vision that slowly became integrated into a whole. But the experience for the maker would be far different—more physical, more fully embodied, longer, and deeper—than that of the viewer. Space prevents me from exploring this issue, and the questions of differential social power that it raises, but it is one more promising avenue of analysis for future study of the perceptual interface.

In Amazonia, while most men and some women engage in some shamanic practices, and even foreign tourists may dabble in psychotropic drug taking, a few individuals become known as serious students of the religion and, eventually, as respected experts in it. Anthropologists interested in cosmology are often directed to these individuals as worthy interlocutors (Reichel-Domatoff 1971; Whitten 1976, 1985). Similarly, at Chavín today, some visitors are knowledgeable and committed scholars for whom a visit to the site is an important milestone in a long-term research project, while other visitors range from the serious amateur to the merely curious, the dilettante, and the thrill seeker. The success of the site design rests on its ability to fulfill these multiple needs and desires of its users: Now, as in the past, Chavín offers a thought-provoking sensory experience that is both shared and individual.

## Summary

Line drawings, maps, and plans are useful and necessary archaeological tools, but there are material aspects of artifacts and buildings that these tools do not capture. Study of the sensory interface between the human body and archaeological sites and artifacts focuses our attention on data that is otherwise overlooked; brings our thinking down to a human scale; and may produce data that more closely approximates the lived experience of past actors and makes intentionality more visible in the archaeological record. This focus may be especially useful in the study of non-Western, precapitalist societies, in which perceptual practices may differ markedly from our own. In the case of the carved stone monuments and site plan at the temple complex of Chavín, attention to the sensory interface allows us to recognize the following: the "poor visibility" of the carved stones as an intentional practice on the part of their makers; the lopsided site plan as a strategy to introduce unpredictability; and the site plan as a processional structure that intentionally directs—but also breaks up—movement through the site. Parallels between the perceptual interface created by architecture and monumental art at the site point to recursive, intentional practices on the part of the site's builders and may provide clues for developing an actor-oriented analysis that differentiates between different groups at the site, including residents and visitors. This analysis suggests that close attention to the sensory interface may provoke archaeologists to ask new questions and provide a useful tool kit to try to answer them.

## Acknowledgments

The author would like to thank Jo Day and the archaeologists at Southern Illinois University Carbondale for inviting me to participate in this project; John and Rosa Rick for their kindness and generosity during my visits to Chavín and Stanford; and my colleagues at Northwestern University for their encouragement and support: Liz Brumfiel and Mark Hauser for their invaluable comments and suggestions on drafts of the paper and Jorge Coronado, Ann Gunther, and

Michelle Molina for listening to and commenting on an earlier form. All errors of fact and interpretation are, of course, entirely my own responsibility.

## Notes

1. *Strombus* shell trumpets of this kind are still used at Andean festivals to produce a loud, discordant cacophony rather than to perform any sort of structured song or musical composition.

2. An important caveat is the possibility that some or all of these surfaces were originally brightly colored; however, even if this were the case, it does not affect the other factors or the overall argument.

3. A comparison with large-scale designs plastered on the walls of contemporaneous coastal sites provides an illuminating contrast: There, deep bas-relief, simple designs, and abundant use of modeling create imagery that can be easily seen from anywhere with a clear sight line.

4. I discuss Sechín Alto only because it is the example chosen by Moore, not to contradict hypotheses about particular cultural affinity between Chavín and specific regions of the coast (cf. Burger and Salazar 2008).

5. Joanne Pillsbury kindly pointed out that no New World construction is technically a "pyramid," but in the absence of a suitable replacement word (*mound* suggests an unstructured pile of dirt, and other terms, such as *temple*, imply particular uses), I have continued to use it here.

6. The building sequence is currently under dispute; see Rick 2008 and Rodriguez Kembel 2008 for newer interpretations and Rowe 1977 and Burger 1992 for what until recently has been the standard view. However, all authors agree that the section of the site containing the Lanzón is probably the oldest; Rick and Rodriguez Kembel differ from Rowe's original interpretation primarily in asserting that the older part of the site was never abandoned but continually repaired and augmented.

7. Like *U*-shaped configurations elsewhere, slight differences—such as unequal lengths of lateral mounds—are found at Chavín.

8. I do not mean to imply that all indigenous Amazonians do so; contemporary residents of the rain forest are just as likely to be Evangelical Protestants, Catholics, or pragmatic atheists.

9. The modern life of the site and adjacent community is an evocative parallel to ancient times: The Peruvian residents of Chavín have been working at the site as guards, maintenance crews, and archaeological excavators for generations and take pride in their extensive, intimate knowledge of the place. With archaeologists playing the role of specialist priests and the small but steady stream of tourists as pilgrims, all the roles are still being played. However, this comparison also puts a check on our assumptions about power: Despite their inherited knowledge and status as the presumed heritage population, it would be difficult to argue that the current residents of Chavín have greater status than the international visitors from Peru's capital, Japan, Europe, or the United States do.

10. The term *artist* is inherently problematic when used in conjunction with premodern material practices that predate the concept of "art" and "artists." However, avoiding its use creates the impression that premodern material practices were lesser than, rather than simply different from, our own. For my purposes, whenever someone made something that we would today recognize as "art," I call that person an "artist."

## References


Ashmore, Wendy, and A. Bernard Knapp

1999 *Archaeologies of Landscape: Contemporary Perspectives*. Blackwell, Oxford.

Ayres, Fred D.

1961 Rubbings from Chavín de Huantar, Peru. *American Antiquity* 27:239–245.

Berger, John

1980 *About Looking*. Pantheon, New York.

Brown, Michael F.

1987 *Tsewa's Gift: Magic and Meaning in an Amazonian Society*. University of Alabama Press, Birmingham.

Burger, Richard L.

1984 *The Prehistoric Occupation of Chavín de Huantar, Peru*. University of California Publications in Anthropology Vol. 14. University of California Press, Berkeley.

1992 *Chavín and the Origins of Andean Civilization*. Thames and Hudson, New York.

Burger, Richard L., and Lucy C. Salazar

2008 The Manchay Culture and the Coastal Inspiration for Highland Chavín Civilization. In *Chavín: Art, Architecture, and Culture*, edited by William J. Conklin and Jeffrey Quilter, pp. 85–106. Cotsen Institute of Archaeology, University of California, Los Angeles.

Conklin, William J., and Jeffrey Quilter

2008 *Chavín: Art, Architecture, and Culture*. Cotsen Institute of Archaeology, University of California, Los Angeles.

Contreras, Daniel A.

2010 A Mito-Style Structure at Chavín de Huantar: Dating and Implications. *Latin American Antiquity* 21:1–19.

Contreras, Daniel A., and David A. Keefer

2009 Implications of the Fluvial History of the Wacheqsa River for Hydrologic Engineering and Water Use at Chavín de Huántar, Peru. *Geoarchaeology: An International Journal* 24:589–618.

Cordy-Collins, Alana K.

1977 Chavín Art: Its Shamanic/Hallucinogenic Origins. In *Pre-Columbian Art History: Selected Readings*, edited by Alana Cordy-Collins and Jean Stern, pp. 353–362. Peek, Palo Alto.

1980 An Artistic Record of the Chavín Hallucinatory Experience. *The Masterkey for Indian Lore and History* 54:84–93.

Cummins, Tom

2008 Felicitous Legacy of the Lanzón. In *Chavín: Art, Architecture, and Culture*, edited by William J. Conklin and Jeffrey Quilter, pp. 279–304. Cotsen Institute of Archaeology, University of California, Los Angeles.

Ferguson, Edna

1931 *Dancing Gods: Indian Ceremonials of Arizona and New Mexico.* University of New Mexico Press, Albuquerque.

Gregor, Thomas A., and Donald Tuzin (editors)

2001 *Gender in Amazonia and Melanesia: An Exploration of the Comparative Method.* University of California Press, Berkeley.

Hall, Martin

2000 *Archaeology and the Modern World: Colonial Transcripts in South Africa and the Chesapeake.* Routledge, New York.

Harner, Michael

1984 *The Jivaro: People of the Sacred Waterfall.* University of California Press, Berkeley.

Howes, David (editor)

2005 *Empires of the Senses.* Berg, Oxford.

Hugh-Jones, Stephen

1988 *The Palm and the Pleiades: Initiation and Cosmology in Northwest Amazonia.* Cambridge University Press, Cambridge.

Isbell, William H.

1997 *Mummies and Mortuary Monuments: A Postprocessual Prehistory of Central Andean Societies.* University of Texas Press, Austin.

Kennard, Edward

2002 [1938] *Hopi Kachinas.* Kiva, Walnut, California.

Kuechler, Suzanne

2002 *Malanggan: Art, Memory, and Sacrifice.* Berg, Oxford.

Lathrap, Donald W.

1973 Gifts of the Cayman: Some Thoughts on the Subsistence Basis of Chavín. In *Dumbarton Oaks Conference on Chavín,* edited by Elizabeth P. Benson, pp. 73–100. Dumbarton Oaks Research Library and Collection, Washington, D.C.

Llobera, Marcos

2007 Reconstructing Visual Landscapes. *World Archaeology* 39:51–69

Lumbreras, Luis

1977 Excavaciones en el Templo Antiguo de Chavín (sector R); informe de la sexta campaña. *Ñawpa Pacha* 15:1–38.

Lumbreras, Luis G., Chacho González, and Bernard Lietaer

1976 *Acerca de la función del sistema hidraúlico de Chavín.* Museo Nacional de Antropología y Arqueología, Lima.

Merleau-Ponty, Maurice

1964 [1945] Cezanne's Doubt. In *Sense and Non-Sense.* Translated by Hubert L. Dreyfus and Patricia Allen Dreyfus, pp. 9–25. Northwestern University Press, Evanston.

2002 [1945] *Phenomenology of Perception.* Translated by Colin Smith. Routledge Classics, London.

Moore, Jerry D.

1996 *Architecture and Power in the Ancient Andes: The Archaeology of Public Buildings.* Cambridge University Press, Cambridge.

2005 *Cultural Landscapes in the Ancient Andes: Archaeologies of Place.* University Press of Florida, Gainevsille.

Morinis, Alan

1992 *Sacred Journeys: The Anthropology of Pilgrimage.* Greenwood, New York.

Murphy, Yolanda, and Robert Francis Murphy

2004 [1985] *Women of the Forest.* Columbia University Press, New York.

Parsons, Elsie Clews
1923 The Hopi Buffalo Dance. *Man* 23:21–27.
Peters, Francis Edward
1995 *The Hajj: The Muslim Pilgrimage to Mecca and the Holy Places.* Princeton University Press, Princeton, New Jersey.
Pozorski, Shelia, and Thomas Pozorski
2002 The Sechín Alto Complex and Its Place Within Casma Valley Initial Period Development. In *Andean Archaeology I: Variations in Sociopolitical Organization,* edited by William H. Isbell and Helaine Silverman, pp. 21–51. Kluwer Academic/Plenum, New York.
Reichel-Domatoff, Gerardo
1971 *Amazonian Cosmos: The Sexual and Religious System of the Tukano Indians.* University of Chicago Press, Chicago.
Richards, Audrey
1982 [1956] *Chisungu: A Girl's Initiation Ceremony among the Bemba of Zambia.* Routledge, New York.
Rick, John W.
2004 The Evolution of Authority and Power at Chavín de Huántar, Peru. In *Foundations of Power in the Prehispanic Andes,* edited by Kevin J. Vaughn, Dennis Ogburn, and Christina A. Conlee, pp. 71–89. Archaeological Papers of the American Anthropological Association, No. 14. Wiley-Blackwell, Malden, Massachusetts.
2008 Construction and Ritual in the Development of Authority at Chavín de Huantar. In *Chavín: Art, Architecture, and Culture,* edited by William J. Conklin and Jeffrey Quilter, pp. 3–34. Cotsen Institute of Archaeology, University of California, Los Angeles.
Rodning, Christopher
2009 Place, Landscape, and Environment: Anthropological Archaeology in 2009. *American Anthropologist* 112:180–190.
Rodriguez Kembel, Silvia
2008 The Architecture at the Monumental Center of Chavín de Huantar: Sequence, Transformations, and Chronology. In *Chavín: Art, Architecture, and Culture,* edited by William J. Conklin and Jeffrey Quilter, pp. 35–84. Cotsen Institute of Archaeology, University of California, Los Angeles.
Roe, Peter G.
2008 How to Build a Raptor: Why the Dumbarton Oaks "Scaled Cayman" Callango Textile Is Really a Jaguaroid Harpy Eagle. In *Chavín: Art, Architecture, and Culture,* edited by William J. Conklin and Jeffrey Quilter, pp. 181–216. Cotsen Institute of Archaeology, University of California, Los Angeles.
Rowe, John H.
1977 [1962] Form and Meaning in Chavín Art. In *Peruvian Archaeology: Selected Readings,* edited by John H. Rowe and Dorothy Menzel, pp. 72–103. Peek, Palo Alto.
Sharon, Douglas
2000 *Shamanism and the Sacred Cactus: Ethnoarchaeological Evidence for San Pedro Use in Northern Peru.* San Diego Museum Papers No. 37. San Diego Museum of Man, San Diego.
Silverman, Helaine
1999 Archaeology and the 1997 Peruvian Hostage Crisis. *Anthropology Today* 15(1):9–13.
Smith, Adam T.
2003 *The Political Landscape: Constellations of Authority in Early Complex Polities.* University of California Press, Los Angeles.

Smith, Mark
2007 *Sensory History.* Berg, Oxford.
Tilley, Christopher
1994 *A Phenomenology of Landscape: Places, Paths, and Landscapes.* Berg, Oxford.
Torres, Constantino Manuel
2008 Chavín's Psychoactive Pharmacopoeia: The Iconographic Evidence. In *Chavín: Art, Architecture, and Culture,* edited by William J. Conklin and Jeffrey Quilter, pp. 239–260. Cotsen Institute of Archaeology, University of California, Los Angeles.
Turner, Victor
1967 *Forest of Symbols: Aspects of Ndembu Ritual.* Cornell University Press, Ithaca.
Turner, Victor, and Edith Turner
1978 *Image and Pilgrimage in Christian Culture: An Anthropological Account.* Columbia University Press, New York.
Urton, Gary
2008 The Body of Meaning in Chavín Art. In *Chavín: Art, Architecture, and Culture,* edited by William J. Conklin and Jeffrey Quilter, pp. 217–238. Cotsen Institute of Archaeology, University of California, Los Angeles.
Van Gennep, Arnold
2004 [1960] *The Rites of Passage*. Translated by Monika B. Vizedom and Gabrielle L. Caffee. Routledge and Kegan Paul, London.
Vivieros de Castro, Eduardo
1992 *From the Enemy's Point of View: Humanity and Divinity in an Amazonian Society.* University of Chicago Press, Chicago.
Weismantel, Mary
2011 Obstinate Things. In *The Archaeology of Colonialism: Intimate Encounters,* edited by Barbara L. Voss and Eleanor Conlin Casella, pp. 303–320. Cambridge University Press, Cambridge.
Whitten, Norman E., Jr.
1976 *Sacha Runa.* University of Illinois Press, Urbana.
1985 *Sicuanga Runa: The Other Side of Development in Amazonia.* University of Illinois Press, Urbana.
Zuidema, R. Tom
1983 Hierarchy and Space in Incaic Social Organization. *Ethnohistory* 30:49–75.

# 7. The Sensory Experience of Blood Sacrifice in the Roman Imperial Cult

*Candace Weddle*

*Abstract:* The field of classical scholarship has been too often reliant on sterile approaches to analyzing the sensory aspects of ancient sacrificial rites. Mute mosaics of choirs and silent reliefs of flute players serve as evidence for the sounds of worship, and ancient descriptions of burning incense suggest the odors of divine rites. Certainly such archaeological and literary sources provide vital evidence, but it is nevertheless difficult for scholars to conceive of the sensory impact of the sacrificial spectacle. I suggest that we may achieve a more thorough understanding of the experience through an autoethnographic investigation of modern religious sacrifice. I analyze my experience of the slaughter of large numbers of bovines during the Islamic Kurban Bayram sacrifices in Istanbul to make suggestions concerning the sensory elements of Roman imperial cult sacrifices and, by extension, of ancient blood sacrifice in general. This is not a comparative religion project but rather an attempt to understand the sensory impact of ancient sacrifice in a way that exceeds the limitations of traditional research.

> Monte Albán, among the heights surrounding a valley, is a complex of ruins: temples, reliefs, grand stairways, platforms for human sacrifice. Horror, sacredness, and mystery are consolidated by tourism, which dictates preordained forms of behavior, the modest surrogates of those rites. Contemplating these stairs, we try to imagine the hot blood spurting from the breast split by the stone axe of the priest.
>
> —Italo Calvino, *Under the Jaguar Sun*

*Making Senses of the Past: Toward a Sensory Archaeology,* edited by Jo Day. Center for Archaeological Investigations, Occasional Paper No. 40.  ISBN 978-0-8093-3287-8.

## Ancient Roman Sacrificial Practice

When the ancient Romans sacrificed to their gods, the sights, sounds, and smells of the rites permeated the city. The smoke from altars filled the air with incense, the voices of choirs were raised in song to the accompaniment of flutes and drums, and prayers were intoned by priests. If the offering included live victims, the smells of slaughtering and butchering the beasts and roasting flesh and hides on wood fires were notable. Whether resulting from a small private offering of incense on a home altar or a large public rite in which one hundred or more bovines were sacrificed, the visual, auditory, and olfactory by-products of sacrifice were a daily presence in the ancient city. The proper control of these sensory elements of sacrifice was vital to correct ritual practice. Roman sacrifices were understood as providing sustenance to the gods through the vehicle of smell; the "savor" of offerings was delivered to the gods on the smoke of sacrifices, and smells thus symbolized the connection of humans with the divine. Things that were heard during the course of sacrifice were also of immense importance. A misspoken word or an unexpected sound, such as the bellow of an animal in distress, could negate an entire ritual, necessitating that it be started again from the beginning.

A significant body of scholarship has been produced on the ancient evidence for the ritual control and ritual meaning of various sensory elements of Roman sacrifice (for example, Fless 1995; Fless and Moede 2007; and Quasten 1983 on cult music and Harvey 2006 and Yerkes 1952 on incense and other scents in worship). However, Roman sources are concerned primarily with the effect of ritual sensory elements within the context of correct accomplishment of specific rites. The sensory impact of cult ritual on the worshippers and on the urban environments in which the rites were often carried out—how far the sounds and smells carried, how they may have affected daily life, whether and how they might have played a role in reactions and responses to particular cults—received little attention in antiquity, nor have these issues been taken up extensively by modern scholars. It is my intention here to raise questions that are, perhaps, of a more mundane nature than those that scholars of religious anthropology and classical culture have often grappled with so eloquently but are, nevertheless, of importance for advancing our understanding of the sensory experience of sacrifice within the ancient city.

Our ancient evidence for sensory elements of Roman sacrificial rites is extensive but limited in scope, and in the field of classical scholarship, we have been too often reliant on sterile approaches to analyzing the sensory aspects of cult worship. Our mental images of what a Roman worshipper would have witnessed at a sacrifice are largely based on artistic representations of the rites, of which many survive in various media, most incorporating a standard visual vocabulary of actors and actions identifiable from literary sources that deal with the rites.[1] An exemplary image is a historical relief now in Florence that depicts one moment of a sacrifice in honor of the emperor Hadrian on his *vicennalia*, the twentieth anniversary of the beginning of his reign (Figure 7-1). The scene, with some variation in details, survives in several other examples, ranging in size and

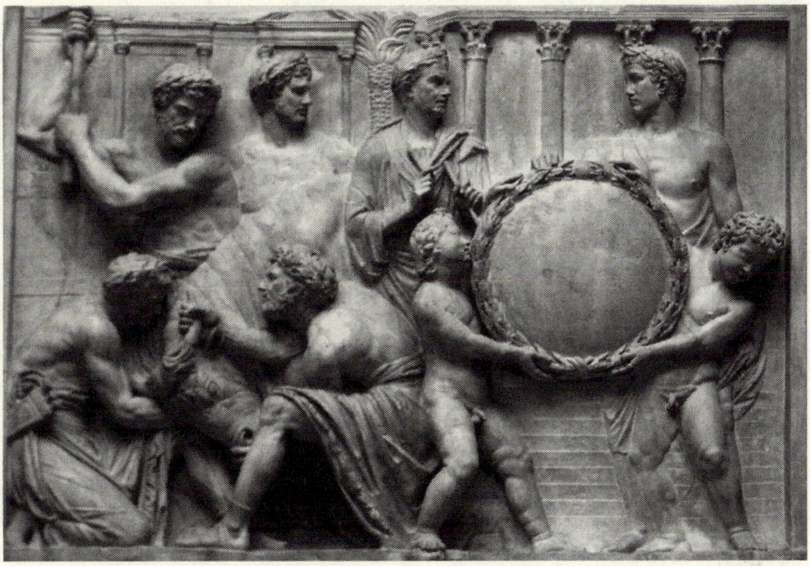

**Figure 7-1.** *Relief showing a sacrifice on the occasion of the twentieth anniversary of Hadrian's reign (137 C.E. Rome, now in Uffizi Gallery, Polo Museale Fiorentino, Florence. Photograph © Nicholas Cipolla; used with permission.)*

medium from an image on a coin struck during the reign of Domitian in 88 C.E. to a fine, small-scale representation on a silver cup from Boscoreale dated to circa 7 B.C.E. to monumental public reliefs such as a panel on the Arch of Trajan at Beneventum (114 C.E.).

In Figure 7-1, bare-chested *victimarii* (slaves responsible for handling sacrificial animals) are portrayed in the moment before the sacrifice of a bull or an ox. Two of them force the head of the animal down while a third man prepares to make a powerful swing with a weapon. The blow, aimed at the back of the neck, is almost certainly not intended to kill the animal. The man wielding the weapon is the *popa,* a Roman ritual actor whose function was to stun large animals prior to their slaughter.[2] Speaking in physiological terms, a significant blow to the atlas vertebra at the base of the skull (or to the next vertebra below it, the axis, between the two of which the end of the brainstem is located) would have stunned an animal, bringing it down and facilitating the slaughter, which was accomplished by slitting the animal's throat with a knife. The formulaic nature of Roman art depicting ritual actions prevents a strictly literal interpretation of such scenes, as if they were a photographic record of sacrificial practice. Nevertheless, within the Roman tradition of artistic representation of ritual activity, this image and others like it are instructive about the practice of Roman sacrifice and may be safely used to imagine, in a general sense, one moment of what an ancient participant might have witnessed during a sacrifice that included the slaughter of a large animal.

Significant methodological difficulties arise when we begin to consider senses other than sight. Given the limits of our evidence, we must employ visual sources to investigate invisible, ephemeral aspects of ritual, such as sound. For example, when we consider the music that was a part of many of the rites, we study images such as a Flavian period (69–96 C.E.) mosaic in honor of the goddess Diana Tifatina that depicts a cult choir (Pollini 2003:Figure 24)[3] or reliefs such as Figure 7-2, which shows the emperor Marcus Aurelius (with covered head) making a sacrifice, while a flute player (*tibicen*) standing to his left plays accompaniment. Of course, mosaics are mute, and the relief is silent. Nevertheless, scholars must use these important but sensorially insufficient sources as primary evidence for the sounds of sacrifice. They may be considered in tandem with archaeological evidence such as inscriptions that tell us, for instance, that a certain temple had a cult choir associated with it, how many members made up its ranks, the genders and ages of the singers, and even sometimes details of their membership dues or benefits they received (see Price 1984:90, 209), but little or nothing about the hymns themselves.

The same holds true of the evidence for the smells of sacrifice. Again, reliefs depicting the use of incense are commonly employed as evidence showing how the act of making a burnt offering of those precious materials was carried out. In Figure 7-2, for example, a young attendant standing beside the emperor holds open the lid of an *acerra*, a box for incense. This detail indicates that the emperor will place a few costly lumps of aromatics on the fire of the small folding altar (*foculus*) when he has completed the action he is shown performing, pouring a libation from a shallow dish called a *patera*. This liquid offering hints at yet another olfactory element of the ritual—the burning of what is probably undiluted wine, a substance that would have produced its own heady fragrance. To supplement the visual evidence, which cannot begin to evoke the actual smells, we may turn to ancient descriptions of the aromas of worship. One that is commonly taken up by ancient authors is the scent of burning incense, which is often described as a "sweet" smell.[4] However, as evocative as some ancient descriptions of incense may be, they fall far short of enabling us to really understand the experience of smelling that incense. Given such difficulties, it is necessary that we consider other avenues by which we may arrive at less "senseless" examinations of ancient sacrifice.

## *Ancient Imperial Cult and Modern Sacrificial Practice*

In order to narrow the scope of this inquiry, it is first necessary to take as a focus a specific type of Roman sacrifice, of which there were many. For the purposes of this paper, I shall concentrate on the Roman imperial cult, a cult for which we have significant archaeological and epigraphical evidence on which to build (see especially Burrell 2004; Fishwick 1987, 1992, 2005; Friesen 2001; Price 1984). *Imperial cult* is a modern term used by scholars to designate the practice of worshipping the Roman emperors and certain members of the royal family. It was a development in Roman religion and politics that occurred as the empire extended eastward to include the Greek-speaking world, an area in which hero worship and the divinization of rulers had long been practiced. Elements of this worship included constructing temples, appointing priests and priestesses, and conducting sacrifices. Though the range of sacrifices considered appropriate in the context of the imperial cult was fairly broad, we know from inscriptional and

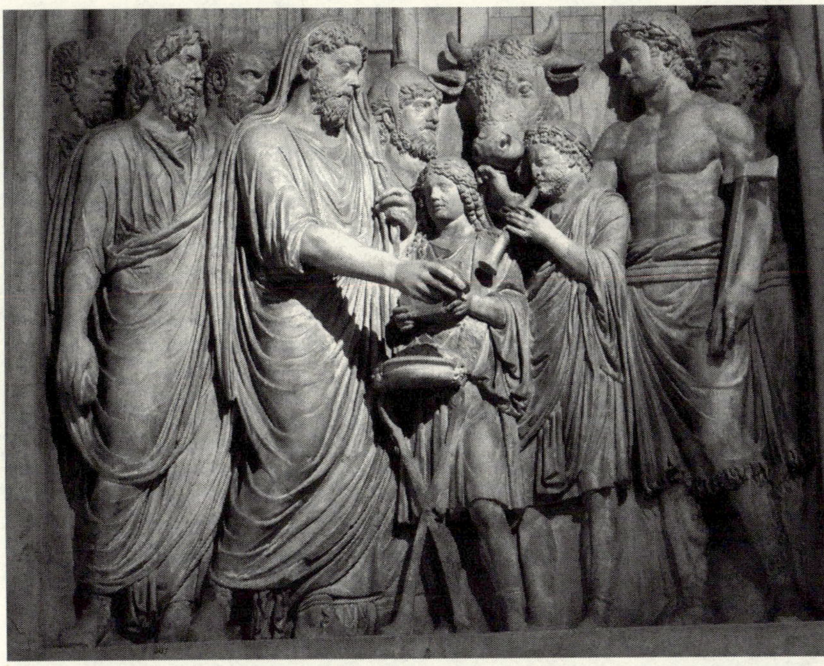

**Figure 7-2.** *Detail of a relief from an honorary monument to Marcus Aurelius: sacrifice to Capitoline Jupiter. (176–180 C.E. Rome, Capitoline Museum. Photograph © John Pollini; used with permission.)*

literary evidence that it included the slaughter and immolation of bulls on a scale up to and including a traditional *hekatomb* (Price 1984:208, Note 7), a Greek term that literally indicates 100 bulls but was used since the time of Homer to refer in general to a large number of cattle for sacrifice.

It is difficult for modern scholars to conceive of the sensory impact of the ancient *hekatomb*. Like Calvino's (1988) character visiting the ruins of a Zapotec temple, we may find ourselves attempting to create in our mind's eye (and nose) an image of sacrifice as we stand at the foot of an ancient altar. However, just as Calvino's character, inspired by the steep and daunting staircase of a pyramid, could only *try* to imagine the axe of the priest and a fountain of sacrificial human blood, based on his experience of the archaeological site (perhaps with the aid of images from the art of the culture), we too are unable to experience the rites of ancient blood sacrifices with their rich panoply of sights, sounds, and odors. We do, however, have the opportunity to experience modern sacrificial rites, and our understanding of ancient sacrifice may benefit from a judiciously applied and self-conscious analysis of such an experience.

In what follows, I will supplement the evidence of ancient sacrifice from literary and archaeological sources with an investigation of a modern sacrificial ceremony to make suggestions regarding the sensory experience of blood sacrifices in the Roman imperial cult. Let me be clear: I am not suggesting any direct comparisons between these modern sacrifices and the ancient practice of cult in terms of either process or meaning. Though some technical similarities are present—both rituals center on the same action of slaughtering a large animal by non-mechanized means—my intention in this study is not to identify or comment on the similarities or differences between the two traditions; this is not a comparative religion project.[5] Rather, I will demonstrate that careful analysis of my own experience of large-scale modern sacrificial rites has allowed me to develop important questions and considerations concerning the sensory elements of sacrifice at imperial cult temples, although the majority of the observations are applicable to any Greek or Roman sacrifice involving the offering of large animals.

My methodological approach in considering my personal experience of sacrificial slaughter may be termed autoethnographic. It is not possible to unpack here the myriad meanings of the term *autoethnography* as it has been pressed into service to distinguish between different forms of texts, different genres of writing, different types of method, and even between traditional written ethnographies and the production of material objects (see Denzin 1989; Dorst 1989; Pratt 1994; Strathern 1987; Van Maanen 1995). However, it is necessary to address my usage of the term and to explain how I intend to employ it to analyze ancient sacrifice.

There is no single methodology designated by the term autoethnography. Since the word was first coined in the 1970s,[6] it has been assigned a wide variety of definitions by ethnographers (see Reed-Danahay 1997:1–17). The following description of sacrifices I attended is autoethnographic in its most basic sense: It is based on my personal experience of blood sacrifice in a contemporary Muslim context. Coming from a Western (Christian) tradition, I am not part of the social or religious culture whose sacrifices I observed, but my role was not that of the traditional ethnographer attempting to analyze the socioreligious practices of another culture. Rather, since the intent of the exercise was to record and analyze the sensory elements of the sacrifices, I may be considered a participant in the group experience because I share the same sensory processes as the other observers of the rites and employ these shared traits as my primary tools of analysis. What follows, then, is an autoethnographic record of my experience of modern rites comparable in type and scale to an ancient *hekatomb.*

## An Autoethnographic Experience of Islamic Sacrifices[7]

I attended the Kurban Bayram sacrifices on December 8, 2008, in the Halıcıoğlu neighborhood of Istanbul. Kurban Bayram (literally, "Sacrifice Holiday") is a Muslim religious holiday that commemorates the intended sacrifice of Ishmael by Abraham and a similar event in which the father of Mohammed was offered up as a sacrifice by *his* father; as with Ishmael, he was also rescued from that fate by Allah at the final moment.[8] For a period of several days, sacrifices of various animals are carried out, as well as communal meals at which the meat from those sacrifices is consumed. The sacrificial area I visited was designated for the slaughter of large animals—that is, cows and bulls. This allows me to make the most salient suggestions about the blood sacrifices in the imperial cult.

I arrived at the sacrificial area about noon. By that time, the sacrifices had been ongoing since the conclusion of the dawn prayer, approximately 7:00 A.M. at that time of the year. The day was overcast and fairly cool, between 44° and 48°F. The location for the sacrifices was an open lot in which several stations for dealing with the animals had been erected; the entire area of the lot was approximately 5 × 10 m. Five or six cows and bulls were tied in various spots around the area. Most of the animals were marked with numbers painted on their hides identifying the owners of the animals, and about half of the cattle had blindfolds, in most cases composed of a type of plastic fiber, probably portions of feed bags, tied over their eyes and secured behind their ears with rope. Interestingly, there was no separation between the people and the animals; the animals were not corralled in pens.

I did not see where the rest of the animals were being held but assume they were kept nearby, with only a few brought into the area at a time. There had already been a significant number of sacrifices before I arrived—the fourth or fifth animal I saw slaughtered was announced as *doksan,* or 90—and the number waiting remained steady while I was there. The number of animals that were dealt with prior to and during my observation of the ceremonies was, therefore, directly comparable to that offered in a true ancient *hekatomb*.

Contrary to my expectations, the animals were extremely docile. The smells of the slaughtering did not seem to agitate them in any way, nor were the ones with their eyes uncovered bothered by the activity around them. Occasionally, an animal would become confused or panicked, as was the case when one of the blindfolded animals stepped into and caught its foot in a wheelbarrow, but in general, the waiting animals were calm and made only the normal sounds of animals in proximity to one another; the people produced far more clamor than the animals.

To facilitate the large number of victims, an enclosed trailer about the size and height of a standard 20-foot shipping container had been brought into the area. The slaughter was being carried out at one open end, and the carcasses were being skinned and chopped into large pieces inside the body of the trailer before being passed out the other end to people waiting to complete the butchering. The trailer was equipped with a makeshift drainage system composed of a single PVC pipe carrying blood from the floor of the trailer into a refuse pit. My location was about 3 m from the end of the trailer where the animals were being killed. I was standing directly next to the refuse pit (Figure 7-3). It was approximately 6 m deep and served as a receptacle for the blood being drained from the floor of the trailer as well as for the waste portions of the animals' bodies. It had been dug adjacent to a concrete retaining wall, which served as one wall of the pit.

The only portions of the bodies that were being discarded consistently were hooves and tails. Much of the waste material in the pit was the contents of the digestive systems of the animals. As the stomachs and intestines were removed, they were carted to the edge of the pit by wheelbarrow. Two women cut the organs open, removed the waste material from them and pushed it into the pit, and then set the viscera aside for later consumption or other use. Some stomachs and

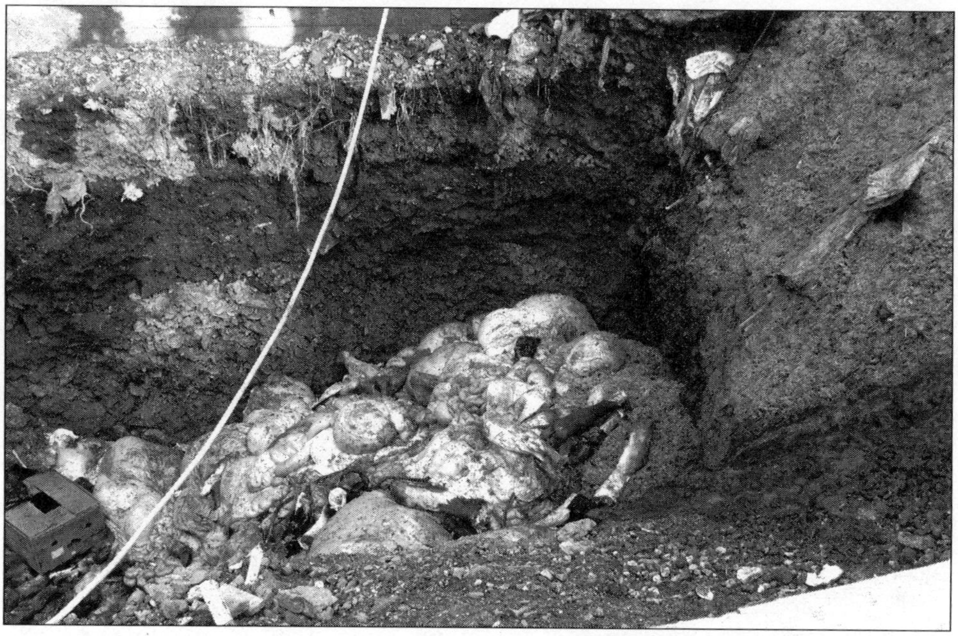

**Figure 7-3.** *Refuse pit containing entrails, hooves, blood, and waste at the Istanbul Kurban Bayram sacrificial area. (Photograph © Candace Weddle.)*

entrails were being discarded, as can be seen in Figure 7-3, but a significant number were salvaged. The concrete wall forming one side of the refuse pit was covered in blood and fecal and intestinal matter (Figure 7-4). The smell of the offal, excrement, and the contents of the animals' stomachs greatly overpowered the scent of the blood. In fact, the fresh blood coming from the throats of the animals produced very little scent, but presumably as it sat in the open air in the pit or on the ground around the sacrificial area the smell would increase, exponentially on days with warmer temperatures. In general, the smells of slaughter and butchering were milder than I had anticipated, especially considering the number of animals sacrificed prior to my arrival.

The process of sacrifice was as follows: An official announced through a handheld electric megaphone the number of the animal to be sacrificed, and the designated victim was led up a ramp to the floor of the trailer. This was the point at which the animals were most likely to balk or struggle. When the animal reached the floor of the trailer, which was about 2 m high, the sacrifice was carried out.

In order to force the animal into a prone position, a chain was looped around one back leg. The chain was attached to a hydraulic mechanism that lifted the animal into the air. Once suspended, the cow or bull was slowly lowered headfirst until it was lying on its side, with its neck pointing away from the crowd. At this point, the prayers dedicating the animal to Allah were pronounced. An assistant then grasped the head of the animal and pulled it backward to expose the throat, and the sacrificant used a very sharp knife to slice the neck deeply. Sacrificial regulations dictate that the cut should sever both main arteries in the

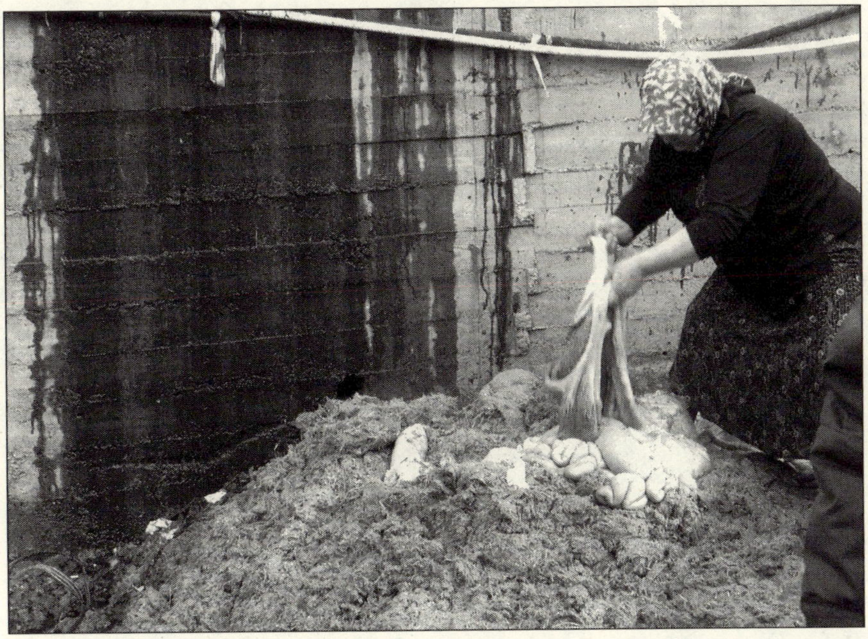

**Figure 7-4.** *A woman cleans entrails in front of a blood-covered concrete wall at the Kurban Bayram sacrificial area. (Photograph © Candace Weddle.)*

neck as well as the gullet and windpipe. This symbolically destroys the means of breath, of ingestion, and of circulation (Siddiqi 2000:39). More pragmatically, it also results in a quick death.

In most cases, the animal struggled very little. The severing of the two main arteries in the neck releases a massive amount of blood, which is thicker and of a more vibrant red color than I had expected. Due to the low temperature of the air, a fair amount of steam was also produced. Again, the smell of the blood was minimal, but the *sound* of it was something that I was not prepared for. Because of the height of the trailer from the ground, the flowing blood pouring down through the PVC pipe and also off the back of the trailer sounded like falling water and was quite striking (Figure 7-5). The animal was left to bleed for about 30 seconds before the butchering process began.

The bodies were skinned and two men with axes then chopped them in half from tail to neck. At this point, the pieces were removed to tables where a number of men broke them down further into smaller pieces that were then packed into large plastic bags and distributed to the owners of the animals. The entire process of butchering the animal and dispersing the meat was extremely quick and efficient. Although I was not able to track the progress of a single animal, I estimate that it took no more than 30 to 45 minutes from the time of the sacrifice to the distribution of the meat and disposal of the refuse.

The slaughtering and handling of the bodies of the victims—that is, all the sacrificial treatment of the animals brought to this location, from the moment of death through butchering—were confined to the officially designated area.[9]

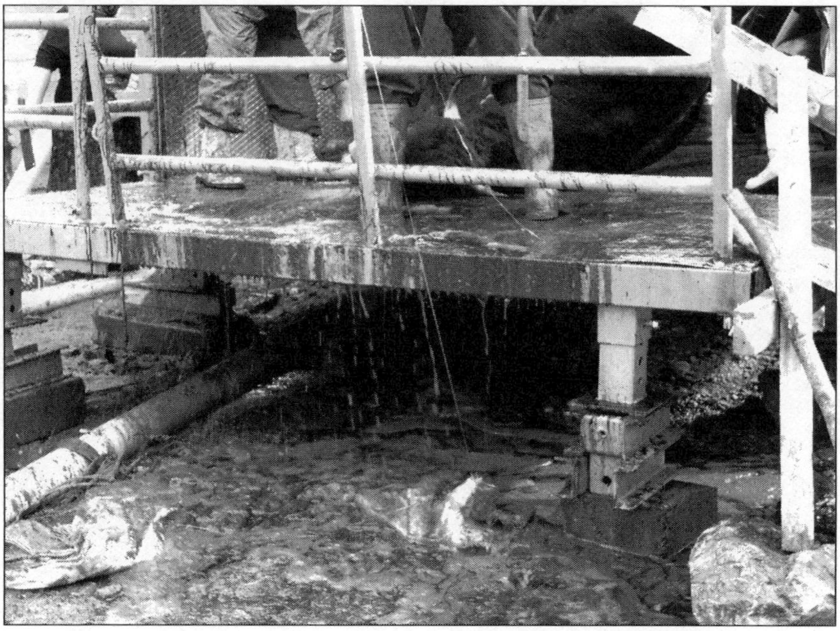

**Figure 7-5.** *Blood falling from the Kurban Bayram trailer platform following slaughter of a bull. The pipe routing most of the blood to the refuse pit can be seen below the trailer. (Photograph © Candace Weddle.)*

The refuse pit was to be covered at the end of the three-day sacrificial period. The results of the sacrifices, however, had an impact on the entire neighborhood around the sacrificial center. Even the culmination of the religious festivities did not bring the sensory impact of the sacrificial process to an end; further research conducted at a later date at the slaughter site illustrates this fact.

I returned to the site of the Bayram sacrifices on January 27, 2009, 50 days after the rites had taken place. The temperature was around 60°F and there was a light breeze. The weather had warmed in the preceding days, following several weeks of cold weather and almost continual precipitation, including snow. By the time of my return, the refuse pit had been filled in with dirt and chunks of concrete. Several meters of fill insulated its contents from the air and from scavenging animals (Figure 7-6). Despite this, the smell of the animals did linger fairly strongly; it was not offensive but was definitely noticeable. The strongest odor was manure, due in part to the fact that some of the waste the animals produced while awaiting slaughter had not been cleared away. However, when I walked to the area of the covered refuse pit, I could smell the slightly metallic scent of blood. The odor was particularly strong closest to the concrete retaining wall on the far side of the area, which had been coated in a considerable amount of blood and other material at the time of the sacrifices. Although from its appearance it seemed that the wall had been heavily cleaned following the sacrificial period, the smells of the blood and waste products lingered more strongly there than elsewhere.

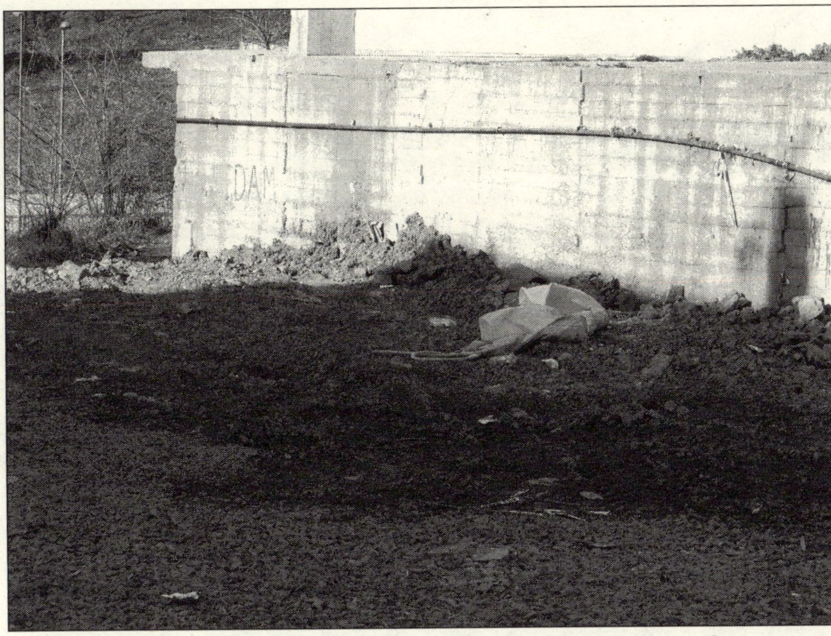

**Figure 7-6.** *The Kurban Bayram refuse pit, filled with dirt and concrete, 50 days after the sacrifices. (Photograph © Candace Weddle.)*

## Applications of the Experience of Modern Rites in Analyzing Ancient Sacrifice

My experience of the Kurban Bayram sacrifices was a powerful one and changed my understanding of the processes of ancient sacrifice in several fundamental ways. A particularly useful result of this exercise has been my new-found awareness of aspects of the process of sacrifice, in many cases things that went on before and after the sacrificial acts themselves, that are often absent from the primary ancient and archaeological evidence. These elements would have had a great impact on the experience of the rites, but because of the pedestrian nature of some of them, they are neither discussed in ancient literary sources nor included in art commemorating the events. However, if we ignore such aspects of the proceedings, we overlook a major source of information, not only on the greater sensory experience of the rituals, but also in some cases on details of the performance of the rites. I will discuss here some of the aspects of sacrifice to which I had given little thought prior to my observation of Kurban Bayram and will propose how they might have affected the sensory experience of ancient sacrificial rites. Restrictions of space do not allow me to address every aspect of the rites. For example, I will not consider elements that would have acted on the sense of touch at sacrificial ceremonies, though one can easily imagine, for instance, the effects of a pressing crowd. I am also aware that some of my suggestions must remain speculative, but I wish to push the boundaries of the evidence.

*The Animals: Sensory Effects of and on the Sacrificial Victims*

One of the aspects of the sensory experience of sacrifice that is often ignored in both ancient and modern sources is the impact of the animals themselves, especially prior to the moment of sacrifice. Preparations carried out on the animals in order to make them ritually acceptable, or to designate them as such, are described in some detail in ancient sources (especially within the Greek tradition), but other facets of their presacrificial existence, and their impact on ritual spaces, have been less discussed by modern scholars. As with many aspects of ancient sacrifice, this is a result of the lack of direct evidence. By drawing on my own experience of the Bayram sacrifices and considering certain types of scientific data not often put to work in this context, I will suggest some areas in which our inquiry may reasonably be expanded.

In antiquity, many aspects of the presacrificial treatment of animals must have differed from cult to cult, even possibly from temple to temple within one cult, as a result of factors such as size and layout of the temple grounds or wealth of the temple treasury. Furthermore, I know of no evidence related specifically to the presacrificial treatment of animals in the context of the imperial cult. It will have to suffice to make inferences, based on data drawn from other Greek and Roman cults, which may reasonably be assumed to apply also to the imperial cult. The unique nature of that cult, which was an element of official Roman state religion that developed in the Hellenistic world out of long-standing practices of hero and ruler worship, was such that it drew heavily on both traditional Greek and Roman practices in instituting its rites.

Evidence such as "shopping lists" enumerating the expenses earmarked for the important festivals of the Posideia and Eileithyaia on the Greek island of Delos in the first decades of the second century B.C.E, both of which included public sacrifice and banquets, indicates that animals were often purchased in advance; in fact, the temple records for the Posideia even include the shipping costs incurred for importing a sacrificial bull, an animal that apparently was not available on the island (Linders 1994:74).[10] It is possible that many such prepurchased animals were simply designated and set aside by cattle merchants and kept in holding pens until retrieved on the day of sacrifice, but a significant number of inscriptions from Greek sanctuaries—such as Delphi, the sanctuary of Hera at Tegea, and Ios, among others—either state regulations against storing and grazing animals within the sacred precincts (indicating that the practice was common enough to require legislation to discourage it) or specifically allow for short-term gathering and grazing of animals on-site prior to sacrificial rites (Dillon 1997). It is possible that similar practices were common at Roman sanctuaries, especially those in the Hellenistic East.

Regardless of whether the animals were kept on sanctuary grounds prior to the rites or only escorted there on the day of their death, their presence would have had a significant impact on the environment of the sanctuary. Sensorially speaking, the olfactory elements in particular would have been notable. The animals themselves produced an animal smell, of course, but by far the greatest olfactory signature of their presence would have been caused by the waste products they produced, an aspect of the experience that will be discussed in some detail below.

Ritual preparation of the victims would have enhanced their odors. On the day of an ancient sacrifice, the animals were often decorated with garlands, sometimes made of plant material, sometimes of wool.[11] Another common decorative element was a long sash, probably also constructed of wool, called a *dorsuale*. In some instances, these ritual objects passed completely around the animal's back and under its belly in the form of a band, and in other cases they were laid across the back of the animal and allowed to hang down on both sides; they figure prominently in many images of ancient sacrifice. In addition to visually signaling the special status of the animal, any type of garland or sash, whether composed of flowers, leaves, or wool, would have imparted its own scent, with the smell of wool being particularly heightened on warm days when the animals perspired; the impact of the decorations was, therefore, both visual and olfactory.

It is also of interest to consider not only the sensory elements that were produced *by* the animals but also the possible effects of other sensory elements of the process *on* the animals. In antiquity, the behavior of the animals in the moments leading up to the sacrifice was extremely important. Any mistake, mishap, or unusual event that occurred during a sacrifice could necessitate that the entire process be started again from the beginning, perhaps wasting a costly animal or even resulting in negative ritual consequences. The actions of a panicked animal had the potential to ruin the rites, and many aspects of the victims' sensory surroundings could have influenced their behavior.

Though it may seem reasonable to assume that animals involved in large-scale rites would have been negatively affected by the presence of crowds, my experience of the general docility of the Bayram animals, as well as research on domestic-animal behavioral patterns, indicates that this was likely not the case. As with the Turkish bulls, the ancient animals would have been used to existing in close quarters with one another and well acquainted with being tended to by people. According to animal-behavior expert Temple Grandin, a pig accustomed to being in proximity to a human for as little as 15 seconds per day is demonstrably easier to handle during slaughter. In addition, bulls and other cattle that have been acclimated to being near people on foot (as opposed to on horseback or in vehicles) are less excitable and less dangerous to handle in slaughterhouses (Grandin 2007:413).

Sounds, also, would have affected the demeanor of the animals. There was no music at the modern sacrifices as there would have been in antiquity; therefore, I cannot provide personal evidence of its effect on animals in a comparable situation. However, in her study of the behavior of cattle raised in the beef industry, Grandin has noted, "High-pitched sounds from hydraulic systems are very disturbing to cattle . . . [in Grandin (1980), I] discussed the use of music to help mask disturbing noises. The cattle became accustomed to the music in the holding pens and it provided a familiar sound when the animals approach [*sic*] noisy equipment" (2007:334). Though there was nothing in the ancient environment to compare with the screech of modern machinery, any loud and sudden noise during the course of a sacrificial ceremony could have startled an animal, with adverse ritual consequences. It seems likely that ancient animal handlers would have been aware of the effect of music on their stock; therefore, this modern scientific data would lend credence to the suggestion that music at the sacrificial ceremonies may have served at least in part to soothe the animals. It is also interesting to consider whether the Greeks and Romans may have played music for the animals prior to the ceremonies or, if one is uncomfortable with such a suggestion, for which I know of no supporting evidence, whether the music that was a feature of presacrificial processions would have been sufficient to successfully acclimate the animals to those types of sounds and thus to prevent extreme reactions to sudden noises closer to the time of slaughter.

Another environmental element with the potential to frighten or panic the animals, perhaps causing them to vocalize, would have been the presence of slick surfaces.[12] The majority of Greek and Roman temple precincts, including those of the imperial cult, were laid out with an exterior altar in front of the temple building. In many instances, the plaza between the temple and the altar was fully paved in slabs of marble. This surface, especially when wet with sacrificial blood, would have been extremely treacherous for hoofed animals.

The first century B.C.E. Roman poet Virgil, describing a sacrifice during a time of plague, notes that "the knife beneath the throat is scarce stained with blood, and only the surface sand (*harena*) is darkened with the thin gore" (*Georgics* 3.493, trans. Rushton Fairclough 1999). In Latin literature, *harena* is employed to refer both to areas of natural sand (such as a desert) and specifically to premises marked off for gladiatorial combat or other events (such as an amphitheater or arena). This passage raises the question of whether sand may also have been scattered in sacrificial areas.[13] If this was the case, the temporary surface would have provided two benefits: traction for the animals and a decrease in the olfactory effects of all animal by-products including gore, feces, and especially, urine.

We should also consider the effects of sensory elements on the animals and their behavior when investigating the actual moment of sacrifice. The docility of the cattle and other animals portrayed in ancient sacrificial scenes may seem to be an idealized representation of the behavior of victims, but barring loud unexpected noises, as addressed above, there was in fact no impetus for an animal to panic in the moments just before slaughter. One issue that is often of concern to modern animal-rights activists investigating slaughtering methods, and that must also have been of great importance to ancient ritual attendants responsible for managing the behavior of the animals up to the moment of their killing, is the reaction of the animals to blood. All but the first victim at an ancient sacrifice would have been led to stand at a spot covered in gore from prior victims, and it is natural to assume a reaction on the part of the animals to the sight or smell of that blood. However, as I noted in my description of the Bayram rites, this does not seem to be the case. The relative calm of those animals when exposed to the blood of their fellow victims is explained by modern science.

Grandin notes that although cattle may balk when confronted with a puddle of blood, a similar reaction can be elicited by tossing a piece of balled-up paper into their path (2007:416). The reaction is, therefore, to the novelty of the object rather than to fear of it. However, in environments that are relatively covered in blood, such as restraining boxes in kosher slaughterhouses, bovines may be observed to walk calmly into the area and willingly place their heads in restraining devices, and in some cases, they will lick or even drink the blood (Grandin 2007:417).

A caveat to this observation is that if one animal should become panicked for some reason prior to slaughter, the animals that follow will often become agitated by the scent of *that* animal's blood. Grandin reports, "An entire slaughter day can turn into a continuous chain of excited animals. The next day, after the equipment has been washed, the animals will be calm. The excited animals may be smelling an alarm pheromone from the blood of severely stressed cattle. Blood from relatively low-stressed cattle may have little effect" (2007:417). A similar response has been documented in other mammals. For instance, a rattrap that instantly kills a rat may be used again, whereas a trap that has injured a rat prior to its death will repel other rats (Eibl-Eibesfeldt 1970:136). This type of chain reaction, which ancient *victimarii* had ample opportunity to observe, provided another compelling reason to maintain the calm of the animals at all steps of the process in order to ensure the correct accomplishment of the rites.

### *The Human Sensory Experience of Ancient Sacrifice*

In the process of discussing the experience of the animals, I have covered much of what made up the visual experience of the audience at a Roman bovine sacrifice. Based on evidence in ancient literature and art, we may also enrich our mental images of the sacrifices with a good deal of knowledge about the appearance of the ritual actors. We are familiar with the costume of the *popa* and *victimarii* from Roman reliefs, such as the ones considered above. They were clad in the *limus*, a loincloth-type or wrapped garment that left them naked from the waist up, a practical arrangement considering the quantity of blood and other material they would be exposed to during the slaughtering process. Although this detail is not suggested in sacrificial art, the *victimarii* must have been thoroughly doused in the blood of their victims.

As in the Muslim sacrifices I witnessed, the man who carried out the actual killing in Roman ceremonies would have been a highly trained specialist, who no doubt had the same goal of severing the arteries, gullet, and windpipe. Not only is this the quickest and most humane approach, it would also have lessened the possibility of adverse reactions on the part of the animal—even the body of a stunned animal can react violently to extreme trauma, but the ideal cutting described above effectively discourages that. Since in antiquity the behavior of the sacrificial victim was of vital importance, killing the animal quickly and with the minimum amount of struggle must have been a primary goal.

When the sacrificant in a Roman ritual made the fatal cut, the sight of the bright, gushing—and steaming, if the sacrifices were performed early in the morning or on days in the cold seasons of the year—blood would have been an arresting element of the experience for those in attendance. However, as noted in my description of the modern sacrifices, we should not limit our sensory analysis of the bloodletting to the visual realm but should consider also both the scent and the sound of the blood. My experience of the smell of the fresh blood, and even the blood in the Bayram refuse pit, was that it was surprisingly limited and inoffensive. However, my sacrificial experience took place during the winter, on a day with low ambient temperatures. Greek and Roman cult rites were practiced year-round and, in the case of the imperial cult, many of the ceremonies were tied to important dates, such as imperial birthdays and ascension days. The probable environmental conditions and temperature at various times of the year and their potential impact on the experience of the rituals may therefore be suggested in certain individual cases. To put it bluntly, the warmer the weather at the time of year of the prescribed date of the rites, the more odoriferous those sacrifices and their by-products would have been. One may imagine that Hadrian's *vicennalia* sacrifice (see Figure 7-1), which would have taken place on or around August 11, 137 C.E., at the height of a Roman summer, must have produced smells considerably more intense than those I experienced during an Istanbul winter.

The sound of the sacrificial blood also should not be underestimated as a rich and evocative element of the proceedings. During the Bayram rites, I was forcefully struck by the sound of blood gushing from the animal onto the floor of the trailer and falling from there to the ground below (see Figure 7-5). We may assume that a similar sound was created by the blood of victims striking the ground at Greek and Roman sacrifices, a sensory aspect perhaps especially notable at rites conducted on a common monumental altar type, raised on a series of steps to approximately the same height as the Bayram trailer in relation to the spectators. Standing near the killing trailer at the Bayram rites, the sound of the blood was marked despite the other ongoing noises, such as those made by the crowd. It is not possible to say whether the music accompanying ancient sacrificial rites would have overwhelmed the sound of the blood for many of the participants, but it is likely that it would have been noticeable to those closest to the proceedings.

### *The Remnants*

One final element of the sacrificial experience that has not been addressed in detail to this point, and that is often omitted from studies on the subject, is the sensory effect of the waste produced by the sacrificial animals, and more broadly, the procedures for dealing with the detritus of sacrifice. Handling and disposing of the waste associated with large-scale sacrifices would have had a tremendous sensory impact, especially in terms of olfactory elements.

László Bartosiewicz, in his study of odors associated with the cattle trade in a late medieval town, includes a chart of the average waste production of bovines (2003:178). He estimates the mean daily output of urine for a 250–275 kg creature to be 7.5 L per day and the production of manure to just top 32 kg per animal. In one day, the individuals necessary for a true *hekatomb* would therefore have produced 3,200 kg (7,000 lb) of solid waste, roughly the capacity of an average modern dump truck!

Though Bartosiewicz was dealing with medieval cattle that as a result of breed type and differences in feed and care practices may have had a higher or lower average body weight than those offered in Roman cult scenarios, these numbers provide a basic point of consideration for ancient cattle as well. Furthermore, the strict ritual requirements for blemish-free young adult animals for Roman sacrificial purposes would likely have situated the bulls offered to the emperor in the top of their weight class. Even if we suppose that the cattle were brought to the sacrificial site only on the day of the rites, it is safe to say (based both on common sense and on my experience of the Bayram slaughter area) that a fair amount of their daily output of excreta would have ended up in the cult area.

In addition, we must factor in a further related source of waste and odor: the undigested or partially digested material that remained in the animals at the moment of death. The disposal of the waste in the stomach and intestines of the bulls and oxen must surely have been an important and immediate part of ancient sacrifice, as it was at the Bayram rites. The manure and the material that had not yet exited the animals combined to produce by far the most overpowering source of smell at the sacrifices I attended.

In addition to the waste outside and inside the animals, some portions of the body may have been discarded in antiquity. As is the case in modern Islamic sacrifices, the greater part of a sacrificial bull would have been put to use by the Romans. Following Greek tradition, the meat was divided between the priests and those participating in banquets associated with the sacrifices. After being examined by ritual specialists for imperfections that could negate the sacrifices or serve as omens of the future, certain internal organs were eaten. Some were also immolated, depending on the particulars of the rites being conducted. Mythological narratives suggest that the bones were wrapped in the hide of the animal and burned as part of the gods' portion (the ur-source on which this theory is based is found in the story of Prometheus's sacrifice to Zeus [Hesiod *Theogony* 535–555]), but as we lack either clear ancient ritual directives or firm material evidence for this practice, we should exercise caution in accepting it as a literal description of sacrificial practice. In any case, this apportioning leaves parts of the animal unaccounted for, including the hooves, tail, and what must have been a significant amount of blood that did not make it onto the altar. All of these materials would have had to have been disposed of, along with the other waste described above.

There are a great many possibilities for how the Romans may have disposed of such materials in ways that would have left little or no archaeological trace: The hooves could have been used in the manufacture of glue, and some of the manure was undoubtedly used for fertilizer. Indeed, an inscription from the Greek sanctuary of Hera at Tegea explicitly directs that the manure from sacrificial animals be sold, presumably for this purpose (Dillon 1997:126). Inedible portions of the animals not burned as part of the sacrifice might have been fed to dogs or pigs, and by the same token any parts not utilized would have had to have been disposed of in such a manner that they were protected from scavenging animals. This is not the place to pursue an exhaustive list but rather to make some suggestions regarding the sensory impact of the sacrificial waste and its disposal.

Upon my return to the Bayram site seven weeks after the sacrifices, I noted that the smell of manure lingered more strongly than did that of blood. This odor may also have been an ever-present one at frequently used ancient sacrificial sites, though it is a fair assumption that the grounds of a temple warranted more thorough cleaning than did the empty Istanbul lot. Nevertheless, it is likely that the smell was present to some degree much of the time at temples where large-scale rites were carried out.

More interesting, however, was the fact that the smell of blood was clearly distinguishable in the vicinity of the concrete retaining wall, which, as I noted, had been cleaned thoroughly. This suggests to me that the smell of blood may linger quite some time in certain hard surfaces. This has interesting implications for ancient altars and paving surfaces comprised of marble, a very porous stone that would have soaked up and retained all types of sacrificial liquid. Even if cleaned assiduously, it seems likely that the smells of sacrifice would have been in evidence near an altar long after completion of the slaughter.

There is a further issue that should be addressed in relation to waste disposal and the handling of sacrificial by-products. Though we often think of the grounds of ancient temples as clean areas, such considerations underscore the importance of contemplating whether our modern concept of "clean" affects our understanding of the condition of ancient temple areas. To keep an area free of *miasma,* or ritual taint, may very well have entailed a great deal of work on the part of temple wardens and servants, but we should not necessarily assume that it resulted in the sort of hypercleanliness that we often now picture, which is based at least partially on our experience of the ultraclean areas as they stand in archaeological sites, stripped of their human and animal inhabitants and even of their color.[14] To give only one example, it seems natural to assume that the manure produced by sacrificial animals (a by-product that falls squarely into the category of things we consider to be "dirty") would have been cleared away from sacred areas. However, ancient epigraphical evidence suggests that such waste was not necessarily considered a tainting material.

Inscriptions from a number of Greek sanctuaries explicitly spell out restrictions against, and considerable sanctions for, spreading manure (*kopros*) within their sacred boundaries. In a few cases, the wording seems to imply that the primary goal of the restriction is to preserve cleanliness—decrees from the sanctuaries of Dionysos and Leto on Delos are of this type (Dillon 1997:125). However, in other instances the restrictions seem to have had a purpose beyond the purely aesthetic or hygienic. In several cases, they appear to have been put in place in order to prevent the fertilization of sanctuary grounds for cultivation, since growing and harvesting crops was prohibited in many sacred areas. This interpretation is strengthened by the fact that other inscriptions have survived that dictate allowing *kopros* to be spread in order to facilitate the cultivation of sacred precincts. In fact, a regulation from Delphi specifically prohibits the *removal* of *kopros* from the precinct, possibly because it was either to be used for fertilizer on-site or sold to raise revenue (Dillon 1997:126). Though the practice of fertilizing temple grounds with the waste produced by sacrificial animals was probably most common at sanctuaries located outside cities, especially those with large holdings of arable land or sacred groves, such directives serve as cautionary evidence against assuming that all manure was removed from temple areas after the conclusion of sacrifice.[15]

### *The Broader Sensory Impact of Sacrificial Spaces*

Attending a modern sacrificial ceremony has allowed me to think more broadly about the range of elements that would have affected the sensory experience of cult spaces, with special attention to elements that are invisible in the evidence of ancient art and literature. This in turn has led not only to a more comprehensive understanding of the various steps involved in the sacrificial process and of the potential logistical details and complications inherent in the completion of large-scale slaughter and its cleanup, but also to an increased realization of the fact that the sensory experience of ancient cult included not only things seen, heard, smelled, tasted, and touched during the active practice of cult but also the ways in which the spaces used for sacrifice had an impact on their surroundings even in periods devoid of active sacrifice. Repeated use of the same spot for sacrifice over and over again, year after year, would have had a great and lasting impact on the cult spaces, an impact that would have spilled over into surrounding urban areas.

When considering possible responses to the impact of cult spaces on the populations of ancient cities, it should be recognized that the ancient Greeks and Romans would have perceived the sensory by-products of sacrifices somewhat differently than would a modern observer. They were accustomed to certain sights, scents, and sounds, in particular those produced by the care and sale of large domestic animals and in the context of religious sacrifices, that would be striking in modern urban settings. When repeatedly exposed to such sensory cues, individuals may become inured to them to the point that such stimuli recede into the sensory background and no longer elicit a conscious response; it is certainly true that a modern urbanite may tune out the sound of constant car traffic or that a dairy farmer may live in close proximity to cattle without being negatively affected by the scent of their waste. This amazing capacity of humans to involuntarily select the cues that require response from the vast range of sensory elements with which we are constantly bombarded should certainly be taken into consideration when formulating hypotheses about the reactions of ancient Greeks and Romans to the sensory results of sacrifice. However, it should also be noted that many of the ancient temples at which sacrifices were performed were not located close by the butcher shops, cattle stalls, and other areas where the people accustomed to related sounds and smells lived and worked on a daily basis but rather were sited in important civic locations, such as public squares, and even in or near fora and agorae, the seats of municipal business.

The sensory landscape of Greek and Roman cities may have been replete with scents that are unfamiliar to us today but that were commonplace to their inhabitants, but they were also organized in such a way that certain categories of sights, sounds, and smells were relegated in large part to carefully circumscribed areas. In contrast, when large numbers of bovines or other sacrificial animals were led to a temple in an important public area to be slaughtered and offered to the gods, sensory elements normally associated with other parts of the city were introduced into an unfamiliar context and would thus have been very notable, even if we factor in the ways in which the sense palette of those ancient societies differed from our own. As Bartosiewicz suggests, when analyzing the sensescapes of human environments, "It is worth distinguishing between acute or dynamic smells (that carry new information and influence human decisions) and chronic or static smells (a constant and unavoidable part of the cultural landscape)" (2003:188). By virtue of their location, the sacrificial odors produced at many Greek and Roman temples did not, in fact, fall into the category of "chronic" smells.

The degree of the odors should also be taken into account when analyzing the impact of the sacrifices. Offerings on such an overwhelming scale as a *hekatomb* were by no means a daily occurrence. They were costly illustrations of the power and prominence of a deity (or of the emperor) and would have been limited to special occasions. Even those individuals living in close proximity to the temples, who may have "tuned out" the smells, sounds, and sights of smaller scale, more common rites, would have felt (and smelled, heard, and been visually affected by) the impact of a sacrifice on the scale of a *hekatomb*. Therefore, while cultivating an awareness of the ways in which the sensescape of ancient cities differed markedly from our own experience of city living, we may also acknowledge that the sensory impact of large-scale ancient sacrifice, including all the elements discussed above, would have been notable and impressive in an urban setting.

By considering the full range of sensory experiences that accompanied ancient cult rites—visual and auditory cues, things smelled, tasted, and touched—we may construct a more robust and provocative picture of Greek and Roman sacrifice. The value of such a study lies not in re-creating the sensory experience of an ancient worshipper, an exercise that in any case would yield ultimately untestable hypotheses. Rather, given the enormous ritual importance of the sensory products of ancient sacrifice, a deeper analysis of those elements of the rites may lead to a more nuanced understanding of the processes and meanings of the sacrifices. I have illustrated here some ways in which an autoethnographic analysis of modern sacrificial practice, an approach not heretofore applied to the study of Greek and Roman sacrifice, may be combined with traditional historical and archaeological inquiry to enhance our understanding of some sensory elements of ancient ritual and their effects within the ancient city.

## Acknowledgments

Research in Turkey was generously supported by a Fulbright Full Grant for dissertation research (2008–2009), administered by the U.S. Department of State, and a Junior Residential Fellowship at the Koç University Research Center for Anatolian Civilizations in Istanbul (2008–2009). I wish to express particular thanks to Professor Sait Özervarlı of Yıldız Teknik Üniversitesi for arranging my attendance at the Kurban Bayram sacrifices and to Ilhan Bey, the representative from the Department of Health for the Beyoğlu Municipality who escorted me to the event and facilitated my photography and filming of the proceedings.

## Notes

1. For an overview, see Ryberg (1955).

2. We know the ritual title and role of the *popa* from the Roman authors Suetonius (*De Vita Caesarum* 4.32) and Servius (*Ad Aeneid* 12.120).

3. Pollini does not discuss the mosaic as an image of a choir.

4. See, for example, the Roman writer Claudian (*De Consulatu Stilichonis* 1.58).

5. Such research has been carried out in studies of neo-Greek sacrifice. See Georgoudi (1989) for an analysis of modern *Kourbánia* in Greek Orthodox practice and their relationship to ancient Greek sacrificial rites.

6. The ethnographer Karl Heider (1975) was perhaps the first to use the term, in an article on the Dani culture of the highlands of West Papua New Guinea.

7. As stated above, the intent of this exercise is not to draw direct comparisons between the ancient and modern rites. For this reason, I will provide few theological explanations of Muslim practices except in instances in which explanations are material to the analysis of the sensory elements of sacrifice. For a thorough explanation of the process of Islamic Kurban and its Koranic bases, see Siddiqi (2000).

8. In Islamic tradition it is the "true firstborn" of Abraham (that is, Ishmael his son by his handmaiden Hagar) who is the intended sacrifice, not Isaac as in the biblical narrative.

9. For reasons of public hygiene, residents are required to bring their sacrifices to a designated location within each neighborhood where the ritual is to be performed. There are some who ignore this directive and carry out the slaughter in the street, on playgrounds, even on apartment balconies, but as a result of increased pressure from the city government, the largest numbers of animals are now sacrificed in city-designated areas.

10. For a brief discussion of the stock-rearing industry in relation to sacrifice, see Rüpke (2007:152–153).

11. See, for example, Virgil *Georgics* 3.487.

12. Grandin notes that slippery floors increase agitation in cattle and are a source of additional animal stress in almost 20 percent of the beef plants she studied (Grandin 2007:420).

13. It is also possible that Virgil is describing a surface in an area other than the grounds of a large temple.

14. In Roman cult practice, prior to the slaughter of an animal a symbolic cleansing was effected by sprinkling water around the altar, an action that may have resulted in ritual cleanliness when physical cleanliness was not possible, given the waste produced during sacrifice.

15. The presence of significant amounts of manure, deposited for even a relatively short period of time, leaves a recognizable chemical signature in soil. It is regrettable that all known imperial cult sanctuaries were first excavated prior to the most recent archaeological advances in soil collection and chemical analysis, which might have yielded evidence of the treatment of this type of sacrificial detritus.

## References

Bartosiewicz, László
2003 "There's something rotten in the state . . .": Bad Smells in Antiquity. *European Journal of Archaeology* 6:175–195.
Burrell, Barbara
2004 *Neokoroi: Greek Cities and Roman Emperors*. Brill, Leiden.
Calvino, Italo
1988 Under the Jaguar Sun. In *Under the Jaguar Sun*. Translated by William Weaver, pp. 1–30. Harcourt Brace Jovanovich, San Diego.
Denzin, Norman
1989 *Interpretive Biography*. Sage, Newbury Park, California.
Dillon, Matthew P. J.
1997 The Ecology of the Greek Sanctuary. *Zeitschrift für Papyrologie und Epigraphik* 118:113–127.
Dorst, John D.
1989 *The Written Suburb: An American Site, An Ethnographic Dilemma*. University of Pennsylvania Press, Philadelphia.
Eibl-Eibesfeldt, Irenäus
1970 *Ethology: The Biology of Behavior*. Holt, Reinhart, and Winston, New York.
Fishwick, Duncan
1987–2005 *The Imperial Cult in the Latin West: Studies in the Ruler Cult of the Western Provinces of the Roman Empire*. 3 vols. Brill, Leiden.
Fless, Friederike
1995 *Opferdiener und Kultmusiker auf stadtrömischen historischen Reliefs: Untersuchungen zur Ikonographie, Funktion und Benennung*. Philipp von Zabern, Mainz.
Fless, Friederike, and Katja Moede
2007 Music and Dance: Forms of Representation in Pictorial and Written Sources. In *A Companion to Roman Religion*, edited by Jörg Rüpke, pp. 249–262. Blackwell, Oxford.
Friesen, Steven J.
2001 *Twice Neokoros: Ephesus, Asia, and the Cult of the Flavian Imperial Family*. Brill, Leiden.
Georgoudi, Stella
1989 Sanctified Slaughter in Modern Greece: The "Kourbánia" of the Saints. In *The Cuisine of Sacrifice among the Greeks*, edited by Marcel Detienne and Jean-Pierre Vernant, pp. 183–203. University of Chicago Press, Chicago.
Grandin, Temple
1980 Livestock Behavior as Related to Handling Facility Design. *International Journal of the Study of Animal Problems* 1:33–52.
2007 *Livestock Handling and Transport*. 3rd ed. CABI Publishing, Cambridge, Massachusetts.
Harvey, Susan Ashbrook
2006 *Scenting Salvation: Ancient Christianity and the Olfactory Imagination*. University of California Press, Berkeley.
Heider, Karl G.
1975 What Do People Do? Dani Auto-Ethnography. *Journal of Anthropological Research* 31:3–17.
Linders, Tullia
1994 Sacred Menus on Delos. In *Ancient Greek Cult Practice From the Epigraphical Evidence*: Proceedings of the Second International Seminar on Ancient Greek Cult,

Swedish Institute at Athens, 22–24 November 1991, edited by Robin Hägg, pp. 71–79. Svenska Institutet i Athen, Stockholm.

Pollini, John

2003 Slave-Boys for Sexual and Religious Service: Images of Pleasure and Devotion. In *Flavian Rome: Culture, Image, Text,* edited by Anthony J. Boyle and William J. Dominik, pp. 149–166. Brill, Leiden.

Pratt, Mary Louise

1994 Transculturation and Autoethnography: Peru 1615/1980. In *Colonial Discourse/Postcolonial Theory,* edited by Frances Barker, Peter Holme, and Margaret Iverson, pp. 24–46. Manchester University Press, Manchester, United Kingdom.

Price, Simon R. F.

1984 *Rituals and Power: The Roman Imperial Cult in Asia Minor*. Cambridge University Press, Cambridge.

Quasten, Johannes

1983 *Music and Worship in Pagan and Christian Antiquity*. National Association of Pastoral Musicians, Washington, D.C.

Reed-Danahay, Deborah E.

1997 Introduction. In *Auto/Ethnography: Rewriting the Self and the Social,* edited by Deborah E. Reed-Danahay, pp. 1–17. Berg, Oxford.

Rüpke, Jörg

2007 *Religion of the Romans.* Translated by Richard Gordon. Polity, Cambridge.

Ryberg, Inez Scott

1955 *Rites of the State Religion in Roman Art*. Memoirs Vol. 22. American Academy in Rome, Rome.

Siddiqi, Muhammad I.

2000 *The Ritual of Animal Sacrifice in Islam.* Kazı, Lahore, Pakistan.

Strathern, Marilyn

1987 The Limits of Auto-Anthropology. In *Anthropology at Home,* edited by Anthony Jackson, pp. 16–37. Tavistock, London.

Van Maanen, John

1995 An End to Innocence: The Ethnography of Ethnography. In *Representation in Ethnography,* edited by John Van Maanen, pp. 1–35. Sage, London.

Virgil

1999 *Georgics.* Translated by H. Rushton Fairclough. Harvard University Press, Cambridge.

Yerkes, Royden K.

1952 *Sacrifice in Greek and Roman Religions and Early Judaism.* Adam and Charles Black, London.

# 8. Embodying the Divine: The Sensational Experience of the Sixth-Century Eucharist

*Heather Hunter-Crawley*

*Abstract:* Through sensory analysis of a set of sixth century C.E. Syrian Eucharistic silverware, the Riha Hoard, an alternative understanding of Christian material culture for the period is proposed. Current interpretations impose a semiotic framework on this material, an approach founded on Cartesian dualism, yet Cartesianism postdates Christianity and its implication must be questioned. Introducing a sensory archaeology (here understood as the investigation of multisensory *affordances* [Knappett 2005]) liberates objects from symbolism, thus rematerializing them, revealing the centrality of embodiment to Christian identity and experience and uncovering a more interrelated notion of body and soul than semiotics allows. My approach suspends uni-sensory analysis and questions about hierarchies, instead presupposing that the body is a synthesized sensorium and, furthermore, implicating sixth-century ideas about sensing. This sensory archaeology, I suggest, offers an opportunity to reinstate as material culture art objects that, like this hoard, are aestheticized because they lack a clear archaeological context.

Christian material culture is traditionally interpreted as symbolic and exegetical in nature; images, like semiotic language, are "read" as didactic signifiers of particular scriptural truths or meanings. The archetypal sign is the cross, understood to signify the scriptural truth of Christ's sacrifice and its salvational meaning for individual Christians, but the model extends to all Christian products, from architecture to liturgy. Within this framework, all material culture acts as a

*Making Senses of the Past: Toward a Sensory Archaeology,* edited by Jo Day. Center for Archaeological Investigations, Occasional Paper No. 40.  ISBN 978-0-8093-3287-8.

referent to a Christian text and can only be interpreted inside the parameters of that text. The function of Christian material culture is therefore understood to be didactic, or exegetical: a physical means to the superior intellectual truth of scripture.[1]

There can be no doubt that scripture has always been a central component of Christianity. However, the imposition of semiotics does not automatically ensue from an interest in text; rather, because it necessitates a disembodied intellectualization of meaning, the relationship between text and semiotics is predicated on modern notions of Cartesian dualism, which assume a stark division between the intellectual and physical levels of human activity. While early Christians quite clearly were concerned with the relationship between body and soul, it would be a mistake to correlate those terms precisely with the entirely separable Cartesian categories of body and mind.

The implementation of Cartesian categories in contemporary interpretations of premodern Christian art is not surprising; Descartes's philosophy was, after all, a product of the same Reformation, and subsequently Enlightenment, movement that gave birth to Protestant Christianities that advocate text over image, scripture over ritual, and language over experience. But early Christians were not modern Protestants, and academia, itself founded on Enlightenment philosophy, must be mindful of assumptions of sameness rather than of difference (cf. Howes 2005).

Disregarding the supposition that Christian soul and body were understood as separable entities means the assumption that early Christians were opposed to the body and were, therefore, immaterialists must be readdressed. The relationship between soul and body for early Christians was a lot more nuanced and complex, and a lot less distinct, than traditional interpretations allow. The importance of embodiment to early Christianity cannot be dismissed.

Importantly, recent influential studies of early Christian art have begun to consider embodiment, but this movement has been limited. For example, although it emphasizes the importance of the viewer, Jaś Elsner's work (1995, 1998) is still primarily concerned with the symbolic and exegetical, and while considering the viewer is a progressive step, it is one that still enforces the Enlightenment paradigm of an ocularcentric sensory hierarchy. Studies by Susan Ashbrook Harvey (2006) and Patricia Cox Miller (2009), meanwhile, have begun to investigate the role of smell and the sensorium, but only in terms of discourse (that is, on a disembodied intellectual and literary level). In these studies, texts are the only source material used, to the neglect of material culture (excepting its limited consideration as an alternative form of discourse).[2] To "read" material culture as discourse is a semiotic process whereby intellectual activity in fact denies material culture its own materiality. Yet, in the absence of materiality, there can be no embodiment and no sensing.

Indeed, the semiotic paradigm as a whole denies ancient Christian material culture its materiality. As a result, the evidence is valued only for intellectual, and not material, qualities—either for its aesthetics (as art) or perceived signification (as discourse). The signifier is superseded in importance by the signified, rendering objects purely as encoded ideas to be deciphered. As art, the object is desensitized, placed in a glass museum case to satisfy the isolated visual pleasures of the modern rational eye. This is especially the case for objects that have been orphaned from a clear archaeological context (the means by which archaeology can claim art objects as artifacts).

A prime example of this is the Riha Hoard, a set of Byzantine Eucharistic equipment from the sixth century C.E.[3] Through a case study of this well-known example of Byzantine art, I will suggest that sensory archaeology offers an opportunity to resensitize such "orphaned" objects and to make new insights about early Christian material culture. I will illustrate how the material properties of these objects enable particular sensory engagements and uses. Carl Knappett's (2005) concept of the *affordances* of objects informs this approach; he proposes that artifacts should be interpreted through the functions and uses enabled by their form and construction (a teacup's qualities afford it being held by the handle and sipped from, for example). I extend this to imply potential sensory interactions afforded by objects—how they invite kinesthesia, interoception, being heard, tasted, touched, and so on. Advantageously, this method enables the derivation of archaeological information that is not reliant on context, and by marrying these sensory affordances with probable contextual information (provided by comparable and related finds), we can gain new insights about function and use.

A further aspect of my approach responds to recent sensory studies that are predominantly concerned with the question of sensory hierarchies (e.g., Classen 1993; Harvey 2006). This involves breaking down the sensorium into component sensory capacities that are independently considered, yet human existence is not about isolated sensory experiences felt in turn but rather about the constant synthesis of channels of experience within the body as a unified sensory organ (cf. Howes 2005). It is therefore more indicative of past lived experiences to consider conjunctions of sensations and this is the approach I adopt here, exploring not just the sensory affordances offered to each sense but how a multiplicity of sensations is concurrently afforded.

Finally, while critical of the overuse of discursive source material, this study does not advocate its neglect but rather checks its predominance in scholarship. Because we have discursive evidence for some ancient Christian ideas about sensory experience, there is an added opportunity to engage sensory affordances through the lens of ancient Christian cultural thought rather than purely through the modern cultural idea of the five senses, which can be as distorting as dualist assumptions (Hurcombe 2007). That is, the full range of sensory affordances is not restricted to "biological" capacities for sensing (as defined by contemporary science) but can also incorporate cultural constructions of sense experience (for example, the synesthetic mapping of touch onto sight through extramission theory) as expressed in written sources. Where relevant, therefore, discursive evidence and its analyses are introduced into my investigation of sensory affordances, but they are nowhere dealt with in isolation from the material. In this way, both discourse and materiality can be brought together to reveal the embodied experience of ancient Christian ritual practice and its central importance to a religion that did not make sharp distinctions between the spiritual and the material.

## The Riha Hoard

The Riha Hoard is considered the finest of Syria's several sixth- and seventh-century hoards of church silver, of which other examples include the Ma'aret en-Noman, Beth Misona, and Phela Treasures. It consists of a silver paten, chalice, and fan (Figures 8-1 through 8-3). Patens and chalices are common among the other Syrian hoards that include a number of stylistically parallel examples, but the fan, despite its liturgical importance, is one of only two extant sixth-century examples in silver. The collective survival of these principal liturgical implements makes them an apt case study for Eucharistic ritual as a whole since they probably constituted a set for performing the Eucharist in a particular church in Syria. Imperial control stamps date the objects to the sixth century, and an inscription acknowledges a wealthy patron who donated them for liturgical use.

Beyond this, our knowledge of their context is patchy; the hoard's modern history is abstruse, and its reconstruction is tenuous. It was probably unearthed in 1908 from a tilled field near Stuma in northern Syria, along with around 53 other pieces of sixth- and seventh-century liturgical silverware, now collectively termed the Kaper Koraon Treasure (Mango 1986). The majority of these pieces instantly entered the art market and passed, in different groupings, through numerous collections during the twentieth century. They are currently housed in around eight collections under varying names (the Stuma, Hama, and Antioch Treasures), with the Riha set comprising a key part of the Dumbarton Oaks Collection in Washington, D.C. Because the silverware had such immediate cultural capital as art objects, their true archaeological context is long lost (though reconstructions have been attempted from old photographs and museum cleaning records, the results are inconclusive [Mango 1986]). As a result, most analyses focus on art historical concerns such as iconography and style, occasionally complemented by technical information such as metallurgical analysis (Mango 1986; Ross 1962). Where the objects' functions and meanings are considered, these are filtered through a narrow range of textual sources relating to liturgy, predominantly the *Apostolic Constitutions* and Germanos's *Historia Mystagogica*, none of which are truly contemporary or geographically consonant (Boyd 1998; Doig 2008:53–83; Mango 1986:147–154). This practice constricts analysis to a symbolist interpretative framework that denies the objects their materiality. Can a sensory archaeology rematerialize the Riha Hoard?

### *The Paten*

The paten is particularly celebrated as a paragon of early Byzantine art and as iconographic evidence for Eucharistic ritual practice of the period (Figure 8-1). It depicts the communion of the Apostles, with Christ officiating twice over the bread and wine. Though this is the ideal and original Eucharist, it takes place in the context of a sixth-century church, as architectural features such as the shell niche, columns, and altar indicate. However, rather than dwell on the iconography of this dish, I turn to an aspect that has not yet been addressed: its sensory affordances.

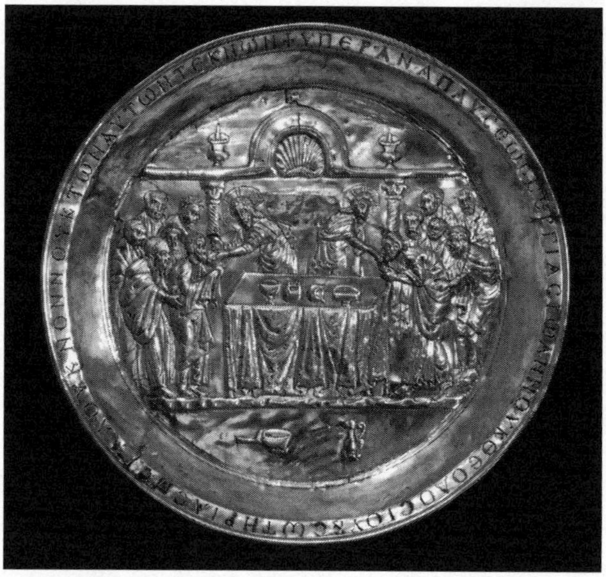

**Figure 8-1.** *The Riha paten. (Dumbarton Oaks Collection, Washington, D.C., BZ.1924.5. Diameter 35 cm, weight 904 g.* © Dumbarton Oaks, Byzantine Collection, Washington, D.C.)

From the fourth century, Christians had what is termed a "jeweled" aesthetic. An increase in wealth enabled a proliferation of sacred objects in gold, silver, jewels, glass, enamels, and rich colors produced from expensive dyes (Miller 2009; Roberts 1989). In tandem, Christianity developed a concept that light reflective surfaces contained spiritual properties. Christ was viewed as a god of light, on a par with Sol and other solar deities, which may have been the religion's main attraction to new converts ("God is light," 1 John 1:5; Jensen 2000:41–44). Gold and silver surfaces were understood not to reflect the light of the sun but to emit a divine light of their own (Franses 2003). In his description of the sixth-century Hagia Sophia cathedral, the historian Procopius notes, "You might say that the [interior] space is not illuminated by the sun from the outside, but that the radiance is generated within" (*On Buildings* 1.1.23, trans. Mango 1972:74), and Paul the Silentiary comments similarly that "no words are sufficient to describe the illumination in the evening: You might say that some nocturnal sun filled the majestic temple with light" (*Description of Hagia Sophia* 806, trans. Mango 1972:89). The presence of light *is* the presence of God inside this space, making the building almost heaven on earth. The Riha paten depicts a comparable architectural space clothed in silver, and the divine figures of Christ and the apostles are highlighted in gold—a metal in which divine light was understood to reside the most (Franses 2003). In this respect, the act of looking at the paten affords bearing witness to the epiphanic presence of the divine in the form of golden and silver light, a light that rebounded from the surfaces of ritual objects and architectural space in which the paten was used.

It is important to note here that vision, in this period, was understood to be a tactile phenomenon. Georgia Frank has shown that early pilgrims gazed on holy sites and relics with "eyes as hands" (2000:109), by extramission. This philosophical theory, current in the sixth century, proposed that the eyeball emits rays that touch objects and bring back a "skin," or physical property, of what they encounter to be experienced by the eye. Vision was, in effect, an extension of the sense of touch. In the context of this cultural understanding of sight, we can appreciate that the act of looking at a material object with spiritual qualities entailed a profound physical encounter with divinity. In the spiritual light of precious metals, the sixth-century Christian was afforded visual-tactile contact with God.

The paten, as a dish for a ritual feast, also affords tactile contact with the skin. Late Antique feasting involved the sharing of a central dish from which diners would take food with their hands. There is an observable trend for such dishes to feature decoration on their interior rather than exterior surfaces, usually in relief.[4] Diners' primary engagement with such decoration would be tactile, in taking food, rather than visual because the image would only be visible when the dish was empty. Bringing this mnemonic feasting practice with them to church, participants in the Eucharist who took bread from the paten were afforded a tactile encounter with the cool repoussé figures of Christ and his disciples. Gradually, with each piece of bread taken, a little more gleaming gold would become visible, reflecting the portion of eternal life achieved by each individual through his or her participation in the ritual. Once empty, Christ could be seen within the paten by "eyes as hands," complementing the tactile contact made with his body, as image and as Eucharistic bread, which occurred while the relief was covered.

The paten is inscribed around the rim in Greek: "For the repose [of the soul] of Sergia, [daughter] of John, and of Theodosios, and [for] the salvation of Megas and of Nonnous and of their children" (trans. Mango 1986:166, brackets in original). Unlike the rest of the decoration, this is executed in niello (blackened silver sulfide paste), which was packed into the engraved letters. Although composed of precious metal, niello lacks the divine gleam of the central figures, indicating a difference between the words and the image here. The inscription's words are a votive prayer from the paten's donors. Votive offerings served to embody and immortalize a request because the dedicant's prayer would be reembodied, that is, vocalized and made audible, with every reading. In studying texts, classicists can forget that in antiquity reading was an embodied act; to read was to speak aloud and to make heard not necessarily to observe silently in private contemplation. Furthermore, speech could be understood as a form of sense in antiquity (Classen 1993:2), so the act of reading was a twofold sensory experience involving both mouth and ears. The donors of this paten no doubt hoped that their salvation would be ensured through the perpetual embodiment of their prayer, as sound and speech, each time the dish was used.

### *The Chalice*

By contrast, the words inscribed on the Riha chalice functioned as an important auditory and spoken part of the Eucharistic ritual itself (Figure 8-2). The only other decoration is two bands of gold that frame the letters and indicate their sanctity. They read: "Thine own of Thine own we offer Thee, O Lord"

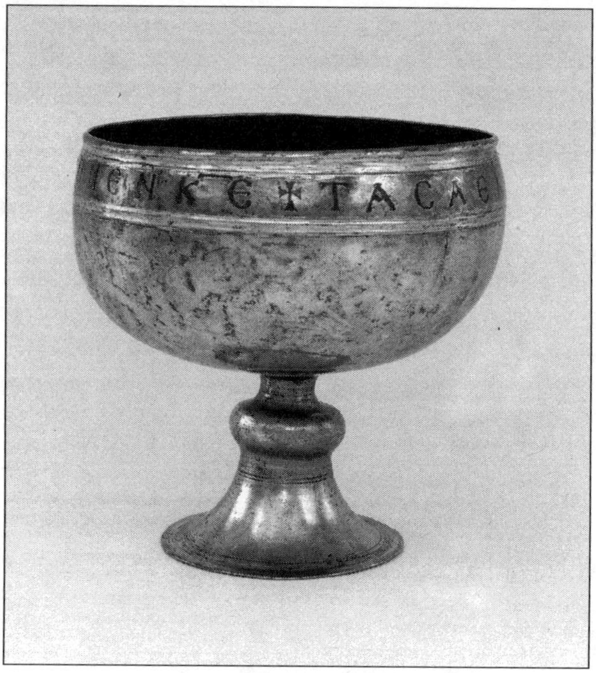

**Figure 8-2.** The Riha chalice. *(Dumbarton Oaks Collection, Washington, D.C., BZ.1955.18. Height 17.5 cm, weight 528 g.* © Dumbarton Oaks, Byzantine Collection, Washington, D.C.)

(trans. Ross 1962:11). This spoken statement articulated the process of exchange within the Eucharist and made it materially real through its afforded embodiment as speech and sound. It reveals the idea that body and soul are entangled, for this process of exchange involves the materialization of the divine in the wine and the divinization of the human body through ingestion of divine substance. It is impossible to make sharp distinctions between the divine and the material, or the soul and the body, in this process. This speech act was an integral part of the ritual of preparing the gifts (Doig 2008:76), and it is likely that it occurred at the miraculous moment of transubstantiation—when ordinary wine transformed into the divine substance of Christ's blood.

Significantly, the act of reading the chalice's inscription demands movement of the vessel, by rotation. Turning it would enhance the light effects of the silver and gold, emphasizing their brilliance as they sparkled and dazzled, because the surface of the chalice would undulate with subtle textures in the beaten surface of the bowl and the gentle striations on the foot. The kinesthetic experience of moving the object would bring the divine light to life, enabling watching eyes to witness divinity by means of movement. In fact, it is possible that the kinesthetic-visual–oral-aural experience of this object *caused* transubstantiation to take place. In ritual use, then, the chalice—courtesy of its sensory affordances—could become the agent for a meeting of humanity and divinity.

The iconography on the Riha paten indicates the rules of engaging with the chalice; while the officiant on the left is allowed to make contact with the vessel, the recipient respectfully covers his hands and allows himself to be fed from it. Along with the lack of tactile relief decoration afforded by the chalice, this indicates that for the congregation who used the Riha set the cup was not to be touched by hands in the act of receiving; instead, contact was made only with the lips. The act of kissing relics and icons, or *proskynesis*, was an intimate way of honoring and touching divine substance throughout this period; indeed, pilgrims to the Holy Land sought this experience as the ultimate goal of their journey. The fourth-century report of the pilgrim Egeria informs us that in the presence of the True Cross "one by one the people pass by, they prostrate themselves and touch the cross, first with forehead, then with eyes, and then they kiss it, but no one puts out a hand to touch it" (*Travels* 37.3; trans. author). We might associate lip contact with the act of embodying the chalice's sacred inscription with the mouth, both of which are ultimately linked to the experience of the divine substance of Christ's blood as the Eucharistic wine that entered the body through the mouth, an experience made sensuously possible by the chalice as container.

### *The Fan*

The third and final piece of the Riha treasure, the fan (Figure 8-3) like the chalice, had an important kinesthetic affordance. Fans were a central element of the Eucharist at this time and were used in pairs. This is usually accounted for as a symbolic hangover from their practical use in earlier days when they were made of real feathers and wafted flies away from the bread and wine (e.g., Boyd 1998:163). Besides the Riha example, there is only one other surviving sixth-century silver fan, and biblical four-winged angels appear on both.[5] Because the Riha's tetramorph has four heads (that of a man, an ox, a lion, and an eagle) it was associated with the four writers of the Gospels (Irenaeus *Against Heresies* 3.11.8), so these fans are presumed to symbolically represent a scriptural parallel between the Old and the New Testaments (Boyd 1998:177–178). This explanation of the fan's primary function seems unsatisfactory, particularly in light of the offertory prayer of the contemporary Syrian liturgy, which calls these objects in use not fans but *hexapteryga* ("six-winged creatures"), that is, actual, not represented, angels (Mango 1986:154). I propose, instead, that the act of waving the fan would reenact, or reembody, the kinesthetic affect of a biblical creature's beating wings; participants could actually feel the waft of air from a hovering being that was understood to herald the presence of God. The fan does not just depict a tetramorph in its design; rather, its silver scalloped peacockfeather border affords the materialization of that being's sacred wing as both divine light and wafted air: It makes a tetramorph present. That fans, like real wings, were used in pairs supports this view. In addition, besides the fan's sensory effect, at this time flies and other pests were understood to embody demonic forces (Maguire et al. 1989:26), so the embodiment of a divine force seems an effective way to counteract their potential to corrupt.

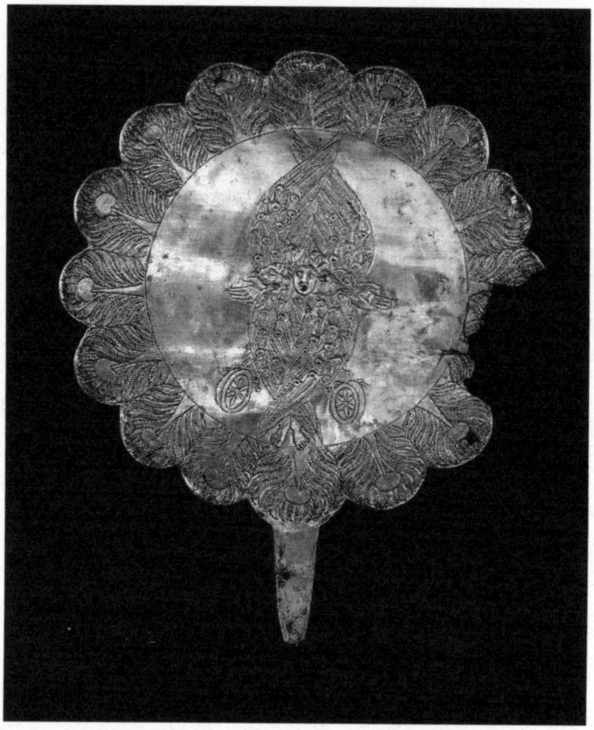

**Figure 8-3.** The Riha fan. *(Dumbarton Oaks Collection, Washington, D.C., BZ.1936.23. Width 25.5 cm, weight 485 g.* © Dumbarton Oaks, Byzantine Collection, Washington, D.C.)

The tetramorph appears in the Old Testament in Ezekiel's divine vision announcing God's presence (Ezekiel 1). The book of Ezekiel powerfully evokes multisensory experiences and forms a moralizing rebuke on the misuse of senses—which are a gift from God—while asserting the incredible power of God's own sensory effects. It is pertinent that sixth-century Christians should have felt the need to create ritual objects that make reference to a book from the Bible that is so strongly interested in sensation. This testifies to the centrality of a coherent sensory cosmology for the Eucharistic ritual and Christianity in this period. It also demonstrates that scripture was not a departure from the material world but a means of reengaging with it; it informed embodiment.

The fan would also have interacted with another important sensory experience during the Eucharist because it was used to waft incense. In antiquity, smells had the power to affect the recipient for good or evil. Beautiful smells heralded, or even embodied, divine presence and could also transport prayers as well as protect against evil; bad smells were demonic forces with the power to corrupt, by causing disease and sinfulness (Caseau 1994; Harvey 2006).[6] In a Eucharistic context, a cloud of incense could embody the sensory presence of the divine, communicate prayers, and serve as a protective or apotropaic shroud around the gifts and participants—indeed, around the whole rite itself. The kinesthetic interaction between protective incense and the waft of the fan as divine wings would have enriched this effect. Furthermore, it is possible that there was a functional link between incense and angelic wings as media for communicating prayer heavenward (Green 2006).

## The Hoard in Context

### *Liturgical Objects*

The question of incense leads us to consider the broader ritual context of the Riha Hoard and certain other important liturgical objects with which the paten, chalice, and fan were used.[7]

The Riha treasure did not include a censer but other hoards did.[8] Most of these censers are made of precious metals, are bowl shaped, have feet for upright placement, and afford being swung by chains for the movement of smoke. Swinging a censer would activate a metallic clinking sound, which may have been considered apotropaic, as was the tinkling of bells in antiquity (John Chrysostom *Homily on 1 Cor.* 12.7). The incense used took the form of granules of fragrant resins, often frankincense, scattered over hot coals. Before use, these grains were probably stored in an ivory *pyxis* (a small lidded box). An example from the Metropolitan Museum of Art, New York, (*Pyxis Depicting Women at the Tomb of Christ*, 17.190.57), makes a connection with its function through an engraved relief of the two Marys, who are swinging censers as they approach an altar. The tactile depiction of the contents in use, accompanied by the aroma of the grains inside this box, would have acted as a mnemonic device that evoked the potential sensory experiences actualized in the Eucharistic ritual itself.

An interesting bronze example of a censer from sixth-century Syria is worth special mention (Figure 8-4). While typically designed in most respects, this example also has a lid and open-worked sides to allow the incense to waft out. On the lid are four anthropomorphic faces that, while the censer was in use, would give the impression of fragrant smoke emerging from eyes and mouths; the lid would literally breathe incense. This exemplifies the sensory effects for the devotee in the shared act of inhaling and exhaling (and also seeing) the powerful incense smoke. In light of contemporary Syrian ideas about the breath of God as the ultimate source of life (Ephrem *Commentary on Genesis* 2.4; Harvey 2006:64), the censer might also have embodied or materialized a form of fragrant divine breath as incense and would have been powerfully effective in combination with other liturgical implements, such as the fan as divine wings. At the very least, it expresses a cultural interest in sensory encounters with incense.

Like censers, lamps also afforded emission of fragrance because their oil was often perfumed, especially in sacred contexts. Perfume fragrance differed from incense because it was relatively smokeless and therefore invisible, a quality that gave it a powerful mystique. In Roman literature, the epiphany of a deity as invisible perfume was a common trope; Apuleius, in his second-century novel *The Golden Ass*, describes the epiphany of the goddess Isis as "breathing out the spices of Arabia" (11.47, trans. author). It is probable that the invisible fragrance

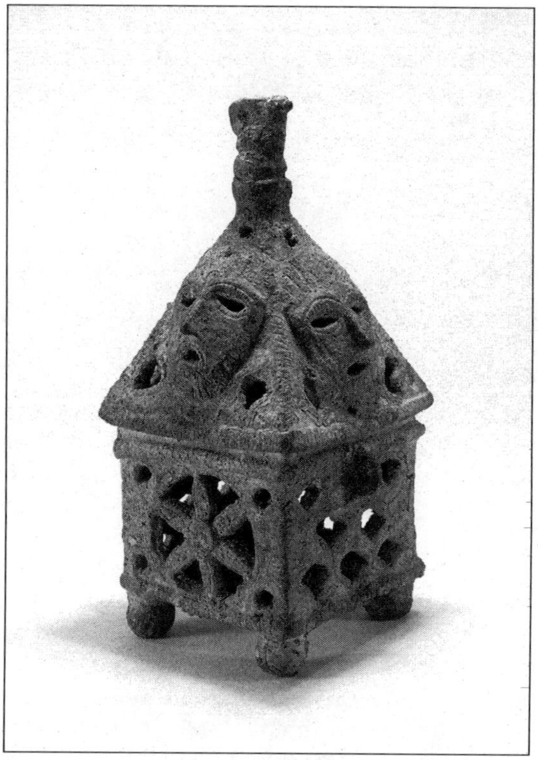

**Figure 8-4.** Bronze incense burner. *(Dumbarton Oaks Collection, Washington, D.C., BZ.1950.33. Sixth century* C.E. *Height 20 cm.* © Dumbarton Oaks, Byzantine Collection, Washington, D.C.)

of scented oils embodied divine presence in the Eucharist even more than did the visible and clinking clouds of incense, which were primarily apotropaic, thus creating subtle differences in function according to degrees of intersensibility. Harvey (2006) suggests fragrance was superior in offering access to the divine because it lacked intersensibility and was, therefore, close to immateriality. However, invisibility and immateriality are not equivalent, and as discussed, no sense operates in true isolation (see note 6).

The other important function of lamps was, of course, the emission of light, particularly since, as mentioned above, light was understood to have sensorally epiphanic qualities. It is no coincidence, therefore, that Christian lamps were designed with their light effects in mind. Metal lamps are frequently openwork and could be either portable and freestanding or large permanent fixtures (*polycandela*) that lit churches by holding quantities of small lamps, usually in glass cups (Figure 8-5). Openwork, particularly in combination with glass, afforded the casting of enlarged shadows over surrounding surfaces, and crosses featured heavily in openwork lamp designs (*polycandelon* chains were sometimes embellished with designs of colored glass to complement the effect [e.g., Benaki Museum, Athens, ΓΕ 11481]). Rather than the standard interpretation that a shadowy

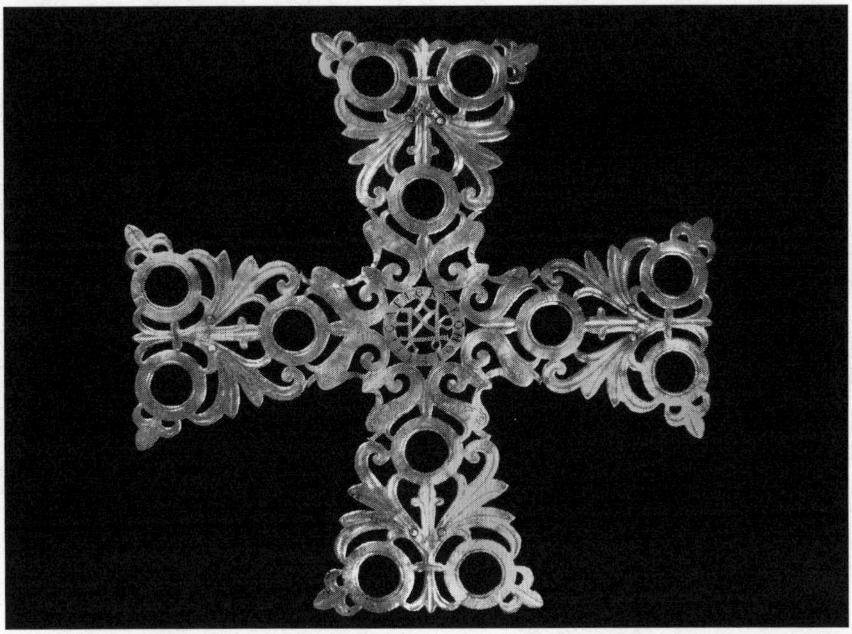

**Figure 8-5.** Cross-shaped polycandelon. *(Dumbarton Oaks Collection, Washington, D.C., BZ.1965.1.1. Sixth century* C.E. *Height 56.6 cm.* © Dumbarton Oaks, Byzantine Collection, Washington, D.C.)

cross "would have emphasized its Christian symbolism" (Metropolitan Museum of Art 2006), I suggest instead that it created a powerful visual presence of Christ.

Apocryphal Christian writings were considered important by many Christians in the sixth century, despite the lack of such texts' canonization. The apocryphal *Acts of John* include a particularly influential description of the crucifixion in which the disciple John does not witness Christ being crucified but instead, while in a cave, sees an apparition of Christ as a cross made of light:

> He showed me a cross of light set up . . . and in the cross was one form and one likeness. And the Lord himself I beheld above the cross, not having a shape, but only . . . a sweet and kind voice and one truly divine, and it said to me; . . . . This cross of light is sometimes called the Word by me for your sakes, sometimes Mind, sometimes Jesus, sometimes Christ, sometimes Door, sometimes Way, sometimes Bread. [*Acts of John* 98, translated by Elliott (1993:320)]

This tangible cross of light embodies everything that Christ is, while language is inefficient in its attempts to quantify him. It seems highly significant, then, that Christians in the sixth century were striving to create ritual objects that projected crosses of light. Should the *Acts of John* have been read aloud in the presence of a lit open-worked lamp, the result would have been a powerful visual, olfactory, and auditory multisensory materialization of the text, indeed of Christ himself. It is likely that through such an affective process the sacred text gained its power, rather than through semiotic intellection alone. Conversely, the memory of John's *Acts* would have informed the embodied experience of a cross of light whenever it occurred, with or without an accompanying recital of the text.

A final object involved in the Eucharistic ritual, and perhaps the most profound, was the gift of bread and wine, which offered the ultimate sensory experience of Christ's presence by transubstantiating into his body and blood. These items afforded the most intimate engagement of all for Christians; they could be seen, smelled, and touched (bread was textured with stamped sacred images or lettering that differentiated it from secular bread [e.g., *Bronze Stamps*, Benaki Museum, Athens, ΓΕ 11473]), but ultimately they were to be tasted and consumed—taken into the body to become one with it. Because they leave no direct archaeological trace, it is difficult to reconstruct these objects. However, it is sufficient to our understanding of the role of the senses in the Eucharist to know that it culminated in interoception. This does not mark a sensory hierarchy topped by taste but instead reveals that the whole experience was layered—building in levels of bodily intimacy from the more remote visual touch of divine sparkle to the complete interiorization of divine substance in the act of ingestion.

### *Performative Context*

To complete a more detailed picture of the sensory experience of the Eucharist in sixth-century Syria, we are obliged to look further afield than liturgical equipment. Literary sources as well as excavated and standing remains of churches can tell us more about the broader ritual and performative context of the Riha Hoard. Other studies have considered these aspects at length (Doig 2008; Mathews 1971), and it is sufficient to summarize a few key points here.

Northern Syrian church architecture was marked by a triple sanctuary at the apse end, which afforded storage of the gifts and vessels as well as a structure for their liturgical procession around the building prior to Communion. Access to this most holy area was restricted to clergy, since hierarchical access was latitudinal, with clergy in the sanctuary cordoned off from a congregation arranged according to rank (those highest in rank closest to the sanctuary barrier) (Mathews 1971:120).

The whole ritual of the Eucharist operated a play of movement and stillness and of concealment and revelation. The gifts were probably prepared in the sanctuary, hidden from view of lay Christians, and only processed (in their vessels, underneath veils) in the main part of the building once the Catechumens, or Christians in training, had been dismissed from the service. (The first part of the service, which they were permitted to attend, involved only scriptural readings.) This is not to say that nonvisual and nontactile experiences of the preparation of the gifts, such as the smell of incense and the sound of chant, were concurrently restricted, but our evidence is unfortunately inconclusive on the precise details of the procedure and, moreover, would not convey regional variations in practice.

After the gifts were processed, they were unveiled and communion took place in the vicinity of the altar; then the congregation was dismissed following a blessing. The congregation and clergy sang psalms throughout the ritual (Doig

2008; Mathews 1971). Our evidence is not clear on the regularity of Eucharistic services and can vary from specifying every Sunday to only special occasions (Mathews 1972:173). At the least, it was a practice only revealed after a degree of preparation, both personal, by becoming Christian, and communal, by attending scriptural services throughout the week or year.

We can conclude, therefore, that there were different levels of access to the ritual sensory experience of the Eucharist for sixth-century Christians. Indeed, the interactive full-body experience of the divine, for which purpose the Riha Hoard was designed, was the culmination of Christian liturgy over and above the reading of scripture to which all were allowed access, whether fully Christian or not. Eucharistic practice defined Christian identity, and that practice was fully embodied, not intellectually abstract.

## Conclusion

Through an investigation of sensory affordances for a set of representative objects, it has become clear that an overlapping and layered multisensory experience was integral to the sixth-century Eucharist. Its performance enabled Christian worshippers to physically experience divine presence—in the cross of light, the shining silverware, the movements of the objects, the divine perfume, the apotropaic incense, the tactile relief of Christ and the apostles, the spoken and heard ritual formulae inscribed on the objects, the waft of angelic wings, and most importantly, in the taste and interoceptive consumption of ordinary bread and wine transubstantiated into Christ's body and blood—aspects all experienced through intermingled sensations like tactile-sight, speech-hearing, and kinesthetic-smell.

Through the implication of a sensory archaeology, then, it is possible to repeople the Christian past and to rematerialize Christian material culture. Evidence that is consigned to art history and aesthetics as a result of being orphaned from a clear archaeological context has been revealed as central for understanding Christian material practice, and as a result, Christian ritual has been revealed as central for understanding the ancient religion itself. This indicates that sensory experience of the much-neglected embodied practice of Christianity, encouraged and emphasized through ritual, was a central means of accessing the divine. Over and above text, the ritual practice of material culture was where Christianity *happened* for ancient Christians. While discursive analysis of text has here contributed to the range of culturally constructed sensory affordances, in isolation it imposes a constrictive interpretative framework that is detrimental to our understanding of both material and literary evidence and, thus, of Christian ritual and culture. The need therefore becomes apparent for the function of text itself to be readdressed as an auditory, spoken, and visual phenomenon with mnemonic potential to plug in to all the senses, indeed as an embodied experience.

Because material culture was a vital agent in the congruence of humanity and divinity for ancient Christians, a much more complex understanding of the interaction between the divine and the material becomes apparent than current interpretations allow. A sensory archaeology for this period enables progression from the impasse of symbolist and Cartesian frameworks and, instead, provides us with a glimpse of the incredibly rich world of the senses that sixth-century Christians inhabited.

It now remains to be seen what important new insights a multisensory archaeology of affordances for "orphaned" finds can offer to studies of other cultures. The results of this study suggest that a great deal of potential information might be sitting in the storerooms and galleries of museums and collections, yet to be realized or, indeed, embodied.

## Notes

1. This is an entrenched tradition with a long history. Exemplary studies include those of André Grabar (1969:xlvi), who viewed Christian material culture as an "iconographic language," Jaś Elsner (1995, 1998), for whom "the [Christian] image relied on a prior text—a scripture—for its meaning" (1998:251), Robin M. Jensen (2000:6, 30), who considers art and text to be parallel modes of (primarily) symbolic and exegetical discourse, and most recently, Gérard-Henry Baudry's (2009) catalog of Christian symbols in art and text.

2. Miller's only sustained recourse to material evidence is an analysis of sarcophagi iconography for characterizing the discursive phenomenon of a fragmentary aesthetic (2009:42–61); while Harvey mentions that it is inappropriate to imply Cartesian dualism in Late Antique Christian understandings of soul and body, she does not acknowledge the Cartesian entrenchment of her own study in its neglect of material evidence (2006:170–171). Interestingly, her discursive findings lead her to conclude that ritual was an important means of accessing the divine. However, she does not explore this in terms of lived experience (ritual in practice rather than in discourse), and as mentioned above, discourse and materiality become meaningless in isolation.

3. All dates mentioned in this chapter are C.E.

4. A typical example can be seen in the Byzantine Collection of Dumbarton Oaks, Washington, D.C., in a fifth-century shallow silver bowl with a hunting scene (BZ.1947.12).

5. The almost identical Stuma fan in the Istanbul Archaeological Museum, 3759, is probably the pair of the Riha fan (Mango 1986:159–164; Ross 1962:16).

6. Harvey (2006) argues that fragrance enabled Late Antique Christians to encounter the divine in a way unparalleled by other senses. However, as discussed above, a segregating approach can distort, and in actuality, a powerful experience of smell could only have occurred in a multisensory context.

7. The objects selected for discussion here are by no means an exhaustive representation of the implements and materials used in the sixth-century Eucharist, and those implements not chosen warrant further study.

8. For example, the Attarouthi Treasure (Metropolitan Museum of Art, 1986.3.1–15) contains three censers; the Sion Treasure, a hexagonal peacock censer (Dumbarton Oaks, BZ.1965.1.5).

## References

Baudry, Gérard-Henry
2009 *Simboli Cristiani delle origini: I-VII secolo.* Jaca Book, Milan.
Boyd, Susan A.
1998 Art in the Service of the Liturgy: Byzantine Silver Plate. In *Heaven on Earth: Art and the Church in Byzantium,* edited by Linda Safran, pp. 160–63. Pennsylvania State University Press, Pennsylvania.
Caseau, Béatrice
1994 *Euōdia:* The Use and Meaning of Fragrances in the Ancient World and Their Christianization (100–900 A.D.). Ph.D. dissertation, Department of Classics, Princeton University, Princeton, New Jersey.
Classen, Constance
1993 *Worlds of Sense: Exploring the Senses in History and across Cultures.* Routledge, New York.
Doig, Allan
2008 *Liturgy and Architecture: From the Early Church to the Middle Ages.* Ashgate, Aldershot.
Elliott, James K.
1993 *The Apocryphal New Testament: A Collection of Apocryphal Christian Literature in an English Translation.* Clarendon, Oxford.
Elsner, Jaś
1995 *Art and the Roman Viewer: The Transformation of Art from the Pagan World to Christianity.* Cambridge University Press, Cambridge.
1998 *Imperial Rome and Christian Triumph: The Art of the Roman Empire, A.D. 100–450.* Oxford University Press, Oxford.
Frank, Georgia
2000 The Pilgrim's Gaze in the Age before Icons. In *Visuality before and beyond the Renaissance: Seeing as Others Saw,* edited by Robert S. Nelson, pp. 98–115. Cambridge University Press, Cambridge.
Franses, Rico
2003 When All That Is Gold Does Not Glitter: On the Strange History of Looking at Byzantine Art. In *Icon and Word, the Power of Images in Byzantium: Studies Presented to Robin Cormack,* edited by Antony Eastmond and Liz James, pp. 13–24. Ashgate, Aldershot.
Grabar, André
1969 *Christian Iconography: A Study of Its Origins.* Routledge and Keagan Paul, London.
Green, Nile
2006 Ostrich Eggs and Peacock Feathers: Sacred Objects as Cultural Exchange between Christianity and Islam. *Al-Masaq: Islam and the Medieval Mediterranean* 18:27–66.
Harvey, Susan Ashbrook
2006 *Scenting Salvation: Ancient Christianity and the Olfactory Imagination.* University of California Press, Berkeley.
Howes, David
2005 Introduction: Empires of the Senses. In *Empire of the Senses: The Sensual Culture Reader,* edited by David Howes, pp.1–17. Berg, Oxford.
Hurcombe, Linda
2007 A Sense of Materials and Sensory Perception in Concepts of Materiality. *World Archaeology* 39:532–545.

Jensen, Robin M.
2000 *Understanding Early Christian Art*. Routledge, New York.
Knappett, Carl
2005 *Thinking through Material Culture: An Interdisciplinary Perspective*. University of Pennsylvania Press, Philadelphia.
Maguire, Eunice Dauterman, Henry Maguire, and Maggie J. Duncan-Flowers
1989 *Art and Holy Powers in the Early Christian House*. University of Illinois Press, Urbana.
Mango, Cyril A.
1972 *The Art of the Byzantine Empire, 312–1453: Sources and Documents*. Prentice-Hall, New Jersey.
Mango, Marlia Mundell
1986 *Silver from Early Byzantium: The Kaper Koraon and Related Treasures*. Trustees of the Walters Art Gallery, Maryland.
Mathews, Thomas F.
1971 *The Early Churches of Constantinople: Architecture and Liturgy*. Pennsylvania State University Press, Pennsylvania.
Metropolitan Museum of Art
2006 Polycandelon with Crosses [Byzantine] (2002.483.7). In *Heilbrunn Timeline of Art History*, Electronic document, http://www.metmuseum.org/toah/works-of-art/2002.483.7, accessed July 8, 2010.
Miller, Patricia Cox
2009 *The Corporeal Imagination: Signifying the Holy in Late Ancient Christianity*. University of Pennsylvania Press, Philadelphia.
Roberts, Michael J.
1989 *The Jeweled Style: Poetry and Poetics in Late Antiquity*. Cornell University Press, Ithaca, New York.
Ross, Marvin
1962 *Metalwork, Ceramics, Glass, Glyptics, Painting*, Vol. 1. *Catalogue of the Byzantine and Early Mediaeval Antiquities in the Dumbarton Oaks Collection*. Dumbarton Oaks Research Library and Collection, Washington, D.C.

# 9. A Sense of Touch—the Full-Body Experience—in the Past and Present of Çatalhöyük, Turkey

*Ruth Tringham*

*Abstract:* In this paper I come to the more general issues of a sensuous archaeology through the sense of touch—the haptic sense. Using data from the Neolithic site of Çatalhöyük, Turkey, I stress that the sense of touch involves far more than just fingers and skin, far more than the obvious haptic sensations, such as surface, form, pressure, pain, temperature, and texture. It involves the full-body sensations of balance and the sense of movement in any part of the body. I anchor my investigation of touch and movement in the past in the archaeological data using existing methodologies such as contact trace analysis and human kinetics. I argue that the concept of taskscapes enables us to think about the temporality, events, and rhythms of the body's haptic responses, which themselves are essential elements for understanding social practice. I suggest that another anchor to investigating sensory responses in the past is to research the process by which practices that started as new and unfamiliar experiences became familiar and "enactive knowledge." I end with an exploration of the potential of digital technologies to transform the sharing of archaeological interpretations of past multisensorial experience that include the sense of touch.

## Sensing Place Through Practice

The potential of a sensuous archaeology pursued through the exploration of ideas of embodiment and landscape perspectives and through the embrace of phenomenology (for example, Bender 1993; Bender et al. 2007; Joyce and Lopiparo 2005; Tilley 1994, Tilley 2008) is gaining momentum.

*Making Senses of the Past: Toward a Sensory Archaeology,* edited by Jo Day. Center for Archaeological Investigations, Occasional Paper No. 40.  ISBN 978-0-8093-3287-8.

My concept of place and its multisensorial experience is very much in line with the practice-based concepts of place as expressed by cultural geographers. Tim Cresswell (2004), for example, summarizes a view of place by incorporating remembered or imagined fragments of practices and events triggered through movement, sound, and visual media, which is very different from the traditional "visualizing" of past places by archaeologists. The connection between place and the senses has been made by a number of other writers (Gibson 1968; Ingold 2000; Merleau-Ponty 2003; Porteous 1990; Rodaway 1994; Tuan 1993).

My aim in this chapter is to address the more general issues of a sensuous archaeology and sensing place as embodied social practice through the sense of touch—the haptic or tactile-kinesthetic sense. In our practice as archaeologists, we are highly sensitive to touch; you might say that our discipline is inherently as tactile as it is visual. Moreover, the sense of touch provides a key component for an archaeologist to empirically experience the sensuous nature of past places. And yet explicit reference to the tactile-kinesthetic sense is so subverted as to be wholly unconscious in the discipline of archaeology. Likewise, Paterson draws attention to a similar situation in general when he points out that "within an academic climate that celebrates visual cultures, and the popular media's infatuation with visuality, touch remains largely neglected, forgotten" (Paterson 2007:1).

## Touch and the Haptic Experience: Thinking about Taskscapes

The tactile-kinesthetic sense is the most fundamental, immediate, intimate, and erotic of all the senses and is important in structuring space and thus in interpreting a person's relationship to others and to the physical and built environment (Ackerman 1990; Classen 2005; Paterson 2007; Porteous 1990:6). The connection between touch deprivation and violence is well documented by experimental and observational research (Kennebrew 2010; Synnott 2005). Touch is far more than just fingers; it includes the whole skin surface (Montagu 1971). The tactile-kinesthetic sense includes not only the more obvious haptic sensations, such as surface, form, pressure, pain, temperature, and texture, but also those full-body sensations of balance and the sense of movement in any part of the body (Gold 1980; Ingold 2000; Merleau-Ponty 2003; Porteous 1990:5). Constance Classen (2005) does not have a chapter on movement and kinetics in her *Book of Touch* but suggests that it is a theme that runs throughout the book. In this paper, I am forefronting this aspect and giving less attention to pain, pleasure, and the erotic issues.

As I was writing my final research report (Tringham 2012) about the senses of place in the present and the past at Çatalhöyük, Turkey, I was forced to step back and think about how we create and experience this place (Figure 9-1). To this end, I was especially attracted by the concept of taskscape-landscape central to Ingold's (2000:195) perception of place and according to which each actor's place is created through an embodied multisensorial experience, as part of her or his rhythmic repetition of sets of movements and activities. We call these "tasks" and participate in them (consciously or subconsciously) every minute of

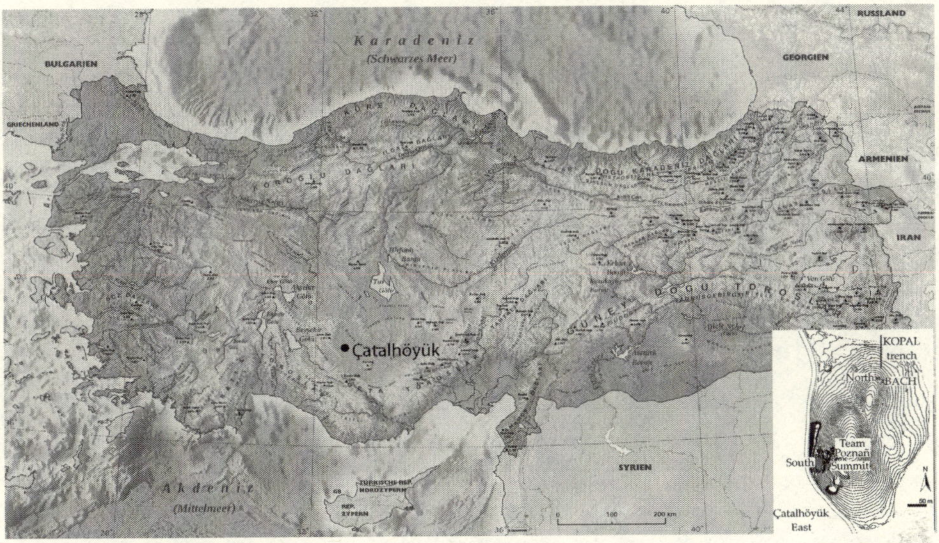


**Figure 9-1.** *Map of the location and excavation areas (Archive Report 2002) of Çatalhöyük, Turkey. (Map is a screenshot from the tool in Flickr.com (fair use); map of the site is from Çatalhöyük Archive Report 2002 © Çatalhöyük Research Project, some rights reserved; licensed under a Creative Commons License http://creativecommons.org/licenses/by-nc-sa/2.0/.)*

our waking day, alongside and aware of other people in our social group (Hodder 2006a:126, Hodder 2006b; Ingold and Vergunst 2008a).

Whereas Seamon's (1980) concept of "body-ballets" and "place-ballets" has been developed from time-space geography, Ingold's (2000) concept of taskscape grew out of an interest in labor as social practice, the value of which is measured in terms of time (hence temporality). Thus a task is "any practical operation, carried out by a skilled agent in an environment as part of his or her normal business of life" (Ingold 2000:195). Moreover "every task takes its meaning from its position within an ensemble of tasks, performed in series or in parallel, and usually by many people working together" (Ingold 2000:195). Ingold calls this ensemble of mutually interlocking (entangled) tasks a "taskscape."

Each taskscape can be conceived of as a place, but it is a place that is hard to grasp in the imagination and to describe since its nature is constantly changing. With repetition and habituation of tasks, some aspects may be grasped, but as Ingold—following Merleau-Ponty (2003)—mentions, a taskscape by its very complex nature cannot be perceived but is to be participated in; that is, it is to be lived in order to experience the multisensorial embodied social interaction. The challenge for an archaeologist trying to imagine taskscapes (places) of the past, then, seems to be—but, I will argue, is not quite—insurmountable. My argument (and starting point) in this paper is that taskscapes, or *place-ballets* as they have elsewhere been termed (Seamon 1980), are the expression of the full-body, haptic-tactile-kinesthetic sensual experience and, thus, create a commonality of experiencing present and past places.

## Movement and Contact: Anchoring the Tactile-Kinesthetic Sense in Archaeological Analysis

The sense of touch can be approached in a number of ways: the internal effect of touch on the human skin (such as pain and pleasure); the kinetics of human-to-human touch contact, human-to-external materials contact, and human-to-animal contact; and the touch of atmospheric and environmental features on the human body (Figure 9-2).

One anchor to the construction and multisensorial experience of place by multiple actors of the present and the past is the idea that body movement and the temporal aspect, events, and rhythms of the body's haptic responses and movement are essential elements of social practice and the construction of sensed places. Although such an anchor has been discussed in geography and anthropology (Bourdieu 1990; de Certeau 1984; Giddens 1979:201–210; Ingold 2000; Thrift and Pred 1981), it has rarely been problematized in archaeology.

Thousands of sensory experiences, events, ballets, and taskscapes contributed to the growing of the East Mound at Çatalhöyük during the 1,400 years of its life nine millennia ago. I can become overwhelmed by the endless questions that need to be asked and answered, and I am not alone in this. For those who take up the challenge of illustrating the constructed past, such as John-Gordon Swogger (2000) and Katherine Killackey (2010) do at Çatalhöyük, the enormity of the task becomes even more obvious (Phillips 2005; Swogger 2000). Did Çatalhöyük's inhabitants' skin and hair become caked with dust and sweat for months on end in the summer, creating in fact a protective layer against insects, sun, dust, and wind? Or did they protect themselves with layers of clothing, as we do when we excavate outside the shelters? Did they wash themselves and their clothes in the river, or was this not regarded as a priority? What did they wear on their feet? A key to constructing or imagining these experiences of everyday practice in the past is to ground them in the empirical remains of these ephemeral events and performances. In the next section of the chapter, I outline how this might be done.

### *Variables Involved in Movement and Touch*

One direction for reconstructing or imagining the taskscape is to reduce the haptic events and experience of the past to their most basic physical elements: contact between two materials and the traces they might leave in the archaeological record. First expounded by French forensic scientist Edmond Locard in 1918 and later by Soviet archaeologist Sergei Semenov, the main premise of contact trace studies in archaeology (sometimes called "microwear" and "use-wear traces") and in criminal investigation laboratories is that any contact between two materials will leave traces (physical abrasions or chemical changes including residue additives) that can be identified by observation with or beyond the naked eye (Houck 2009; Semenov 1964). Known as Locard's Exchange Principle, it has been adapted in archaeology especially to identify the use of stone and bone tools, the contents of ceramic vessels, and a few other materials (Barnard

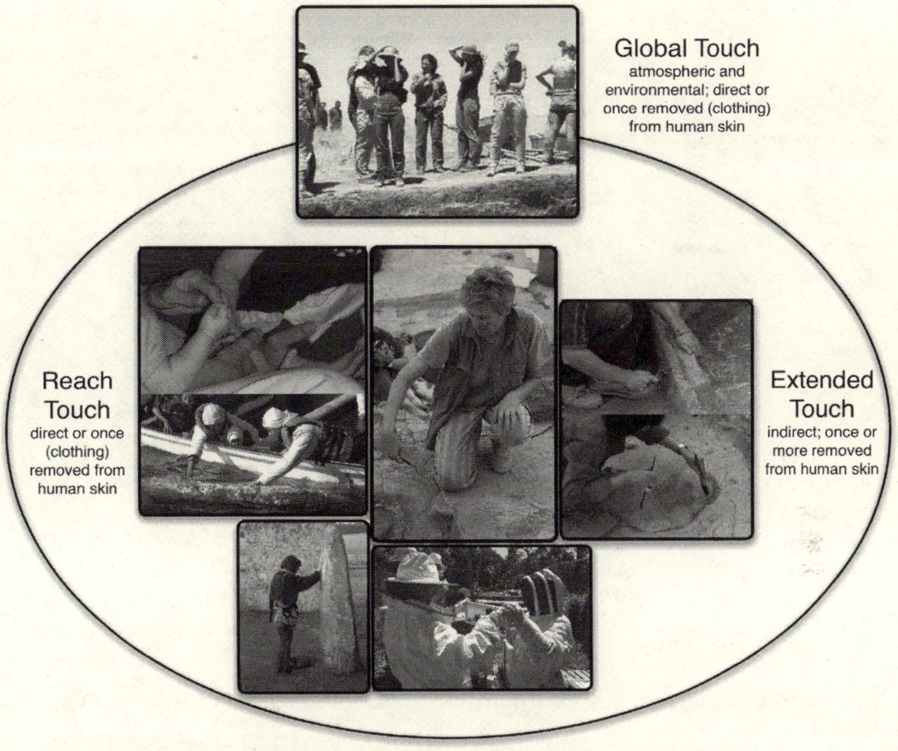


**Figure 9-2.** *Three different kinds of touch: global touch, reach touch, and extended touch. (© Ruth Tringham and the Çatalhöyük Research Project; some rights reserved; licensed under a Creative Commons License http://creativecommons.org/licenses/by-nc-sa/2.0/.)*

and Eerkens 2007; Keeley 1980; Kooyman 2000:151–166; Middleton et al. 2005; Schiffer and Skibo 1989; Tringham 1978).

In the full-body sensual experience, however, many of the contact situations we are interested in—for example, human skin surface with other human skin or with softer or harder materials—leave traces that are extremely challenging, if not impossible, to identify because of their poor archaeological preservation (Figure 9-3). With human remains, after soft tissue has disappeared, traces of contact are limited to bone deformation as a result of injury or illness, muscle indentation, or indirect traces on bone through specific activity; occasional residues of substances that were originally inside the internal organs; and, of course, wear on teeth—the most direct of the contact traces on the human body (Hager and Boz 2012; Molleson et al. 2005). So when thinking about the haptic experience of past taskscapes in terms of movement and contact, we are directed to materials that may have made body contact, including tool surfaces (which themselves may not have survived but can be inferred), and to surfaces that act as intermediaries between skin and the outside world or material, such as clothing, bags, sheaths, handles, and hafts.

| Touch | Contact with human body | Materials leaving traces of contact archaeologically | Kinetics of Contact | Traces of Contact |
|---|---|---|---|---|
| Extended: once or more removed from human skin | handle<br>haft<br>shaft<br>container | wood<br>soil<br>macrocrystalline rocks<br>microcrystalline rocks<br>clays/bricks/ceramics<br>bone/antler/teeth<br>metals | pressure<br>percussion<br>additives<br>heat damage | residues<br>abrasions<br>fractures<br>polish/fine abrasion |
| Reach: direct or once removed from human skin | clothing<br>shoes<br>soil | bone/antler/teeth<br>soil | | |
| Global: direct or once removed from human skin | clothing<br>shoes | | | |

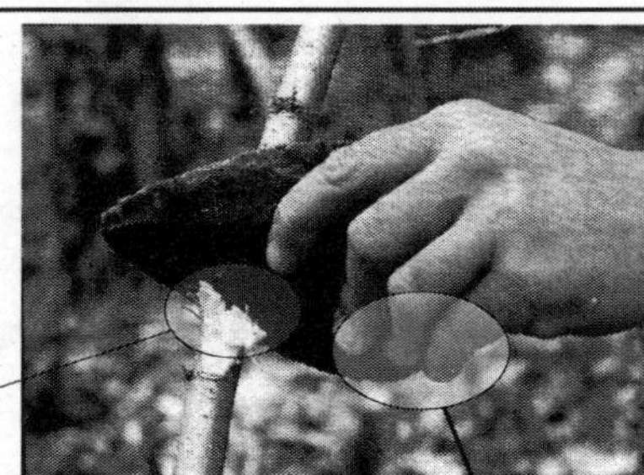
visible traces of contact will survive on the stone tool
no visible traces of contact will survive

**Figure 9-3.** *Contact traces that might survive archaeologically from the different kinds of touch. (Chart and photograph © Ruth Tringham.)*

In contact trace studies, the nature of the materials is but one aspect of a contact situation. The other important aspect comprises the kinetics of the contact—including percussion, pressure, variable force, and so on, and its direction, speed, and friction—between two inanimate materials and between inanimate material and human agent. Which part(s) of the human body are involved and the kinetics of the human body itself are significant factors in the traces created. As mentioned above, the bioarchaeologists analyzing the Neolithic human remains at Çatalhöyük remarked on the trauma and degeneration of the body caused by repetitive tasks in the house interiors, such as those that resulted from the preferred squatting position (Hager and Boz 2012; Molleson et al. 2005:288). They also suggested that a common haptic experience for the Neolithic residents was probably pain, which was hopefully ameliorated by strong, good-tasting potions. Through experimental replication and vicariously through ethnographic observation or historic description, we archaeologists can experience the kinesthetic details of taskscapes from fine, fiddly hand movements required in tasks such as bead making and obsidian knapping to movements of the whole body in tasks such as threshing, digging, brick making, and hammering. Through the same means—what I have earlier termed *educational experiments* (Tringham 1978)—we can share with the Neolithic residents of Çatalhöyük the sensation of touching and working with clay, plaster, obsidian, flint, andesite, straw, bone, wood, reeds, grasses, other plant materials, live animals, dead animals, fire, and so on.

What tends to be taken for granted in our construction of contact situations in the past are the environmental haptic experiences: heat, cold, the wind that carries stinging dust in the summer, rain, and other sensations that we have sampled during our field seasons. Another environmental context of haptic sensation is the changing ground surface underfoot—an important consideration in the Neolithic when pedestrian transport dominated every movement. At Çatalhöyük, we include not only traffic across the mound and beyond but also across and inside the houses (the built environment). What amounts to contact trace information in these contexts has been provided by micromorphological and microstratigraphic analyses (Matthews 2005a, 2005b) and analyses of a variety of residues on the occupational surfaces of the plastered mud-brick buildings (Middleton et al. 2005). Moreover, as archaeologists working primarily during the summer, we have almost no experience of the place during other seasons—for example, when snow lies on the ground—but all seasonal factors need to be taken into consideration when constructing taskscapes of the past.

## Haptic Aspects of Neolithic Taskscapes at Çatalhöyük

In a single context excavation, each archaeological unit that is excavated represents a depositional event in the life of a building. Each depositional event can be related to others chronologically and spatially and can be represented, for example, in the Harris Matrix. The "unit" comprises soil and / or building matrix and its associated materials and samples. From this foundation of contact trace evidence in the archaeological record, it is up to the archaeologist to bring all his or her powers of inference and imagination to construct the wealth of tactile contact that was experienced, the everyday repetitive practices—tasks, rhythms, and activities—that were carried out by the different actors.

In his book *The Leopard's Tale,* Ian Hodder (2006a) carries out the exercise of imagining the everyday entanglements of tasks within a complex tapestry of domains of domestic, symbolic, and spiritual practices. Rob Swigart in *Stone Mirror* (2007) also imagines daily routines. Rather than reiterate their excellent narratives here, I shall offer some fragments that focus exploration of Neolithic multisensorial experiences through the sense of touch.

### *Rhythmic Repetitions*

The rhythmic repetition of a task is emphasized by all who write about taskscapes and social practice. Information about it can be winkled out of the ground, but such information is often taken for granted (e.g., the carrying of water, the pounding of clay for plaster, the plastering of walls and floors).

The rhythm of movement that lies at the heart of the temporality of taskscapes is multiscalar: rhythm at the pace of contact between human body and material—the footstep, gestures of storytelling, hand on obsidian core, hand stirring soup; the daily rhythms of eating, drinking, and other bodily functions; seasonal rhythms and annual rhythms. All of these can be imagined or inferred against the longer rhythms of the life cycle of people and of the houses and the village(s) themselves, whose debris creates the East Mound at Çatalhöyük (Tringham 2012). Changes in taskscape rhythms can be created by the demographics of an aging population in a building or by accidents, illness, and serendipitous meetings that might occur at a crucial time. Disentangling these different scales of rhythms through the archaeological record is an enormous challenge. Surprisingly, some of the most constructive responses to the challenge at Çatalhöyük have come from the most intimate scale of observation in the microartifactual and microstratigraphic analyses, through which it is possible to plot the shifting locations and intensity of daily tasks during the life history of a building (Cessford 2003; Cessford and Mitrovic 2005; Matthews 2005a, 2012; May 2005; Middleton et al. 2005).

### *Walking, Running, Slipping, Falling, Tripping*

The kinetics of moving, especially on foot, has been extensively and engagingly explored by Tim Ingold and his colleagues, opening up the topic of the tactile-kinesthetic sense and movement in very interesting ways (Ingold 2000, 2007; Ingold and Vergunst 2008b). There are many general aspects of movement that we can infer from our own experience. From the time we are born, we never stop moving. Daily we engage repeatedly in tasks to produce, maintain, and store food, tools, containers, and clothing, whether in solitude or in company, and while moving in various ways: walking, squatting, sitting, and standing. We know that the body can be both adversely and positively affected by movement, and we have seen this in the human remains that show the result of long-term squatting in Neolithic Çatalhöyük. Evidence shows that "[t]he habit of squatting in one form or another and working from the ground has resulted in the presence of extended kneeling articulations on the first metatarsals of most individuals, both male and female" (Molleson et al. 2005:289).

Moreover, the world moves—or, rather, places are created and re-created—as we move. At Çatalhöyük, we thought often about moving and creating places. There is still lively discussion as to mapping the surface of the mound at different times in its prehistoric past (Hodder 2007; Matthews 1996). For example, both Building 1 and Building 3, which are dated in the middle of the occupation of the East Mound, were excavated at its modern surface. So the question is, How much earth has been lost through erosion, and as a result, how close to that of Neolithic people is our experience of walking across the mound? For the purpose of this and my other papers on the same topic, I have assumed that the surface of the East Mound was probably very similar to what it is today, minus perhaps a meter of earth (Tringham 2012). The Remediated Places project (Tringham et al. 2007), whose first location was the East Mound at Çatalhöyük, forefronts the process of walking and moving in the present and past as a process of thinking about prehistoric topography and constructing place. Ingold (2007) distinguishes between a goal-oriented ("navigation") mode of movement and an exploratory ("wayfaring") mode in which the process of the journey takes priority. The Remediated Places Project forefronts the latter mode of walking, focusing on what people were thinking and saying as they moved rather than on what the goal of their destination was.

But the goal of the movement and by what path it was reached are also important elements to consider. We imagine that movement in the house interior and across rooftops between houses was regulated by rules and prohibitions that permitted pathways and destinations that changed during the lifetime of the house and the lifetime of a man or a woman. The data from the archaeological excavations at Çatalhöyük lead us to ask many questions about movement, most of which cannot be answered definitively but which nevertheless inspire the creative imagination. What kind of choreography allowed multiple residents of Building 3 to move around its main room (which started off 6 × 5.5 m and ended its life 6 × 4 m), while avoiding hazards such as open fires (Stevanović 2012a)? Who was allowed to tread on the platforms under which the dead were buried? Who moved in crouch-walking fashion through crawlways to reach stored items? Was the ceiling of the Neolithic rooms high enough to allow residents to move and stand with upright posture? If we assume that entry was predominantly from the roof by ladder, can we also assume that at certain points in a person's life cycle and under certain conditions it became too hard to climb the ladder (i.e., when a person was too young or too old or injured or when the ladder was too slippery or broken)? Did people ever fall down the ladder or off the roof? At this point we can ask ourselves, How did the mature woman identified as F.634, who is buried under platform F.162, dislocate her hip and break her ribs (Hager and Boz 2012)?

As a result of recent excavations in the northern part of the East Mound at Çatalhöyük, Ian Hodder has suggested that the densely packed buildings were actually grouped into small neighborhoods or zones (Hodder 2006a:101, Figure 40) separated by alleyways. Thus, to travel from one zone to another, a walker would be required to go down from the roof to ground level. Movement from house to house within the neighborhood may very well have been across the rooftops, as has been surmised by the majority of authors. But it would be remiss not to imagine that alleyways between houses at ground level were also accessed from at least some of the buildings. Hodder (2006a:101), Matthews (2004), and Eddisford (Farid et al. 2007:52), however, have argued that the surfaces in these alleys do not show the fragmentation and trampling evidence that would indicate their use by humans or animals for walking. I have argued, however, that to imagine a soft-footed walker not minding or noticing the smells and picking his or her way between the larger obstacles in order to escape the confines of the neighborhood is not unfeasible (Tringham 2012). All of this speculation becomes irrelevant if, as my colleague Colleen Morgan has mused (personal communication, March 2009), the outside walls of the Neolithic buildings were not exposed at all but were buried in the matrix of the mound with only their "roof and roof structures" showing above the surface!

To walk up the northern end of the mound on a path takes us four minutes. We are walking along a dusty path that rises at a steady rate; it is summer and we are wearing shoes. The path is covered in soft, very fine dust, which makes our tread almost soundless. How different is this modern path in winter or spring, with snow and rain? How different would it have been for the Neolithic residents and visitors? Would they have had a clearly defined path 9,000 years ago? Would there have been grass- or weed-covered slopes on each side, or would there have been buildings in various stages of decay, construction, and occupation? Did the path rise gradually across the mound's surface as it does now, or did it wind its way along streets, rising in steps, similar to the Plaka on the slopes of the Athenian Acropolis?

The question of footwear is important and has implications both for haptic contact, between foot and path and movement across the mound and beyond to the fields or salt lakes, and for hearing the movements of other people. We can draw ideas of possible footwear from the fortunate remains of leather and fiber "shoes" that have been found in other (later) archaeological contexts, such as that on the frozen iceman, "Ötzi," found in the Similaun glacier in the Alps (Goubitz et al. 2001:380–381) or that in the Areni-1 cave in Armenia (Pinhasi et al. 2010), both of which were leather and 5,500 years old, or the 8,000-year-old fibrous sandals from the North American Midwest (Kuttruff et al. 1998). Perhaps because no such remains of footwear have been found at Çatalhöyük, illustrator John Swogger in his visualizations—maybe unintentionally—tends to cut off any views of the feet of the residents. In fact, however, what was covering the feet (or not) can be investigated and inferred through the anatomical changes that are effected by footwear, such as narrowing of the feet and higher peaking at the heel and metatarsals (D'Aout et al. 2009). No such investigation, however, has been carried out on the human remains at Çatalhöyük.

I keep coming back to the multisensorial whole-body experience of walking because I believe that, whether we think of their paths as taking place in Ingold's (2007) goal-oriented "transport" mode or his exploratory "wayfaring" mode, this was as essential a part of social practice as was the more traditionally studied sitting or squatting still. As the Neolithic residents of Çatalhöyük walked through the village or across the mound from one village to another, their attention may well have been on the immediate landscape of houses and people (just as ours, as archaeologists, tends to be on the excavation). But they may also have been much more in touch with life, views, and sounds beyond the mound than we are today.

Whereas we see a boundary around the base of the East Mound and around the modern archaeologists' compound, to the residents of Çatalhöyük the boundary between the familiar and the unfamiliar may have been much farther away, perhaps even chronological: walking at dawn in the surrounding marshland may have been familiar, whereas doing so at night entered the realm of unfamiliar. Walking to the fields—a short walk of an hour or two—would have been very different from a longer overnight adventure. For example, obsidian was acquired from Cappadocia in the mountains to the northeast—many days' walk from Çatalhöyük—where it was reduced to workable pieces (Carter et al. 2005). In his book *Stone Mirror* (2007), Rob Swigart imagines the long journey to Cappadocia in the kind of detail that I find valuable for considering the multisensorial experience of Neolithic walking: How many stops were made along the way? Were the walkers nervous in the dark of the Central Anatolian night? Did they appreciate the numerous and bright stars in the night sky?

In their quest for materials—stone, timber, and exotics—it is clear that the Neolithic villagers of Çatalhöyük did not exist in a social vacuum (Asouti 2005; Baird 2005). Visits to and by distant villagers and relatives in the mountains or on the seacoast must have been at least an annual event, in addition to more frequent visits to friends, allies, or relatives close by. All these visits in 7000 B.C.E. involved walking.

There is much more to think about walking (Ingold 2007; Ingold and Vergunst 2008b). For example, in addition to its mechanics, some of the less considered topics include whether walks were taken in groups or in solitude, what group members might have been talking about as they walked, and what they might have been thinking about. Did they look at the ground but not see beyond their memories and imaginations? Did they hear voices and birdsong but not listen? Were they aware of the wind or heat or wet or cold or their tired, painful feet? As Vergunst (2008) points out, when you walk and don't pay attention accidents happen: among them falling, slipping, tripping, and losing your way. The demise of F.634 at Çatalhöyük (mentioned above) might have been precipitated by just such an accident.

### *Carrying*

In addition to movement and walking, daily routines almost always involved some kind of carrying. "'A woman carries three corners of the farm and helps her husband hold the fourth' is a saying often heard in Croatia," writes Eva Skold Westerlind at the beginning of her book *Carrying the Farm on Her Back* (1989). We archaeologists tend to carry heavy loads (e.g., flotation samples, finds) *down* the mound; the Neolithic residents would have carried heavy loads (water, bricks, or building materials) *up* the mound. They would have climbed up the mound wearily at the end of the day, whereas we archaeologists, probably less tired than they, stagger down the mound at the end of the day.

Early morning rhythms were all about carrying: carrying water, carrying firewood or dung, carrying waste to its various dedicated places, carrying food to animals. And all of these tasks were much harder in winter and in rain. Whole-body labor in the fields, marshes, and forests was always accompanied or followed by carrying stuff: for example, raw materials, including wood, reeds, dead animals, and plants for food and a multitude of other purposes, were toted back to the village every day.

The idea of the life cycle of places, people, and things has drawn us to focus on the formation of the tell itself, on house life histories and human burials. House construction and maintenance involved a good deal of walking and carrying from locations away from the mound (Stevanović 2012b). Such tasks at Çatalhöyük included finding clay, choosing clay, walking to the clay and other construction materials; carrying tools for digging clay and for cutting reeds and wood; digging clay; cutting reeds and wood; and carrying clay, reeds, and timber to the base of the mound. Once the necessary supplies were at the base of the mound, work included mixing plaster, mixing mortar, mixing packing, making bricks, making the roof, and carrying it all from the base of the mound to the house site (see Stevanović 2012b for a discussion of the empirical data to support this inference). These were complex tasks, involving organization and planning, and were unlikely to be performed on a daily basis or when people were occupied with other duties. It is likely, as has been argued by Mirjana Stevanović, that these tasks were combined and collaborative, involving more than one household.

## Learning, Apprenticeship, Habituation

I suggest here a third anchor to investigating sensory responses in the past, that is, researching the process by which practices that started as new and unfamiliar experiences became familiar, "enactive knowledge." It is unusual for a practice to become familiar to a learner by its repetition in social isolation. It is more likely for observation of, communication with, and even instruction from others who are further along the learning curve to provide the context of the growing familiarity. This process of familiarization or learning—as described, for example, by Jean Lave in her "apprenticeship" model (Lave and Wenger 1991) or by Lev Vygotsky (1978) in his "zone of proximal development"—is the process of acquiring *enactive* knowledge "that is stored in bodily sensori-motor responses" rather than acquired through symbolic or iconic means (Bennett and O'Modhrain 2007). We tend to apply this model of learning to childhood development, but I believe that it can be constructively applied to learning throughout a lifetime.

To think about how and why a practice becomes "embodied," or as some think of it "internalized," leads us beyond the practice itself to its historical contingency and to its entanglement in other practices. Let us consider a practice as "simple" as bringing water to the 9,000-year-old Building 3 at Çatalhöyük. Imagine it is a young person performing the action; at some point he or she was shown the container, how to hold it to collect water, where to fill it, how to carry it filled with water, and which the best path by which to carry it. In most cases, we think of these skills as already learned and not objects of investigation. But, in fact, each step in the task had to be learned by observation, discovery, imitation, and demonstration, each of which is an important social practice contributing to a multitude of experiences in an endless process of learning.

## Transposing the Haptic Experience of the Past to Digital On-Screen Environments

I want to end with a short discussion of the use of the on-screen environment to address the challenge of sharing ideas about the past (prehistoric or historic) whole-body haptic and kinetic sensuous experiences. The explosion of digital consumer products that provide changing contexts of haptic sensation (e.g., the iPodTouch, iPhone, and now iPad) is just the tip of the iceberg of ways that digital technology is fast revolutionizing how we can incorporate the sense of touch into our digital archaeological interpretations.

Mark Paterson (2005, 2007), embarking on what he calls an archaeology of the technologies of touch, describes the many different ways the ability of the body and its extremities to move, manipulate, inspect, and explore within a space and a dynamically changing environment (with other people) and with all senses cooperating has been used to trigger tactile experience for a digital audience. These are haptics, or technologies of touch. He has given a foundation to his "archaeology" in the philosophical discussion of haptics and tactile sensation. He contrasts haptics, or technologies of touch, with multimedia technologies in which visual and audial senses are stimulated: "Whereas the keyboard is a passive mechanical channel between the computer and user, haptics enables a more active exploration, is programmable according to the type of data or object to be manipulated, and allows the user not just to see three dimensional shapes on the screen visually but also to feel them and mould them through the haptic interface" (Paterson 2007:128). Currently, haptics technologies are designed for specific industries, such as medicine, engineering, or architecture, and for consumers of computer games and simulation experiences (e.g., as provided by Nintendo Wii). Archaeological applications are very few, but it is only a matter of time before incorporating haptic technologies in the exploration of artifacts, sediments, residues, etc., becomes commonplace.

Even without the use of haptics, however, digital media can contribute to vicariously experiencing a haptic sensation. Digital media—photography and video—can provide audiovisual cues that might trigger a haptic metaphorical response in the viewer: for example, sweat dripping off an excavator's forehead might engender a feeling or memory of heat in the viewer. The audiovisual "multimedia" exploration of archaeological remains and cultural heritage sites and buildings through Quick Time Virtual Reality (QTVR) and virtual reality (VR) interfaces has long been favored by presenters and viewers of past reconstructions. Even though digital media can now express first-person movement through space at a wandering human, exploratory pace instead of the stomach-sickening fly-through pace much favored by VR reconstructionists, such presentations have been quite heavily criticized as encouraging passive acceptance of the presented reconstruction (Morgan 2009).

In the Remediated Places Project, we aimed to confound—and thus to enhance—the body's haptic experience by requiring the user to swing from virtual touch and movement to physical movement and touch (Tringham et al. 2007). We are currently seeking ways to increase the bodily haptic experience: for example, by giving instructions to the participant to move his or her hands in certain ways or remove his- or herself from the screen and move his or her feet. Meanwhile, we can be content with the awkward virtuality of Çatalhöyük at Okapi Island in Second Life (Morgan 2009).[1] Even the challenges of building and gesturing through the medium of an avatar, however, can set one to use the imagination to experience moving around in a Neolithic village, where entry into buildings is through the roof. Moreover, on our virtual replica, the Remediated Places videowalks have been mirrored so that a virtual walker can—through a personal avatar—walk along a virtual path while holding a virtual iPod on which he or she views a video that ultimately mediates a real event.

It cannot be repeated enough that the meaning of a sensuous experience, and even the experience itself, would be very different for us than it would be for people living 9,000 years ago or for people living now but at a location 9,000 miles away from our own (Classen 1993, 2005; Howes 2005). Other researchers, such as Pink (2009) and Stewart (2007), would argue it is different for each contingency and for each person. However hard we imagine, we of the Now situation are the filter through which we construct the rhythms and taskscapes of the Then situation; hence, the close attention paid to how we experience East Mound now is warranted. In contradiction to what our intuitions tell us, it is only by being aware of our experiences of the Now that we can begin to find our way to the event-filled everyday of prehistory.

## Note

1. See http://okapi.wordpress.com/projects/okapi-island-in-second-life/ and http://www.ruthtringham.com/Ruth_Tringham/Okapi_Island.html. However, due to the doubling of land rent in Second Life, Okapi Island itself became archaeological in May 2012.

## References


Ackerman, Diane

1995 *A Natural History of the Senses*. Reprinted. Vintage Books, New York. Originally published 1990, Random House, New York.

Asouti, Eleni

2005 Group Identity and the Politics of Dwelling at Neolithic Çatalhöyük. In *Çatalhöyük Perspectives: Reports from the 1995–1999 Seasons,* Vol. 6, edited by Ian Hodder, pp. 75–91. British Institute of Archaeology at Ankara and McDonald Institute for Archaeological Research, Cambridge.

Baird, Douglas

2005 The History of Settlement and Social Landscapes in the Early Holocene in the Çatalhöyük Area. In *Çatalhöyük Perspectives: Reports from the 1995–1999 Seasons,* Vol. 6, edited by Ian Hodder, pp. 55–74. British Institute of Archaeology at Ankara and McDonald Institute for Archaeological Research, Cambridge.

Barnard, Hans, and Jelmer Eerkens (editors)

2007 *Theory and Practice of Archaeological Residue Analysis*. BAR International Series 1650. Archaeopress, Oxford.

Bender, Barbara (editor)

1993 *Landscape—Politics and Perspectives*. Berg, Oxford.

Bender, Barbara, Sue Hamilton, and Chris Tilley

2007 *Stone Worlds: Narrative and Reflexivity in Landscape Archaeology*. Publications of the Institute of Archaeology, University College London. Left Coast, Walnut Creek, California.

Bennett, Peter, and Sile O'Modhrain

2007 Towards Tangible Enactive-Interfaces. In Enactive/07 Proceedings, edited by Annie Luciani and Claude Cadoz, pp. 37–40. ACROE, Grenoble, France.

Bourdieu, Pierre

1990 *The Logic of Practice*. Polity, Cambridge.

Carter, Tristan, James Conolly, and Ana Spasojevic

2005 The Chipped Stone. In *Changing Materialities at Çatalhöyük: Reports from the 1995–99 Seasons,* Vol. 5, edited by Ian Hodder, pp. 221–284. British Institute of Archaeology at Ankara and McDonald Institute for Archaeological Research, Cambridge.

Cessford, Craig

2003 Microartefactual Floor Patterning: the Case at Çatalhöyük. *Assemblage* 7. Electronic document, http://www.assemblage.group.shef.ac.uk/issue7/cessford.html, accessed March 3, 2012.

Cessford, Craig, and Slobodan Mitrovic

2005 Heavy-Residue Analysis. In *Changing Materialities at Çatalhöyük: Reports from the 1995–99 Seasons*, Vol. 5, edited by Ian Hodder, pp. 45–65. British Institute of Archaeology at Ankara and McDonald Institute for Archaeological Research, Cambridge.

Classen, Constance

1993 *Worlds of Sense: Exploring the Senses in History and across Cultures*. Routledge, London.

2005 *The Book of Touch*. Berg, Oxford.

Cresswell, Tim

2004 *Place: A Short Introduction*. Blackwell, Oxford.

D'Aout, Kristiaan, Todd C. Pataky, Dirk De Clercq, and Peter Aerts

2009 The Effects of Habitual Footwear Use: Foot Shape and Function in Native Barefoot Walkers. *Footwear Science* 1:81–94.

de Certeau, Michel

1984 *The Practice of Everyday Life*. University of California Press, Berkeley.

Farid, Shahina, Daniel Eddisford, Anies Hasan, Marina Lizaralde, Simon McCann, Freya Sadarangani, James Taylor, and Lisa Yeomans

2007 Areas of Excavation 2007: 4040 Area, Foundation Trenches. *Çatalhöyük Archive Reports 2007*:23–75.

Gibson, James J.

1968 *The Senses Considered as Perceptual Systems*. Allen and Unwin, London.

Giddens, Anthony

1979 *Central Problems in Social Theory: Action, Structure, and Contradiction in Social Analysis*. University of California Press, Berkeley.

Gold, John

1980 *An Introduction to Behavioral Geography*. Oxford University Press, Oxford.

Goubitz, Olaf, Carol Driel-Murray, and Willy Groenman-van Waateringe

2001 *Stepping through Time: Archaeological Footwear from Prehistoric Times until 1800*. Stichting Promotie Archeologie, Zwolle, The Netherlands.

Hager, Lori, and Başak Boz

2012 Death and Its Relationship to Life: Neolithic Burials from Building 3 and Space 87 at Çatalhöyük, Turkey. In *Last House on the Hill: BACH Area Reports from Çatalhöyük, Turkey* (Çatalhöyük Vol. 7), edited by Ruth Tringham and Mirjana Stevanović, pp. 297–330. Cotsen Institute of Archaeology Publications, University of California, Los Angeles.

Hodder, Ian

2006a *The Leopard's Tale: Revealing the Mysteries of Çatalhöyük*. Thames and Hudson, London.

2006b The Spectacle of Daily Performance at Çatalhöyük. In *Archaeology of Performance. Theaters of Power, Community, and Politics*, edited by Takeshi Inomata and Lawrence Coben, pp. 81–102. Altamira, Lanham, Maryland.

2007 Summary of Results. In *Excavating Çatalhöyük: South, North, and KOPAL Area Reports from the 1995–99 Seasons*, Vol. 3, edited by Ian Hodder pp. 25–37. British Institute of Archaeology at Ankara and McDonald Institute for Archaeological Research, Cambridge.

Houck, Max

2009 *Trace Evidence (Essentials of Forensic Science)*. Facts on File, New York.

Howes, David (editor)
2005 *Empire of the Senses: The Sensual Culture Reader*. Berg, Oxford.

Ingold, Tim
2000 *The Perception of the Environment : Essays on Livelihood, Dwelling, and Skill*. Routledge, London.
2007 *Lines: A Brief History*. Routledge, London.

Ingold, Tim, and Jo Vergunst
2008a Introduction. In *Ways of Walking: Ethnography and Practice on Foot*, edited by Tim Ingold and Jo Vergunst, pp. 1–20. Ashgate, Aldershot, United Kingdom.
2008b *Ways of Walking: Ethnography and Practice on Foot*. Ashgate, Aldershot, United Kingdom.

Joyce, Rosemary, and Jeanne Lopiparo
2005 Postscript: Doing Agency in Archaeology. *Journal of Archaeological Method and Theory* 12:365–374.

Keeley, Lawrence
1980 *Experimental Determination of Stone Tool Uses*. University of Chicago Press, Chicago.

Kennebrew, Versandra
2010 Touch Deprivation Articles and Research. Electronic document, http://www.touchisgreat.com/pb/wp_0ac8b62c/wp_0ac8b62c.html, accessed July 26, 2010.

Killackey, Katherine
2010 Electronic document, http://killackeyillustration.com/about.html, accessed March 3, 2012.

Kooyman, Brian
2000 *Understanding Stone Tools and Archaeological Sites*. University of New Mexico Press, Albuquerque.

Kuttruff, Jenna T., S. Gail DeHart, and Michael J. O'Brien
1998 7,500 Years of Prehistoric Footwear from Arnold Research Cave, Missouri. *Science* 281:72–75.

Lave, Jean, and Etienne Wenger
1991 *Situated Learning: Legitimate Peripheral Participation*. Cambridge University Press, Cambridge.

Matthews, Roger
1996 Surface Scraping and Planning. In *On the Surface: Çatalhöyük 1993–95*, edited by Ian Hodder, pp. 79–101. British Institute of Archaeology at Ankara and McDonald Institute for Archaeological Research, Cambridge.

Matthews, Wendy
2005a Life-Cycle and Life-Course of Buildings. In *Çatalhöyük Perspectives: Reports from the 1995–1999 Seasons*, Vol. 6, edited by Ian Hodder, pp. 125–150. British Institute of Archaeology at Ankara and McDonald Institute for Archaeological Research, Cambridge.
2005b Micromorphological and Microstratigraphic Traces of Uses and Concepts of Space. In *Inhabiting Çatalhöyük: Reports from the 1995–1999 Seasons*, Vol. 4, edited by Ian Hodder, pp. 355–398. British Institute of Archaeology at Ankara and McDonald Institute for Archaeological Research, Cambridge.
2012 Household Life-Histories and Boundaries: Microstratigraphy and Micromorphology of Architectural Surfaces in Building 3 of the BACH Area. In *Last House on the Hill: BACH Area Reports from Çatalhöyük, Turkey* (Çatalhöyük Vol. 7), edited by Ruth Tringham and Mirjana Stevanović, pp. 205–222. Cotsen Institute of Archaeology, University of California, Los Angeles.

Matthews, Wendy, Lisa-Marie Shillito, and Matthew Almond
2004 Micromorphology: Investigation of Neolithic Social and Ecological Strategies at Seasonal, Annual and Life-Cycle Timescales. In *Çatalhöyük Archive Reports 2004*. Electronic document, http://www.catalhoyuk.com/archive_reports/2004/ar04_22.html, accessed March 3, 2012.

May, Sarah C.
2005 Statistical Integration of Contextual Data. In *Changing Materialities at Çatalhöyük: Reports from the 1995–99 Seasons,* Vol. 5, edited by Ian Hodder, pp. 23–44. British Institute of Archaeology at Ankara and McDonald Institute for Archaeological Research, Cambridge.

Merleau-Ponty, Maurice
2003 *Phenomenology of Perception*. 2nd ed. Routledge, New York.

Middleton, William, Douglas Price, and David Meiggs
2005 Chemical Analysis of Floor Sediments for the Identification of Anthropogenic Activity Residues. In *Inhabiting Çatalhöyük: Reports from the 1995–99 Seasons,* Vol. 4, edited by Ian Hodder, pp. 399–412. British Institute of Archaeology at Ankara and McDonald Institute for Archaeological Research, Cambridge.

Molleson, Theya, Peter Andrews, and Başak Boz
2005 Reconstruction of the Neolithic People at Çatalhöyük. In *Inhabiting Çatalhöyük: Reports from the 1995–99 Seasons,* Vol. 4, edited by Ian Hodder, pp. 279–300. British Institute of Archaeology at Ankara and McDonald Institute for Archaeological Research, Cambridge.

Montagu, Ashley
1971 *Touching: The Human Significance of the Skin*. Columbia University Press, New York.

Morgan, Colleen
2009 (Re)Building Çatalhöyük: Changing Virtual Reality in Archaeology. *Archaeologies: Journal of the World Archaeological Congress* 5:468–487.

Paterson, Mark
2005 Digital Touch. In *The Book of Touch,* edited by Constance Classen, pp. 431–436. Berg, Oxford.
2007 *The Senses of Touch: Haptics, Affects, and Technologies*. Berg, Oxford.

Phillips, James
2005 "To Make the Dry Bones Live": Amédée Forestier's Glastonbury Lake Village. In *Envisioning the Past: Archaeology and the Image,* edited by Sam Smiles and Stephanie Moser, pp. 72–91. Blackwell, Oxford.

Pinhasi, Ron, Boris Gasparian, Gregory Areshian, Diana Zardaryan, Alexia Smith, Guy Bar-Oz, and Thomas Higham
2010 First Direct Evidence of Chalcolithic Footwear from the Near Eastern Highlands. *PLoS ONE* 5(6):e10984. doi:101371/journal.pone.0010984.

Pink, Sarah
2009 *Doing Sensory Anthropology.* Sage, Thousand Oaks, California.

Porteous, Douglas
1990 *Landscapes of the Mind: Worlds of Sense and Metaphor.* University of Toronto Press, Toronto.

Rodaway, Paul
1994 *Sensuous Geographies: Body, Sense, Place*. Routledge, London.

Schiffer, Michael, and James Skibo
1989 A Provisional Theory of Ceramic Abrasion. *American Anthropologist* 91:101–115.

Seamon, David
1980 Body-Subject, Time-Space Routines, and Place-Ballets. In *The Human Experience of Space and Place*, edited by Anne Buttimer and David Seamon, pp. 148–165. St. Martin's, New York.

Semenov, Sergei A.
1964 *Prehistoric Technology*. Cory, Adams & McKay, London.

Stevanović, Mirjana
2012a Summary of the Results of the Excavation in the BACH Area. In *Last House on the Hill: BACH Area Reports from Çatalhöyük, Turkey* (Çatalhöyük Vol. 7), edited by Ruth Tringham and Mirjana Stevanović, pp. 49–80. Cotsen Institute of Archaeology, University of California, Los Angeles.
2012b Building and Caring for the House at Çatalhöyük. In *Last House on the Hill: BACH Area Reports from Çatalhöyük, Turkey* (Çatalhöyük Vol. 7), edited by Ruth Tringham and Mirjana Stevanović, pp. 173–204. Cotsen Institute of Archaeology, University of California, Los Angeles.

Stewart, Kathleen
2007 *Ordinary Affects*. Duke University Press, Durham, North Carolina.

Swigart, Rob
2007 *Stone Mirror: A Novel of the Neolithic*. Left Coast, Walnut Creek, California.

Swogger, John-Gordon
2000 Image and Interpretation: The Tyranny of Representation? In *Towards Reflexive Method in Archaeology: The Example at Çatalhöyük*, edited by Ian Hodder, pp. 143–152. BIAA Monograph No. 28. McDonald Institute for Archaeological Research, Cambridge.

Synnott, Anthony
2005 Handling Children: To Touch or Not to Touch. In *The Book of Touch*, edited by Constance Classen, pp. 41–47. Berg, Oxford.

Thrift, Nigel, and Allan Pred
1981 Time-Geography: A New Beginning. *Progress in Human Geography* 5:272–286.

Tilley, Chris
1994 *A Phenomenology of Landscape*. Berg, Oxford.
2008 *Body and Image: Explorations in Landscape Phenomenology* 2. Left Coast, Walnut Creek, California.

Tringham, Ruth
1978 Experimentation, Ethnoarchaeology, and the Leapfrogs in Archaeological Methodology. In *Explorations in Ethnoarchaeology*, edited by Richard Gould, pp. 169–199. University of New Mexico Press, Albuquerque.
2012 Sensing the Place of Çatalhöyük: The Rhythms of Daily Life. In *Last House on the Hill: BACH Area Reports from Çatalhöyük, Turkey* (Çatalhöyük Vol. 7), edited by Ruth Tringham and Mirjana Stevanović, pp. 531–552. Cotsen Institute of Archaeology, University of California, Los Angeles.

Tringham, Ruth, Michael Ashley, and Steve Mills
2007 Senses of Places: Remediations from Text to Digital Performance. Electronic document, http://chimeraspider.wordpress.com/2007/09/19/remediated-places-final-draft/, accessed March 3, 2012.

Tuan, Yi-Fu
1993 *Passing Strange and Wonderful: Aesthetics, Nature, and Culture*. Island Press, Washington, D.C.

Vergunst, Jo
2008 Taking a Trip and Taking Care in Everyday Life. In *Ways of Walking: Ethnography*

*and Practice on Foot*, edited by Tim Ingold and Jo Vergunst, pp. 105–122. Ashgate, Aldershot, United Kingdom.

Vygotsky, Lev
1978 *Mind and Society: The Development of Higher Psychological Processes.* Harvard University Press, Cambridge.

Westerlind, Eva Skold
1989 *Carrying the Farm on Her Back*. Rainier Books, Kirkland, Washington.

# 10. Musical Space and Quiet Space in Medieval Monastic Canterbury

*Joe Williams*

*Abstract:* In this chapter, the background noises, or *belles noiseuses*, of everyday mid-thirteenth century C.E. life at a Benedictine monastery and an Augustinian house of regular canons, both in Canterbury, England, are studied by focusing on the movement of people through the buildings and on artifacts found during excavations. The significance of sound to studies of monastic sites is evident when one considers the emphasis placed on silence in monastic rules. Musical space and quiet space are not considered here as dichotomous but rather as similar qualitative types in that both require a relative lack of external sound to function as desired by their users. The idea of copresence is significant in this regard, as it is often through sound that we are aware of the proximity of another. An interpretive approach, utilizing access analysis and considering copresence zones in conjunction with the archaeological context of artifacts, suggests that the background noises of these two sites were somewhat dissimilar in terms of amount, character, and spatial distribution. On the basis of data generated by access analysis, the reasons for such variation can be said to relate to the layouts of the main claustral buildings, but elements of the artifactual evidence suggest that differences between the rules followed by the two monastic orders may also have played a part.

It has been suggested by numerous commentators that there is significantly less silence in the modern world than there was in the past. Luigi Russolo, in a manifesto of Futurist music (Apollonio 1973:74), wrote that "[a]ncient life was all silence. In the nineteenth century, with the invention of the machine, Noise was born." Bruce Davis (1990:1), writing with a less enthusiastic attitude toward noise, states that "[t]he twentieth century may go down in history as the one in which we

*Making Senses of the Past: Toward a Sensory Archaeology*, edited by Jo Day. Center for Archaeological Investigations, Occasional Paper No. 40.  ISBN 978-0-8093-3287-8.

lost the silence. Since the industrial revolution, the noise of machines has increasingly filled our homes, cities, farms, skies, and earth." One aim of this chapter is to challenge this idea. While it would be fair to say that the noises of automobiles, aircraft, and electrical devices were absent from medieval life, the assertion that in their absence what results would be silence is spurious. As Christopher Witmore (2006:274) observes, "To hear noise is to hear things. Indeed, some background noise is resistant to the 'flow' of time. [He gives examples of sounds, including rain and cicadas, which] are transient and yet recurrent. These are philosopher Michel Serres' *belles noiseuses*. These background noises are . . . fundamental, not simply to our experiences of place, they are fundamental to our very being."

The examples given by Witmore are predominantly sounds of nature, but the inclusion of the above quote in this chapter should not be taken to imply that the present author subscribes to the idea of the ancient world as an age before machines; such an idea is misleading, for one could certainly refer to as machines such objects as carts, pulley systems, and winepresses, which are known to have existed for many centuries. Even if these sources of noise are discounted, there are many other possible places from which sound could emanate. Jonathan Hill (2006:181) explores the concept of silence by discussing John Cage's *4'33"*, in which the music is in fact the "incidental sounds in a performance environment, whether a creak or a cough," occurring during the silence of the performer. In an atmosphere of attempted silence, "previously insignificant and familiar sounds assume importance" (Hill 2006:181–182).

This chapter presents findings of an archaeological study of sound at two medieval monastic sites in Canterbury (Figure 10-1): St. Augustine's Abbey, a Benedictine foundation, and St. Gregory's Priory, a house of Augustinian canons. These sites were chosen as case studies on the basis of their excavation reports, which are of a sufficient standard to enable extensive analysis. As something that does not tend to leave direct material traces, sound is not often considered in archaeological work outside the subdiscipline of archaeomusicology (Witmore 2006:268–276; see also Coles 1973:158–167; Megaw 1968; Megaw and Longworth 1981). It is, however, an important aspect of life that can be investigated using an interpretive approach to the archaeological remains. In order to form a comprehensive understanding of a site used by people, it should be remembered, for example, that their movements can result in sounds such as those of footsteps, opening and closing doors (at some sites), and clothing fabric moving over the body.

## Medieval Monasticism

Medieval monasticism had its origins in the thought of late antique Christian theologians; most notable is St. Benedict, whose Rule, written in the sixth century C.E., "was the foundation upon which the entire structure of medieval monasticism in Western Europe was eventually built" (Greene 1992:2). This Rule represented a shift in the setting of monastic existence, from desert hermitages to communities more integrated with contemporary society, and its contents dictated (among other things) the organization of the monastic liturgical day, based

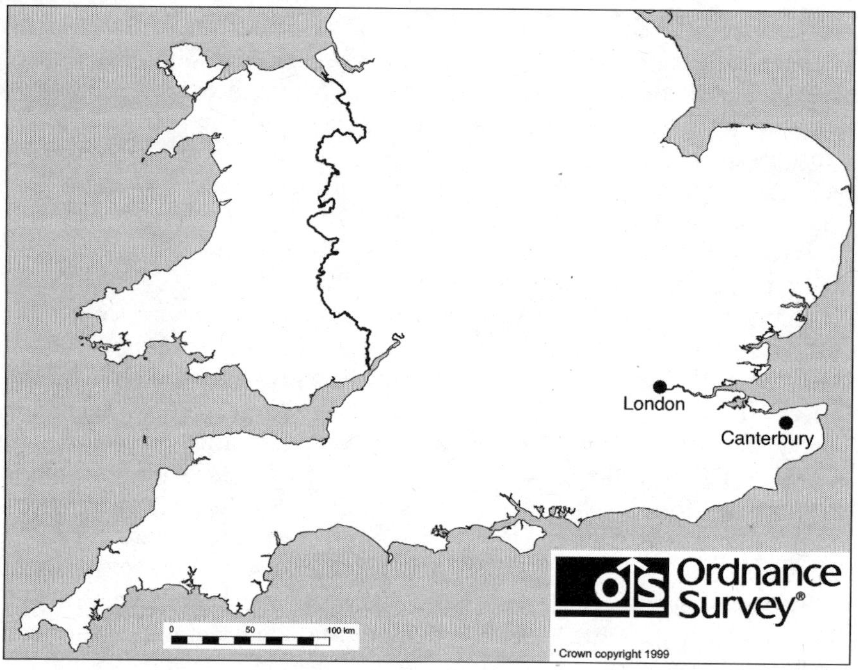


**Figure 10-1.** *Map showing location of Canterbury in the United Kingdom.*

around the seven "offices," or services, recited at regular intervals from soon after midnight until dusk (Butler and Given-Wilson 1979:15). The Benedictine order directly spawned numerous related orders of monks and nuns, examples being the Cistercian order (which followed a more puritanical interpretation of Benedict's Rule) and the Cluniac order (which focused to a much greater extent on the liturgy [Butler and Given-Wilson 1979:32–35]). However, the Benedictine Rule also had a significant influence on monastic orders with other lineages. In the context of urban monasticism in England, the order of Augustinian canons was the most prominent of these (see Greene 1992:15); its Rule was based primarily on the thought of Augustine of Hippo but also borrowed from that of Benedict and could be adapted by individual institutions (Butler and Given-Wilson 1979:44).

The broad similarities between monastic orders also extended to the physical arrangement of their institutions. While it would not be quite accurate to state that the buildings of monastic sites were constructed to standardized plans, the importance of set locations for particular activities prescribed by the monastic rules does give these sites a distinctive signature. The most prominent building, and that which the monastic day revolved around, was the church. Connected to the church was the cloister, which was surrounded by buildings fulfilling other needs, some primarily domestic (such as the lavatory, or rere-dorter; the kitchen; the cellar; and the dormitory), some ritual (such as the chapter house, in which daily readings from the Rule took place), and some a combination of the two (in particular the refectory, in which the daily meal was eaten in silence while readings from scripture were recited). In many cases, a house for the abbot or prior also adjoined the cloister, allowing for the reception of guests. In general, the cloister and associated buildings lay to the south of the church, but in practice this was dependent upon limitations of the site, and both St. Augustine's Abbey and St. Gregory's Priory had cloisters to the north.[1]

### *Monastic Sound*

Music was an important aspect of the religious lives of those who followed the Augustinian and Benedictine Rules (and continues to be so today). Benedict's Rule is identified by Andrew Wilson-Dickson (1992:33) as having been "most influential in shaping monastic [musical] tradition" on the basis of its division of the monastic day into the liturgical offices. Augustine of Hippo studied and wrote about music and recognized its power as an element of religious experience (Brennan 1988:268–269). The position of music in archaeological studies could be said to suffer from problems similar to those of many artifact types: the focus is more on the intrinsic value of the instruments, or artifacts, rather than on what they can tell us about the lives of the inhabitants of the sites at which they were found.

In seeking to understand music in medieval monasteries, however, there can be little focus on evidence of instruments, for they did not feature to any great extent in the liturgy—use of the organ in this context was rare (Caldwell 1967:12; Wilson-Dickson 1992:76–77). There is a wealth of evidence relating to chant traditions in the forms of text and notated music, allowing study of musical style and the development of polyphony among other things (see, for example, Caldwell 1992), but the scant nature of artifactual evidence for the performance of such music is unsurprising when one considers that little equipment is necessary. This is not to say, though, that material evidence cannot inform interpretations of medieval Christian music: Laura Moretti (2004), for example, studies the development of polyphonic double choir music in sixteenth-century Venice by focusing on changes made to the architectural spaces of St. Mark's Basilica.

As the title of this chapter suggests, its main focus will be on how sound is experienced in the spaces of the sites, with an emphasis on musical spaces and quiet spaces. It should be clarified here that *musical space* and *quiet space* are not being considered as dichotomous but rather as related phenomena. Indeed, the two types of space are similar in that both require a relative absence of external aural stimuli in order to function as desired by their users. A musical space, while being ostensibly an area of considerable noise, could therefore be referred to as a quiet space. Thus, the research question of this work could be phrased, How quiet were the quiet spaces of these two monasteries? This question must be informed by some consideration of why quietness was valued at medieval monastic sites. Linguistically, *quiet* is not only an opposite of *loud*, but it can also be thought of as antonymous with *busy* (Kirkpatrick 1995:90). As such, an understanding of quiet space at a monastery can be informed by consideration of the movement of people around the site.

*Case Studies: St. Augustine's Abbey and St. Gregory's Priory*

This study of the two sites focuses on a particular point in their lives—specifically, the mid-thirteenth century, circa 1250 C.E. This time period was selected as both sites had been substantially rebuilt following fires in the mid- to late twelfth century—and so are comparable in that each had a new arrangement of space in an already-established monastic setting—but were not then undergoing major building modifications (which occurred at both sites after the mid-thirteenth century [Hicks and Hicks 2001:31; Tatton-Brown 1991:69]). As such, it could perhaps be expected that they would exhibit spatial manifestations of the social needs of the communities using them (Steadman 2000:171–172). The analytical element of this work involves the use of two methods of spatial analysis—access analysis and the study of copresence zones. Both methods must be informed by an understanding of the sites as they existed in the mid-thirteenth century.

These methods rely predominantly on the architectural remains at the sites, an approach that has been selected partly as a result of the specific circumstances surrounding the creation of the archaeological record relating to English monastic sites. While the events of Henry VIII's dissolution of the monasteries can be said to have reduced the possibility of applying some archaeological approaches—those based solely on artifact study being particularly affected—the survival of foundations and walls, along with less high-status artifacts and features that escaped removal or destruction in the sixteenth century, means that investigation of the lives of these sites does not suffer to a great degree. A comparison of these two sites can be seen to some extent as work within the field of local history, but it also relates to the broader fields of monastic studies and sensory studies as the people living at the two institutions subscribed to different monastic rules—that of St. Benedict in the case of St. Augustine's Abbey and that of St. Augustine at St. Gregory's Priory. Thus, such a study can provide some idea of how these rules affected the sensory lives of those who followed them.

## Built Space

*Spatial Analysis*

A central tenet of the work of Bill Hillier and Julienne Hanson is the idea that built space, when allowed to develop organically over time, reflects the social structure of the people using the space (Hillier and Hanson 1984:1–25)—the inner logic of buildings and settlements corresponding with the "inner social logic of society" (Kent 1990:127). Their methods of access analysis form a framework by which, it is argued, one can study such spatial arrangements to find the principles that govern them. However, consideration of the movement of people through spatial systems is here used not so much to form judgments about the organization of monastic society as to interpret sensory experiences of monastic spaces.

Access analysis, despite its nonarchaeological origins, has been successfully applied to archaeological evidence with informative results (Foster 1989;

Grahame 2000; Steadman 2000). Sharon R. Steadman (2000:167–169) refers to access analysis and proxemics as "resulting from the broader perspective of architectural semiotics." Space syntax theory, from which access analysis developed (Lawson 2001:241–246), views space as a language, with clues about social organization encoded in its "grammar"—or the relationships between individual spaces. Proxemics can also be said to view space, or rather human interactions within space, in such a way, with Edward Hall's (1963) notation system being equivalent to the grammatical lexicon used by linguists in the study of sentence structure.

An important aspect of proxemics for the sensory archaeologist is the notion of the *field of copresence*: "an entire spatial extent which is . . . accessible to unaided human sensory processing and which offers an adequately strong and rich sensory input. . . . [It] is made of five *zones* corresponding to the five basic manners in Man's transactions with his *environment*" (Ciolek 1983:63, emphasis in original). According to Donald Sanders (1990:48), "Each zone is roughly one-ninth the area of the previous, ranging in decreasing size through vision, hearing, smell, reach-with-a-tool, and contact zones." In Sanders's study of Cretan Bronze Age houses, he predominantly makes use of the three smallest zones, along with consideration of views, in order to evaluate social interaction (Sanders 1990:59–63), but in the present work the hearing zone shall be the focus.

### *Monastic Space as Sensory Experience*

With reference to the linguistic discussion of the introduction to this chapter, it will be remembered that both *loud* and *busy* are antonyms of *quiet*. The second of these terms highlights the effect that a relative absence of other people has on the amount of sound one experiences when in a place. Peter-Damian Belisle (2003:85–86) discusses the connection between silence and solitude in Benedictine communities at some length:

> To create an atmosphere of silence in the Benedictine community is crucial—an atmosphere within which every monk or nun can do the "work" of solitude, maintaining a mindfulness of divine presence. By cultivating this silence . . . Benedict's followers help to create, in effect, solitude within communal life. Benedictines form community to experience solitude together. . . . To enable others around oneself to do so, it is important not to disturb others. The Rule regulates silence to promote contemplative union and communion.

The mention here of solitude within communal life is of particular relevance to this chapter, as to some extent its aim is to investigate whether the desire for solitude in a community is manifested spatially *and* socially or purely socially. In the case of the former, which is called sociospatial solitude here, both interior and exterior solitudes (see below) are involved, with exterior solitude enabling interior solitude to be more easily achieved; in the case of social solitude, the attainment of interior (social) solitude is more of a personal challenge as it is not facilitated by the provision of exterior (spatial) solitude.

Monastic space should not be thought of as homogeneous across space (i.e., geographical areas) and time; indeed, it is the heterogeneity of monastic spaces that makes them fertile ground for this study. Christopher Brooke (1971:163), in a discussion of the work of Edmund Bishop, makes the point that "in every substantial variety in church design one may find an attempt to solve a problem in a church's function, to follow this and that new or old fashion, and to reflect in an appropriate way some of the religious sentiments of the age." If this notion is extended to include the claustral buildings of monasteries, it would also seem reasonable to expect to find significant differences in the designs of spaces used by different orders. As John Teahan (1982:524) has identified, Thomas Merton distinguished between exterior solitude and interior solitude. In Merton's words, "the truest solitude is not something outside you, not an absence of men or of sound around you; it is an abyss opening up in the center of your own soul" (Merton 1950:31). If such an attitude can be extrapolated to medieval Christian monasticism (a potentially dangerous exercise considering the recent date of Merton's work and the evolution of Christian traditions), it may perhaps be found that there is less of a design for solitude apparent in the spatial arrangements of medieval monastic sites than could at first be expected.

## Methodology

### *Access Analysis*

Gamma analysis is a form of access analysis developed by Hillier and Hanson (1984:143–175) for the study of buildings. It encompasses a number of different methods for the analysis of spatial systems, of which some are more useful than others when studying archaeological remains. These methods generate data that can form the basis of interpretations of human movement and social interaction at the sites being analyzed. Justified access maps for each site (Figure 10-2) were used to obtain these data, in the forms of control values and relative asymmetry (RA) values for the individual spaces. The former relate to the control each space has over access to its neighbors, with a higher value indicating a greater degree of control. The latter values are indicators of each space's level of accessibility relative to the system of spaces as a whole, with a lower value representing a more accessible space. As the spaces of larger spatial systems tend to have smaller RA values and in order to allow comparison between sites, the RA values are calibrated using a table produced by Hillier and Hanson (1984:112); the resulting values measure "real relative asymmetry" (RRA).

When considered together, control and RRA values can be used to assess the levels of presence availability of the sites' spaces (see below; see also Grahame 1997:150; Putzeys et al. 2003). The processes involved in the undertaking of access analysis as a part of archaeological research have been discussed at length elsewhere (Foster 1989; Grahame 2000), so they are not presented in detail here. Tables 10-1 and 10-2 show control and RRA values for St. Augustine's Abbey and St. Gregory's Priory. The production of two data sets for each site, one including the exterior space and the other discounting it, allows spatial solitude to be

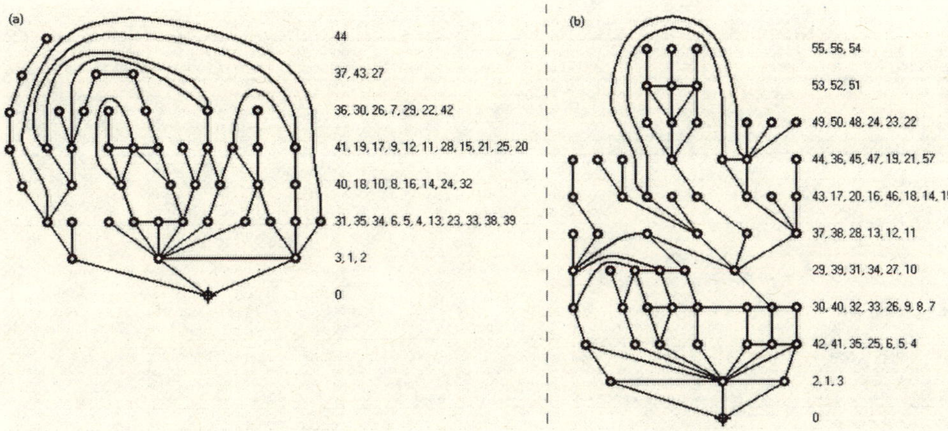


**Figure 10-2.** *Justified access maps of (a) St. Gregory's Priory and (b) St. Augustine's Abbey.*

considered in terms of encounters between inhabitants and visitors and between inhabitants and inhabitants (Hanson 1998:29–30). This aspect of the analysis is particularly important for this project, as inhabitants are monastics living by monastic rules while visitors are not bound by such rules. In general, the boundaries between spaces correspond to known walls or other architectural features, such as colonnades. However, in the exceptional cases of the cloisters, the use of different criteria for the identification of spatial boundaries was necessary. As an architectural element or a setting for activities, the monastic cloister can be said to be a single thing, but in terms of space, it is not a homogeneous area. An immediately obvious distinction is that between the garth (the central courtyard or garden of the cloister) and the covered area surrounding it; the garth is the least problematic aspect of the cloister, and it can be considered as a single space. The area between the garth and the claustral buildings is traditionally referred to either as four separate places—north, east, south, and west walks (Greene 1992:6)—or occasionally as a single passage (Butler and Given-Wilson 1979:65). However, these architectural conventions do not seem adequate when considering the cloister as spatial experience; there are significant areas of overlap between the walks. In order to arrive at a more satisfactory interpretation of claustral spaces, it was necessary to consider plans of cloisters, informed by visits to standing and ruined cloisters. The resulting (and admittedly subjective) decision was that the cloister can be presented as nine spaces: garth, walks, and corners (Figure 10-3). These triangular corner spaces are the areas of overlap between walks, including areas within the field of view around the corners at the meetings of colonnades; it is therefore possible to enter the garth from the spaces of the walks but not from the spaces of the corners.

While RRA and control values can be useful on their own, it is when they are considered together that they are most informative for this project. This allows the identification of levels of presence availability for each space in the system (Putzeys et al. 2003); these indicate the relative likelihood of an encounter (which

**Table 10-1.** *St. Augustine's Abbey: Access Analysis Data for Quiet Spaces*

| | *Control value* | | *Control rank* | | *RRA value* | | *RRA rank* | | *PA level* | |
|---|---|---|---|---|---|---|---|---|---|---|
| Space | 0 | θ | 0 | θ | 0 | θ | 0 | θ | 0 | θ |
| 12 (choir) | .700 | .700 | 25 | 22 | .860 | .855 | 4 | 3 | 4 | 4 |
| 27 (study area) | .833 | .833 | 20 | 19 | .953 | .924 | 10 | 7 | 4 | 4 |
| 36 (vestry?) | .333 | .333 | 30 | 28 | 1.429 | 1.425 | 35 | 32 | 2 | 2 |
| 39 (refectory) | .333 | .333 | 30 | 28 | 1.667 | 1.684 | 41 | 38 | 1 | 1 |
| 43 (dormitory) | 1.500 | 1.500 | 10 | 9 | 1.440 | 1.441 | 36 | 33 | 6 | 6 |
| Mean (site as a whole) | | | | | 1.26081 | 1.25813 | | | 4.0862 | 4.1930 |

*Note:* Data in columns headed "0" and "θ" are taken from data sets resulting from analysis of spatial systems respectively including and excluding the exterior (space 0).

**Table 10-2.** *St. Gregory's Priory: Access Analysis Data for Quiet Spaces*

| | *Control value* | | *Control rank* | | *RRA value* | | *RRA rank* | | *PA level* | |
|---|---|---|---|---|---|---|---|---|---|---|
| Space | 0 | θ | 0 | θ | 0 | θ | 0 | θ | 0 | θ |
| 9 (choir) | 1.833 | 1.833 | 4 | 3 | 1.236 | 1.307 | 29 | 25 | 6 | 6 |
| 20 (study area) | 1.083 | 1.083 | 12 | 11 | 1.072 | 1.084 | 21 | 15 | 5 | 5 |
| 21 (study area) | 1.166 | 1.166 | 11 | 10 | .931 | .961 | 13 | 7 | 8 | 8 |
| 32 (refectory | .833 | .833 | 17 | 15 | 1.102 | 1.138 | 34 | 27 | 5 | 5 |
| 43 (dormitory) | 1.000 | 1.000 | 14 | 13 | 1.347 | 1.492 | 33 | 29 | 6 | 6 |
| Mean (site as a whole) | | | | | 1.11068 | 1.18764 | | | 5.2222 | 5.1364 |

*Note:* Data in columns headed "0" and "θ" are taken from data sets resulting from analysis of spatial systems respectively including and excluding the exterior (space 0).

need not necessarily involve verbal communication) between people occurring in any particular space compared to the other spaces in the system. This measure is therefore important in the consideration of sound at the sites, as a person is likely to be aware of another's presence in a space through use of his or her senses, including hearing. Presence availability (PA) is a relative measure based on the rank orders of control and accessibility of the spaces in the systems. In order to convert these rankings into levels of PA, they were plotted on a scatter graph divided into sections, as seen in Figure 10-3.

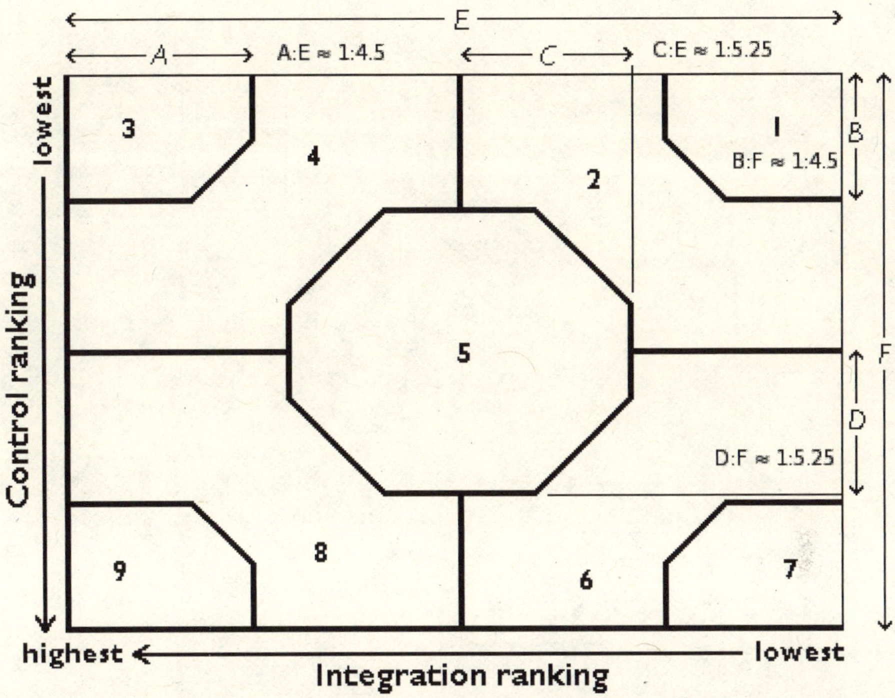


**Figure 10-3.** *Format of graph used to obtain levels of presence availability for spaces in a system. The numbered sections of the plot area represent the levels of presence availability of spaces appearing within them when plotted on the graph, from 1 (very low) to 9 (very high).*

The division of this graph is based on a table produced by Mark Grahame (1997:150). For the purposes of this investigation, it was decided that the four PA levels presented in this table, while sufficient when dealing with small systems of spaces, would not allow for fine enough distinction in larger systems, such as those of the two monastic sites studied here. As such, further divisions were added within the four sections to enable the identification of nine levels of presence availability. It should be noted that the method used in this work to obtain presence availability values does not take into account the sizes and shapes of spaces, and is therefore closer to that detailed by Toon Putzeys and colleagues (2003) than it is to that detailed by Grahame (2000:56–57); a reassessment of the sites using the latter method is a possibility for future research. Figures 10-4 and 10-5 show schematic representations of each site with shading to show the PA levels for each space when the exterior is included in the analysis.

A multiphase plan of St. Augustine's Abbey (Bennett 1987:82–83) and a single-phase plan of St. Gregory's Priory (Hicks and Hicks 2001:25) were used to distinguish the individual spaces of each site. The directors of the rescue excavations at the priory site highlight the exceptional preservation of the sequence of building phases—from Lanfranc's original foundation to the last modifications before the dissolution—and occupation deposits in the introduction to their report (Hicks

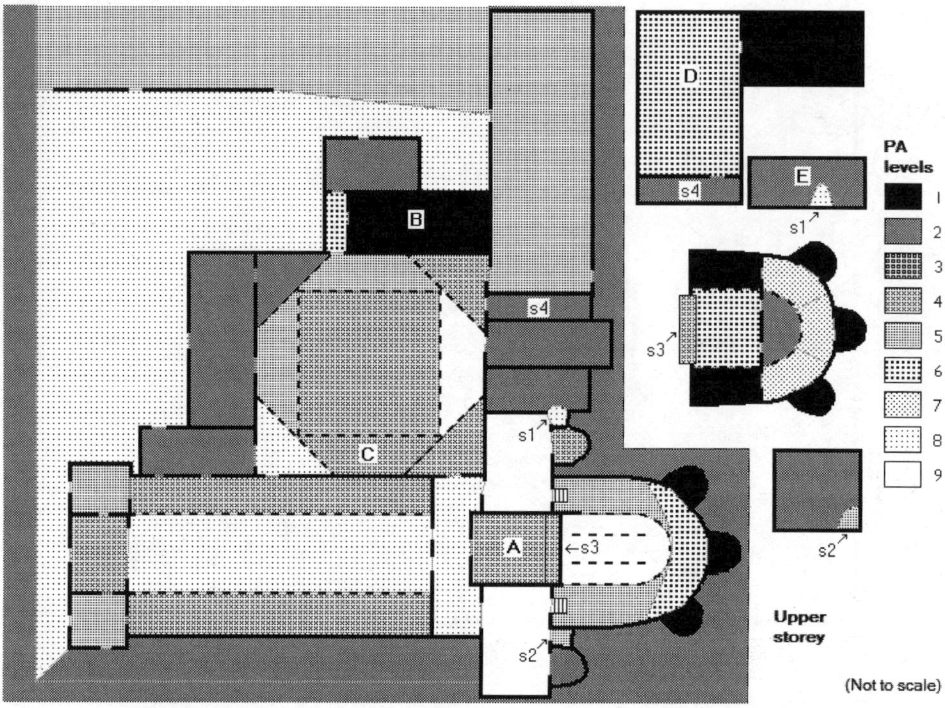


**Figure 10-4.** *Presence availability diagram of St. Augustine's Abbey, including exterior (space 0). Spaces labeled with an s represent staircases; each label appears twice, once for the lower story and once for the upper. Numbered spaces are referred to in the text. Key to other labeled spaces: A – choir; B – refectory; C – cloister study area; D – dormitory; E – possible vestry.*

and Hicks 2001:xxiii). The latter are of considerable importance for this study, as they are a valuable resource for the formation of an interpretation of sound at the priory. As the architectural remains at the sites survive only at ground-floor level, some speculation was necessary regarding first-floor rooms; only those known to have existed have been included, and their representations have been kept as simple as possible. The construction of a royal palace at the abbey site following the dissolution means that there is some uncertainty as to the appearance of the western claustral range in the mid-thirteenth century (Tatton-Brown 1991:71). Thus, only two spaces are shown, representing the cellarer's range as a whole, with no internal divisions and no upper story (space 35), and a space joining the inner court to the cloister (space 25), which may have been either a parlor or similar room or a part of the inner court close to the cellarer's range. The focus of much of the archaeological literature and excavation has been on the Anglo-Saxon churches (Tatton-Brown 1991:62), with the result that the visitor to the abbey today may experience difficulty visualizing the abbey church as it appeared in the post-Conquest period—however, positions of the rood and *pulpitum* screens within the church are known from early twentieth-century plans made before the destruction of these features to expose part of an earlier church (Tatton-Brown 1991:63).

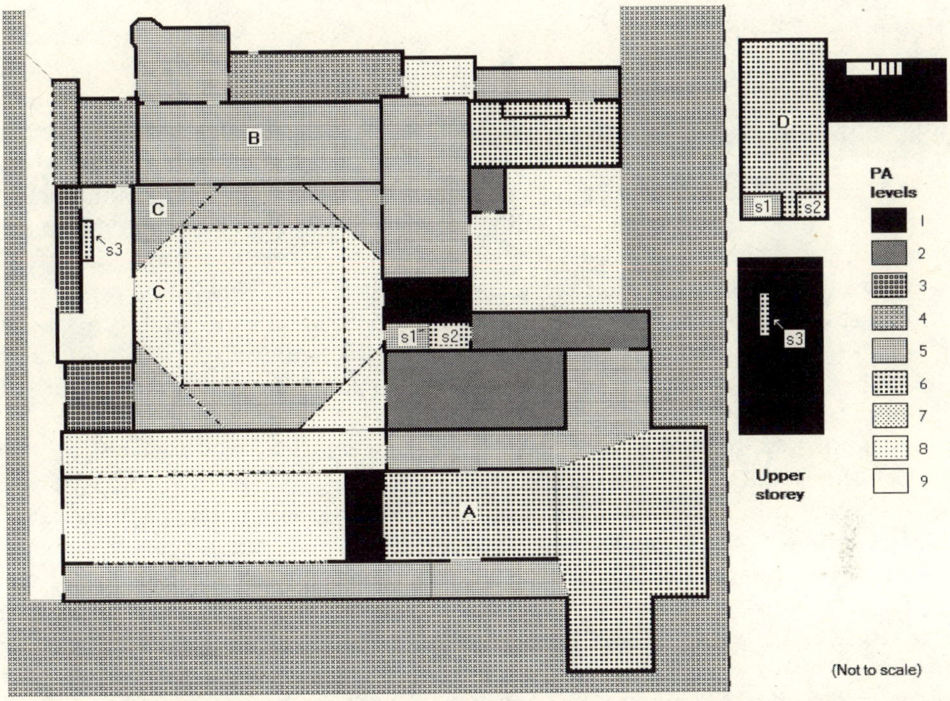


**Figure 10-5.** *Presence availability diagram of St. Gregory's Priory, including exterior (space 0). Spaces labeled with an s represent staircases; each label appears twice, once for the lower story and once for the upper. Numbered spaces are referred to in the text. Key to other labeled spaces: A – choir; B – refectory; C – cloister study area; D – dormitory.*

In the case of the priory, the extent of excavation meant that the representation of the east end of the church was also conjectural. Permeability of the boundary between the north transept and the passage to the north of it has been assumed, as the night stairs led into this passage (Hicks and Hicks 2001:72). The infirmary buildings were also outside the excavated area; the excavators' interpretation is that these were connected to the main claustral buildings by the passage perpendicular to the east claustral range (space 41; Hicks and Hicks 2001:91). This passage has been shown on the schematic representation with a closed east end, and the decision was made to focus only on the main claustral buildings and churches at both sites in order to allow a more accurate comparison between the two. Thus, the abbey's infirmary and the spaces connecting it to the east claustral range were excluded from this study.

### *Study of Copresence Zones*

Michele George (2002:239), reviewing Grahame's study of Pompeian houses, writes that the author's conclusion "demands justification beyond the numerical results of a formula." Lawrence (1990:75) also presents a criticism of

Hillier and Hanson's access analysis, accusing the authors of determinism on the grounds that they "[consider] only the graphical representation of buildings, while overlooking the growing volume of research in the social sciences." It is true that in archaeological terms, while analysis of the spaces of buildings can be a valuable endeavor on its own, its usefulness is increased dramatically when artifactual evidence is considered alongside it. A number of scholars, notably Penelope Allison (1997), as well as Bradley A. Ault and Lisa C. Nevett (1999), have in recent years encouraged archaeologists to adopt a more assemblage-focused view of finds, in the hope that more can be learned from excavation reports. In both cases (Allison 1997:81; Ault and Nevett 1999:51–52), the authors propose modes of presentation that enable simultaneous consideration of artifacts and architecture—and, thus, built space—in order to gain a better understanding of life at the site.

The second method used in this project was study of copresence zones, or CPZs (Ciolek 1983:63). The concept of CPZs utilizes an approach to space that is somewhat different from access analysis. While gamma analysis focuses on representational spaces, or lived space, without considering representations of space, or measured space (Lefebvre 1991:39), the methods used in the study of CPZs in this work rely heavily on representations of space. In order to undertake this study, the 30.2 m CPZs of hearing (Sanders 1990:59) surrounding the mid-thirteenth century musical and quiet spaces of the sites were superimposed upon plans of the sites. Excavation reports were then consulted to identify possible disturbances of peace that could have been heard from these spaces. It was not necessary to note everything in these areas but rather to identify significant features and artifacts from mid-thirteenth-century contexts.

At St. Gregory's Priory, the hearing CPZs surrounding the quiet spaces encompass the entire excavated area, so all finds from the rescue excavations were considered. At the larger St. Augustine's Abbey, however, a number of excavations have taken place over a much longer period and in various parts of the abbey precinct; finds from those not within the area of the quiet spaces' hearing CPZs have generally been excluded from this study. It should be noted that application of this method is subject to some weaknesses: Most obviously, the buildings themselves would have had an effect on the audibility of sounds (Sanders 1990:62), but without a suitable degree of knowledge of the building materials used beyond the extant remains, it would be unwise to assume too much about this. The 30.2 m hearing CPZ is, therefore, used for this study, with the possibility of further research at a later date.

## Discussion

### *Access Analysis of Sites—General Observations*

Two data sets were produced for each site, the first including the exterior, or carrier, space (space 0) and the second set excluding this space; this enables consideration of what Hanson (1998:29) refers to as "the relative importance of inhabitant-inhabitant and inhabitant-visitor relationships for the planning and organization of the [building]." The main aspects of the access-analysis data used in this consideration are the mean real relative asymmetry (RRA) values—where a low value represents a high level of integration and vice versa—of each site and the rank orders of integration of the spaces of each site. According to Hanson (1998:29), in complexes of spaces in which disregarding the exterior has little effect on mean integration or the rank order of integration of individual spaces, "configuration is principally organized so as to structure interior relations, and hence the inhabitant-inhabitant interface." Conversely, when "the way in which each cell features within the configuration is strongly affected by the way the complex relates to the exterior, the inhabitant-visitor interface is implicated in the sociogram of [the] building at least as much as the relations among its inhabitants" (Hanson 1998:29).

Such consideration is of particular relevance to this investigation of quiet space at medieval monastic sites because, as was mentioned above, there is a significant difference between the inhabitants of these sites and the majority of visitors to them. The main claustral buildings were the domains of monks or canons ostensibly following a monastic rule (including its specifications about silence), and it is these people who were the inhabitants. The consideration of only these buildings in this work excludes lay people living and working elsewhere in the precinct (as well as monastics in the infirmary living for a period under a relaxed version of the rule) from the subset inhabitants. These lay people, along with others such as traders and pilgrims, comprise the subset visitors (Hillier and Hanson 1984:146); their presence within the claustral buildings creates a potential for disturbance in the inhabitants' quiet spaces.

The effect on the access analysis data for the abbey of disregarding the exterior is fairly minimal: The mean RRA of the complex decreases slightly, from 1.26081 to 1.25813, meaning that as a whole it becomes slightly more integrated, and there are few changes in the rank order of integration of individual spaces (see Table 10-1); the changes in position of a small number of spaces are noteworthy, however, and these are discussed in greater detail below. However, the effect on the data for the priory is more dramatic; the complex becomes significantly more segregated, as the mean RRA increases from 1.11068 to 1.18764, and the rank order of integration of individual spaces changes significantly (see Table 10-2). In light of Hanson's statements quoted above, these observations tell us that the claustral buildings of the priory structured relations between inhabitants and visitors to a greater degree than those of the abbey, which could be said, in the words of Hanson (1998:29), to "structure interior relations." This should perhaps be expected, considering the far greater number of inhabitants at the abbey: Timothy Tatton-Brown (1997:126) suggests, on the basis of dormitory floor area, that the abbey could accommodate at least one hundred monks, compared with approximately ten canons at the priory (Hicks and Hicks 2001:375).

If one were to forget for a moment that only the main claustral buildings are being considered, these observations could appear surprising, as it could be supposed that the combination of the abbey's status as an important pilgrimage site with the material requirements of a large number of monks would bring a considerable number of visiting pilgrims and traders, thus requiring a greater degree of structuring of inhabitant-visitor relations. Remembering, though, that the abbey's precinct included more than just these buildings, the observations are rather less surprising; there were other structures to provide for the needs of many visitors, but the presence of a large number of monks within the claustral buildings would create a requirement for some degree of structuring of the relations between the inhabitants. At the smaller establishment of St. Gregory's Priory, where (it is supposed by the excavators [Hicks and Hicks 2001:133]) guests were often entertained at the prior's lodge within the western claustral range, it can perhaps be concluded that more structuring of relations between inhabitants and visitors was required.

### *Quiet Spaces*

While an idea of monasteries in their entireties as being quiet places can be said to exist, certain spaces within a monastery can also be identified as being particularly quiet in relation to the entire precinct. Identification of such spaces is based predominantly on the monastic rules and on information from secondary sources. The main quiet spaces examined here, in terms of named rooms or spaces, are the dormitories, refectories, monastics' choirs, and study areas in cloisters. Site-specific quiet spaces must also be taken into account. The choirs are included in this list because, as discussed in this chapter's introduction, the production of music in these spaces requires a low level of external noise. While the liturgical east ends of the churches could be thought of as quiet spaces because they also require similar low levels of noise for the saying of masses and other services, the lack of information about the east end of the priory's church means that they cannot be included in this study.

In order to compare the sites' quiet spaces, a diagram showing quiet space presence availability genotypes (based on Hillier and Hanson's notion of building genotypes; Hanson 1998:35) was produced (Figure 10-6). The concept of building genotypes will not be discussed at length here; it is sufficient to know that it relates to the spatial system of a building, as distinguished from a building phenotype, which relates to the building's form (Hillier and Hanson 1984:12–13). The spaces are presented in order of presence availability levels, giving us some idea of the relative likelihoods of encounters occurring in quiet spaces both within a single site and across both sites. One of the first things that is noticeable about this diagram is that the quiet spaces of the priory in general have significantly higher levels of presence availability than those of the abbey. At the abbey, all but one (the dormitory) of the quiet spaces have levels below 5, the medium level, and the dormitory is only slightly above this at level 6. However, at the priory, all quiet spaces have levels of 5 or higher, with one (part of the cloister study area) being significantly higher at level 8, one of the highest PA levels at the site. At the abbey, only the refectory has a PA level higher than the averages for the site (4.0862 in terms of inhabitant-visitor relations and 4.1930 for inhabitant-inhabitant relations); whereas, at the priory, the majority of the quiet spaces have higher-than-average PA levels (the averages being 5.2222 for inhabitant-visitor relations and 5.1364 for inhabitant-inhabitant relations). Having considered this, we can suggest

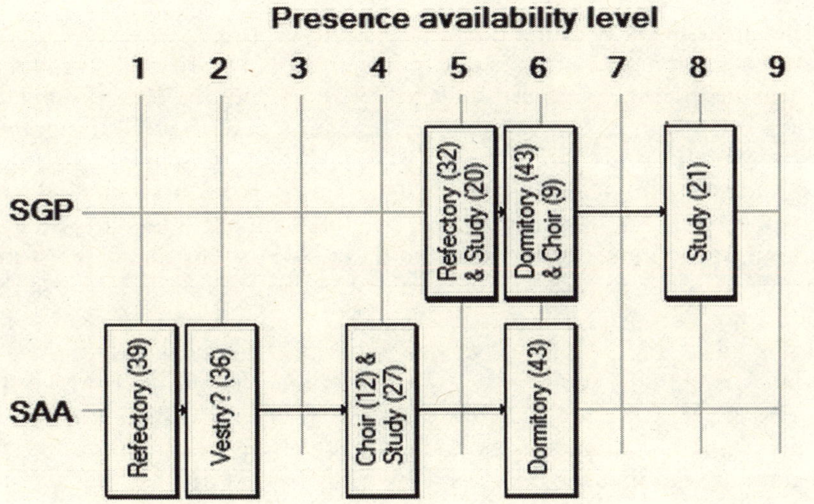


**Figure 10-6.** *Quiet space presence availability genotypes of St. Gregory's Priory (SGP) and St. Augustine's Abbey (SAA).*

that the quiet spaces of the priory would have been noisier than those of the abbey on the basis that encounters between people were more likely in these spaces. The example of sounds created by people's movement should be remembered here; these encounters need not be thought of as including verbal communication.

The nature of the music that would have been heard in medieval monastic choirs is the subject of extensive scholarship and cannot be explored in any detail in a study of this length; to state that the majority of this music would have been unaccompanied chant (Wilson-Dickson 1992:76–77) will suffice here. However, the sound of the organ should also be taken into account. According to George Smith (1883:5), it is likely that Canterbury Cathedral came into possession of an organ during the archbishopric of Theodore (668–690 C.E.) (Brooks 1984:71–76). Organs, then, had been known in Canterbury in a Christian religious—though not necessarily liturgical—context (Bowles 1962:13–14) for some centuries by the period of focus of this study. The abbey is known to have had an organ; a thirteenth-century customary mentions its use, but it should not be supposed that such was a frequent occurrence at the abbey. The instrument was only used in the liturgy some ten to twelve times per year, the number being dependent upon when Easter fell, and it is more likely to have been played in alternation with the choir than it is to have accompanied it (Harrison 1980:205–206). Use of the organ in this manner means it is likely that, on these special occasions, it would not have been of much concern to the monks whether or not the sound of the instrument traveled throughout the monastery as they would all have been involved in the liturgy. Nonetheless, the sound of the organ may have been heard at other times, as it would surely have been necessary for at least one monk to have learned to play the instrument at times outside the liturgical hours. No extant documentary evidence suggests that the priory possessed an organ (Hicks and Hicks 2001:371–376).

The study areas within the cloisters are also worthy of further discussion. While these are treated here as quiet spaces, it should be remembered that when study was taking place in these spaces they would not have been silent: "Reading was a process that involved the pronunciation of each word, if not out loud, at least distinctly enough for the reader himself to be conscious of it" (Meyvaert 1973:54). Even so, this should not be taken to mean that sounds created by things other than people reading would have been welcome in the study areas. Thus, it is important to consider the surroundings of these areas. At the priory, the study area (benches against the western wall of the cloister and against the west end of the northern wall) is in spaces 20 and 21 on the schematic representations. Adjoining these spaces to the west was the prior's house, which has been identified as a potentially noisy space. A mid-eighteenth-century engraving of the prior's house, on which the roofline of the west cloister walk appears to be visible, shows that there do not seem to have been any windows at ground level in the section of wall that the benches would have stood against; this would have gone some way toward preventing sounds in the house from being heard in the study area, as the masonry walls would have muffled more sound than a glass window would have.

If the presence availability diagrams for the cloister at the priory (Figure 10-7) are consulted, it is apparent that encounters were fairly likely in the spaces of the study areas and in the cloister as a whole—more so in terms of inhabitant-inhabitant relations, as spaces 14 and 17 increase in PA level when the exterior is disregarded. At the abbey, where the study area was in space 27, the cloister as a whole had lower levels of PA, but the east walk and the south-west corner space (adjoining the study area) have very high PA levels in terms of both inhabitant-visitor and inhabitant-inhabitant relations, with that of the east walk being one of the highest at the site. However, the location of the study area in the south walk, rather than the east (Tatton-Brown 1991:66), may have alleviated to some degree any possible problems with noise from the cellarer's range (space 35). This space can be assumed to have been an area of interaction between inhabitants and visitors, on the basis of its function and the PA diagrams; the PA level of this space is significantly reduced when the exterior space is disregarded. At the priory, the cellarer's range did not directly adjoin the cloister, and its PA level is the same whether inhabitant-visitor or inhabitant-inhabitant relations are being considered. The fact that this range is adjacent to the quiet space of the refectory may not be too significant, as it seems reasonable to assume that business dealings would not have been taking place in the range during mealtimes.

One final point relating to the study areas in the cloisters is raised by the relationship between the extent of the hearing copresence zone and the size of each cloister. The diagonal distance across the priory's cloister was less than 30.2 m, so the hearing CPZ of a person standing anywhere within the cloister would extend beyond the cloister. However, the abbey's cloister was larger, and the distance across the garth was only slightly smaller than the radius of the hearing CPZ; parts of the cloister were thus outside the hearing CPZ of the study area, which was situated against the southern wall. As such, the study area of the abbey can be said to have been slightly more peaceful with reference to sound events in the

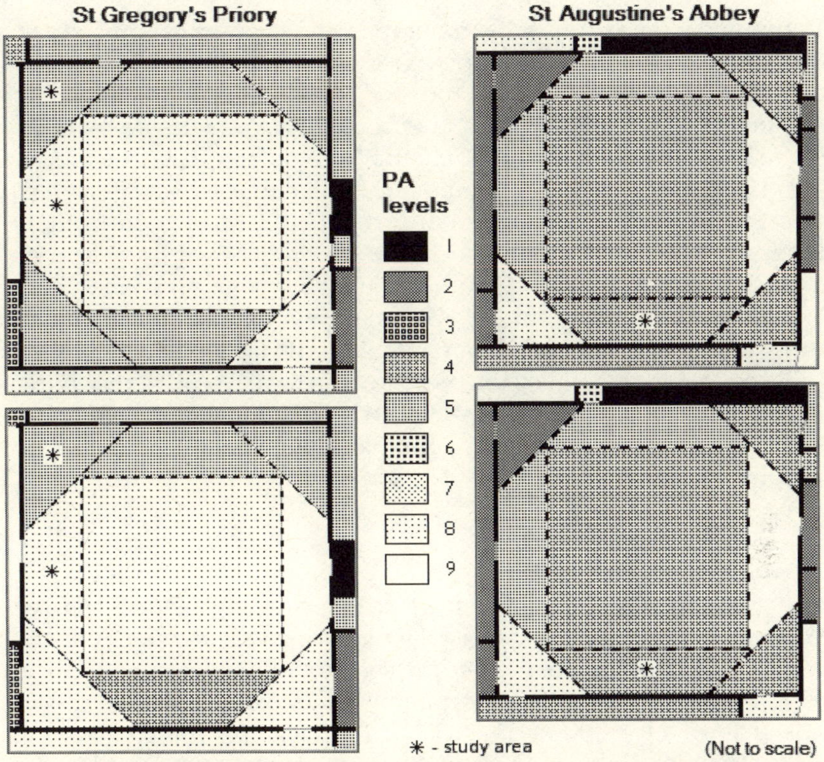


**Figure 10-7.** *Details of PA diagrams of St. Gregory's Priory and St. Augustine's Abbey, showing cloisters and neighboring spaces. For both sites, the upper image represents inhabitant-visitor interactions and the lower represents inhabitant-inhabitant interactions. Study areas are shown with asterisks.*

cloister. It should be remembered, though, that the abbey had an organ that is likely to have been located in the area of the choir (space 12), which was within the study area's hearing CPZ and could have created some disturbance if played outside the temporal context of the liturgy—if being practiced on, for instance.

A further quiet space that could have been affected by the sound of the organ, or other sounds in the area of the monks' choir at the abbey, is the possible vestry (space 36). This is a site-specific quiet space, identified as such not by reference to a monastic rule but from a secondary source relating to the site. Tatton-Brown (1991:66) writes of the space, "Since it had no doors in its east and west walls and could only be approached by a stair from the north transept, it was clearly not a parlor or a passage but some sort of place of safety. It may have been a vestry or treasury, or a library." The isolation of this space, which leads Tatton-Brown to call it a place of safety, would have presumably resulted in its being quiet; this can certainly be said to be true on the basis of its low PA level (level 2). However, as its only access was from the north transept and it was well within the hearing CPZ of the choir, it seems possible that sounds in the choir that would have affected the cloister study area would also have reached this space through the stairway.

Returning to the spaces of the monastics' choirs, we must consider the structuring of movement within the church as an important element of the creation of quiet space. At St. Gregory's Priory, the rood screen not only creates a psychological division between monastics and lay people, it also creates a physical division that prevents the use of the canons' choir and retrochoir (spaces 9 and 7, respectively) as transitional spaces for movement along the east-west axis of the church, somewhat reducing the likelihood of disturbance. It is worth noting, though, that the westward extent of the canons' choir's hearing CPZ at St. Gregory's Priory corresponds almost exactly with the length of the nave, so sounds in the nave would be heard from the choir. At St. Augustine's Abbey the arrangement is significantly different; the monks' choir (space 12) is an important thoroughfare, as it is the only space through which the presbytery in the east end of the church can be accessed. The position of the monks' choir within the spatial system of St. Augustine's Abbey highlights the importance of considering these spaces as ritualized and temporal (see below).

### *Loud Objects*

Marilyn Y. Goldberg, in an article investigating gendered space in Classical Athenian houses, uses evidence relating to so-called women's objects (particularly loom weights) to argue that the idea of "exclusively male and female spaces in Classical Athenian households" is unfounded (Goldberg 1999:149–158). It seems plausible that a similar approach to artifacts and features could be informative in this study. The identification of quiet objects would be rather challenging, but it would certainly be reasonable to classify some objects at the two sites as loud. This can be illustrated by using the hypothetical example of a barrel. Barrels would have been fairly common at monastic sites, as ale was an important part of the medieval monastic diet (Hicks and Hicks 2001:251). While a barrel standing in a rack in an undercroft would not be a loud object, the same barrel being transported, by rolling, into and out of this storage area would certainly make a great deal of noise.

#### Loud Objects at St. Augustine's Abbey

A shaft in the nave, excavated by Stuart Rigold in 1965, has a *terminus ante quem* of the early to mid-fourteenth century (Sherlock and Woods 1988:30–32). This shaft contained weights that, Rigold suggested, came from a mechanical clock; Sherlock and Woods (1988:30–32) suggest an alternative interpretation: that these were counterweights for a lifting mechanism. It may thus be supposed that some mechanical noise would have been occasionally heard within the hearing CPZs of the monks' choir and the cloister, but without a firm *terminus post quem,* it is difficult to make judgments about the sounds of the church in the mid-thirteenth century based on this evidence. However, a find from this shaft, part of a folding balance, is compared by Sherlock and Woods to a similar item from a mid-thirteenth-century context elsewhere (1988:185), so there is a possibility that such noise would have been heard at the time in question.

Whetstones were found in a number of places by excavators, but none appear to have come from mid-thirteenth-century contexts within hearing CPZs of the quiet spaces (cf. Sherlock and Woods 1988:74, 199, 226). However, it is reasonable to suppose that whetstones were used by monks at the abbey and, thus, that the sound of knives being sharpened would have been heard; it is also possible that there may have been prohibitions about where this was allowed to occur—which was certainly the case at Barnwell Abbey (Greene 1992:116).

Paul Bennett's excavations in 1983 and 1984 took place in an area of the outer court some distance away from the hearing CPZs of any of the quiet spaces (Bennett 1987:82–83), and finds from these excavations are therefore not considered here. Note, however, that Dom Basil Watkins (2009) states that the outer court "would have been rather like a large farmyard" and that parts of this court were within the hearing copresence zone of the dormitory; as such, it is possible that the noises usually associated with farmyards would have been heard by the monks in the mid-thirteenth century from the dormitory. Similarly, sounds from the undercroft beneath the dormitory, such as noises created by the movement of barrels as discussed above, would also have been heard from the dormitory, refectory, and cloister, though there are no specific artifacts to which the loud label can be attached listed in relevant finds catalogs.

### Loud Objects at St. Gregory's Priory

The rescue excavations by Martin and Alison Hicks at the priory were the only excavations at the site (Hicks and Hicks 2001:xxiii), and as such, all finds considered in this work are published in their report. As mentioned above, the hearing CPZs of the quiet spaces extend across the entire excavated area, so all artifacts in the catalog of finds that could be described as loud must be considered. The first object mentioned in the catalog that could be firmly associated with a particular sound is a copper alloy tap "found in a post-medieval context but . . . undoubtedly of late medieval date" (Hicks and Hicks 2001:227–228). The necessary ambiguity of the term *late medieval* means that we cannot firmly connect this object with the mid-thirteenth century. However, the excavators suggest, on the basis of the presence of a twelfth-century drain found beneath a fourteenth- or fifteenth-century laver against the north wall of the cloister, that there was also a laver in the same position prior to this later feature (Hicks and Hicks 2001:94). The sound of running water can, therefore, be concluded to have been one of the *belles noiseuses* of the cloister, a sound produced close to the study area but within the hearing CPZs of all quiet spaces.

At least one knife was found in the refectory, and knives were found in thirteenth-century contexts (Hicks and Hicks 2001:276). While the use of knives at meals would have made some sounds, we should not presume that these would be comparable to those made by modern cutlery and crockery, as wooden bowls and platters are often found at medieval monastic sites (Greene 1992:150) and the excavators note that "the thirteenth- to sixteenth-century [pottery] assemblages at the priory are dominated to an unusually high degree by jugs . . . taken to indicate that the main function of pottery in the later phases of the priory was as vessels for drinking and possibly water carrying" (Hicks and Hicks 2001:250–251). As such, sounds created by the scraping of a knife against a wooden food-serving vessel may have been of a somewhat dull quality, compared with those of a modern dining room. A whetstone was found in the western courtyard (Hicks and Hicks 2001:281). Details of its context are limited to "occupation deposits," but as was the case with St. Augustine's Abbey, it is reasonable to suppose that the sound of knives being sharpened would have been heard at the priory at the time in question. A small copper alloy pellet bell was found in "a late medieval context in the infirmary cloister," but the excavators note that such bells "first occur in thirteenth-century contexts and become common by the end of the century . . . [and can] occur as dress fittings" (Hicks and Hicks 2001:281). It is also noted here that these bells are fairly common finds in Canterbury (one was also found at St. Augustine's Abbey, though not within the hearing CPZs of the quiet spaces [Sherlock and Woods 1988:216]), and the sounds created by them may therefore have occasionally been heard at both sites in the mid-thirteenth century.

Animal bone from the priory site included mammal bones (regular canons were not prohibited from eating meat [Greene 1992:147]), with "a moderate degree of dog-gnawing" (Hicks and Hicks 2001:291). Much of the bone was found in sealed occupation deposits in the northern courtyard adjoining the kitchen, "strewn across the occupation horizons" (Hicks and Hicks 2001:35), suggesting that waste was thrown from the kitchen into the yard and leading to the excavators' suggestion that this was "a squalid service court roamed by at least one scavenging dog" (Hicks and Hicks 2001:146). Watkins (2009) writes that "dogs in monasteries were considered an abuse," but also comments that this applies with more force to lapdogs and hunting dogs and that the animals may have been kept as ratters or guard dogs (Dom Basil Watkins, personal communication 2009). Whatever the reason for a dog's presence at the priory, it is likely that it would have created a considerable amount of noise (particularly if it was not the only dog at the site), which is very likely on the basis of gnawed bones having been found within the hearing CPZs of the cloister, refectory, and dormitory. As Mary Weismantel (personal communication 2010) observes, dogs are omnivorous and vegetable waste is also likely to have attracted them; however, the nature of such waste means that, unlike with the bones, evidence of canine gnawing is not preserved and one can only speculate as to the presence of dogs at St. Augustine's Abbey. Animal-bone evidence also suggests the presence of domestic fowl at the priory and such birds would have created noise, but the presence of skeletal remains within hearing distance of the quiet spaces does not necessarily indicate the presence of live birds in these areas and it may be that they were, in fact, kept some distance away in the precinct.

### *The Temporality of Sound*

To conclude this discussion, it is important to briefly consider again the fleeting nature of sounds; they cannot be considered as purely spatial phenomena. Time has a significant influence on the sounds heard in a place, whether this time is the rhythm of the monastery's liturgical day, with prescribed periods during which talking is allowed or singing is compulsory, or of the changes of season throughout a year, resulting in less frequent but equally regular sound events, such as the creaking of wooden winepresses after grape harvest. These events can be fairly reliably predicted, but other unscheduled phenomena also have an impact on the sounds heard at a site, an impact that is perhaps more noticeable by virtue of its unexpectedness. Weather-related events are a good example of this, perhaps in the form of rainwater running into a drain or of a flock of seagulls driven inland by a storm at sea—the sounds of which can be reasonably expected to have been heard at both sites, considering Canterbury's proximity to the coast. Indeed, seagulls often gather in the skies over the city today. Wild birds may also have been heard on the ground at these sites, scavenging in areas in which refuse was deposited. Unpredictable sound events relate to humans as well as to nature in general, as a specification in *The Rule of St. Benedict* (Parry, trans. 1990:84)—one that does not appear to have had an effect on the arrangements of St. Augustine's Abbey or St. Gregory's Priory in the mid-thirteenth century—makes clear: "The kitchen for the Abbot and guests should be separate, so that when guests arrive at unforeseeable times (and they are always coming to a monastery) they may not disturb the brethren." The likelihood of more unusual sound events having occurred must thus be remembered, but it is clear that only general patterns can be observed using the methods applied here if such events left no material trace.

## Conclusions

In the introduction to this chapter, it was suggested that consideration of sound at St. Augustine's Abbey and St. Gregory's Priory could give an idea of the effects that the different monastic rules had on the lives of those following them. While the majority of differences between the sounds heard at the two sites—for example, the mechanical sounds that may have been heard only at St. Augustine's Abbey—do not relate directly to the rules, there is one important point that does have a direct connection to the differences between the rules. This point is the evidence for the presence of dogs near the claustral buildings at St. Gregory's Priory, in the form of gnawed mammal bones outside the kitchen, which suggests that the sounds of barking dogs may have been more likely to have been heard at this site. These bones indicate a type of sound that relates to the Augustinian order's permission of the eating of meat in everyday monastic life, and therefore suggest that if this type of sound was heard at Benedictine monasteries it would have been more likely to have occurred near the infirmary buildings than near the main claustral ranges.

This chapter was not so much an argument that monastic claustral buildings were constructed specifically to enable the creation of quiet spaces but rather an investigation of how the arrangement of the buildings affected the level of noise in certain spaces. One of the reasons for the choice of the sites studied here was that historically St. Gregory's Priory has been considered a somewhat unruly monastery in comparison to others, such as St. Augustine's Abbey, and it was hoped that study of the quiet spaces at both could increase our understanding of why this was the case. If monasteries are thought of as dwelling places, they can be seen to have been structuring structures (Bourdieu 1977:91; Donley-Reid

1990:119). Thus, the relatively bad reputation of St. Gregory's Priory (at least in relation to the observance of the rule of silence) could be linked to the way its buildings structured relations between the people using them, in that, as Figure 10-6 demonstrates, its quiet spaces were not places of sociospatial solitude to the same extent as were those of St. Augustine's Abbey.

Such an interpretation must be subject to a caveat, in the form of an idea expressed by Linda Donley-Reid (1990:115): "Objects and spaces are a part of culture. They are not the sole determinants of social organization. Studying how spaces and objects are given meaning and how that meaning helps to shape a society is a means to understanding the pattern of a specific social order." It should be remembered that, even if the spatial arrangement of St. Gregory's Priory's claustral buildings could be blamed for the failure of its quiet spaces, there are also human reasons for its relatively low standing as a monastery: The state of the "bad beer" served to a visitor (Page, ed. 1926:158) is an example of something that cannot be attributed to the plan of the buildings, and the decision whether to observe the rule of silence would similarly have been more a matter of personal or social choice than of spatial inevitability. However, this is not to say that these decisions were not influenced by the difficulty of attaining social solitude in a place where spatial solitude was rare, and they may reflect an element of giving up one's personal attempts at solitude in the face of a community that seemed superficially to be unable to provide for it. It could be argued that archaeology cannot fully grasp the metaphysical aspects of monastic life and that studies can only go so far with material remains alone. The wealth of evidence available to those studying the sensory experience of monastic sites during this period means that further exploration of this topic can benefit from research based on texts and images. Nevertheless, it is hoped that this chapter will have contributed to an understanding of such sensory experience, in addition to having demonstrated the possibilities presented to the sensory archaeologist by analytical methods that may not immediately appear to be associated with the human sensorium.

## Note

1. For further information, see Andrews 2006:120–139; Butler and Given-Wilson 1979; Greene 1992:1–56.

## References

Allison, Penelope M.

1997 Why Do Excavation Reports Have Finds' Catalogues? In *Not So Much a Pot, More a Way of Life*, edited by Christopher G. Cumberpatch and Paul W. Blinkhorn, pp. 77–84. Oxbow Monograph 83. Oxbow Books, Oxford.

Andrews, Frances

2006 *The Other Friars: The Carmelite, Augustinian, Sack and Pied Friars in the Middle Ages*. Boydell, Woodbridge, United Kingdom.

Apollonio, Umbro (editor)

1973 *Futurist Manifestos*. Thames and Hudson, London.

Ault, Bradley A., and Lisa C. Nevett

1999 Digging Houses: Archaeologies of Classical and Hellenistic Greek Domestic Assemblages. In *The Archaeology of Household Activities*, edited by Penelope M. Allison, pp. 43–56. Routledge, London.

Belisle, Peter-Damian

2003 *The Language of Silence: The Changing Face of Monastic Solitude*. Darton, Longman and Todd, London.

Bennett, Paul

1987 Rescue Excavations in the Outer Court of St. Augustine's Abbey, 1983–84. *Archaeologia Cantiana* 103:79–117.

Bourdieu, Pierre

1977 *Outline of a Theory of Practice*. Translated by Richard Nice. Cambridge University Press, Cambridge.

Bowles, Edmund A.

1962 The Organ in the Medieval Liturgical Service. *Revue belge de Musicologie/Belgisch Tijdschrift voor Muziekwetenschap* 16(1/4):13–29.

Brennan, Brian

1988 Augustine's 'De musica.' *Vigiliae Christianae* 42(3):267–281.

Brooke, Christopher

1971 *Medieval Church and Society*. Sidgwick and Jackson, London.

Brooks, Nicholas

1984 *The Early History of the Church of Canterbury: Christ Church from 597 to 1066*. Leicester University Press, London.

Butler, Lionel, and Chris Given-Wilson

1979 *Medieval Monasteries of Great Britain*. Michael Joseph, London.

Caldwell, John

1967 The Organ in the Medieval Latin Liturgy, 800–1500. *Proceedings of the Royal Musical Association*, 93rd Sess., 1966–1967, pp. 11–24.

1992 Plainsong and Polyphony 1250–1550. In *Plainsong in the Age of Polyphony*, edited by Thomas Forrest Kelly, pp. 6–31. Cambridge University Press, Cambridge.

Ciolek, T. Matthew

1983 The Proxemics Lexicon: A First Approximation. *Journal of Nonverbal Behavior* 8:55–79.

Coles, John M.

1973 *Archaeology by Experiment*. Hutchinson, London.

Davis, Bruce

1990 *Monastery Without Walls: Daily Life in the Silence*. Authors Choice Press, Lincoln, Nebraska.

Donley-Reid, Linda W.

1990 A Structuring Structure: The Swahili House. In *Domestic Architecture and the Use of Space: An Interdisciplinary Cross-Cultural Study*, edited by Susan Kent, pp. 114–126. Cambridge University Press, Cambridge.

Foster, Sally M.

1989 Analysis of Spatial Patterns in Buildings (Access Analysis) as an Insight into Social Structure: Examples from the Scottish Atlantic Iron Age. *Antiquity* 63:40–50.

George, Michele

2002 Review of *Reading Space: Social Interaction and Identity in the Houses of Roman Pompeii*, by Mark Grahame. *Journal of Roman Studies* 92:238–239.

Goldberg, Marilyn Y.
1999 Spatial and Behavioural Negotiation in Classical Athenian City Houses. In *The Archaeology of Household Activities*, edited by Penelope M. Allison, pp. 142–161. Routledge, London.
Grahame, Mark
1997 Public and Private in the Roman House: The Spatial Order of the *Casa del Fauno*. In *Domestic Space in the Roman World: Pompeii and Beyond*, edited by Ray Laurence and Andrew Wallace-Hadrill, pp. 137–164. JRA Supplementary Series, No. 22. JRA, Portsmouth, Rhode Island.
2000 *Reading Space: Social Interaction and Identity in the Houses of Roman Pompeii—A Syntactical Approach to the Analysis and Interpretation of Built Space*. BAR International Series 886. Archaeopress, Oxford.
Greene, J. Patrick
1992 *Medieval Monasteries*. Leicester University Press, London.
Hall, Edward T.
1963 A System for the Notation of Proxemic Behavior. *American Anthropologist*, n.s. 65:1003–1026.
Hanson, Julienne
1998 *Decoding Homes and Houses*. Cambridge University Press, Cambridge.
Harrison, Frank Llewellyn
1980 Music in Medieval Britain. 4th ed. Knuf, Buren.
Hicks, Martin, and Alison Hicks
2001 *St. Gregory's Priory, Northgate, Canterbury: Excavations 1988–1991*. The Archaeology of Canterbury, n.s., Vol. 2. Canterbury Archaeological Trust, Canterbury.
Hill, Jonathan
2006 *Immaterial Architecture*. Routledge, London.
Hillier, Bill, and Julienne Hanson
1984 *The Social Logic of Space*. Cambridge University Press, Cambridge.
Kent, Susan
1990 A Cross-Cultural Study of Segmentation, Architecture, and the Use of Space. In *Domestic Architecture and the Use of Space: An Interdisciplinary Cross-Cultural Study*, edited by Susan Kent, pp. 127–152. Cambridge University Press, Cambridge.
Kirkpatrick, Betty
1995 *Oxford Concise Thesaurus*. Oxford University Press, Oxford.
Lawrence, Roderick J.
1990 Public Collective and Private Space: A Study of Urban Housing in Switzerland. In *Domestic Architecture and the Use of Space: An Interdisciplinary Cross-Cultural Study*, edited by Susan Kent, pp. 73–91. Cambridge University Press, Cambridge.
Lawson, Bryan
2001 *The Language of Space*. Architectural Press, Oxford.
Lefebvre, Henri
1991 *The Production of Space*. Translated by Donald Nicholson-Smith. Blackwell, Oxford.
Megaw, John V. S.
1968 Problems and Non-Problems in Palaeo-Organology: A Musical Miscellany. In *Studies in Ancient Europe*, edited by John M. Coles and Derek Douglas Alexander Simpson, pp. 333–358. Leicester University Press, Leicester.
Megaw, John V. S., and Ian Longworth (editors)
1981 Archaeology and Musical Instruments. *World Archaeology* 12(3).

Merton, Thomas
1950 *Seeds of Contemplation*. Rev. ed. Burns and Oates, London.
Meyvaert, Paul
1973 The Medieval Monastic Claustrum. *Gesta* 12(1/2):53–59.
Moretti, Laura
2004 Architectural Spaces for Music: Jacopo Sansovino and Adrian Willaert at St. Mark's. *Early Music History* 23:153–184.
Page, William (editor)
1926 *The Victoria County History of the County of Kent*, Vol. 2. St. Catherine Press, London.
Parry, Abbot David (translator)
1990 *The Rule of St. Benedict*. Gracewing, Leominster.
Putzeys, Toon, Marc Waelkens, Jeroen Poblome, Wim Van Neer, Thijs Van Thuyne, and Nathalie Kellens
2003 *Contextual Analysis at Sagalassos: Developing a Methodology*. Electronic document, http://perswww.kuleuven.be/~u0038677/logboek/roct_pres.html, accessed July 27, 2009.
Sanders, Donald
1990 Behavioral Conventions and Archaeology: Methods for the Analysis of Ancient Architecture. In *Domestic Architecture and the Use of Space: An Interdisciplinary Cross-Cultural Study*, edited by Susan Kent, pp. 43–72. Cambridge University Press, Cambridge.
Sherlock, David, and Humphrey Woods
1988 *St. Augustine's Abbey: Report on Excavations, 1960–78*. Monograph Series of the Kent Archaeological Society, No. 4. Kent Archaeological Society, Maidstone.
Smith, George
1883 *Chronological History of Canterbury Cathedral*. H. S. Claris, "Kent Herald" Office, Canterbury.
Steadman, Sharon R.
2000 Spatial Patterning and Social Complexity on Prehistoric Anatolian *Tell* Sites: Models for Mounds. *Journal of Anthropological Archaeology* 19:164–199.
Tatton-Brown, Timothy
1991 The Buildings and Topography of St. Augustine's Abbey, Canterbury. *Journal of the British Archaeological Association* 144:61–91.
1997 The Abbey Precinct, Liberty and Estate. In *English Heritage Book of St. Augustine's Abbey, Canterbury*, edited by Richard Gem, pp. 123–142. B. T. Batsford, London.
Teahan, John F.
1982 Solitude: A Central Motif in Thomas Merton's Life and Writings. *Journal of the American Academy of Religion* 50:521–538.
Watkins, Dom Basil
2009 *St. Augustine's Abbey at Canterbury—Layout*. Annotated drawing on file, St. Augustine's Abbey Museum, Canterbury.
Wilson-Dickson, Andrew
1992 *The Story of Christian Music: From Gregorian Chant to Black Gospel*. Lion, Oxford.
Witmore, Christopher L.
2006 Vision, Media, Noise, and the Percolation of Time: Symmetrical Approaches to the Mediation of the Material World. *Journal of Material Culture* 11:267–292.

# 11. Sustenance, Taste, and the Practice of Community in Ancient Mesopotamia

*Marie Hopwood*

*Abstract:* Archaeological food studies have long been relegated to either analyses of power manipulation through feasting or issues of production and domestication. Yet, by doing this, the importance of daily consumption is muted. Archaeological explorations of commensality are often viewed with reticence, as if commensalism were sybaritic and not worthy of research. It is through our senses, however, that we experience the world around us, and the same was true in the past. The preparation of food is a total sensory experience: feeling the texture of the raw food itself, stirring it in a pot, smelling it cooking across an open space, tasting it for seasoning and "doneness," even hearing its sounds as you go about another task. In this chapter, I explore food preparation at the Halaf period site of Fıstıklı Höyük, Turkey. This exploration will build off a discussion of food-preparation practices utilized at the site as evidenced by the etched surfaces of ceramic food preparation vessels. The goal is to explore the powerful humanity of the past as people cooked for each other, sustaining themselves both in body and in community.

In cultural anthropology, food is recognized as a powerful material used to actively and purposefully create personal, familial, ethnic, and even national identities (e.g., Appadurai 1981; Counihan and Van Esterik 2007; Gaytan 2008; Harbottle 1997; Siskind 1992; Suen 2007; Wilk 2006). It is intimately entwined within taste, identity, social class, and gender. Food goes well beyond our physical need for sustenance, shaping ideas of taboo, propriety, celebration, mourning, and human rights, to name only a few possibilities. Yet, with archaeology, food

*Making Senses of the Past: Toward a Sensory Archaeology*, edited by Jo Day. Center for Archaeological Investigations, Occasional Paper No. 40.  ISBN 978-0-8093-3287-8.

loses many of these meanings and nuances. Owing to the broken and fragmentary nature of the material data, discussions of food in archaeological research are often relegated to topics of production; the analysis of presence and absence of foodstuffs; whether it is domesticated or wild; and rituals involving feasting or commensality. It is as if talking about food, imagining ancient people having the same depth of feeling, enjoyment and memory associated with food that we have today, is to catch them in a private act; it is treated as if unseemly. It is also somehow embarrassing to archaeologists as researchers, therefore becoming archaeologically unimaginable, and what is lost is the humanity of the past (Hamilakis 2002:123; Hayden 2001:24).

Therefore, one is left to ask whether it matters if food and its consumption (beyond feasting) are undertheorized in archaeology. Does that hinder our understanding of the past? When dealing with prehistoric remains in particular, or other situations in which there are no texts or accurate depictions of specific dishes, archaeological research may not be able to explore those nuances of food introduced above. In my own research into the Halaf period (sixth millennium B.C.E) of ancient Mesopotamia, there are no texts; the floral and faunal studies are still under way for the site under discussion here; and the lipid analyses of cook pots (although preliminary) have not been able to distinguish between the types of foodstuffs prepared in the vessels (Hopwood 2010; Hopwood and Mitra 2012). So what can a discussion of food and taste add to our understanding of life at Fıstıklı Höyük during this period?

By way of beginning to answer the above questions, let me relate an experience concerning a student's writing assignment for a colleague. The assignment was to write about a day in the life of an imagined person from one of the ancient cities discussed in class. The student wrote a well-thought-through paper in all respects but one. The imagined woman woke up in the morning, climbed down the ladder into her home, and began to prepare breakfast for her family. The breakfast described was simply emmer wheat and water. This was not cooked into porridge or flavored in any way; it was simply a species of wheat with a tasteless liquid served as a meal. That the student could imagine fantastic details of other aspects of life—from clothing to religion to work—but not with respect to food was discouraging. Yet, on further reflection, the discouraging aspect of this experience lies not in the student's lull in imagination but in our abilities as archaeologists, researchers, and teachers to pass knowledge on to our students and to the rest of our discipline through our research. A basic aspect of humanity is the meaning we place on food and the relationships surrounding its preparation and consumption. This is as true today as it was in the past. To mute this importance is to ignore an integral part of the intricacies of the lives that we study.

The exploration of the experiences of food in the past is not purely imaginary nor is it based on fiction. The materiality of food preparation opens avenues of exploration into the cultural construction of food—the practicing and sharing of habitual actions—and into the sensing of the past. This chapter begins with a discussion of creating a sensuous past. Our senses shape how we experience and interact with the world, and thus should be an important part of archaeological interpretations of the past. Following this is a discussion of the cultural importance of food, touching on its creation, transformation, and meaning in consumption. The third section discusses the repetition, practice, and creation of habitual actions of food preparation. These repetitive actions can result in evidence of use wear on artifacts, and these traces of wear in turn can be interpreted through ceramic use alteration methodologies to explore vessel use, even from a sherd-based assemblage. Finally, the evidence of food preparation at the Halaf period site of Fıstıklı Höyük, Turkey, is discussed.

## Sensing the Past

As stated by Houston and Taube (2000:261), "sight, sound, touch, hearing, and smell are not ordinarily the concern of archaeologists, since the senses do not leave vestiges that can readily be accessed." We cannot excavate scent, we cannot dig up the sound of lost music, nor can we interpret what tasted good to a person in the past. Intriguingly, similar arguments were once made as to why archaeologists could not study gender. Yet gender has become a major focus of much archaeological research for the very reason that it is so important in human culture. As archaeologists, we can explore senses as the ways that people in the past experienced and interacted with the world around them (Classen 1997; Hamilakis 2002:122; Howes 1991a:4; Howes and Classen 1991).

The senses, as described by Classen (1991, 1997:401), are experienced perceptions that are both physical as well as cultural. There is no denying the bodily expressions and reactions to the senses, but it must also be realized that such experiences are not entirely natural or biological. Our senses are shaped by culture, and thus the ways that we perceive the world around us are also culture specific (Dawson et al. 2007:18; Frieman and Gillings 2007:12; Gosden 2001:166; Houston and Taube 2000:289). What is important in the anthropology of the senses is to recognize this potential for difference, even in something that at face value can seem so "natural" and universal. The idea that different societies and cultures perceive senses differently is applicable not only to modern peoples but also to past societies (e.g., Classen, Howes, and Synnott 1994; Dawson et al. 2007; Hamilton and Whitehouse 2006; Houston and Taube 2000; Howes 1991a). We must be able to imagine the past as something inherently alien from our own comprehension.

In the West, sensory experiences have been divided according to five senses: smell, sight, hearing, taste, and touch (MacGregor 1999). This division has created a false idea of the science of the five separate senses, something that has shaped our own cultural experiences. We often describe these senses on their own, as if sight or smell is experienced separately from the others. This unimodal method of describing the senses is also represented in our interpretations of the past where vision tends to be privileged at the expense of the others (MacGregor 1999:264). Recent anthropological work has pointed to the possibilities of plurisensorial experiences, in which people of different cultures have been taught to experience multiple senses at once, such as hearing-smelling together.

Such a division of the senses has also been applied very specifically to taste, with the "scientific" division of our taste buds into salty, sour, bitter, and sweet.

It was deemed scientific fact that we could only recognize combinations of these four elements of taste perception. In 1908, when Japanese chemist Kikunae Ikeda announced the discovery of a fifth taste, *umami*, Western scientists rejected this idea, stating that umami was unique to the Japanese and that scientific knowledge had determined that the tongue was full; there was no room for a fifth taste (Lehrer 2008:57). It was not until the year 2000 that Western scientists validated Ikeda's claim and made room in our science of the body to fit in umami, a savory taste that had been recognized by the Japanese for centuries but for which the West had no word. Even now, trying to explain umami to Western audiences is difficult, but some foods that have been described as embodying this savoriness include mushrooms, asparagus, and soy sauce.

As artifacts are perceived through the senses, their very sensuality should be a part of archaeological discussions (Brumfiel 2005:225). In her study of the materiality of Aztec feasting, Brumfiel (2005:231) argues that the use of specially painted vessels as receptacles for food and drink at these events is one of the things that made the ceremonies possible at all. Without the vessels and without the food and the drink contained within, the ceremonies themselves could not have taken place nor would the special meaning of the food, drink, and pottery have been possible.

The experience of taste is one of the most sensuous of the senses (Howes 1991b:168; Jonaitis 2006:162). Eating, preparing, and sharing food evoke all the senses: sight, smell, hearing, touch, and taste. Food has also been found to evoke memories—to remind a person of an event, another person, or even a feeling (Holtzman 2006; Mintz and DuBois 2002). As such, the vessels used in these practices also are affected by the sensuousness of the food contained within (Brumfiel 2005). Therefore, the artifacts used in food preparation and consumption are lines of evidence to understanding the ways people in the past experienced food, as well as to all the incumbent relationships surrounding its preparation, presentation, and consumption. Food is not, nor was it ever, only about sustenance.

## Importance of Food

The power of food derives from the inherent and unending need for food and drink, both relatively plastic materials that can be combined in myriad ways (Appadurai 1981:494; Dietler 1990, 1996:89; Pollock 2003). Pollock (2003:18) describes the nearly infinite possibilities of food manipulation through the types of things eaten, the methods of preparation, the social contexts of consumption, and the cultural meanings applied. The culinary combinations possible are vast, accounting for the incredible diversity in global food practices, as well as the depth of meaning, comfort, and memory associated with food (Hamilakis 2002:124; Holtzman 2006; Mintz and DuBois 2002; Stoller 1989). Atalay and Hastorf (2006:284) go so far as to describe food as the "original social glue," forming and strengthening bonds between and within family and community.

Food can also serve as a means of distinction (Barnes 2001:17; Bourdieu 1987; Jonaitis 2006:142). The foods that characterize specific groups of people can serve as markers of identity but also work as markers of difference. In her exploration of the changes in food practices of the Kwakwaka'wakw of the northwest American coast from precontact to modern times, Jonaitis (2006) focuses on the use of *t'lina*, or fermented fish oil, in creating both unity within and difference between groups. This condiment, often served with fish, defies attempts to describe its taste, beyond the fact that most nonnatives find it repulsive at best. Yet, this is a prized condiment among the Kwakwaka'wakw, one that makes a meal complete. Jonaitis describes *t'lina* as a food that distinguishes the Kwakwaka'wakw from their colonizers, one that sets them apart and creates difference.

It must also be acknowledged that the meaning of food only exists within social contexts. The transformation of something that is *edible* into something that is *good to eat* happens within culture (Douglas 1997; Harris 1987; Lévi-Strauss 1966, 1969). Therefore, archaeological analyses of food-related practices can lead to information about the social contexts in which these activities were carried out (Blitz 1993:81). Hamilakis (1999) discusses our need as archaeologists to move beyond describing ancient people as having been as preoccupied as we are with food as sustenance, sources of vitamins, and essential to health. This is not to say that people in the past were not aware of or concerned with foods that were good for their bodies, but this is not necessarily how foods were primarily comprehended.

A powerful aspect of food lies in its sensuousness (Holtzman 2006). Food's ability to draw on multiple senses has led to its role in discussions of memory. The scent of food can "conjure" up memories, bringing us back to different places, times, and even feelings. The word *conjure* implies an almost magical quality of food: a power much stronger than its constituent parts. This power seems to lie in food's ability to simultaneously utilize multiple senses linked to memory (Holtzman 2006). The simple sound and aroma of food cooking can bring us back to good or bad times, and while this remembrance is not always pleasant, without our conscious effort it can link us to our past for better or for worse.

## Shared Knowledge

Practices of food preparation can be explored archaeologically specifically because they are repetitive, patterned, and habitual. The practices used to create edible food, from starting a cooking fire in the hearth to placing a vessel over the heat to adding foodstuffs and serving, are all learned and repeated. It is not necessary to re-create how to boil water every day, but these tasks are taught, practiced, and repeated. They are patterned. This is the habitus of Bourdieu (1987), as pointed out by Atalay and Hastorf (2006:283); they are practices that structure the lives of the people preparing the meals, as well as those who consume them.

Habitual food-preparation practices are not thoughtless but thoughtful (Barnes 2001:20). They involve both action and conscious thought, combining as shared knowledge. Another way to think of this, as discussed by Barnes (2001), is as practicing embodied knowledge. The task itself does not need to be re-created but instead is "done because it is traditionally done, or routinely done, or done because it is part of the practice of the collective" (Barnes 2001:21). As part of collective action, shared knowledge, such as in the practices of food preparation, can be used to explore the community in question. This shared knowledge involves information about how to correctly prepare specific dishes, the types of flavors and textures desired by that group of people, and in short, all aspects of that particular society and culture that relate to food, its preparation, and its consumption. That is no small role and is something that cannot be carried out by one person alone but rather by the collective whole of the community (Barnes 2001:23).

Creating certain meals requires following prescribed movements and activities that are, in a sense, performed. These performed actions are carried out with specific tools for specific functions. Within the variety of shapes and sizes of vessels available for food preparation, a person will choose the one that best suits the purpose at hand. Particular types of vessels, consequently, become materially inscribed in distinctive ways based on functions that they are considered best suited for. Hence, by linking use wear patterns with certain sizes and shapes of vessels, the larger picture of food preparation within a community can be made apparent. Thus, the materiality of food preparation, with the archaeological traces of these activities, can be used to explore the broader social relationships associated with food.

## Materiality of Cooking: The Case of Fıstıklı Höyük

The Halaf period falls within the sixth millennium B.C.E., from 6100 to 5300 B.C.E., and includes areas of the modern nations of Syria, Turkey, and Iraq (Figure 11-1). The site (Figure 11-2) of Fıstıklı Höyük, Turkey, was established on a low-lying, naturally occurring rise, flanked to the west by the Euphrates River, which today passes approximately 1 km to the west of the site, and to the south by a small stream rushing westward to join the river (Bernbeck et al. 2002, 2003:20; Campbell 2007; Pollock et al. 2001; Pollock and Bernbeck 1998). The settlement encompassed .5 ha at the top of the rise and at the height of its occupation consisted of at least five tholoi, or living structures, with associated storage structures, hearths, ovens, and earthen constructions. Over the course of 50–100 years, the site was occupied and then slowly abandoned.

The settlement at Fıstıklı Höyük began as a temporary encampment with minimal modification and underwent many changes over the course of its few generations of occupation. This occupation has been divided into four phases within the Early Halaf period (Table 11-1), beginning with the earliest Phase IV and moving through IIIc and IIIb, with IIIa as the latest Halaf occupation (Bernbeck et al. 2003:20). By approximately 5750 cal B.C., the last tholos of Fıstıklı Höyük was abandoned and no extensive occupation is seen again until the Hellenistic/Roman period (Bernbeck et al. 2003:25). Sometime after abandonment, however, visitors returned to the site and constructed a windbreak associated with a hearth within Earthwork II, during what has been named Phase IIIx (Bernbeck et al. 2003:25).

At this small hamlet, I conducted research on the ceramic coarse ware assemblage, with the goal of exploring community function through the inhabitants' food preparation practices. A focus on community moves beyond distinct

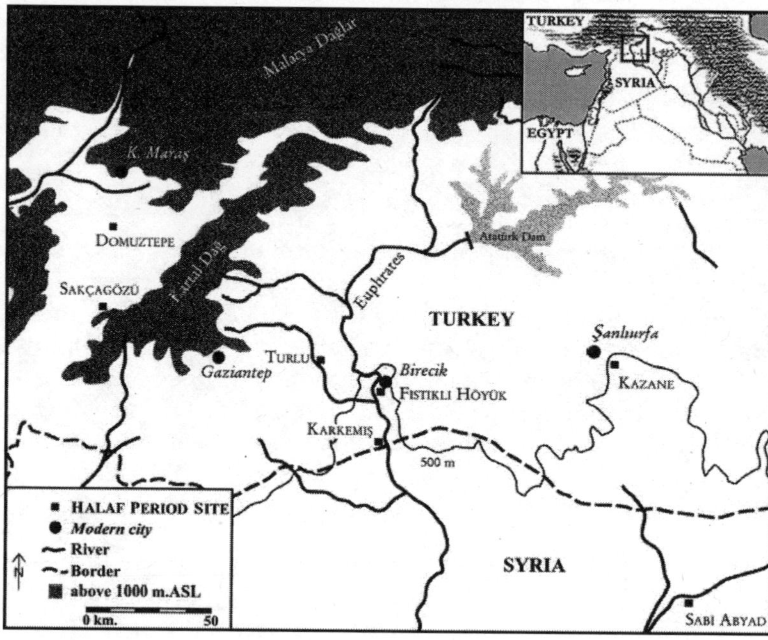


**Figure 11-1.** *Regional map of the modern nations of Turkey and Syria, showing the location of Fıstıklı Höyük in southeastern Turkey (Bernbeck 2008: Figure 3.1). Used with permission.*

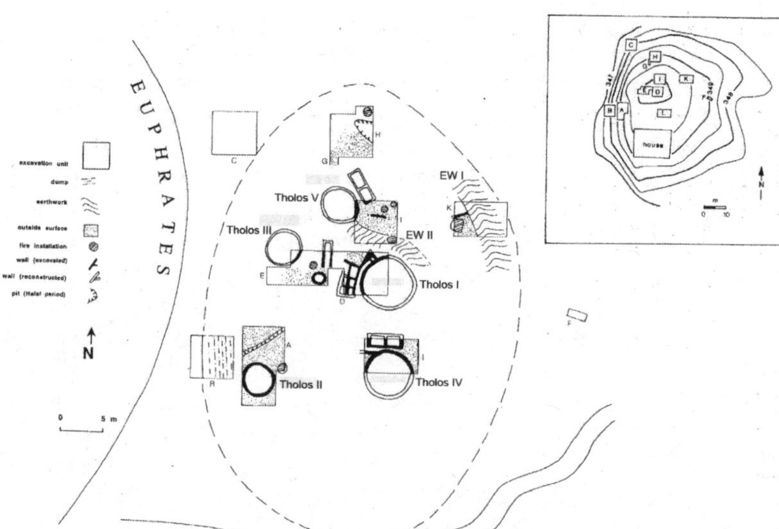


**Figure 11-2.** *The Fıstıklı Höyük settlement as it existed at the height of occupation in Phase IIIa (Bernbeck et al. 2003:Figure 2). Note that the Euphrates River is drawn very near the site but was likely farther away during the Halaf period. Used with permission.*

**Table 11-1.** *Dates and Descriptions for Fıstıklı Höyük Occupational Phases*

| *Phase* | *Date Ranges* (B.C.)[a] | *Phase Duration* | *Description* |
|---|---|---|---|
| IV | - | | Temporary encampment. Site modification only at the most basic level. People as visitors. |
| IIIc | Beginning 7566–6087<br>Ending 5902–5757 | 35 yr. | Investing in the site. Construction of permanent storage not based on pottery. |
| IIIb | Beginning 5902–5757<br>Ending 5832–5744 | 35 yr. | Creation of domestic space. Households with walls take shape. |
| IIIa | Beginning 5832–5744<br>Ending 5811–5711 | 30 yr. | Expansion of community to its apex. Varied population and food preparation needs. |
| IIIx | - | | Slow abandonment and community moves elsewhere. |

*Note:* Dates based on Campbell's (2007:Figure 3) reevaluation of Halaf chronologies.
[a]Date ranges shown represent an agreement index of 94.5%.

actors, unlike agency studies in which the larger group can be silenced in pursuit of the individual. Instead, analysis of community allows the data to be explored for evidence of groups of actors, focusing on the practices and actions of groups of people working toward community creation and re-creation. Richards (1932) described the need to eat as the most basic, most powerful drive that people experience (cf. Mintz 1996:35). Its unique ability to embody rich cultural consequences, while at the same time being incessantly bound to human physiology, grants it this position. Thus, change in food preparation can be used to infer other changes within a group as well. In other words, community can be made manifest by daily practices, such as food preparation (Bawden 1982:181; Ingold 1983:555).

This research was carried out through a ceramic use-alteration analysis of the coarse ware assemblage (Figures 11-3 and 11-4), details of which can be found elsewhere (Hopwood 2010). Of importance is that the relatively soft (in comparison to hard stone or metal) surfaces of coarse ware vessels allow them to be etched or marked with traces of the activities to which they were put to use. These uses can often leave behind traces of wear in the form of scratches, gouges, patches of abrasion, chips, and spalls. As the gestures and activities that created these traces of wear are repetitive, habitual, and patterned, so too are their resultant traces of wear (Skibo 1992). Ceramic use alteration focuses on evidence of cooking fire, wear, and absorbed food residue.

Over time at Fıstıklı Höyük, changes in food-preparation activities at the site highlight changes occurring in the community as a whole (Table 11-2). Utilizing the data collected from the analysis of the Fıstıklı Höyük coarse ware sherds, I divided the assemblage into three categories of vessel used for food preparation. The first category of use, and perhaps the most obvious, is for cooking food. All

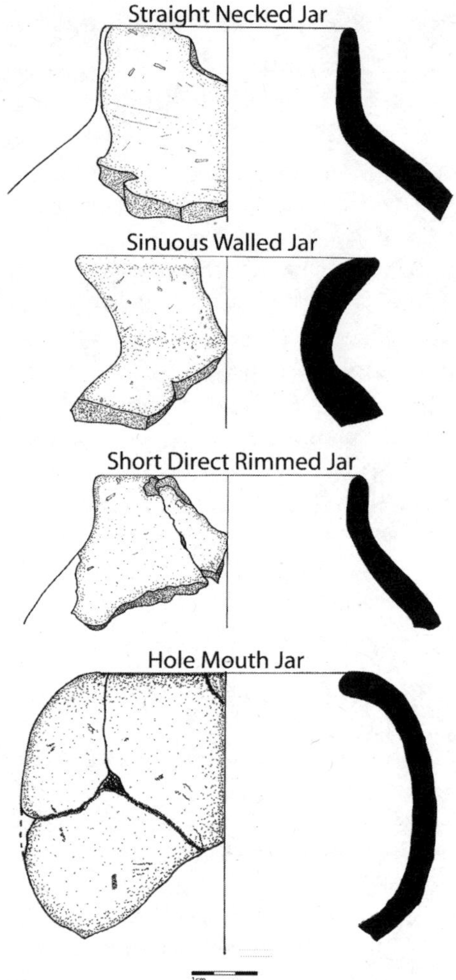


**Figure 11-3.** *Restricted vessel shapes from Fıstıklı Höyük are characterized by openings that are smaller than their body circumference. These restricted orifices can help protect vessel contents from spilling, as well as create a ledge or lip that can be used to secure a soft covering or lid.*

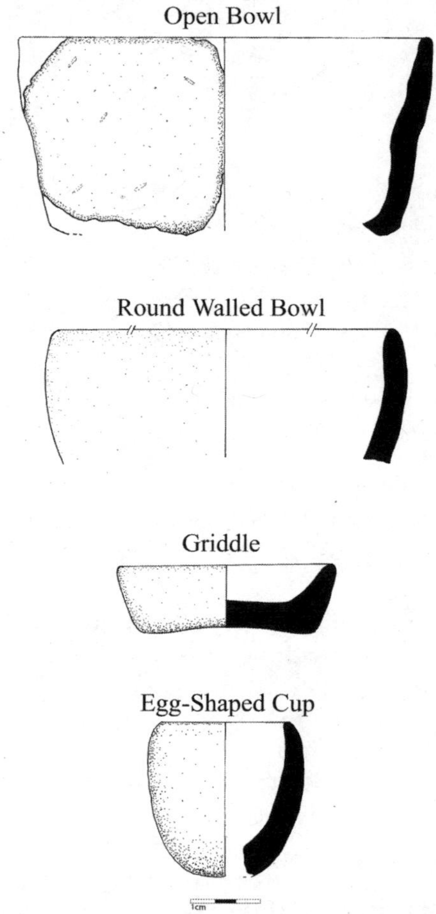


**Figure 11-4.** *Unrestricted vessel shapes from Fıstıklı Höyük are characterized by openings that are as wide or wider than their body circumference. These vessels allow relatively easy access to their contents.*

sherds showing evidence of use over a fire—through sooting, carbonization, or a combination of both—were described as heating/cooking vessels. The second category includes those sherds with evidence of exterior wear suggestive of that of frequently moved containers. These mobile storage containers were used to hold materials, as well as to move them around, and potentially beyond, the site. The transportation of water from the river, the short-term storage of grain before

**Table 11-2.** *Percentages of Coarse Ware Sherds by Categories of Vessel Use across the Four Occupational Phases at Fıstıklı Höyük*

| *Phase* | *Heating/Cooking* | *Mobile Container* | *Stationary Storage* |
|---|---|---|---|
| Phase IV | | | |
| Total no. | 29.0 | 9.0 | 31.0 |
| Total % | 42.0 | 13.0 | 44.9 |
| Phase IIIC | | | |
| Total no. | 68.0 | 43.0 | 61.0 |
| Total % | 39.5 | 25.0 | 35.5 |
| Phase IIIB | | | |
| Total no. | 15.0 | 17.0 | 55.0 |
| Total % | 17.2 | 19.5 | 63.2 |
| Phase IIIA | | | |
| Total no. | 501.0 | 391.0 | 1054.0 |
| Total % | 25.8 | 20.1 | 54.2 |

grinding, or any form of preparation in which movement of a vessel is required could create this pattern of wear. Finally, those sherds with interior wear but little or no evidence of exterior wear are interpreted as stationary storage vessels. These vessels were filled and then left alone, without other objects banging into them and without being dragged across rough surfaces. This absence of wear could be indicative of larger vessels that, when filled, were too heavy to move or of fragile vessels that were handled carefully, as well as of vessels with fragile, perishable, or valuable contents that required careful handling.

### *Phase IV: Tent Encampment*

The earliest evidence of occupation at Fıstıklı Höyük, Phase IV, suggests the site was a temporary encampment and lacked permanent structures. Visitors did not modify the mound to suit occupation beyond construction of a narrow drainage ditch dug into the western slope (Bernbeck et al. 2003:23). Whether the site was utilized with the goal of pasturing flocks, harvesting local foods, or for other functions, it suited the people's needs as it was. Archaeological remains from this phase are limited, but coarse ware sherds from a number of broken vessels were recovered.

From this early occupation phase, the remains of many smaller shattered cooking vessels, a few larger mobile containers, and many moderate-sized stationary containers were recovered. The sizes of cooking vessels suggest the preparation of food for a small number of people. This could suggest an overall small group to be provided for or that subsets of a larger group prepared foods for themselves alone. The production of large quantities of food at any one time in any one vessel was not carried out.

Most of the Phase IV vessels are restricted shapes. Here I use Rice's (1987:212) term *restricted,* rather than *closed,* to refer to vessels whose orifices are smaller than their maximum diameters, since none of these vessels are truly closed. These restricted vessels can easily be covered to provide protection of their contents.

Heating and storing are the prevalent vessel functions in Phase IV. Cooking vessels tend to be small, allowing food preparation for only a limited number of people. This fits the general interpretation of this phase as a small campsite without permanent fixtures. Cooking was carried out by filling the pots and setting them to the side of the fire to heat over long periods of time, thus freeing people to carry out other tasks, as seen in Brumfiel's (1991) discussion of Aztec cooking techniques. The stationary storage vessels also tended to be relatively small and, thus, held only limited amounts of food or other materials. Interestingly, although mobile containers make up the smallest percentage of analyzed sherds, they are the largest in vessel size. Materials were moved within and around the site, as well as potentially to the site from elsewhere.

Thus, the food preparation during Phase IV tended to involve long preparation time but little active labor. Long-term storage in ceramic vessels was limited, with a focus on the preservation of small quantities of potentially special foods, certainly not bulk foodstuffs such as grain. Other resources were either prepared to be transported away from the site or brought in from elsewhere. Unless appreciable quantities of food were stored in nonpottery vessels, such as baskets or leather bags, the ability of the community to support its members at this site would have been limited to short-term occupation.

### *Phase IIIc: Advent of Permanent Storage*

While the site itself was not modified to any great extent during Phase IV, in Phase IIIc changes were made to shape the space to suit different needs, which is primarily evident in the building of a cell-plan storage building. While the nonceramic potential for long-term storage increased drastically, so too did the amount of variation in the shapes and sizes of the coarse ware vessels. In this phase, vessels of different size classes held variable quantities of material and were likely used to prepare not only different amounts but also different kinds of food. The presence of larger vessels in Phase IIIc implies the preparation of food for more people than were present during Phase IV. The percentages of restricted to unrestricted vessels also changed to almost equal proportions of each. Furthermore, unrestricted vessels became the preferred shape for cooking activities. These vessels allow easy access to their contents but are more difficult to cover. Overall, the heating methods are characterized by a variety of heating levels, preparation, and quantities prepared. This is a much more varied array of food preparation than in the earlier Phase IV.

With the creation of the permanent storage units in Phase IIIc, there is a corresponding dearth of large storage vessels. The miniature- to medium-sized stationary storage containers would have held only small quantities of food. If larger volumes of storage were required, cell-plan structures were used for this purpose, as well as nonpottery vessels perhaps.

The mobile storage containers, on the other hand, were larger than in Phase IV and exhibited a variety of wear patterns that indicate multiple types of content manipulation and different types of vessel closure.

A notable change during Phase IIIc is a shift away from heat application to vessels, as well as away from use as stationary storage toward increased use as mobile storage. A further interesting interpretation from this phase is the use of small vessels, like miniature Open Bowls, as scoops. These scoops can be found in subsequent phases of occupation and are the only tool type identified as utensils. With the focus on preserving materials, whether they are preserved in situ or moved around or away from the site, the use of tools to add, manipulate, and remove vessel contents is essential. The community established structures on the site that would allow them to potentially live there year-round, and the coarse ware vessels were used in ways to augment the storage and use of necessary foodstuffs.

### *Phase IIIb: Permanent Domestic Structures*

The site structure changed dramatically in Phase IIIb. At this time, an earthwork was created at the top of the mound, potentially protecting the storage structures and the site itself from floodwaters moving from the slopes to the east, across the site, and toward the stream or river. This construction was followed by the building of two tholoi (domestic structures), more storage units, and a trash area on the western edge of the site.

A further change for Phase IIIb that manifests archaeologically is a distinct shift in pottery use to a primary focus on stationary storage containers, with appreciably less evidence of heating as food preparation, as well as somewhat less mobile storage. Heat applications are less prevalent during this phase among all types of coarse ware vessels. Those vessels that were in use tended to be small to medium in size and, based on the degree of sooting and carbonization present, when exposed to heat, the temperatures tended to be high. Thus, as evidence of more-permanent settlement at the site increases, heated food preparation activities decrease. It is possible that consumption of heated foods was simply practiced much less frequently than today or that other cooking techniques were utilized.

The vessels used for mobile containers were also found in both small and medium sizes with a focus on content protection in the form of covering or capping of vessels. Scoops were recovered from this phase as well. Most coarse ware vessels, however, served as stationary storage. Intriguingly, large storage vessels were not found in this phase, other than one example of a very large Open Bowl; all other storage vessels were medium to small in size. It is possible that with the increased nonpottery storage available there was less need for vessels to fulfill these functions. Thus, most of the pottery storage was for small quantities of materials. Some examples of foodstuffs that could have been stored in such small quantities are flavoring agents, such as oils, fats, and herbs, whose importance should not be undervalued. Larger quantities of food that would have supported the population during lean times of the year would have been stored in cell-plan buildings and potentially in baskets that did not survive in the record.

### *Phase IIIa: Height of Community Occupation*

Finally, with Phase IIIa, Fıstıklı Höyük was occupied to its greatest extent with multiple domestic structures, storage structures, ovens, hearths, and many work surfaces both exterior and interior to the buildings—indicating a sharp demographic increase. A good number of these work surfaces show evidence of intense food preparation activities. The expansion in construction on the site, as well as the increased variety in coarse ware materials, suggests growth in the number of people living in a more enduring fashion at the site. Based on their construction, which required regular and at times extensive repairs, the Fıstıklı Höyük tholoi and other structures were not designed for permanent occupation, but there was an intensification of living at the site during this phase. The Phase IIIa coarse ware assemblage was varied in available vessel shapes and sizes, as well as in evidence of use wear. The sheer amount of variation signifies that there was a need for variable quantities of food to be stored, manipulated, and prepared for consumption, as well as varied methods of preparation. This situation suggests a more varied population to be provided for. Different age groups can require different types of food, as both the very young and very old often benefit from relatively soft foods. With a larger population living at the site, there could also be more opportunities for meals of different levels of importance, ranging from daily consumption to special celebratory meals, even to meals designed to create or reinforce relationships both within the community and beyond.

The focus of food preparation in Phase IIIa was on stationary storage, with heating and mobile-container use being less important. As in Phase IIIb, coarse wares may not have been used as often to heat food as in earlier phases. As opposed to Phase IIIc, during which storage units are first constructed on the site and a drop in ceramic stationary storage occurs, in Phase IIIa the intensity of use of coarse ware for storage is highest, even though there are also many cell-plan buildings in use. The vessels used for stationary storage tended to be medium to large in size, thus holding larger quantities of material than in earlier phases. This could indicate the need to support the larger population living at the site, but as this is also the apogee of the Halaf period occupation, it may indicate the provisioning of another site or sites elsewhere that the population moved to later. An interesting change seen in these storage vessels is an increase in wear suggestive of vessel weakening from applications of wet or liquid materials, such as would be the case in soaking, leaching, pickling, or even fermenting. Finally, a variety of scoops were recovered from this phase, again representing important tools for food preparation, as well as for the utilization of stored materials.

## Food Preparation at Fıstıklı Höyük

At Fıstıklı Höyük, food preparation was carried out both inside and outside the domestic structures, or tholoi. At the height of its occupation, each tholos was associated with an oven and a storage unit (Bernbeck 2008:Table 3.3). Consequently, each residential unit had access to individual places located in open, public space in which to prepare and store food. A few of the tholoi were large enough to have had one or more hearths inside of their walls, and exterior fire installations were also found at the center and western borders of the settlement. The open spaces between the tholoi are often filled with work areas stretching from one tholos wall to another. Extensive work areas were located at the northern portion of the site, which also contained the remains of two hearths embedded within the deep lithic, ceramic, and faunal detritus. This pattern suggests that members of multiple residential units could choose to pool labor for some tasks, while at the same time carry out other activities in public, but exclusively used, areas.

Thus, the activities of food preparation were both public and private: potentially communal and restricted to labor within a residential unit. The preparation of food to support the community had a focus on individual residential units supporting themselves but was also under public surveillance. For those working away from the site, the scent of foods cooking would have been apparent long before the sounds and sights of these preparations were recognized. Methods of manipulating hot pots and hot contents would have been devised out of materials that did not survive in the archaeological record. All but one vessel shape, and this one is speculative, lacked handles of any kind and thus required some form of hand protection to remove them from the fire and utensils to remove the contents from the pots. And above all, the food preparation practices as cultural creations were repeated, passed on, and changed as different food types fell in and out of favor. Food preparation can be imagined as a possibly dreaded, possibly enjoyed, required daily task; it was quotidian for most purposes but also infinitely mutable to fit different occasions of joy or sorrow, of coming together or separation. These are traces of the lives lived, not simply of tools created and utilized.

However, to leave this discussion with the food bubbling away in a pot is to leave too soon. Food preparation moves into consumption through the serving of the food, and as Hamilakis (1999) states, this transference from one vessel to another is also a form of transformation of cooked food into food that is to be eaten. The food changes meaning as it is offered up for consumption. In the Halaf period context of Fıstıklı Höyük, this also implies the use of intricately painted vessels for serving (see Figure 11-5). While a detailed discussion of the vessels used for consumption is forthcoming (Hopwood 2013, in press), there are sensorial differences between the coarse ware food preparation vessels and the fine ware serving and consumption vessels that can be introduced here. Three of these differences are the appearance, the tactility, and the sound of the consumption vessels in use.

The appearance of the fine ware vessels can be discussed both in terms of their painted decorations and their shapes. The painted vessels from Fıstıklı Höyük

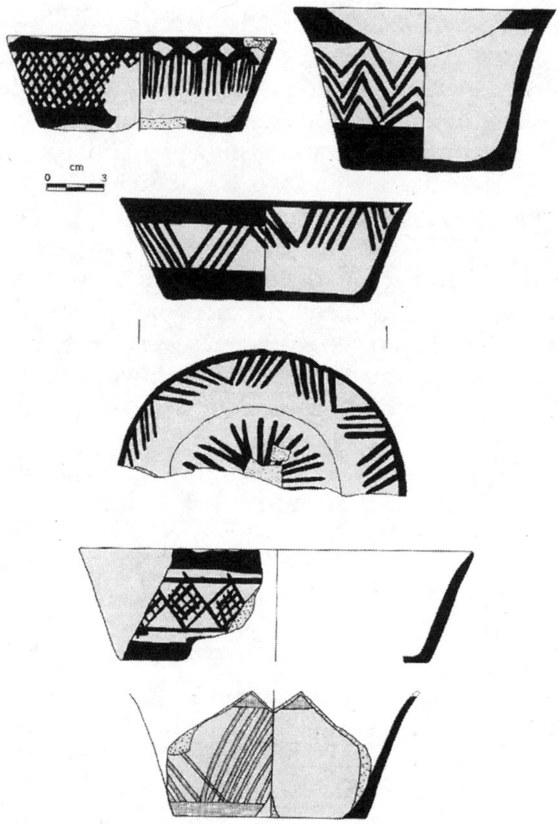


**Figure 11-5.** *Examples of painted pottery from Fıstıklı Höyük. (Bernbeck et al. 2003:Figure 14). Used with permission.*

include shapes such as *Trichterrandschallen*, cream bowls, tall-necked jars, straight-sided bowls, and lugged vessels to name a few (Bernbeck et al. 2003). While further research is necessary, it is possible that specific shapes were used for different types of food. The painted designs are characteristically Halaf period, with the cream to buff background painted with black geometric, anthropomorphic, and zoomorphic designs. Bowser and Patton (2004:176) discuss how exterior designs on pottery vessels for use in public-viewing contexts contain intended meanings that would be understood by the users. The variations in painted designs during the Halaf period could be indicative of specific local meanings understood and transmitted by the people offering and consuming food from the vessels.

These vessels would also have felt different to the hands and mouth. The walls tend to be thinner and smoother, and the vessels do not have the same rough vegetal voids and mineral inclusions found in the coarse wares. We can also imagine that the sound of using the painted vessels to eat from would have been different. If wooden, bone, or horn utensils were used to serve food in the vessels or to eat from them, the thinner walls would have sounded different. If vessels were purposefully or accidentally struck together, the walls would have made a more hollow clinking noise, like the sound we associate with striking thin-walled ceramics. Therefore, the entire sensorial experience of using the painted vessels would have been very different from the experience of using the thicker-walled, heavy, and undecorated food-preparation vessels.

Crucially, not only is the bowl meaningful in its design, but so too is the food it contains. The food itself was affected by the serving vessel and vice versa. It is the act of serving, offering, and consuming that transforms the prepared food, giving it a new meaning. Hamilakis (1999:39) describes food consumption as primarily an act of incorporation, which involves emotions, pleasures, and feelings (e.g., Becker 1995; Falk 1994). We can also view food preparation in a similar fashion. Not all food preparation is special, just like not all eating is special. However, the most special eating experiences are often wrapped up in memories of food preparation, of the person or people creating the food, of the aromas and sounds that fill the cooking space, and of the memories that these senses can evoke. The power of food, though likely quite different in the ancient past, was still emotive. It moved beyond simply cooking and eating for sustenance and was ripe with culture, tradition, and communication, all of which were transmitted and experienced through the senses.

## Conclusions

Exploring the senses involved in food preparation can open up different insights into the lives of those people whose material remains we study. Kopytoff (1988) suggests the interpretation of material studies as the social life of things, particularly the biography of an object. When dealing with a sherd-based assemblage, it can be difficult to expound on the social life of a shattered pot. While the final deposition of a midden can say something about the end of its use life, the earlier functions can be more difficult to uncover. Building off Kopytoff, MacGregor (1999:259) suggests that a change in an artifact's context also implies a change in its meaning. How then does one resuscitate a potsherd not only from the dregs of the excavated past but also from the midden heap of ancient refuse? Ceramic use alteration is one way to work toward this.

In archaeology, there have been frequent debates about food production, but they stop short of considering preparation. Similarly, consumption has been much discussed but primarily in relation to power and feasting, hence losing track of the quotidian practices of eating. Yet, it is the very fact of the repetitive nature of food preparation that makes it such a powerful tool of archaeological analysis. Repetition suggests habit, which suggests patterned behavior; that which is patterned can leave traces behind in the archaeological record. These traces can be etched into the surfaces of pottery, scattered across work areas, and gathered around certain features like ovens and hearths.

Hayden (2001:24) suggests that archaeologists' lack of focus on food and taste could result from some level of embarrassment: the belief being that taste is somehow too sybaritic to warrant academic consideration. He writes that "perhaps archaeologists have simply written the study of feasting off as a frivolous type of psychological self-gratification that pleasure-loving individuals engage in, but which is not particularly important" (Hayden 2001:24). While Hayden's focus is clearly on feasting, how much more so must this aversion affect the discussion of daily eating if the exercise of power through food is a distasteful study? Hamilakis (2002:123) notes that the consuming body, the body involved in eating and sharing food, is ignored even in archaeological discussions of embodiment. Even at the 27th Annual Visiting Scholar Conference, which highlighted the archaeology of the senses, this was the only paper presented dealing with food. Yet, with the understanding of the importance of food in culture, both past and present, we must shake off these Victorian restraints. As archaeologists and anthropologists, if we are to accurately represent the past we must be able to deal with the world of the senses, the world that marks our own understanding of our surroundings. While we may never be able to truly excavate what it was like to experience these senses in the ancient past or to dig up these ephemeral traces, by recognizing the importance of the sensorial experience and working with our data with these senses in mind we can come "closer to what it was like to smell, hear, speak, see—to live—in" the past that we study (Houston and Taube 2000:290).

## References

Appadurai, Arjun

1981 Gastro-politics in Hindu South Asia. *American Ethnologist* 8:494–511.

Atalay, Sonya, and Christine A. Hastorf

2006 Food, Meals, and Daily Activities: Food *Habitus* at Neolithic Çatalhöyük. *American Antiquity* 71:283–319.

Barnes, Barry

2001 Practice as Collective Action. In *The Practice Turn in Contemporary Theory*, edited by Karin Knorr Cetina, Theodore R. Schatzki, and Eike von Savigny, pp. 17–28. Routledge, London.

Bawden, Garth

1982 Community Organization Reflected by the Household: A Study of Pre-Columbian Social Dynamics. *Journal of Field Archaeology* 9:165–181.

Becker, Anne E.

1995 *Body, Self, and Society: The View from Fiji*. University of Pennsylvania Press, Philadelphia.

Bernbeck, Reinhard

2008 An Archaeology of Multi-sited Communities. In *The Archaeology of Mobility: Old World and New World Nomadism*, edited by Hans Barnard and Willeke Wendrich, pp. 43–77. Cotsen Institute of Archaeology Press, Los Angeles.

Bernbeck, Reinhard, Susan Pollock, Susan Allen, Ana Gabriela Castro-Gessner, Sarah Kielt-Costello, Robert Costello, Melissa Foree, Margarita Y. Gleba, Marie Goodwin, Sarah Lepinski, Carolyn Nakamura, and Sarah Niebuhr

2003 The Biography of an Early Halaf Village: Fıstıklı Höyük 1999–2000. *Istanbuler Mitteilungen* 53:9–77.

Bernbeck, Reinhard, Susan Pollock, Ana Gabriela Castro-Gessner, Robert Costello, Sarah Kielt-Costello, Melissa Foree, Margarita Gleba, Marie Goodwin, Peter Horan, Sarah Lepinski, Carolyn Nakamura, Sarah Niebuhr, and Rasmi Shoocongdej
2002 Preliminary Report on the 2000 Season at Fıstıklı Höyük. In *Salvage Project of the Archaeological Heritage of the Ilisu and Carchemish Dam Reservoirs: Activities in 2000,* edited by Numan Tuna and Jâle Velibeyoğlu, pp. 1–39. METU Centre for Research and Assessment of the Historic Environment (TACDAM)/Middle East Technical University, Ankara, Turkey.

Blitz, John H.
1993 Big Pots for Big Shots: Feasting and Storage in a Mississippian Community. *American Antiquity* 58:80–96.

Bourdieu, Pierre
1987 *Distinction: A Social Critique of the Judgment of Taste.* Harvard University Press, Cambridge.

Bowser, Brenda J., and John Q. Patton
2004 Domestic Spaces as Public Places: An Ethnoarchaeological Case Study of Houses, Gender, and Politics in the Ecuadorian Amazon. *Journal of Archaeological Method and Theory* 11:157–181.

Brumfiel, Elizabeth
1991 Weaving and Cooking: Women's Production in Aztec Mexico. In *Engendering Archaeology: Women and Prehistory,* edited by Joan Gero and Meg Conkey, pp. 224–251. Blackwell, Oxford.
2005 Materiality, Feasts, and Figured Worlds in Aztec Mexico. In *Rethinking Materiality,* edited by Elizabeth DeMarrais, Chris Gosden, and Colin Renfrew, pp. 225–237. McDonald Institute for Archaeological Research, Cambridge.

Campbell, Stuart
2007 Rethinking Halaf Chronologies. *Paléorient* 33:103–136.

Classen, Constance
1991 The Sensory Orders of "Wild Children." In *The Varieties of Sensory Experience: A Sourcebook in the Anthropology of the Senses,* edited by David Howes, pp. 45–60. University of Toronto Press, Toronto.
1997 Foundations for an Anthropology of the Senses. *International Social Science Journal* 49:401–412.

Classen, Constance, David Howes, and Anthony Synnott
1994 The Aromas of Antiquity. In *Aroma: The Cultural History of Smell,* pp. 13–50. Routledge, London.

Counihan, Carole, and Penny Van Esterik (editors)
2007 *Food and Culture: A Reader.* 2nd ed. Routledge, New York.

Dawson, Peter, Richard Levy, Don Gardner, and Matthew Walls
2007 Simulating the Behaviour of Light Inside Arctic Dwellings: Implications for Assessing the Role of Vision in Task Performance. *World Archaeology* 39:17–35.

Dietler, Michael
1990 Driven by Drink: The Role of Drinking in the Political Economy and the Case of Early Iron Age France. *Journal of Anthropological Archaeology* 9:352–406.
1996 Feasts and Commensal Politics in the Political Economy: Food, Power, and Status in Prehistoric Europe. In *Food and the Status Quest: An Interdisciplinary Perspective,* edited by Polly Wiessner and Wulf Schiefenhovel, pp. 87–125. Berghahn, Providence.

Douglas, Mary
1997 Deciphering a Meal. In *Food and Culture,* edited by Carole Counihan and Penny Van Esterik, pp. 36–54. Routledge, New York.

Falk, Pasi
1994 *The Consuming Body*. Sage, London.
Frieman, Catherine, and Mark Gillings
2007 Seeing Is Perceiving? *World Archaeology* 39:4–16.
Gaytan, Marie Sarita
2008 From Sombreros to Sincronizadas: Authenticity, Ethnicity, and the Mexican Restaurant Industry. *Journal of Contemporary Ethnography* 37:314–341.
Gosden, Chris
2001 Making Sense: Archaeology and Aesthetics. *World Archaeology* 33:163–167.
Hamilakis, Yannis
1999 Food Technologies/Technologies of the Body: The Social Context of Wine and Oil Production and Consumption in Bronze Age Crete. *World Archaeology* 31:38–54.
2002 The Past as Oral History: Towards an Archaeology of the Senses. In *Thinking through the Body: Archaeologies of Corporeality*, edited by Yannis Hamilakis, Mark Pluciennik, and Sarah Tarlow, pp. 121–136. Kluwer Academic/Plenum, New York.
Hamilton, Sue, and Ruth Whitehouse
2006 Three Senses of Dwelling: Beginning to Socialize the Neolithic Ditched Villages of the Tavoliere, Southeast Italy. *Journal of Iberian Archaeology* 8:159–184.
Harbottle, Lynn
1997 Fast Food/Spoiled Identity: Iranian Migrants in the British Catering Trade. In *Food, Health, and Identity*, edited by Pat Caplan, pp. 87–110. Routledge, London.
Harris, Marvin
1987 *The Sacred Cow and the Abominable Pig: Riddles of Food and Culture*. Touchstone Books, Kent.
Hayden, Brian
2001 Introduction. In *Feasts: Archaeological and Ethnographic Perspectives on Food, Politics, and Power*, edited by Michael Dietler and Brian Hayden. Smithsonian Institution Press, Washington, D.C.
Holtzman, Jon D.
2006 Food and Memory. *Annual Review of Anthropology* 35:361–378.
Hopwood, Marie H.
2010 The Fed Community: Food Preparation and Community at the Halaf Site of Fıstıklı Höyük, Turkey. Unpublished Ph.D. dissertation, Department of Anthropology, Binghamton University, State University of New York.
2013 More than Just a Pretty Face: The Meaningful Use of Painted Pottery in the Halaf Period. In *Painting Pots, Painting People: Investigating Decorated Ceramics from the Late Neolithic Near East*, edited by Inna Mateiciucova, Olivier Nieuwenhuyse, and Walter Cruells. Ox Bow, Woodbridge, Connecticut, in press.
Hopwood, Marie H., and Siddharatha Mitra
2012 Feeding Households: A Multiproxy Method for Analysis of Food Preparation in the Halaf Period, at Fıstıklı Höyük, Turkey. In *New Perspectives in Household Archaeology*, edited by Bradley J. Parker and Catherine P. Foster, Eisenbrauns, Winona Lake, Illinois, in press.
Houston, Stephen, and Karl Taube
2000 An Archaeology of the Senses: Perception and Cultural Expression in Ancient Mesoamerica. *Cambridge Archaeological Journal* 10:261–294.
Howes, David
1991a Introduction: "To Summon All the Senses." In *The Varieties of Sensory Experience: A Sourcebook in the Anthropology of the Senses*, edited by David Howes, pp. 3–21. University of Toronto Press, Toronto.

1991b Sensorial Anthropology. In *The Varieties of Sensory Experience: A Sourcebook in the Anthropology of the Senses*, edited by David Howes, pp. 167–191. University of Toronto Press, Toronto.

Howes, David (editor)

1991 *The Varieties of Sensory Experience: A Sourcebook in the Anthropology of the Senses.* University of Toronto Press, Toronto.

Howes, David, and Constance Classen

1991 Sounding Sensory Profiles. In *The Varieties of Sensory Experience: A Sourcebook in the Anthropology of the Senses*, edited by David Howes, pp. 257–288. University of Toronto Press, Toronto.

Ingold, Tim

1983 The Significance of Storage in Hunting Societies. *Man* 18:553–571.

Jonaitis, Aldona

2006 Smoked Fish and Fermented Oil: Taste and Smell among the Kwakwaka'wakw. In *Sensible Objects: Colonialism, Museums, and Material Culture*, edited by Elizabeth Edwards, Chris Gosden, and Ruth Phillips, pp. 141–167. Berg, Oxford.

Kopytoff, Igor

1988 The Cultural Biography of Things: Commoditization as Process. In *The Social Life of Things: Commodities in Cultural Perspective*, edited by Arjun Appadurai, pp. 64–94. Cambridge University Press, New York.

Lehrer, Jonah

2008 Auguste Escoffier: The Essence of Taste. In *Proust Was a Neuroscientist*, pp. 53–74. Mariner, New York.

Lévi-Strauss, Claude

1966 The Culinary Triangle. *Partisan Review* 7/6:586–595.

1969 *The Raw and the Cooked*. Harper and Row, New York.

MacGregor, Gavin

1999 Making Sense of the Past in the Present: A Sensory Analysis of Carved Stone Balls. *World Archaeology* 31:258–271.

Mintz, Sidney W.

1996 Tasting Food, Tasting Freedom. In *Tasting Food, Tasting Freedom: Excursions into Eating, Culture, and the Past*, edited by Sidney W. Mintz, pp. 33–49. Beacon, Boston.

Mintz, Sidney W., and Christine M. Du Bois

2002 The Anthropology of Food and Eating. *Annual Review of Anthropology* 31:99–119.

Pollock, Susan

2003 Feasts, Funerals, and Fast Food in Early Mesopotamian States. In *The Archaeology and Politics of Food and Feasting in Early States and Empires*, edited by Tamara L. Bray, pp. 17–38. Kluwer Academic, New York.

Pollock, Susan, and Reinhard Bernbeck

1998 Fıstıklı Höyük 1998: Systematic Survey and Sounding. In *Salvage Project of the Archaeological Heritage of the Ilisu and Carchemish Dam Reservoirs: Activities in 1998*, edited by Numan Tuna and Jean Ozturk. METU Centre for Research and Assessment of the Historic Environment (TACDAM)/Middle East Technical University, Ankara, Turkey.

Pollock, Susan, Reinhard Bernbeck, Susan Allen, Ana Gabriela Castro-Gessner, Robert Costello, Sarah Kielt-Costello, Melissa Foree, Sarah Lepinski, and Sarah Niebuhr

2001 Excavations at Fıstıklı Höyük, 1999. In *Salvage Project of the Archaeological Heritage of the Ilisu and Carchemish Dam Reservoirs: Activities in 1999*, edited by Numan Tuna, Jean Ozturk, and Jâle Velibeyoğlu. METU Centre for Research and Assessment of the Historic Environment (TACDAM)/Middle East Technical University, Ankara, Turkey.

Rice, Prudence M.
1987 *Pottery Analysis: A Sourcebook*. University of Chicago Press, Chicago.
Richards, Audrey
1932 *Hunger and Work in a Savage Tribe*. Geo. Routledge and Sons, London.
Siskind, Janet
1992 The Invention of Thanksgiving: A Ritual of American Nationality. *Critique of Anthropology* 12:167–191.
Skibo, James M.
1992 *Pottery Function: A Use-Alteration Perspective*. Plenum, New York.
Stoller, Paul
1989 *The Taste of Ethnographic Things: The Senses in Anthropology*. University of Pennsylvania Press, Philadelphia.
Suen, Wong Hong
2007 A Taste of the Past: Historically Themed Restaurants and Social Memory in Singapore. In *Food and Foodways in Asia: Resource, Tradition, and Cooking*, edited by Sidney C. H. Cheung and Tan Chee-Beng, pp. 115–128. Routledge, London.
Wilk, Richard (editor)
2006 *Fast Food/Slow Food*. AltaMira, New York.

# 12. The Scent of Status: Prestige and Perfume at the Bronze Age Palace at Pylos, Greece

*Joanne M. A. Murphy*

*Abstract:* The prominent position of the perfume industry at the Mycenaean palace of Pylos has long been known. Both the archaeological remains and textual evidence indicate that perfume was a prestigious commodity at Pylos that was manufactured under palatial control at the palace itself. The finished product was a restricted commodity that was distributed by the *wanax*, the highest ranked individual at the palace. The fragrance of the perfumed oil would have been prominent there, creating both a physical and a sensory connection between the palace—its power, its prestige, and its wealth—and the smell. While the smell of the manufacturing of perfume would have been available to all who lived in and around the palace or even visited it, the finished refined perfume was available to only a limited few. This paper thus connects some well- and long-known data about perfume production at Pylos and combines them with more recent work in sensory anthropology, neuroscience, and biology.

This chapter focuses on the production and consumption of perfume at the Mycenaean palace of Pylos in Messenia, southwestern Greece, at the end of the Late Bronze Age, circa 1200 B.C.E. The archaeological remains from the palatial and nonpalatial sites of Mycenaean Greece afford us a rich understanding of this culture with its site hierarchy, craft specialization, limited access to the production and consumption of elite goods, elaborate burial sites, and contacts with the greater Mediterranean world. Moreover, our knowledge of Mycenaean culture has benefited immensely from the decipherment of the Linear B script in the 1950s. Large numbers of clay tablets inscribed with Linear B were found at major Mycenaean sites such as Mycenae, Tiryns, Thebes, Pylos, Knossos, and Chania (Figure

*Making Senses of the Past: Toward a Sensory Archaeology,* edited by Jo Day. Center for Archaeological Investigations, Occasional Paper No. 40.  ISBN 978-0-8093-3287-8.

12-1). It is thanks to the decipherment and detailed study of these tablets (Figure 12-2) that archaeologists have been able to explore many aspects of the complex economies at these sites. In particular, there is extensive scholarship discussing the likely location of a perfume industry at Pylos, the palatial control of perfume, and the economic importance of scented oils (e.g., Beck and Beck 1978; Bendall 2002; Shelmerdine 1985), all of which we would know little about without the texts. This scholarship, however, has focused mainly on the manufacturing and distributive elements of the perfume industry at Pylos. This chapter builds on this important past work but expands our understanding of perfume in Pylian society by presenting it as a sensory metaphor for power, a social communication device, and an integral perceptual element of wealth finance and commensal activities.

Although many works that deal with smell also include taste, and indeed at Pylos perfume was used at feasts (as discussed below), I have chosen to limit my analysis to perfume and smell to highlight the various and changing impacts perfume would have had in Pylos. In this paper, I discuss perfume as a key to the past experience of the people of Pylos, contributing to a re-creation of dynamic, multisensory life at this site. I explore a parochial expression and manipulation of a universal fact: Smell triggers memory and creates associations. This work brings together biological anthropology and cultural anthropology in an attempt to enhance awareness of the lived experience of individuals in the past (Ingold 2000:1–2).

Both the archaeological remains and textual evidence indicate that at Pylos perfume was a prestigious commodity manufactured at the palace under close palatial control (Shelmerdine 1985). The finished product, moreover, was a restricted commodity distributed by the *wanax*, the highest ranked individual at the palace, to himself and to the main gods and used in religious and commensal feasts (Palaima 1995a, 1995b; Shelmerdine 1985). The fragrance of the perfumed oil would have been prominent at the palace, creating both a physical and a sensory connection between scent and the palace—its power, its prestige, and its wealth. Although the smell of the perfume during its manufacture would have been available to all who lived in and around the palace or even visited it, the finished, refined perfume was only accessible to a limited few; the smell of perfume, therefore, simultaneously united the people of Pylos and emphasized their separation into sociopolitical groups. This chapter thus connects some well- and long-known data about perfume production at Pylos with more recent work in sensory anthropology. By combining biological information about the olfactory system with archaeological evidence from Pylos, I examine the smells of Pylos with a view to highlighting the significance of perfumed oil in the Bronze Age. I stress the Pylian appreciation and manipulation of perfume not just as an economic and political substance but also as a mnemonic, evocative device.

## The Science behind the Proustian Moment

Interpretive archaeology (Hodder 1995; Hodder et al. 1995), developing since the 1980s, strives to embody and populate the past with the feelings and emotions of individuals, with a goal of exploring how people interacted and

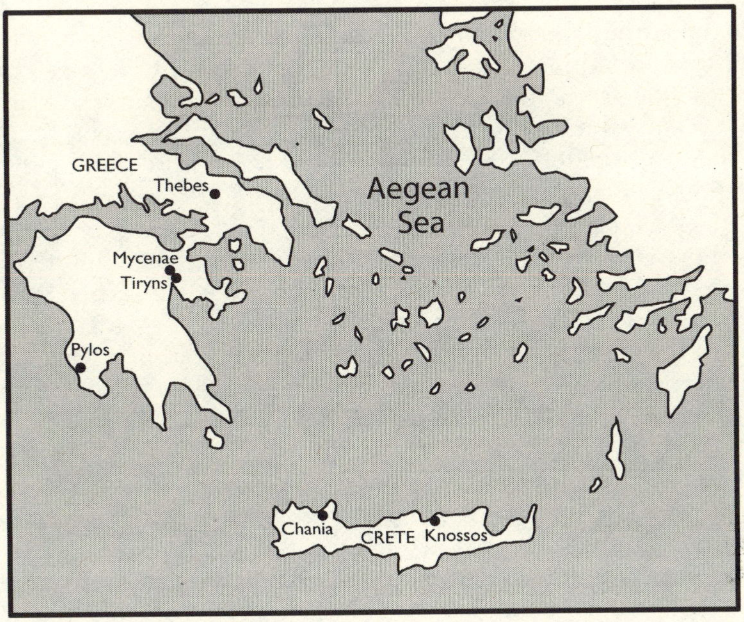


**Figure 12-1.** *Map of Mycenaean sites mentioned in text. (Courtesy of John Wallrodt)*

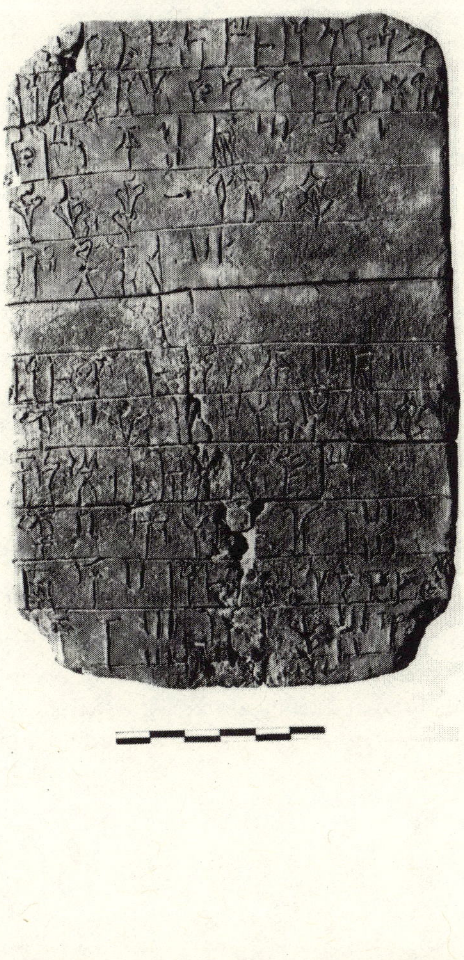

**Figure 12-2.** *Linear B tablet Un 718 (scale in cm). (Courtesy of The Department of Classics, University of Cincinnati.)*

understood themselves in relation to each other. Archaeology has relied on ethnographic and anthropological work to support this cultural research; a wealth of scientific evidence can be added to corroborate these theories (Alaoui-Ismaïli 1997; Jones-Gotman and Zatorre 1993; Ingold 2000). The evocative passage in Proust's (1927) semiautobiographical novel has frequently been cited to support interpretations of the role of the olfactory and gustatory senses; the growing volume of biological, psychological, and neuroscientific research on this topic both confirms and explains the impressionistic assessment of the importance of those senses. Recently, both biological and cultural studies have reached the same conclusion: Humans understand the world through the senses. Identity and the relationship of the individual to others are experienced through feeling, taste, and smell, as well as through sight and hearing (e.g., Carrithers et al. 1985; Descartes 1995). Furthermore, studies in the psychology of olfactory perceptions demonstrate that humans and animals do not entrust their assessment of the world and their place in it to any one sense but, rather, use all their available senses to live and interact with the world around them. However, scientists argue that the senses that physically influence the body, such as smell, taste, and touch, play a greater role in socialization. Olfactory stimuli, in particular, evoke a higher level of emotion in the amygdala (Figure 12-3) than auditory and visual stimuli do (Lledo et al. 2005:305; Royet et al. 2000), and the epithelieum, of which the internal section of the nose is made, has a more direct impact than other sensors such as the skin (Lledo et al. 2005:305). These studies suggest that smell is a primary and most immediate sense for connecting with the outside world.

Although the connection between the olfactory system, emotions, and memory has long been known, biologists have only recently been able to explain the processes of these connections. Recent studies demonstrate that the stimuli from scent are processed, identified, classified, and responded to through the olfactory system. The physical structure of the nose and brain results in a privileged connection between the olfactory system and the limbic system that manages emotions, behavior, and memory (Lledo et al. 2005:305). The olfactory bulbs are, in fact, extensions of the brain tissue. The primary olfactory cortex projects to the hypothalamus, the amygdala, and the entorhinal area, which in turn projects to the hippocampus (Lledo et al. 2005:305; Zald and Pardo 1997). Thus, the olfactory system directly influences the amygdala, which processes emotional responses to the object being smelled (Zald and Pardo 1997). In sum, the olfactory system is directly connected to the brain in a manner that is not shared with the other senses. Therefore, anything that is smelled instantly has an impact on the brain and creates an immediate and emotional impression there.

Lledo, Ghieus, and Vincent (2005:306) stress that the olfactory system is not static and passive in its reception of odors but rather is active and performs the first stage in creating responses to those odors. Unlike other senses, the olfactory system quickly encodes the identity of an odor and on next encounter if shortly thereafter, even among distracting smells, can recognize and label the first odor (Rabin and Cain 1984). Initially, scents connect with the most basic emotions of good or bad, correlating with safe or unsafe and fear or pleasure, from which more complex reactions are created. Not only does the odor activate the amygdala and

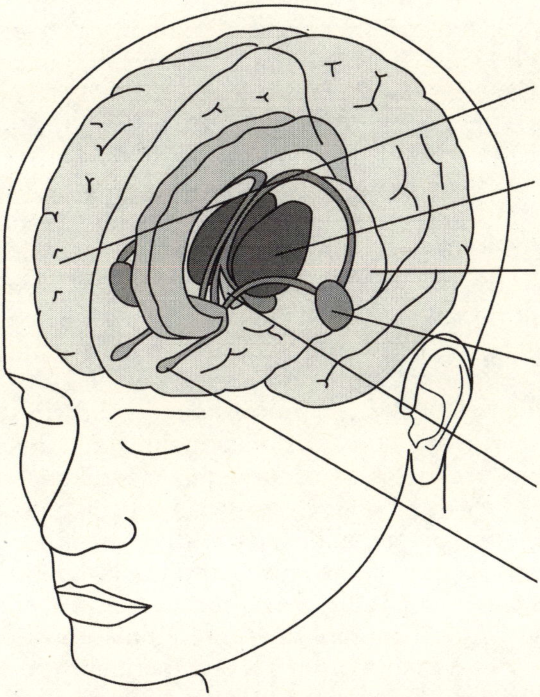


**Figure 12-3.** *Parts of the brain connected with smell and memory (by Tina Ross, after Morris and Maisto 2001).*

thereby evoke emotions, but this activation also facilitates the coding of memories (Lledo et al. 2005:306). Therefore, over time the emotional responses to odors are encoded on the brain and connect memory with the reactions; smells thus have the power to evoke both emotions and memories.

The olfactory system is key in creating sensory and emotional associations, connecting people to the physical and cultural environment. Because of the physical composition of the olfactory system with the epithelium that is a projection of the limbic system, the emotions and memories evoked by smell are powerful and immediate.

## Anthropology of the Senses

While biology provides a detailed empirical evaluation of smell and of the creation of memories, anthropology and sociology have explained the cultural and personal impact of the senses, both in learning to use those senses and in socializing to particular cultural values through them (Classen 1993; Howes 1991, 2003; Howes, ed. 1991). The conclusions reached by anthropological studies of the senses concur with those from biology and neuroscience that smell, unlike the other senses, immediately triggers emotional responses and memories. In contrast to smell, which stimulates emotional or motivational arousal (Engen

1982), visual experiences more commonly result in thought or cognition (Herz and Cupchik 1992, 1995; Porteous 2006:91); vision, moreover, distances the viewer from the object, but smell permeates the body (Porteous 2006:91). The emotions evoked by an odor are more potent than the emotions evoked by other sensory stimuli such as visual or verbal cues (Herz and Cupchik 1995:527). Furthermore, the longevity of memories created through odor has also been demonstrated (Engen 1991); indeed, the ability to remember a scent is less remarkable than the inability to forget it (Engen 1991:81). Cultural anthropologists have also drawn attention to the contexts in which smell is manipulated; based on a variety of examples from diverse cultures and times, an intrinsic connection between olfaction and transition has been established, and smell is used particularly in rites of passage and at the most sacred times during rituals (Howes 1991).

According to Baudrillard's (1983) concept of hyper-reality, the senses are not solely physical components of a human "situated within and defined by the socio-economic, cultural, and technological context of their employment"; he also endorses the widely argued view that the senses socialize people to their world and that senses are a potent part of their interaction with others (Rodaway 1994). While Baudrillard's contention may be universally applicable, definitions of the senses and their categorization and value are culturally defined. Ethnographic research shows that the Western cultural division into five senses is a social construct. Studies of some non-Western groups reveal that they also sense their way in the world but in different manners than Western groups do (Edwards et al. 2006; Scarre and Lawson 2006), frequently differing in their cultural definition and classification of the senses (e.g., the Javanese identify talk rather than taste as the sense associated with the mouth [Howes and Classen 1991:257–258; Watson 2006:15]), the number of senses recognized (e.g., the Hausa only identify two senses [Ritchie 1991:193–195]), and the hierarchy of the senses (e.g., the forest people in Papua New Guinea place sounds at the top of their sensory hierarchy [Gell 1995; Howes and Cassen 1991]).

The Western division of the senses into five (visual, auditory, tactile, olfactory, and gustatory) is not only a cultural construct but also a rather recent classification (Classen 1993:1–4). Sight has been overvalued as the supreme sense at the expense of the others in Western culture in general since the nineteenth century and by archaeologists in particular, as an abundance of scholarly literature illustrates (Classen et al. 1994:82–84; Classen and Howes 2006:199–200; Ingold 2000:155), with the result that the other senses have been left underexplored. As multiple disciplines demonstrate, however, each object encountered in life has some impact on the senses, and associations and judgments are based on that sensory impact. Hurcombe (2007) argues that while the division into five senses is convenient for analysis it does not allow for a holistic reality in which the experience of one sense triggers the other senses (Ingold 2000:268; Merleau-Ponty 1962) nor does it recognize intersensoriality (Classen et al. 1994; Howes 2002; 2006); life is inescapably multisensorial. The sensory hierarchies and divisions of the senses among groups in the past may be beyond our grasp and are definitely beyond the scope of this paper; nevertheless, it is possible to assess Pylian society through a sensory lens and to detect conscious awareness of their sensory interaction with the world and manipulation of the senses by the palatial elite to create and maintain their hierarchy.

## Senses and Pylos

Thus, on the one hand, biologists and anthropologists claim that smell evokes memories, emotions, and connections more readily and strongly than other senses do but, on the other, that such associations are cultural. Evidence from Pylos illustrates the cultural importance accorded to manipulation of many senses; the perfume industry is only one of the ways that the Pylians manipulated and attempted to control sensory relations. The Lyre Player wall painting (Lang 1969; McCallum 1987; Shank 2008), which was the large-scale focal figure in a feasting scene in the Throne Room (Room 6 in Figure 12-4), succinctly illustrates both the multisensorial reality of life in Pylos and the manipulation of the senses by the palatial elite. This and other wall paintings represent elite investments in a high level of craft specialization; directly experienced through the sense of sight, this depiction would have stimulated associations with the sounds of the music and the tastes and smells of the feast—senses that cannot be remembered directly but that can be evoked by images or references (Engen 1991:6; Holley 2002:23). Further depictions of elite activities—such as riding in chariots and hunting—that were portrayed on valuable objects—such as gold rings and decorated weapons—and in other wall paintings would likewise have communicated visually the association between elite individuals, the object, and the activities and would have evoked a ramified reality in which the elite activities were fully and sensorially incorporated into the Pylian world.

The following section discusses evidence for the production of perfume at the palace, the methods of production, the location of production in the palace, perfume's connection with the palatial economy, and its role in creating and maintaining the elite hierarchy.

## Production of Perfume at Pylos

Evidence for the production and consumption of perfume at the palace of Pylos is, as yet, reliant on Linear B and archaeological evidence from the site; thus far, no organic residue analysis has been carried out on the relevant ceramic material, but such analyses could add greatly to our understanding of the perfumery processes. The available evidence does demonstrate clearly that perfume was produced at the palace of Pylos; the palace, furthermore, controlled all aspects of its production and distribution, documenting its ingredients, allocation, and storage. Linear B establishes that it was one of the few commodities directly controlled by the palace (Lupack 2007; Schon 2007; Shelmerdine 1985). The classification of perfume as a high-value item is supported not only by the attention paid to all phases of the industry by the palatial bureaucracy (Shelmerdine 1985:153) but also by the comparative value of the other crafts recorded at

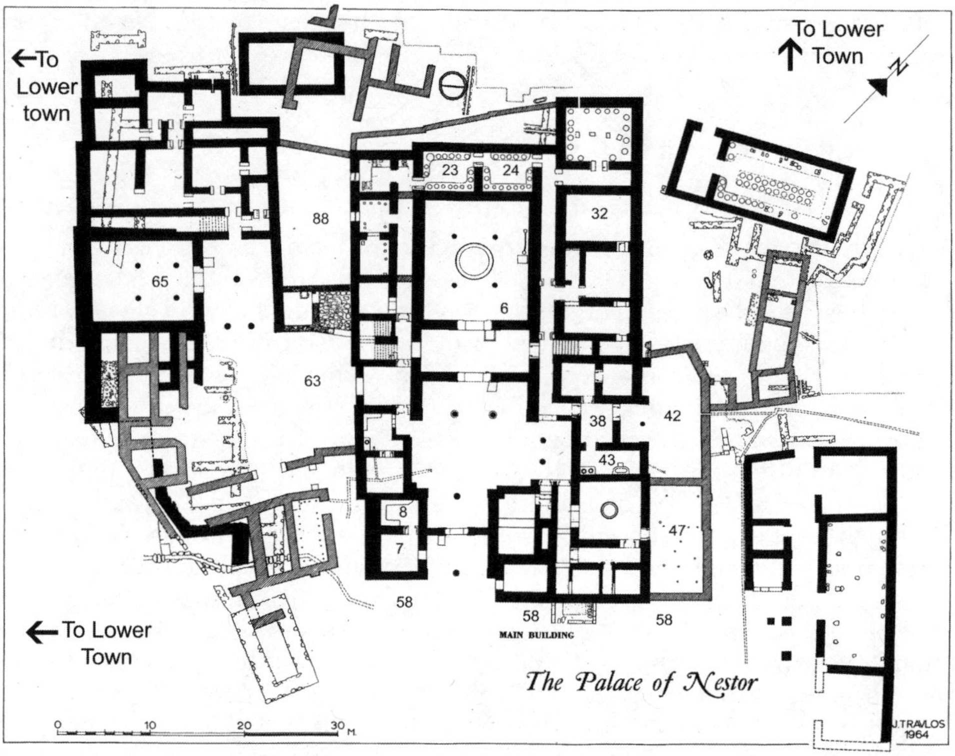


**Figure 12-4.** *Plan of the Palace of Nestor, Pylos, indicating areas of feasting, storage, production, and the lower town. (Blegen and Rawson 1966: Key Plan. Courtesy of The Department of Classics, University of Cincinnati.)*

the palace: bronze working, textile manufacture, weapon production, and chariot assembly (Killen 1995; Lupack 2007; Schon 2007).

According to the Linear B evidence, the perfume produced at Pylos had an olive-oil base that was fragranced by spices, herbs, and flowers. It seems to have had two forms: a more liquid one (OLE which signifies oil) and a thicker unguent type (AREPA) (Shelmerdine 1985:31). Several of the tablets deal with raw materials (An 616r, Un 249, Un 267, and Un 592 kept in Archive room 7-8 [see Figure 12-4]) (Shelmerdine 1985:8). They include references to the basic oil from both palatial stores and from outside the palace; coriander and cyperus, which were lightly scented spices and astringents used to prepare the oil for the final fragrance; and henna (Un 267), which was probably used to dye the oil (Shelmerdine 1985:17–23, 151). In the disbursement tablets (the Fr series), there are references to rose-, sage-, and cyperus-scented oils (Shelmerdine 1985:25).

The procurement of the spices and herbs used in the production of perfumes may mirror the variety of means by which the palace obtained other goods. Lupack (2007:55) has argued, contrary to Killen (1992, 2007), that the spices were imported from overseas; many of the herbs necessary for perfuming oil, however, would have come to the palace through decentralized systems of exchange

(Palaima and Shelmerdine 1984; Palmer 1963; Palmer 1999, 2003). Unlike the Ga series from Knossos (see Foster 1977:20–28), tablets that might record the gathering of plant supplies for perfume have not been found at Pylos (Palmer 1963:300–313; Shelmerdine 1985:108–109). This may be due to the season during which the palace was destroyed, which Chadwick suggests was early spring, a time when most of the fresh plants would have been collected into the palace (Chadwick 1976:191–192; Foster 1977; Shelmerdine 1985:107). This is in contrast to the destruction of the palace at Knossos, which is thought to have occurred after the local herbs used in perfume production had been gathered (Foster 1977).

It has been inferred from Linear B tablets that perfume was made within the palace itself. The theory of on-site production is mainly derived from the contrast in information recorded for the bronze smiths, for which the tablets explicitly refer to a production site outside the palace, compared with that for the perfumers; no similar off-site location is given for the four perfumers. All the supplies and provisions of the perfumers came from the palace; this also strengthens the argument that the palace was the location of production. The main archaeological question regarding the perfume industry in the palace at Pylos, however, is identification of the specific production location; although several rooms in the palace have archaeological remains of appropriate storage jars and tablets referring to perfumed oil, the production area has not been securely identified. The crux of the problem is that production of perfume does not require unique and, therefore, easily identifiable equipment; open vessels for heating, shallow open vessels for steeping, large vessels for storage, and small narrow-mouthed jars for perfume use and distribution (Shelmerdine 1985), like the Mycenaean stirrup jars (Figure 12-5), are all rather common types of vessels. Shelmerdine (1985:59), however, has argued persuasively for perfume production in Courts 42 and 47 (see Figure 12-4) on the northeast side of the palace, based on the large number of stirrup jars in Court 47 along with pithoi, braziers, tripods, basins, dippers, and scoops and the flat pan, basin, several cooking pots, small pithoi, and large jars found in Court 42. Both of these courts afford the ventilation required for perfume production.

The exact procedure for the production of Bronze Age perfumed oil is difficult to ascertain. Linear B tablet Un 267 refers to an unguent that should be boiled, indicating that perfume was produced using a heat process like that depicted on the walls of a contemporary Egyptian tomb and described in some of the later Classical texts (Shelmerdine 1985:17, Note 27). Wine and honey are also included in the process. Because of its alcohol content, wine was most probably used for presoaking the aromatic herbs. Honey may have been used to coat the jars and hands of perfumers and sometimes as an ingredient (Shelmerdine 1985:19). The references to wool in the perfume texts may indicate that it was used to strain the oil as in Classical times (Shelmerdine 1985:17–21) or that it was used an ingredient (Beck and Beck 1978). Parallels for the production process may be sought either in the descriptions of the later Classical authors Theophrastus and Dioscorides or in a contemporary Assyrian procedure. The former is known in greater detail. To a base of oil, a lightly scented astringent was added, which would have both prepared it for the final heavier scent and caused it to thicken

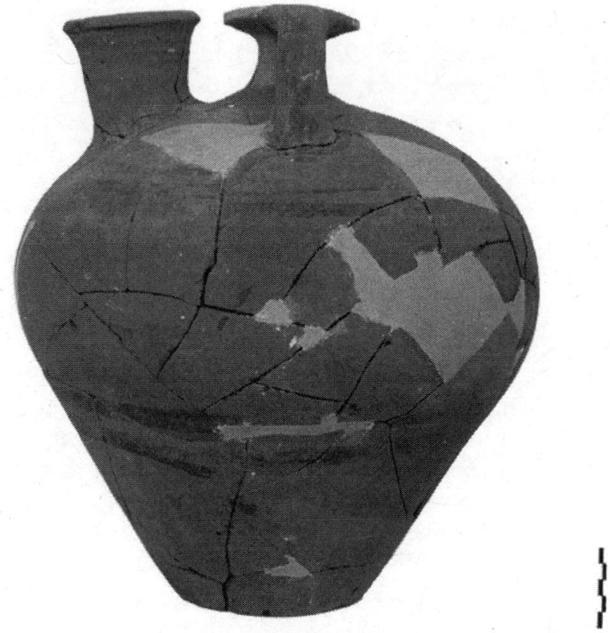

**Figure 12-5.** *Stirrup jar (scale in cm). (Blegen and Rawson 1966:Figure 389. Courtesy of The Department of Classics, University of Cincinnati.)*

(Shelmerdine 1985:13). The spices and herbs were ground and then mixed in, and the mixture was heated with either direct or indirect heat. Finally, the botanical remains were strained from the oil with wool, and fresh spices and herbs were added. In the Assyrian method, the aromatics were put in hot water several times before adding the oil. It is not known which method was used at Pylos; either procedure, however, would have included heating the oil, in agreement with the indications of tablet Un 267, and would therefore have created fragrant vapors.

The vapors produced by either of the manufacturing processes outlined above would have carried the fragrance, which would have wafted around the palatial area and lower town in the diffusing molecules of the oil. The Pylos Regional Archaeological Project has demonstrated that the palace occupied approximately 15,000 $m^2$ of the Englianos hilltop and that the lower town surrounding the palace spread down the ridge to the southwest, southeast, and northwest of the palace (Blegen and Rawson 1966:33; Davis et al. 1997:430). Even on a still day, the fragranced molecules would easily have permeated the area surrounding the palace. The weather conditions would have had a significant impact on the movement of the vapors: A warm, humid day would have amplified the fragrance, while a breeze would have both dictated the traveling direction of the molecules and increased their traveling speed but would have also hastened their dispersal.

Descriptions of the putrid smells of Classical Greek and Roman towns and of medieval cities record the constant assault on the olfactory system by different smells of decay; fetid organics, including human waste; and the fumes of different work places, such as produced by tanneries and laundries (Classen et al. 1994; Corbin 1986). Ancient sources inform us that, while these smells were classed even then as unpleasant, people became inured to them; a new fragrance, however, stands out even in such a cacophony of smells. Similarly, the ambient smells at Pylos must have been overpowering in comparison to modern Western settlements, but they would have been relatively unnoticed by contemporary inhabitants. So also, the initial days of the production of the perfume and the addition of new fragrant organics would have registered with people despite the other smells, although if perfume manufacture were performed frequently at the palace, then its fragrance would eventually have been absorbed into the jumble of odors in the town.

Recent studies have shown that even at undetectable doses, scents in the air can elicit emotional responses (Li et al. 2007), which over time may become encoded in the mind of the inhaler; while the association of a scent is with the production area and source, the more nuanced emotional response varies individually (Almagor 1990:255). The production of perfume at Pylos would have been an inclusive experience that the community and visitors would have associated with the palace, evoking a range of emotions even if the fragrance was not consciously noted. Because of the immediacy of the sense of smell and its biologically and anthropologically demonstrated ability to form associations in the brain and to create long-lasting memories based on the physical connections between the olfactory bulbs and the brain, the pervasive scent of perfume manufacture in the palace and town at Pylos would have recalled emotional associations and memories among the inhabitants.

The presence of the odors, and consequently the emotional encoding and responses, involved with the large-scale production of refined perfume would have been unique to Pylos in this region. Little evidence for large-scale perfumed oil production might be expected in nonpalatial contexts and, indeed, none has been reported elsewhere in Messenia (Galaty and Parkinson 2007:5). Since perfume can be made from easily obtained ingredients and its production needs little in the way of specialized utensils, it is plausible that nonelite members of Pylian society also had perfume, as their counterparts did in the better-documented Classical period. The local homemade perfume would have been distinctly different from the palatial version, not least because it lacked the production expertise of a minimum of four professional perfumers. Nor would the homemade perfume carry the prestige of a commodity distributed by the wanax. Therefore, the perfumes made at the palace and the fragrances of their manufacture are likely to have been distinctive and closely associated with the palace itself; the emotional responses evoked by those scents will also have been intimately associated with the palace.

Perfume was not only manufactured at the palace at Pylos; it was also stored there. Several storerooms for this substance have been identified on the basis of pottery, tablets, or sealings: Rooms 23 and 24 behind the megaron and 32 and 38 to its east (see Figure 12-4). Room 23 has been identified both as a storage area for perfumed oil and as a scribal center for recording its disbursement (Blegen and Rawson 1966:136; Shelmerdine 1985:87–88), since it held 32 of the 49 Fr tablets concerned with storage and disbursement; in addition, one tablet (Fr 1241) refers to oil owed by the palace (Shelmerdine 1985:88). The adjacent oil storeroom, Room 24, had large pithoi in benches around the wall and produced a sealing (Wr 1437) with AREPA on it (Shelmerdine 1985:88) but no tablets; a second sealing had a name on it. The sealings have been interpreted as labels for the oil and the name as that of the person who brought the oil to the palace; therefore, oil from outside the palace was apparently stored with the palace's oil in this room. Rooms 32 and 38 were also storerooms associated with perfumed oil (Blegen and Rawson 1966:156–160, 170–173); the former is better decorated than Rooms 23 and 24 and contained a great variety of ceramic shapes: small pithoid jars, large quantities of decorated pottery, and stirrup jars of various sizes, two of which may have been imported from the Argolid; five other jars may also be from there as well. These may be the only imported vases in the palace (Shelmerdine 1985:89–90). Similar decorated pottery was found in Room 38, which also contained tablets. Although some of the pottery in Room 38 seems to have originally belonged there and may have been used in the adjoining Room 43, a bathroom (Shelmerdine 1985:94–96), the tablets and other vases may have fallen from an upper room in the possible "women's quarter" of the palace, where there is evidence of textile production (Shelmerdine 1985:104–105).

The differences between these storerooms may indicate that various types or categories of perfume were stored in them; unlike Room 32, where all the oil was perfumed, some but not all the oil was treated in Rooms 23 and 24 (Shelmerdine 1985:94). Blegen and Rawson (1966:158) suggest that Rooms 32 and 38 "may have held a refined type of oil" (Shelmerdine 1985:69–96). The various locations of the tablets and of the pottery related to perfumed oil suggest that the oil was stored in different areas in the palace; some oil may have been used within the palace during bathing and for treating other palatial products such as textiles, while other oil may not have been used close to its storage place.

## Pylian Perfume and Power

The palace was as deeply involved in the distribution and consumption of perfume as it was in its manufacture and storage. Although smelling the fragrance of perfume during its production would have been an experience shared by all inhabitants of the palace and town at Pylos, the finished product, in contrast, can be demonstrated to have been distributed differentially among members of society. It therefore would have marked divisions within the populace between the privileged and the disadvantaged; access to perfume would have acted as a sensory reinforcer and creator of the Pylian social hierarchy. Moreover, even with a pervasive undercurrent of the aroma from perfume manufacture, the distinct and stronger scent of perfume on an individual would have been quite noticeable and would have separated that individual from the other members of society.

The wanax was the head of the stratified social and political hierarchy at Pylos, with significant political, economic, and religious authority over diverse aspects of Pylian society, as documented in the Linear B tablets (Hooker 1979; Kilian 1988; Palaima 1995a, 1995b). These textual references indicate that he drew his "funds of power" (Blanton et al. 1996:2; Brumfield 1992:554–555) from the production and distribution of prestige goods, from connections between that production and the deities, and from large-scale social and religious rituals. One of the duties of the wanax was to oversee the distribution of scented oil from the palace storerooms to the divinities and to himself (Fr 1215.1, 12220.2, 1235.1) (Palaima 1995a:131, 134). Perfumed oil was given to Poseidon (Fr 343, 1219) and also to the goddess Potnia (Fr 1231, 1235) (Shelmerdine 1985:124); these were probably the two most important gods in the Pylian cosmology (Palaima 1995a:134). The wanax was the only official to receive perfume as an offering (Fr 1235; Palaima 1995a:134), although he was not the only nondeity to receive the substance, since some servants were also issued perfume (Un 219) (Bendall 2007:258–249; Shelmerdine 2007:44). It is plausible, given the palatial nature of Linear B and the listing of religious personnel and "temple servants" in the tablets (Bendall 2007:59–60, 66–70, 101) that these servants were in some way connected to either the wanax or the deities. The connection between perfume, the wanax, and the local divinities (Palaima 1995a:131–133) places perfume in a distinctly privileged and prestigious position in the Pylian world and creates referential associations between them.

Perfumed oil was not only given to the gods but also used as a dedication in festivals at Pylos (Fr 433, 1217, 1222) (Bendall 2002; Shelmerdine 1985:124). These dedications were made by the palace and, therefore, created a strong association between the gods, the palace, the palace personnel, and the scent of perfume. The adjective *Potnian* (Un 249), referring to the most prominent female deity in the Linear B, was used to describe a perfumer and the perfume intended for the goddess (Lupack 2007:56; Shelmerdine 1985:20). Such epithets connect the production of perfume to the goddess and highlight its elevated status in Pylian society.

Perfumed oil was also used as an ointment for cloths, possibly of the goddess (Fr 1225). Based on the Homeric reference to youths' cloaks gleaming with oil (*Iliad* 18.595–596) and the Linear B record of oil being given to the goddess for chitons, Shelmerdine (1985:124) suggests that putting oil on cloth was a Mycenaean practice. The idea of applying oil to cloth supports the interpretation that the oil that fell into Room 38 was used in textile production.

The issuance of perfume to the gods and to the wanax, its distribution by the wanax, and its use during festivals creates an olfactory association between the gods, the palace, the wanax, and the perfume. Those experiencing the palatial perfume by any degree of participation in or familiarity with these events would make the association between the wanax, the divinities, and the fragrance. The intended limited access to palatial perfumed oils at Pylos accentuates the correlation of scent, power, and religion in the Bronze Age world.

## Pylian Perfume and Feasts

Feasts further create and ramify the sensory connection between perfumed oil and power at Pylos. Recent investigations have identified extensive evidence of frequent large-scale feasts at the palace, demonstrating that food and feasting played significant roles in the creation of group identity and political hierarchy (see Hitchcock et al. 2007; Wright, ed. 2004) and that the Pylians were interested and invested in evoking the more immediate senses of smell and taste. Feasts in the Pylian kingdom were a primary strategy for social cohesion (Palaima 2004:112; Shelmerdine 1998; Wright 2004a, 2004b), linking religion, the wanax, and the palace (Shelmerdine 1998).

The feasts varied in size and function; the smaller ones were private, while the public ones were large enough to feed several thousand people (Stocker and Davis 2004:72). Nakassis (2010), in an estimation of the food and numbers from the Linear B tablets, concludes that the largest feasts could feed 10,000–15,000 people, which according to the population estimates by Whitelaw (2001) would have constituted approximately one-third of the population of Messenia. Several scholars have recently argued that the feasts were tiered, with different groups in the hierarchy feasting at the same time but in different parts of the palace (Bendall 2004; Stocker and Davis 2004:71); Bendall (2004) places the most elite participants in Hall 6, the megaron; the second tier in Hall 65; more general groups in Courts 63 and 88; and the lowest tier in Court 58, in front of the palace. Fox (2008) concurs that Halls 6 and 65 are more private, while the courtyard locations are more public.

Food echoed the social hierarchy that was laid out by the spatial separation of the groups at the feast. Goody's (1982) work on cuisine suggests that in societies that have a strict social hierarchy we should expect to have an haute cuisine for the upper class and a lower, more ordinary type of cuisine for the lower classes. Based on her study of the palatial ceramics at Pylos, Hruby (2008) argues that such a distinct haute cuisine—consisting of a flatbread, grilled meats, and sauces—existed. The smell of the food, both during its preparation and consumption, would have been a prominent factor in the experience of the feast. Fox (2008) comments on the potentially strong smell of herbs and spices—such as cumin, cardamom, and sesame—included in these haute cuisine dishes. She points out that the smell of this food would have been an integral part of the feasting experience and would also have created a sensory boundary between those who could only smell these elaborate dishes and those privileged to eat them (Fox 2008:136). Such restricted access to certain types of food is a common practice among diverse groups to reinforce group division and solidarity among the subgroups (see Marquardt 1987:98).

Perfumed oil and unguents also played a prominent role in these feasts. Bendall (2002:260) argues that at least 86 percent of the Fr tablets refer to perfumed oils in religious contexts and several of these are feasting activities. Bendall (2007:260) also notes that unguents are only recorded in relation to feasts on the Pylos tablets. It is not clear how perfumed oil was used at the feasts. Fappas (2008:369–373) suggests that the Mycenaean use of the perfumed oil may have been similar to that in the contemporary Near East or Egypt. In accounts from the Near East, perfumed oil was used to anoint kings, priests, and priestesses after a feast, while according to Egyptian records, everyone at the feast had oil on their heads. Egyptian perfume in the form of an unguent was previously thought to have melted and flowed down the head of the feaster (Fappas 2008:373; Manniche 1999), although recent work suggests that the cones, which are depicted on the heads of elite Egyptians at feasts, were only symbolic of the perfumed fat or even of odor itself (Meskell and Joyce 2003:56). A song from Egypt celebrated the use of perfume: "Put anitu resin on your head . . . anoint yourself with the true wonders of the divine offering" (Fappas 2008:373; Manniche 1999:7). Fappas further explains the wool on tablet Un 853 from Pylos (which concerns a feast and perfumed oil) as an aspergillum, comparing its use to the Hittite practice of using wool soaked in perfumed oil to sprinkle the scent around in order to attract the deities.

Regardless of how perfumes were used at Pylian feasts, if they were distributed to the elite participants in Rooms 6 and 65 as I suggest, their fragrance would have wafted through the palace to all participants (see Figure 12-4). However, the farther one moved from the upper tiers of diners, the weaker the odor would have been. Fox (2008:136) has argued that the perfumed oil used at feasts would have communicated the stages of the ritual to those not within sight of the most elite areas. However, like the smell of the haute cuisine dishes, the perfume would also have acted as a participatory sensory boundary reinforcing the exclusion of some participants from aspects of the feast. The quantities of perfume for consumption at the feasts as recorded in Linear B tablets (Un 6, Un 718, Un 853, Un 1177), while insufficient for distribution to all the estimated participants, were nevertheless prodigious (approximately 24 L) and would therefore have created a very strong odor; even though it was diluted as it wafted through the palace, it would have had an effect on those participants who were not privileged to consume it directly with their meal.

Most archaeologists understand commensal acts as events that create a connection between the participants. Seremetakis (1994:57) particularly emphasizes the senses in the creation of this shared experience, of emotional responses to it, and of encoded memories of it, defining *commensality* as " the exchange of sensory memories and emotions, and of substances and objects incarnating remembrance and feeling." Feasting at Pylos was not a de-sensified commensal event but rather encompassed a multisensory experience in which the food and smells of the feast imprinted themselves on the memory of the individuals present, regardless of their level of participation. From the prominence of perfume at the feast, along with frescoes, elaborate clothing, and valuable objects and furniture, it is clear that food consumption was not the only sensory element of commensality.

## Pylian Perfume and Wealth Finance

The economic system at Pylos has recently been described as a wealth-finance economy in which gift exchange and the creation of networks were powerful social strategies for negotiating positions in society (Galaty and Parkinson 2007). The power of the wanax, who was head of the wealth-finance economy, was unstable; it rested mainly on controlling the circulation of elite commodities as part of an exclusionary strategy within a network of social relationships established outside the local group (Blanton et al. 1996; Galaty 1999; Galaty and Parkinson 2007; Wright 2004a). Within these networks, access to and consumption of prestige commodities set the elite members of society apart from other groups in the populace. Perfume was clearly a politically charged commodity of this type because of its production at the palace and its association with the wanax and with deities (Brumfield and Earle 1987:5; Stein 1994:14).

Although the gifts given to people visiting the palace are not listed on the Linear B tablets, it is plausible to envision that perfume was given at feasts, based on the reference to special oil "for the guests" (*ke-se-ni-wi-jo*; Fr 1231) (Bendall 2007:101; Shelmerdine 1985:79–80, 2007:44). It is, moreover, easily transportable. Gifts given at palatial feasts would have created relationships of reciprocity and obligation among the social elite. Perfume would have been a compelling gift because it interacts with nonvisual senses; smell is particularly mnemonic and emotionally evocative. Perfume could thus viscerally reinforce the position of power; as a gift it would have been a continuing olfactory reminder of the relationship.

It is possible that Pylos also traded some of its perfume across the wider Mediterranean world. Estimates of the quantity of oil produced at Pylos in comparison to that used in the palace suggest that surplus oil, of which some may have been perfumed, would have been available for trade (Shelmerdine 1985:152). Nevertheless, none of the abundant stirrup jars, which probably held perfume, found in large numbers outside the Aegean world, have been shown by petrographic analysis to come from Pylos (Galaty 2009:3). If Pylos was trading its oil and perfume, therefore, it was doing so indirectly, on an interregional basis or in bulk to merchants who repackaged it.

## Conclusion

Although one can clearly distinguish wealthier people by their clothes and jewelry, this visual experience is a relatively passive one for the viewer. In contrast, perfume is an immediate experience of another individual's wealth; the fumes of an expensive perfume are inhaled and this action brings the inhaler into direct and immediate contact with the unattainable substance and with the marker of affluence. This sensory manipulation through scent enforces the power hierarchy in the most intimate way; one inhales the scent that activates the limbic system and creates powerful memories and associations. Perfume does not communicate wealth and status purely symbolically but provokes physical and emotional reactions in the inhaler, a fact that has been confirmed by biological and anthropological studies. Through association with the scent, the wanax, deities, and other members of the elite class at Pylos all exuded the same message—power and status.

The Linear B tablets and the material remains at Pylos examined in this study demonstrate that the social impact of smell, which is a biological inevitability, was also culturally manipulated through the production of perfume at the palace, its dissemination by the wanax, and its distribution to the wanax and deities. This palatial control and selective distribution of perfume show an awareness of the social potential of the senses and a conscious attempt to evoke sensory reactions among the populace. Perfume was also associated with feasts at the palace, where it was probably issued as a gift to certain guests; at such ceremonies, which reinforce the creation of identities, perfume would have been a sensory continuation of the exclusion of some participants. It is impossible to avoid inhaling, identifying, and reacting to scents as they unravel in the direct connection between the nose and the brain; the unavoidable experience of inhaling perfume at Pylos would thus have manipulated the senses to create and reinforce identity and differential status, so that perfume can be understood as a sensory metaphor for the relationship with the palace elite.

## Acknowledgments

I would like to thank Jo Day for producing a stimulating conference and the participants of the conference for lively discussion. I also thank The Classics Department of the University of Cincinnati for permission to publish the images in this paper. I am grateful to Jack L. Davis, Carol Hersehenson, and Ruth Palmer for their comments on the text and to the UNCG Agraphia group, especially Cheryl Logan, for stimulating ideas and references for this paper.

## References

Alaoui-Ismaïli, Ouafe, O. Robin, H. Rada, André Dittmar, and Evelyne Vernet-Maury
1997 Basic Emotions Evoked by Odorants: Comparison between Autonomic Responses and Self-Evaluation. *Physiological Behavior* 62:713–720.

Almagor, Uri
1990 Odors and Private Language: Observations on the Phenomenology of Scent. *Human Studies* 13:253–274.

Baudrillard, Jean
1983 *Simulations.* MIT Press, Cambridge, Massachusetts.

Beck, Lily Y., and Curt W. Beck
1978 Wi-ri-za Wool on Linear B Tablets of Perfume Ingredients. *American Journal of Archaeology* 82:213–215.

Bendall, Lisa Marie
2002 A Time for Offerings: Dedication of Perfumed Oil at Pylian Festivals. In *A-NA-QO-TA: Studies Presented to J. T. Killen*, Minos 33–34, edited by John Bennet and Jan Driessen, pp. 1–9. University of Salamanca Press, Salamanca.
2004 Fit for a King? Hierarchy, Exclusion, Aspiration, and Desire in the Social Structure of Mycenaean Banqueting. In *Food, Cuisine, and Society in Prehistoric Greece,* edited by Paul Halstead and John C. Barrett, pp. 105–135. Sheffield Academic, Sheffield.
2007 *Economics of Religion in the Mycenaean World, Resources Dedicated to Religion in the Mycenaean Palace Economy.* Oxford University School of Archaeology, Oxford.

Blanton, Richard E., Gary M. Feinman, Stephen A. Kowalewski, and Peter N. Peregrine
1996 A Dual-Processual Theory for the Evolution of Mesoamerican Civilization. *Current Anthropology* 37:1–14.

Blegen, Carl W., and Marion Rawson
1966 *The Palace of Nestor at Pylos in Western Messenia,* Vol. 1, Pt. 1 and 2, *The Buildings and Their Contents.* University of Cincinnati and Princeton Univeristy Press, Princeton, New Jersey.
Brumfield, Elizabeth M.
1992 Distinguished Lecture in Archaeology: Breaking and Entering the Ecosystem—Gender, Class, and Faction Steal the Show. *American Anthropologist* 94:551–567.
Brumfield, Elizabeth M., and Timothy Earle
1987 Specialization, Exchange, and Complex Societies: An Introduction. In *Specialization, Exchange, and Complex Societies,* edited by Elizabeth M. Brumfield and Timothy Earle, pp. 1–9. Cambridge University Press, Cambridge.
Carrithers, Michael, Steven Collins, and Steven Lukes (editors)
1985 *The Category of the Person: Anthropology, Philosophy, History.* Cambridge University Press, Cambridge.
Chadwick, John,
1976 *The Mycenaean World.* Cambridge University Press, Cambridge.
Classen, Constance
1993 *Worlds of Sense: Exploring the Senses in History and across Cultures.* Routledge, London.
Classen, Constance, and Davis Howes
2006 The Museum as Sensescape: Western Sensibilities and Indigenous Artefacts. In *Sensible Objects: Colonialism, Museums, and Material Culture* edited by Elizabeth Edwards, Chris Gosden, and Ruth B. Phillips, pp. 199–222. Berg, Oxford.
Classen, Constance, David Howes, and Anthony Synnott
1994 *Aroma: The Cultural History of Smell.* Routledge, London.
Corbin, Alain
1986 *The Foul and the Fragrant: Odor and the French Social Imagination.* Harvard University Press, Cambridge.
Davis, Jack L., Susan Alcock, John Bennet, Yannis Lolos, and Cynthia W. Shelmerdine
1997 The Pylos Regional Archaeological Project, Part 1: Overview and the Archaeological Survey. *Hesperia* 66:391–494.
Descartes, René
1995 *A Discourse on Method: Meditations and Principles of Philosophy.* Translated by John Veitch. Everyman, London.
Edwards, Elizabeth, Chris Gosden, and Ruth Philips
2006 *Sensible Objects, Colonialism, Museums, and Material Culture.* Berg, Oxford.
Engen, Trygg
1982 *The Perception of Odor.* Addison-Wesley, Reading, Massachusetts.
1991 *Odor Sensation and Memory.* Praeger, New York.
Fappas, Ioannis
2008 The Use of Perfumed Oils during Feasting Activities: A Comparison of Mycenaean and Near Eastern Written Sources. In *DAIS: The Aegean Feast,* edited by Louise A. Hitchcock, Robert Laffineur, and Janice Crowley, pp. 367–377. Aegaeum 29. Université de Liège, Liège.
Foster, Ellen D.
1977 An Administrative Department at Knossos Concerned with Perfumery and Offerings. *Minos* 16:19–51.
Fox, Rachel
2008 Tastes, Smells, and Spaces: Sensory Perceptions and Mycenaean Palatial Feasting.

In *DAIS: The Aegean Feast,* edited by Louise A. Hitchcock, Robert Laffineur, and Janice Crowley, pp. 133–141. Aegaeum 29. Université de Liège, Liège.

Galaty, Michael L.

1999 Wealth Ceramics, Staple Ceramics: Pots and the Mycenaean Palaces. In *Rethinking Mycenaean Palaces: New Interpretations of an Old Idea,* edited by Michael L. Galaty and William A. Parkinson, pp. 49–59. Cotsen Institute of Archaeology at UCLA, Los Angeles.

2009 Review of *Reading Economics of Religion in the Mycenaean World: Resources Dedicated to Religion in the Mycenaean Palace Economy,* by Lisa Bendall. *American Journal of Archaeology*. Electronic document, http://www.ajaonline.org/pdfs/book_reviews/113.2/10_Galaty.pdf, accessed June 11, 2010.

Galaty, Michael L., and William A. Parkinson

2007 Introduction: Mycenaean Palaces Rethought. In *Rethinking Mycenaean Palaces: New Interpretations of an Old Idea II,* edited by Michael L. Galaty and William A. Parkinson, pp. 1–17. Cotsen Institute of Archaeology, Los Angeles.

Gell, Alfred

1995 The Language of the Forest: Landscape and Phonological Iconism in Umeda. In *The Anthropology of Landscape: Perspectives on Place and Space,* edited by Eric Hirsch and Michael O' Hanlon, pp. 232–254. Oxford University Press, Oxford.

Goody, Jack

1982 *Cooking, Cuisine, and Class*. Cambridge University Press, Cambridge.

Herz, Rachel S., and Gerald C. Cupchik

1992 An Experimental Characterization of Odor-Evoked Memories in Humans. *Chemical Senses* 17:519–528.

1995 The Emotional Distinctiveness of Odor-Evoked Memories. *Chemical Senses* 20:517–528.

Hitchcock, Louise A., Robert Laffineur, and Janice Crowley (editors)

2007 *DAIS: The Aegean Feast.* Aegaeum 29. Université de Liège, Liège.

Hodder, Ian

1995 Material Culture in Time. In *Interpreting Archaeology: Finding Meaning in the Past,* edited by Ian Hodder, Michael Shanks, Alexandra Alexandri, Victor Buchli, John Carman, Jonathan Last, and Gavin Lucas, pp. 164–168. Routledge, London.

Hodder, Ian, Michael Shanks, Alexndra Alexandri, Victor Buchli, John Carman, Jonathan Last, and Gavin Lucas (editors)

1995 *Interpreting Archaeology: Finding Meaning in the Past*. Routledge, London.

Holley, André

2002 Cognitive Aspects of Olfaction in Perfumer Practice. In *Olfaction, Taste, and Cognition,* edited by Catherine Rouby, Benosit Schaal, Danièle Dubois, Rémi Gervias, André Holley, pp. 16–26. Cambridge University Press, Cambridge.

Hooker, John T.

1979 The Wanax in Linear B Texts. *Kadmos* 18:100–111.

Howes, David

1991 Olfaction and Transition. In *Varieties of Sensory Experiences: A Sourcebook in the Anthropology of the Senses,* edited by David Howes, pp. 128–147. University of Toronto Press, Toronto.

2002 Nose-Wise: Olfactory Metaphors in Mind. In *Perfumery in Olfaction, Taste, and Cognition,* edited by Catherine Rouby, Benosit Schaal, Danièle Dubois, Rémi Gervias, André Holley, pp. 67–81. Cambridge University Press. Cambridge.

2003 *Sensual Relations: Engaging the Senses in Culture and Social Theory*. University of Michigan Press, Ann Arbor.

2006 Scent, Sound, and Synaethesia; Intersensoriality and Material Culture. In *The Handbook of Material Culture*, edited by Christopher Tilley, Webb Keane, Susanne Küchler, Mike Rowlands, and Patricia Spyer, pp. 161–172. Sage, London.

Howes, David (editor)

1991 *Varieties of Sensory Experiences: A Sourcebook in the Anthropology of the Senses*. University of Toronto Press, Toronto.

Howes, David, and Constance Classen

1991 Sounding Sensory Profiles. In *Varieties of Sensory Experiences: A Sourcebook in the Anthropology of the Senses*, edited by David Howes, pp. 257–288. University of Toronto Press, Toronto.

Hruby, Julie

2008 You Are How You Eat: Mycenaean Class and Cuisine. In *DAIS: The Aegean Feast*, edited by Louise A. Hitchcock, Robert Laffineur, and Janice Crowley, pp. 151–158. Aegaeum 29. Université de Liège, Liège.

Hurcombe, Linda

2007 A Sense of Materials and Sensory Perception in Concepts of Materiality. *World Archaeology* 39:532–545.

Ingold, Timothy

2000 *The Perception of the Environment*. Routledge, London.

Jones-Gotman, Marilyn, and Robert J. Zatorre

1993 Odor Recognition Memory in Humans: Role of Right Temporal and Orbitofrontal Regions. *Brain and Cognition* 22:182–198.

Kilian, Klaus

1988 The Emergence of Wanax Ideology in the Mycenaean Palaces. *Oxford Journal of Archaeology* 7:291–302.

Killen, John

1992 Observation on the Theban Seals. In *Mykenaïka: Actes du IXe Colloque international sur les textes mycéniens et égéens [BCH Supplement* 25], edited by Jean-Paul Olivier, pp. 367–370. Paris.

1995 Some Further Thoughts on "Collectors." In *Politeia: Society and State in the Aegean Bronze Age*, edited by Robert Laffineur and Wolf-Dietrich Niemeier, pp. 213–224. Aegaeum 12. Université de Liège, Liège.

2007 Critique: A View from the Tablets. In *Rethinking Mycenaean Palaces II*. Rev. 2nd ed., edited by Michael L. Galaty and William A. Parkinson, pp. 114–117. Cotsen Institute of Archaeology, Los Angeles.

Lang, Mabel L.

1969 *The Palace of Nestor at Pylos in Western Messenia II: The Frescoes*. Princeton University Press, Princeton.

Li, Wen, Isabel Moallem, Ken A. Paller, and Jay A. Gottfried

2007 Subliminal Smells Can Guide Social Preferences. *Psychological Science* 18:1044–1049.

Lledo, Pierre-Marie, Gilles Gheusi, and Jean-Didier Vincent

2005 Information Processing in the Mammalian Olfactory System: From Odorants to Smell. *Physiological Review* 85:281–317.

Lupack, Susan

2007 Palaces, Sanctuaries, and Workshops: The Role of the Religious Sector in Mycenaean Economics, In *Rethinking Mycenaean Palaces II*. Rev. 2nd ed., edited by Michael L. Galaty and William A. Parkinson, pp. 54–65. Cotsen Institute of Archaeology, Los Angeles.

McCallum, Lucinda R.

1987 Decorative Program in the Mycenaean Palace of Pylos: The Megaron Frescoes. Unpublished Ph.D. dissertation, Department of the History of Art, University of Pennsylvania, Philadelphia.

Manniche, Lisa

1999 *Sacred Luxuries: Fragrance, Aromatherapy, and Cosmetics in Ancient Egypt*. Cornell University Press, Ithaca, New York.

Marquardt, William H.

1987 The Calusa Social Formation in Protohistoric South Florida. In *Power Relations and State Formation*, edited by Thomas C. Patterson and Christine W. Gailey, pp. 98–116. American Anthropological Association, Washington, D.C.

Merleau-Ponty, Maurice

1962 *Phenomenology of Perception*. Translated by Colin Smith. Routledge & Kegan Paul, London.

Meskell, Lynn M., and Rosemary A. Joyce

2003 *Embodied Lives: Figuring Ancient Maya and Egyptian Experience*. Routledge, London.

Morris, Charles G., and Albert A. Maisto

2001 *Psychology: An Introduction*, 11th ed. Prentice Hall, New Jersey.

Nakassis, Dimitri

2010 Reevaluating Staple and Wealth Finance at Mycenaean Pylos. In *Political Economies in Bronze Age Greece: Papers from the Langford Conference, Florida State University, Tallahassee, 22–24 February 2007*, edited by Daniel Pullen, pp. 127–148. Oxbow Books, Oxford.

Palaima, Thomas G.

1995a The Nature of the Mycenaean Wanax: Non–Indo-European Origins and Priestly Functions. In *The Role of the Ruler in the Prehistoric Aegean*, edited by Paul Rehak, pp. 119–142. Aegaeum 11. Université de Liège, Liège.

1995b The Last Days of the Pylos Polity. In *Politeia: Society and State in the Aegean Bronze Age*, edited by Robert Laffineur and Wolf-Dietrich Niemeier, pp. 623–633. Aegaeum 12. Université de Liège, Liège.

2004 Sacrificial Feasting in the Linear B Documents. In *The Mycenaean Feast*, edited by James C. Wright, pp. 97–126. American School of Classical Studies at Athens, Princeton, New Jersey.

Palaima, Thomas G., and Cynthia W. Shelmerdine

1984 Mycenaean Archaeology and the Pylos Texts. *Cambridge Archaeological Review* 3(2):76–89.

Palmer, Leonard R.

1963 *The Interpretation of Mycenaean Greek Texts*. Clarendon Press, Oxford.

Palmer, Ruth

1999 Perishable Goods in Mycenaean Texts. In *Floreant Studia Mycenaea*, edited by Sigrid Deger-Jalkotzy, Stefan Hiller, Oswald Panagl, Georg Nightingale, and Thomas Lindner, pp. 463–485. Austrian Academy of Sciences Press, Vienna.

2003 Trade in Wine, Perfumed Oil, and Foodstuffs: The Linear B Evidence and Beyond. In *ΠΛΟΕΣ. Sea Routes. Interconnections in the Mediterranean 16th–6th c. BC*, edited by Nicholas Stampolidis and Vassos Karageorghis, pp.125–140. Proceedings of the International Symposium held at Rethymnon, Crete September 29–October 2, 2002. University of Crete and the A. G. Leventis Foundation, Athens.

Porteous, J. Douglas
2006 Smellscape. In *The Smell Culture Reader*, edited by Jim Drobnick, pp. 89–106. Berg, Oxford.
Proust, Marcel
1927 *À la recherche du temps perdu*. Grasset and Gallimard, Paris.
Rabin, Michael D., and William S. Cain
1984 Odor Recognition: Familiarity, Identifiability, and Encoding Consistency. *Journal of Experimental Psychology: Learning, Memory, and Cognition* 10:316–325.
Ritchie, Ian
1991 Fusion of the Faculties: A Study of the Language of the Senses in Hausaland. In *Varieties of Sensory Experiences: A Sourcebook in the Anthropology of the Senses*, edited by David Howes, pp. 192–202. University of Toronto Press, Toronto.
Rodaway, Paul
1994 *Sensuous Geographies: Body, Sense, and Place*. Routledge, New York.
Royet, Jean P., David Zald, Rémy Versace, Nicolas Costes, Frank Lavenne, Olivier Koenig, and Rémi Gervais
2000 Emotional Responses to Pleasant and Unpleasant Olfactory, Visual, and Auditory Stimuli: A Positron Emission Tomography Study. *Journal of Neuroscience* 20:7752–7759.
Scarre, Chris, and Graeme Lawson (editors)
2006 *Archaeoacoustics*. McDonald Institute for Archaeological Research, Cambridge.
Schon, Robert
2007 Chariots, Industry, and Elite Power at Pylos. In *Rethinking Mycenaean Palaces II*. Rev. 2nd ed., edited by Michael L. Galaty and William A. Parkinson, pp. 133–145. Cotsen Institute of Archaeology, Los Angeles.
Seremetakis, C. Nadia
1994 Memory of the Senses, Part II: Still Acts. In *The Senses Still*, edited by C. Nadia Seremetakis, pp. 23–44. Westview Press, Oxford.
Shank, Elizabeth
2008 Decorated Dining Halls. In *DAIS: The Aegean Feast*, edited by Louise A. Hitchcock, Robert Laffineur, and Janice Crowley, pp. 97–104. Aegaeum 29. Université de Liège, Liège.
Shelmerdine, Cynthia W.
1985 *The Perfume Industry of Mycenaean Pylos*. Åströms Förlag, Göteborg.
1998 Where Do We Go from Here? And How Can the Linear B Tablets Help Us Get There? In *The Aegean and the Orient in the Second Millennium*, edited by Eric H. Cline and Diane Harris-Cline, pp. 291–298. Aegaeum 18. Université de Liège, Liège.
2007 Administration in the Mycenaean Palaces: Where's the Chief? In *Rethinking Mycenaean Palaces II*. Rev. 2nd ed., edited by Michael L. Galaty and William A. Parkinson, pp. 40–46. Cotsen Institute of Archaeology, Los Angeles.
Stein, Gil
1994 Introduction Part II: The Organizational Dynamics of Complexity in Greater Mesopotamia. In *Chiefdoms and Early States in the Near East: The Organizational Dynamics of Complexity*, edited by Gil Stein and Mitchell Rothman, pp. 11–22. Prehistory Press, Madison.
Stocker, Sharon R., and Jack L. Davis
2004 Animal Sacrifice, Archives, and Feasting at the Palace of Nestor. In *The Mycenaean Feast*, edited by James C. Wright, pp. 59–75. American School of Classical Studies at Athens, Princeton, New Jersey.

Watson, Aaron

2006 (Un)intentional Sound? Acoustic and Neolithic Monuments. In *Archaeoacoustics*, edited by Chris Scarre and Graeme Lawson, pp. 11–22. McDonald Institute for Archaeological Research, Cambridge.

Whitelaw, Todd

2001 Reading between the Tablets: Assessing Mycenaean Palatial Involvement in Ceramic Production and Consumption. In *Economy and Politics in the Mycenaean Palace States, Proceedings of a Conference held on 1–3 July 1999 in the Faculty of Classics, Cambridge*, edited by Sophia Voutsaki and John T. Killen, pp. 51–79. Cambridge Philological Society Supplementary Vol. 27. Cambridge Philological Society, Cambridge.

Wilson, Jennifer

2008 What Were the Women Doing While the Men Were Eating and Drinking? The Evidence of the Frescoes. In *DAIS: The Aegean Feast*, edited by Louise A. Hitchcock, Robert Laffineur, and Janice Crowley, pp. 23–28. Aegaeum 29. Université de Liège, Liège.

Wright, James C.

2004a A Survey of Evidence for Feasting in Mycenaean Society. In *The Mycenaean Feast*, edited by James C. Wright, pp. 13–58. American School of Classical Studies at Athens, Princeton, New Jersey.

2004b The Emergence of Leadership and the Rise of Civilization in the Aegean. In *The Emergence of Civilization Revisited*, edited by John Barrett and Paul Halstead, pp. 64–89. Oxbow Books, Oxford.

Wright, James C. (editor)

2004 *The Mycenaean Feast*. American School of Classical Studies at Athens, Princeton, New Jersey.

Zald, David H., and José V. Pardo

1997 Emotion, Olfaction, and the Human Amygdala: Amygdala Activation during Aversive Olfactory Stimulation. *Proceedings of the National Academy of Sciences of the United States of America*, 94:4119–4124.

# 13. A Whiff of Mortality: The Smells of Death in Roman and Byzantine Beth She'an-Scythopolis

*Emerson Avery*

*Abstract:* Roman tombs were occupied by the dead but experienced by the living. In this paper, I draw on evidence from the Roman and Byzantine chamber tombs of the Northern Cemetery at Beth She'an-Scythopolis to explore the sensory experience of Roman mortuary space. An examination of selected tombs and their contents reveals spaces filled with darkness but redolent with the smell of offered food, the perfume of scented oil, and the fetor of decay. The selective engagement of visitors' senses, as well as the particular range of stimuli provided to each, served to render the tomb a liminal space between the living and the dead, existing outside quotidian experience but eminently sensible to those whose duties brought them there.

The study of Roman mortuary practices in the provinces of Palestine (Figure 13-1) has a long history. At least since the beginning of the twentieth century, when Macalister (1912) uncovered the cemetery at Gezer, the excavation of Roman graves in modern Israel and Palestine has continued practically uninterrupted. So, too, has been publication in a variety of journals and monographs, the result of which is a corpus of archaeological knowledge that is, in some respects at least, fairly comprehensive.

In other respects, however, it leaves something to be desired. Due to the lingering influence of the discipline's early, culture-historical emphasis on the construction of typologies, there remains a powerful interest in classification for its own sake: of material culture, of funerary space, and of mortuary practice (e.g., Avni et al. 2008; Oren and Rappaport 1984; Waterhouse 1998). Alongside such

*Making Senses of the Past: Toward a Sensory Archaeology*, edited by Jo Day. Center for Archaeological Investigations, Occasional Paper No. 40.  ISBN 978-0-8093-3287-8.

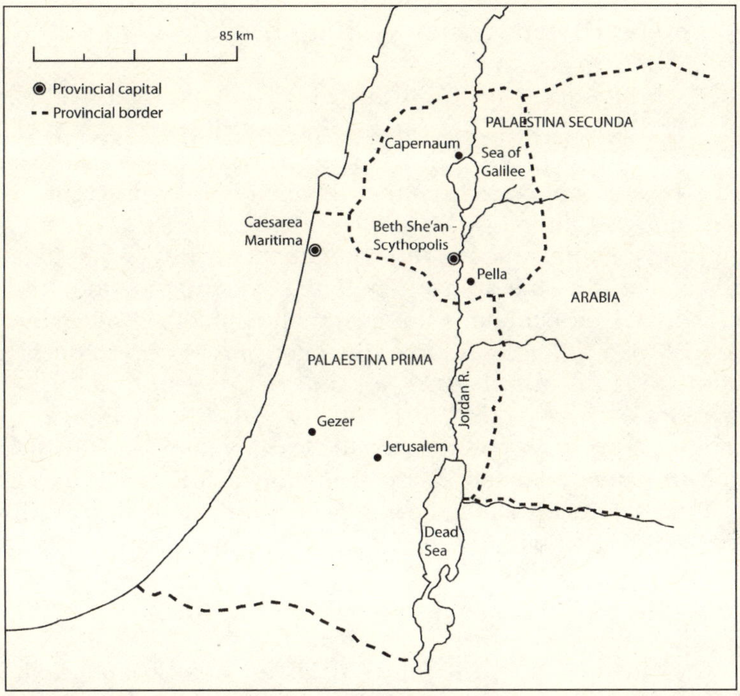


**Figure 13-1.** *Late Roman Palestine, with sites mentioned in the text. (Map by Emerson Avery.)*

studies are others purporting to explore the eschatological import of the practices thus inventoried or the religious identity of the people under study (e.g., Avni et al. 2008; Samellas 2002). Both are obviously important, especially during the several centuries of Roman sovereignty in Palestine. The first six hundred years of the Common Era were a period of remarkable religious diversity, and the dynamic relationships among Roman polytheists, Jews, and Christians are of obvious historical importance. But such studies do not always address the fundamentally *human* character of history. When religious demography is at issue, both the living and the dead are interesting to scholars primarily for their value as representatives of different faith communities. Their carnal reality is, ironically, immaterial to their use as examples of a social abstraction.

The purpose of this paper is to investigate an embodied human experience of death. The material remains of Roman and Byzantine mortuary practice at Beth She'an-Scythopolis are no more or less concrete than the people who (inter)acted with and through them and whose understanding of the significance of funerary ritual was informed, and powerfully reinforced, by the evidence of their senses. As will be demonstrated here, the selective engagement of the "close" sense of smell and the relative unimportance of sight—as well as the particular range of stimuli with which each of these senses was confronted—served to distinguish the tomb and its immediate environs from quotidian space, making it a fitting place for the transition between life and death.

## The Northern Cemetery, Beth She'an

The urban cemetery of Beth She'an-Scythopolis (Figure 13-2), by the beginning of the fifth century C.E. the capital of the Byzantine province of Palaestina Secunda (Tsafrir and Foerster 1997:86, Note 2), was discovered in the early twentieth century by archaeologists from the University of Pennsylvania Museum of Archaeology and Anthropology. Beginning in 1922, a series of four campaigns of excavation were completed there, ultimately documenting more than two hundred tombs dating from the Bronze Age to the Byzantine period. And while information about the earlier tombs was eventually published, albeit by a different hand (Oren 1973), a full accounting of the later graves never appeared. Gerald Fitzgerald's typescript *Excavations in the Northern Cemetery Area, 1922–1931* (University Museum Archive [UMA], 1944), its margins filled with notes in the author's hand but never incorporated into the text, remains in the University Museum to the present day. So, too, do the field diaries, registers, and other records of the dig. The analysis presented here derives from an ongoing restudy of these materials in conjunction with the artifacts retained by the University Museum.

### *The Cemetery and the Tombs*

Broadly speaking, the tombs datable to the Roman and Byzantine periods—that is, the first century B.C.E. through the seventh century C.E. (Magness 1993:11–12; Rowe 1930; Tsafrir and Foerster 1997)—are chamber tombs with a central room from which radiate a variable number of spaces for burial. I have selected a group of eleven such to discuss at greater length. What fraction of the total Roman and Byzantine tombs this sample represents is difficult to tell, since a substantial number of the spaces numbered as tombs cannot conclusively be shown to have served as such. It is, in any event, almost certainly a sample comprising the tombs of the wealthy. Among the many empty cist graves discovered in the Northern Cemetery are surely some from this paper's period of interest, but as most were empty when excavated, it is impossible to date them. Insofar as this paper succeeds in suggesting the contours of a living experience of the space of the dead, it is an experience that was particular to people of a certain status.

Tombs 205, 206, 210, 224, 239, 248, and 260 all belong to Fitzgerald's Class G, or *loculus* tombs (Figure 13-3), which he characterizes as "having small burial places (*loculi*) opening out of a rectangular central chamber" (UMA, *Excavations* 1944). These spaces are oriented perpendicular to the walls of the central room. Tombs 201, 207, and 225, on the other hand, belong to his Class J, *arcosolium* tombs (Figure 13-4), which have arched burial recesses parallel to the walls of the central chamber. Tombs 208a and 208b, so numbered by the excavators to reflect a belated realization that what they had originally thought to be a single tomb was, in fact, two tombs (UMA, 1926 Field Diary [FD], September 22 entry), are also of the arcosolium type. The chronology of these two basic tomb types has been much discussed, particularly with respect to the primacy of one or the other (Avni et al. 2008:107; Hachlili and Killebrew 1999:57–59; Rahmani 1981a, 1981b, 1982a, 1982b;

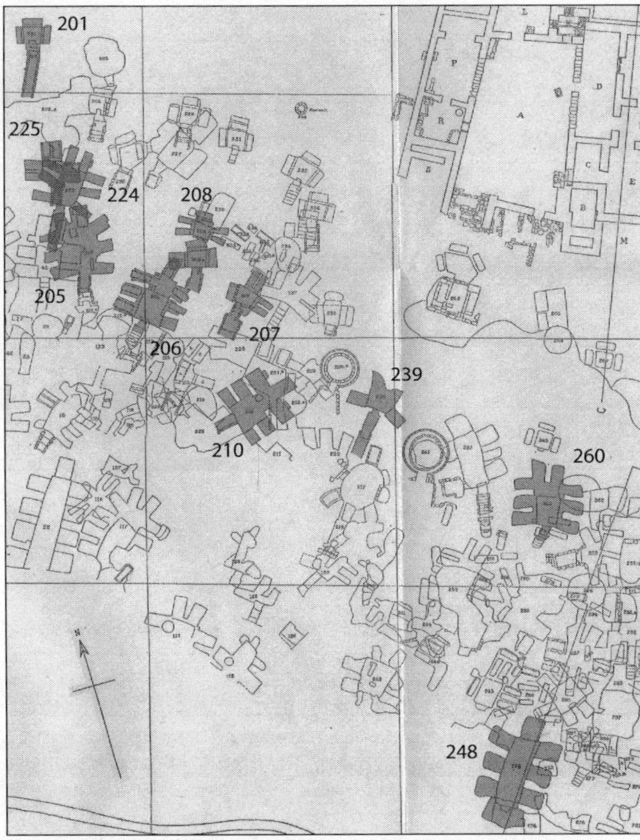


**Figure 13-2.** *Detail of Beth She'an Northern Cemetery, with tombs mentioned in text shaded in grey. (Courtesy of the Penn Museum.)*

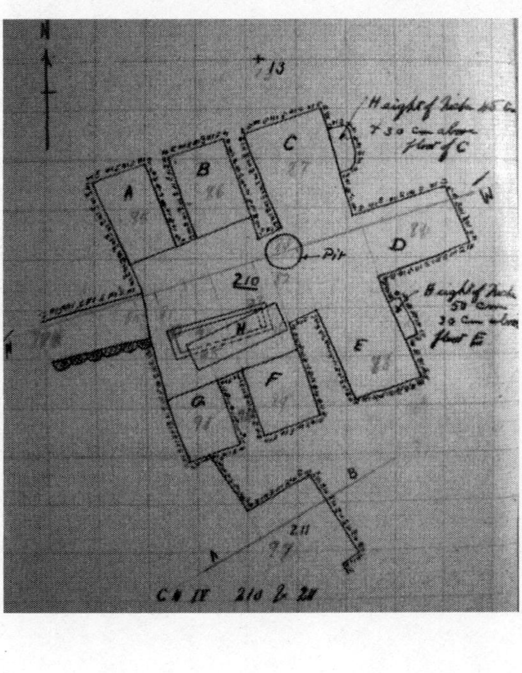


**Figure 13-3.** *Plan, Tomb 210. (Courtesy of the Penn Museum.)*

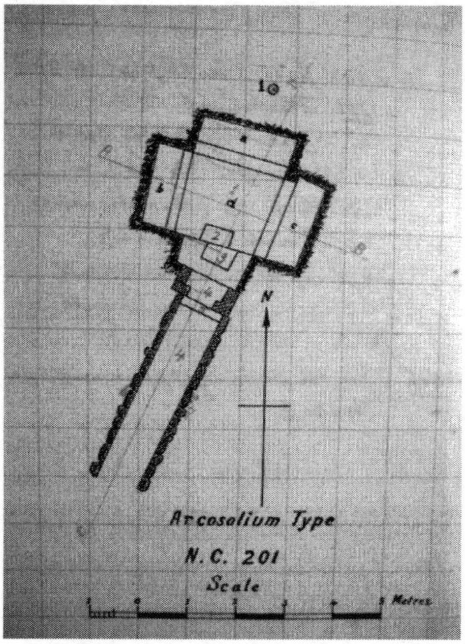


**Figure 13-4.** *Plan, Tomb 201. (Courtesy of the Penn Museum.)*

cf. Avigad 1976; Haddad 2007:74*–75*). In the Late Roman and Byzantine periods, however, both were in regular use in the Galilee (Avni et al. 2008:115–116), and in most respects, such morphological distinction is irrelevant for this discussion.

### *Light and Space*

Far more important is the awareness that each of the spaces under study was both closed and relatively close. The presence of painted decoration in at least some of the tombs—Alan Rowe (1927:43) observed that "[a] certain Christian tomb [231] had crosses in red paint . . . over each grave," and a trough in Tomb 208a was bordered in red (UMA, 1926 FD, September 23 entry)—implies that their interiors were meant to be seen. The discovery of two ceramic mirror plaques, either in Tomb 208a or 208b (the excavators do not specify the findspot more precisely), is similarly suggestive. And inasmuch as both mirrors (Avni and Dahari 1990:310; Rahmani 1964) and painted decoration (cf. Cave 3, Chamber C in the Akeldama tombs [Avni and Greenhut 1996:25–29]) are relatively common in Roman and Byzantine period tombs in Palestine, there are grounds for considering the possibilities of the tomb as a lighted space.

Importantly, however, such possibilities were limited with respect to both light *and* space. The former was only as intense as artificial illumination could procure. Mostly this meant the use of ceramic oil lamps (Figure 13-5), examples of which were found within all the tombs under discussion. The sole exception was Tomb 239, which was incompletely cleared owing to the excavators' fear of its collapse (UMA, 1926 FD, October 31 entry). And while a great many oil

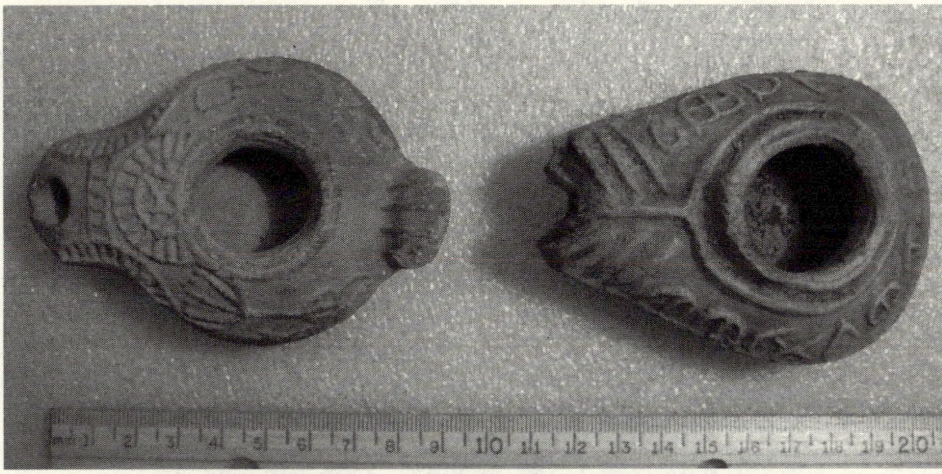

**Figure 13-5.** *Byzantine-period lamps from Tombs 206 (left) and 224 (right). (Photograph © Emerson Avery. Used with permission of University of Pennsylvania Museum of Archaeology and Anthropology.)*

lamps could be brought simultaneously into the tomb (Tomb 210 contained 13, and Tomb 206, at least 9), doing so was insufficient to guarantee the illumination of the space. Instead, it produced a variegated lightscape of shadows shifting in response to both the movement of the lamps and the people who held them (cf. Bille and Sørensen 2007). Different parts of the interior may have been illuminated at different times, but the entirety was unlikely to have been encompassed at a glance.

This was rendered truer by the generally small size of the tomb, which afforded the viewer no great expanse to span with what Hamilakis (2002:122) has called the "distant" sense par excellence. Barring the loculi and arcosolia in which bodies were deposited, the chamber tombs under study have a mean internal area of 8.34 $m^2$. Many, however, were smaller still: Tombs 201, 225, and 207 all have a central chamber measuring less than 5 $m^2$. Tombs 208a and 208b measure 2.84$m^2$ and 2.67 $m^2$, respectively.[1] Even the presence of a very few individuals would have served to crowd the central chamber, potentially breaking lines of sight.

As to the mirrors found in Tomb 208, it hardly need be said that their use required some ambient light. And at first glance, it seems sensible that, by reflecting light, they might serve to magnify it. The mirrors in question, however, cannot have achieved very much in this regard. The inset glass reflective surface on the larger, which is circular, measures only 5.5 cm in diameter (Figure 13-6). These dimensions, as well as the mirrors' morphological characteristics, situate both objects within a class of similar objects dating to the Late Roman and Byzantine period, during which they are found primarily in tombs (Rahmani 1964). The consistently small size of these mirrors—the two from Tomb 208 are among the larger examples of the type—led Rahmani (1964:59) to conclude that they were ill suited to "practical, everyday use," and instead served an "apotropaic"

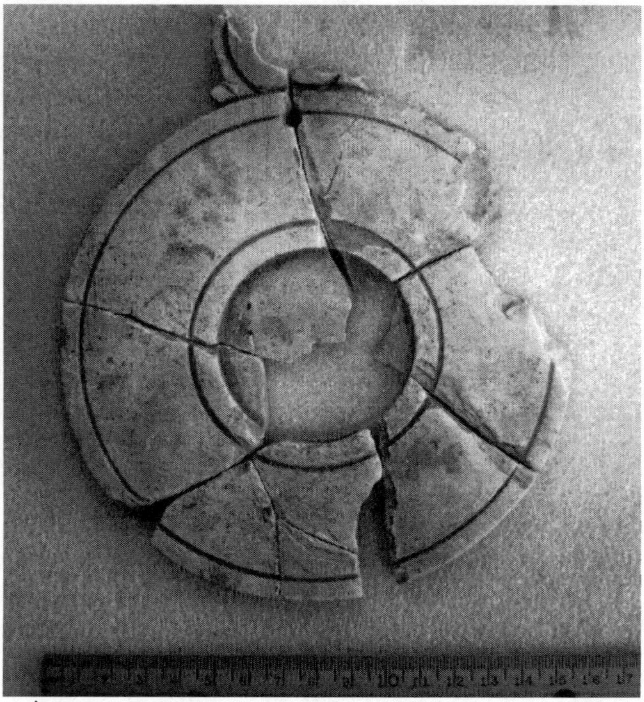

**Figure 13-6.** *Mirror plaque from Tomb 208. (Photograph © Emerson Avery. Used with permission of University of Pennsylvania Museum of Archaeology and Anthropology.)*

function. The latter conclusion is perhaps too anodyne to be really useful, but the former is interesting, particularly in light of evidence for the use of, for example, Etruscan bronze mirrors in habitation contexts as well as in the tombs (De Grummond 2002:309) where they are most often found. Etruscan mirrors were, in the first instance, precisely that, notwithstanding the associations they may have had when employed as grave goods. It is unclear if the objects discovered in Tomb 208 should be regarded in the same way or if, more to the point, their reflective properties were of more than symbolic significance. If indeed they were exposed to light, and not simply buried with the deceased—a question we cannot answer, given the lack of specific information regarding their findspot(s)—it seems most likely that their effect was to contribute to the dim and shifting lightscape, as they were variously illuminated and obscured by moving points of light.

## Material Culture and Olfaction

The relative lack of visual stimuli in the tombs under study, however, did not extend to all the other senses. The objects associated with each tomb make clear that their interiors furnished a powerful variety of stimulants to the sense of smell.

While the range of material culture discovered in and around the tombs under study is relatively wide, there are nevertheless classes of object that are noteworthy for the consistency of their appearance. The ceramic lamps mentioned above are one such. Among the others are vessels that probably served as containers for perfume or comestibles.

### *Unguentaria*

It must be admitted that the identification of a given vessel type with a given sort of content is in some measure speculative. As the discovery of two "finger bones" in a third or fourth century C.E. glass jar from Tomb 1 indicates (UMA, 1922 Field Register [FR], May 16 entry), contents could vary in surprising ways. But both classes are defensible on the strength of the evidence. Vessberg (1952:111) was mostly correct, I believe, in identifying small glass vessels as containers for perfume and similar cosmetics. His stance is in some respects the product of modern scholarly convention, which began, during the French excavations at Carthage, to employ the term *unguentarium* for such vessels and so prejudged their contents (Gauckler 1915:545). But at least some of the vessels in question seem well suited for unctuous, aromatic substances. Common to many is a long, narrow neck, which, as Vessberg (1952:136) notes, "facilitates pouring in very small quantities and which prevents a too rapid evaporation of the contents."

The argument is supported by the few residue analyses that have been undertaken to date (e.g., Alcock 1980:62; Biers et al. 1994; Greenewalt et al. 1985:84–85). Especially relevant, by reason of the vessels' type and chronology, is an analysis of residues discovered within two candlestick unguentaria from the area of Jerusalem, dating probably to the first or second and the second or third centuries C.E., respectively (Barag 1972). The contents were ascertained to be a mixture of oil, probably olive, and an aqueous solution, which Basch (1972:32) hypothesizes may have contained aromatic components. A similar result was obtained by the Biomolecular Archaeology Laboratory for Cuisine, Fermented Beverages, and Health, headed by Patrick E. McGovern of the University of Pennsylvania Museum of Archaeology and Anthropology. This laboratory's analysis of a residue which the author noted in a fourth century C.E. glass vessel from Tomb 206 revealed "an aged pine resin, saturated fatty acids, and glycerol . . . consistent with the vessel having originally contained a wine (perhaps herbal) or a scented oil" (Figure 13-7).[2] Inasmuch as these glass unguentaria seem to have replaced the ceramic variety, which was widespread in the Roman Mediterranean until the first century C.E., it is likely that the earlier sort served a similar purpose (Anderson-Stojanović 1987:113; Camilli 1999:9).

As such, I understand small closed vessels of both ceramic and glass as "unguentaria," the contents of which were more or less powerfully aromatic. Vessels describable as *unguentaria* were found in ten of the eleven tombs under study. The breadth of their chronology is equally impressive. Examples date from all the phases of the tombs' use and, among some of the longest-used tombs, all the phases of an *individual* tomb's. Such is the case in Tombs 206, 207, and 224.

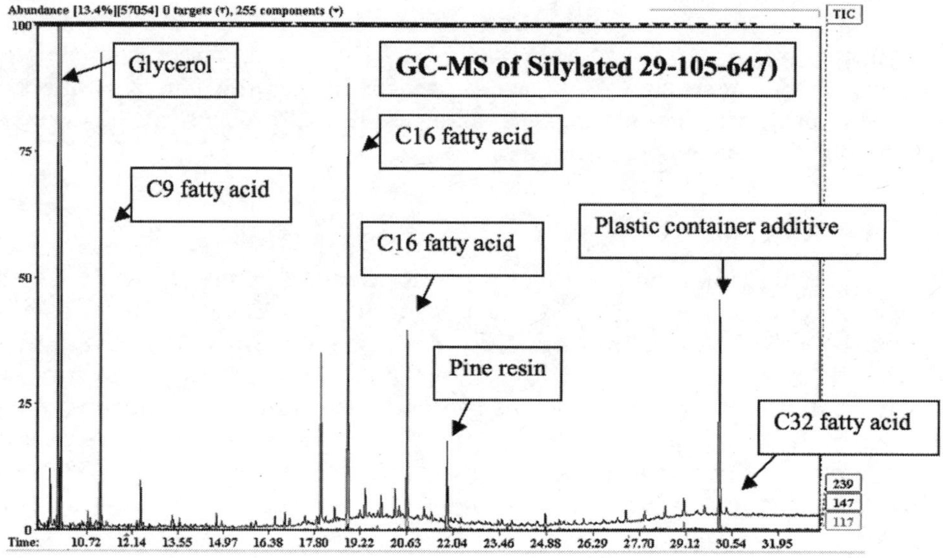


**Figure 13-7.** *GC-MS chromatogram for the silylated sample extracted from unguentarium 29-105-647. The analysis was carried out by G. R. Hall at the Scientific Research and Analysis Laboratory of the Winterthur Museum and Country Estate. (Used with permission of P. E. McGovern, Biomolecular Archaeology Laboratory, University of Pennsylvania Museum of Archaeology and Anthropology.)*

The former two were used in the first through the second centuries C.E. and, after a hiatus that is difficult to explain, again in the fourth through the sixth centuries. Tomb 224, on the other hand, was used continuously from the second through the sixth centuries. With respect to the placement of unguentaria within the tomb, they seem to have been deposited as often in the central chamber as in particular burial loci.

### *Eating and Drinking Vessels*

Vessels relating to the preparation, service, and storage of food and drink were nearly as common. They are present in eight of the tombs under study, and their chronology is as wide as that of the unguentaria. Among the earliest are first century C.E. tablewares from various manufacturing centers in the Eastern Mediterranean. Tomb 206 contained a Cypriot Sigillata cup of Hayes's (1985:85–86) form P28; Tomb 207, a Cypriote Sigillata form X52 jug (Hayes 1985:89–90) and what is probably a Çandarlı-ware plate of form L26 (Hayes 1985:77), the latter made in Pergamon; and Tomb 239, an Eastern Sigillata A cup, form 45 or 47, manufactured in Northern Syria (Hayes 1985:34, 35–36). Later on, especially beginning in the fourth century C.E., vessels for preparation and storage become more common. Chief among these are an assortment of coarse-ware ceramic basins from Tombs 205 and 206 (cf. Bagatti 1967:287, Figure 232:5; Johnson 1988:Figure

7-32:494, 496; Peleg 2004:Figure 26:1, 3; Smith and Day 1989:Plate 52:27); two basalt mortars from 239 and 260 (cf. Hamilton and Husseini 1935:Plate LXXXII:8); a late Roman cookpot from 205 (cf. Ben-Nachum 2007:Figure 6:6; Johnson 1988:Figure 7:43); and a number of fragmentary Palestinian baggy jars from Tombs 205, 206, and 210. (These last—some of which were manufactured in the vicinity of Beth She'an (Landgraf 1980:80)[3]—were employed as foodstuff containers virtually everywhere in Late Roman Palestine.) Tablewares are correspondingly fewer and include a post–fourth century C.E. glass wine goblet of Isings's (1957:139–140) form 111, found in Tomb 207; a Phocaean Red Slip plate from the end of the fifth or the beginning of the sixth century (Hayes 1972:329–338), in 206; and a jug that is generically Late Roman (cf. Covello-Paran and Avshalom-Gorni 2008:Figure 4:5), in 224. It is unfortunate that none of these vessels contained anything at the time of study, especially in light of a tantalizing note regarding a third- or fourth-century glass jug from Tomb 1. When discovered, it had a "spongy brown material" inside (UMA, 1922 FR, May 16 entry; cf. Hayes 1975:96–97, Plate 23:336) that has since been scrubbed away.

## Material Culture and Ritual

The presence of all of these objects in the tomb may be explained, or rather interpreted, in a variety of ways. Traditionally, their value has been as a window into Roman and Byzantine mortuary ritual, some particulars of which may be hypothesized. Vessels for food, and most especially its service, can be related to the practice of feasting with the dead: a pagan Roman custom on the occasion of the funeral, on the ninth day thereafter, and once a year during the festival of Parentalia (Lindsay 1998; Toynbee 1971:50–54, 61–64). The archaeological evidence for tombside banquets in the Northern Cemetery of Beth She'an is not as suggestive as elsewhere in the empire; the stone biclinia (couches) adjoining tombs at Isola Sacra outside Ostia (Gee 2008), and the triclinia in the Nabataean cemetery at Petra (Hachlili and Killebrew 1983:113), are more impressive evidence for the practice. But neither can it be discounted out of hand, as is made clear by the grumbling of Eastern ecclesiastical sources over the pagan "recidivism" of the common folk during the early centuries of the Christian era (Jensen 2008; Rebillard 2009). In any event, there was always a place for offering food and drink to the dead, whether or not the living also partook (Jensen 2008). Graves throughout the Roman Mediterranean were provided with mensae (e.g., Barral i Altet 1978; Giuntella et al. 1985), on which a meal might be set, and libation tubes (e.g., Avner and Gendelman 2007; Slane and Walbank 2006:383), into which liquid offerings could be poured.

The use of unguentaria in mortuary ritual is a little harder to parse, not least because they seem to have possessed a variety of significations, only some of which required that the vessel be opened and its contents exposed. Jars included in the tomb as personal possessions of the deceased or grave gifts from the living may have been left sealed (Green 2008:171–173). Others, however, must have been opened, in order that their contents could be sprinkled on the corpse of the deceased (John Chrysostom *In Joannem* 5, Homily LXXXV); scattered within the tomb (Prudentius *Liber Cathemerinon* 10.169–172); or poured as a libation (Paulinus of Nola *Poemata* 21.590–615). The second and third possibilities, at least, should have taken place at the tomb, but regarding the first, we cannot be sure.

There is, however, a fourth possibility.[4] The Yerushalmi Talmud, redacted in the fourth and fifth centuries C.E., contains a discussion of the various circumstances under which aromatics might be blessed (*y. Ber.* 6.6, 10d). Therein, it states that "oil that is for filth, one does not bless." The reference is to the oil that was used to clean one's hands after a meal, which was part of the Jewish toilet but also part of the generic Roman one as well. If unguents were employed to clean the hands after a funerary feast, they might well be left at the scene, their remaining contents allowed to diffuse into the tomb's atmosphere.

## The Living in the Space of Death

Similar conclusions could be spun out at greater length, but it should already be apparent that, with the exception of the last, they have a great deal more to do with the dead than with the living. The latter's experience of mortuary ritual was powerfully affected, however, by the peculiar sensorium encountered inside the tomb. There, visual stimuli were relatively scanty, and owing to the character of the space, of a particular sort. Olfactory information, in contrast, was abundant and equally particular. The significance of this fact is difficult to overstate. In the absence of ethnographic data pertaining to the culture under study, we must be wary of applying our sensory hierarchy to other societies. But textual evidence from the Roman world—which, following Andrén (1998:156), I read as a variety of "contemporary ethnographic analogy"—provides ground for seeing a degree of continuity between ancient and modern Western views. Conditions within the tomb represented an inversion of the Classical sensorium, which had, since Plato at least, held that vision was the highest of the senses and the truest means of understanding (Synnott 1991). Early Christian writers diverged from their predecessors in considering the moral ramifications of sensation, but they seem basically to have agreed with their forebears' estimation of the senses' relative utility (Synnott 1988, 1991).

None of this, of course, is to say that the ancient world was unaccustomed to olfactory information. Alex Scobie's (1986) study of sanitation in a handful of Italian Roman cities is, among other things, a catalog of the (mal)odors with which city dwellers were confronted on a daily basis. His characterization of urban living does not on all points apply to *Palestinian* Roman cities; as Hirschfeld (1995:103) observes, "[m]ulti-story apartment houses of the type found in the major cities of the Roman Empire," and singled out by Scobie (1986:430–431) as especially noxious places to live, "have not been found in Palestine to date." But his points concerning the ubiquity of human and, especially, animal wastes in the streets; refuse; and perhaps even corpses, both animal and human (Scobie 1986:418–419), are probably more applicable than not. These smells, meanwhile, intermingled with others of a more appealing sort. The use of perfume, incense, and aromatic spices was much more common, and occurred in a much wider variety of contexts, than in current practice (Classen et al. 1994:14–16). But even in situations where such aromas were appreciated—as, for example, at the banquets of the upper class, at least as glimpsed through the lens of Athenaeus's *Deipnosophists*, a literary work of the third century C.E.—they were experienced alongside a variety of visual delights.

Visitors to the tombs under study had a different experience. Their approach entailed a passage from the outdoors to a much smaller and dimmer space (Figure 13-8). Inside, where light was at its weakest, the scents characteristic of the tomb, among them scented oils and food, were at their most powerful. These familiar scents mingled, in turn, with an unfamiliar one: the pervasive smell of human decay. This was an odor Roman administrators strove mightily to exclude from the city (Scobie 1986:409), albeit with mixed success, and one that the wealthy could still afford to avoid. Even in the case of Tombs 210 and 248, which appear to have been used for a only a century or two, generations of individuals were apt to be buried together in what amounted to a very small space.[5]

It is possible to overstate the degree to which this peculiar mix of scents was "unpleasant," since such judgments depend on a changeable cultural logic (Green 2008:167, Note 63). But it is hard to escape the conclusion that the odor of decay, at least, was fairly strong (cf. Green 2008:167–168), especially in the tombs under discussion. The graves in the Northern Cemetery at Beth She'an were excavated in a porous travertine that was very susceptible to infiltration by rainwater (UMA, *Excavations* 1944). Their interiors were likely damp and probably accessible to animal as well as microbial life. This is hardly the sort of environment that would act to retard decomposition. Additionally, the loculi and arcosolia in which bodies were placed seem to have been somewhat indifferently closed. The excavators make occasional mention of tomb doors, usually pushed into the tomb by looters (e.g., Tomb 201 [UMA, 1926 FD, September 18 entry]), but I have yet to come across a reference to stones for sealing the places of deposition, either in situ or pushed aside. Under the circumstances, it is easy to imagine that the odor of decomposition would have been immediately perceptible. Indeed, as Howes (1991:143) has noted, odors are most apparent at boundaries, before their effect is diminished by familiarity. This sudden efflorescence was a powerful indicator that ritual participants were entering another world, one in which the hierarchy of perception was partially inverted.

## Familiar Smells, Unfamiliar Effects

This inversion is crucial to the definition of Foucault's (1986) "heterotopias," a class of places that upend the normal order of things for reasons of social utility; cemeteries, significantly, are explicitly listed among them. Heterotopias, he says, are "something like counter-sites, a kind of effectively enacted utopia in which the real sites, all the other real sites that can be found within

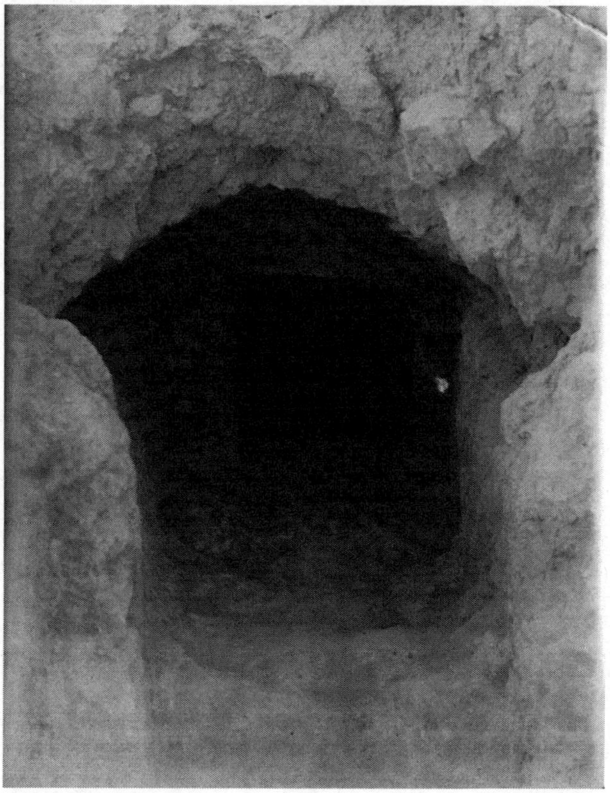

**Figure 13-8.** *Entrance to Tomb 239. (Courtesy of the Penn Museum, image #79607.)*

the culture, are simultaneously represented, contested, and inverted" (Foucault 1986:24). They are not, in other words, quotidian spaces, but they can only be understood *with respect to* quotidian spaces.

This linkage is, I believe, the proper context in which to understand an old but still current trope, inherited by archaeologists from the Romans themselves (Wallace-Hadrill 2008:39–43): that ancient tombs, in the Galilee as elsewhere, were designed as "houses" for the dead, for whom provision was made as it had been in life (e.g., Fleming 1997:53–58). Formulated thusly, this is an idea with a great deal more descriptive than analytical force. It is manifestly the case that the range of objects found within the tombs discussed here would be as much at home in a contemporary Roman house. Stuart Fleming (1999:99), whose study of the Beth She'an glass represents the only other modern work on the materials under discussion, noted that the unguentaria and other glass vessels differed little from the range found in contemporary domestic contexts. The same can be said of vessels for food, especially those employed in its preparation and storage.

Crucially, however, we need not understand the relationship between house and tomb in so simplistic a fashion. It was, rather, a "game of allusion," in which particular resonances could be manipulated to produce a variety of effects

(Wallace-Hadrill 2008:77). The response that conditions inside the tomb might have elicited from the living is admittedly difficult to intuit. But a comparison with conditions in Roman and Early Byzantine period Palestinian houses,[6] which for most people represented a paradigmatically "normal" space, is suggestive. The experience of entering a tomb evoked a limited range of familiar sensations, and so perhaps familiar resonances, brought together in an unfamiliar way.

Houses were lighted by a combination of artificial and natural light. The former was supplied by basically the same range of lamps as is found in contemporary tombs—generally mounted on stands provided for the purpose—as well as by glass lamps in hanging *polycandela,* the latter especially after the fifth century C.E. (Bouras and Parani 2006:20; Ellis 2000:150; Hadad 1998). Natural light, meanwhile, was obviously strongest in the courtyard, which seems to have been an almost indispensable part of the Palestinian house plan (Hirschfeld 1995:290). But it also entered through the door, which was kept open during the day, and the windows, which were generally small and few in number. They tended to be located high up on the exterior walls (Hirschfeld 1995:249–258, 289). In the Golan, the Upper Galilee, and the region of Beth She'an—areas where vernacular construction was typically in the abundant local stone, and two-story dwellings were common (Hirschfeld 1995:264; Tsafrir and Foerster 1997:89–90)—this meant, in practice, that windows were most frequent in the rooms given over to human habitation. In general, the lower floor was used for storage, domestic tasks, and sometimes retail, and the upper and better lit, for the residence proper (e.g., McNicoll et al. 1982:130–139, a Pellan house probably belonging to a wealthy family).

Especially during the day, it is probable that most living spaces were adequately illuminated, if neither so brightly nor so uniformly as now (Ellis 2000:150). Darkness comparable to that within the tomb was experienced primarily at night or in those rooms that the sun could not reach. Among these was the *kiton,* or dormitory, "small" (Hirschfeld 1995:276) examples of which measured some 7–8 $m^2$ (e.g., Hirschfeld 1995:Figure 13, a sixth-century village house at Ḥorvat Susiya). Significantly, these dimensions are comparable with the mean area calculated for our tombs. This seems appropriate, particularly for Christians, for whom the "sleep" of death was precisely that. But in no space was the fetor of human decay normal, and its presence must have been arresting.

The range of quotidian objects found within the tomb was as paradoxically evocative of difference. Cooking for the dead may have been mechanically the same as cooking for the living, but there is literary, and some archaeological, evidence that the recipes were distinct. Festus-Paulus (377L) describes the *silicernium,* the meal taken on the day of the funeral, as consisting of a special type of sausage. The menu at the banquet on the ninth day, the *cena novemdialis,* was also traditional, consisting in a fixed array of eggs, vegetables, beans, salted lentils, bread, and poultry (Lindsay 1998:73). Finally, there is *Kollyva,* a dish made from boiled wheat and prepared to this day in the Levant to commemorate the death of Eastern Orthodox Christians. As Lawson (1910:535) notes, it is of ancient pagan origin; Seyrig (1951:6), writing about the Palmyrene tomb of Iarhai, dated to the second and third centuries C.E., identified a funerary stela as depicting a representation of this dish. The service of similar foods in the necropolis of Beth She'an, and so the presence of their unique aromas, would have served to mark the space of the tomb as even more obviously apart.

## Conclusion

The othering of the tomb space—or, in Foucault's terms, its conversion into a heterotopia—was accomplished primarily through the construction of a particular kind of sensorium, defined in the first instance by the selective engagement of the entrants' senses, and in the second, by the peculiar continuum of stimuli, some familiar and some alien, with which they were presented therein. Heterotopias, however, do not exist without purpose. By way of conclusion, it is worth asking what that purpose may have been, and how the emphasis on olfaction achieved it. A partial answer may be found in the special characteristics of the human sense of smell. Of all the senses, it is the one most effective in stimulating memory (Howes 1991:132), in this case both of the dead, whose living descendants entered the tomb to inter or commemorate them, and of the tomb itself, whose charnel odors clung briefly to the living upon their exit. As such, it made poignant the boundary between life and death. Indeed, the use of scents in rituals marking transitions—from childhood to adulthood, for example, or from life to death—is almost universal (Howes 1991). Whatever their religious profession, the smell of mortality was not one that people might easily forget.

## Acknowledgments

Drs. Sebastian Heath, Jodi Magness, and Deborah Green read and commented on an earlier draft of this paper, improving it enormously thereby. Dr. Patrick McGovern was kind enough to lend his expertise in residue analysis, the results of which I refer to above. Finally, thanks are due to Dr. Jo Day, who organized the conference at which an earlier version of this paper was given, and the conference attendees, whose comments and company proved stimulating throughout.

## Notes

1. All of these dimensions are calculated using the statistics function of ArcGis 9.3. I exclude Tomb 239 from consideration, since, as mentioned above, it was incompletely cleared, and its dimensions cannot therefore be stated with confidence.

2. My thanks to Drs. Patrick McGovern and Gretchen R. Hall for their time and expertise.

3. The shape, in its guise as Late Roman Amphora 6, was particularly well distributed from the fifth through the eighth centuries C.E., but its genesis is almost certainly earlier. Loffreda (2008:132–136) dates its presence at Capernaum to

the beginning of the fourth century C.E. At Beth She'an itself, Johnson (2006:540–541, 549–550) publishes examples with a similar chronology.

4. I owe this idea, as well as the citation and its translation, to Deborah Green.

5. Looters' depredations, and the inconsistency of excavators' records with respect to skeletal remains, have made it impossible to be more quantitatively specific.

6. The residential quarters of Beth She'an are still little known (Tsafrir and Foerster 1997:88, Note 19). There is little reason, however, to expect that these more general remarks do not apply.

## References


Alcock, Joan P.

1980 Classical Religious Belief and Burial Practice in Roman Britain. *Archaeological Journal* 137:50–85.

Anderson-Stojanović, Virginia R.

1987 The Chronology and Function of Ceramic Unguentaria. *American Journal of Archaeology* 91:105–122.

Andrén, Anders

1998 *Between Artifacts and Texts: Historical Archaeology in Global Perspective*. Translated by Alan Crozier. Plenum, New York.

Avigad, Nahman

1976 *Beth She'arim III: Report on the Excavations during 1953–1958*. Vol. 3, Catacombs 12–23. Rutgers University Press, New Brunswick, New Jersey.

Avner, Rina, and Peter Gendelman

2007 *Caesarea: Final Report*. Excavations and Surveys in Israel 119. Electronic document, http://www.hadashot-esi.org.il/report_detail_eng.asp?id=470&mag_id=112, accessed August 10, 2010.

Avni, Gideon, and Uzi Dahari

1990 Christian Burial Caves from the Byzantine Period at Luzit. In *Christian Archaeology in the Holy Land: New Discoveries. Essays in Honour of Virgilio C. Corbo*, edited by Giovanni Claudio Bottini, Leah Di Segni, and Eugenio Alliata, pp. 301–320. Franciscan Printing Press, Jerusalem.

Avni, Gideon, Uzi Dahari, and Amos Kloner

2008 *The Necropolis of Bet Guvrin-Eleutheropolis*. IAA Reports, Vol. 36. Israel Antiquities Authority, Jerusalem.

Avni, Gideon, and Zvi Greenhut

1996 Architecture, Burial Customs, and Chronology. In *The Akeldama Tombs: Three Burial Caves in the Kidron Valley, Jerusalem*, edited by Gideon Avni and Zvi Greenhut, pp. 1–39. IAA Reports, Vol. 1. Israel Antiquities Authority, Jerusalem.

Bagatti, Bellarmino

1967 *Gli scavi di Nazaret. Vol. I: Dalle origini al secolo XII*. Pubblicazioni dello Studium Biblicum Franciscanum, Vol. 17. Tipografia dei PP. Francescani, Jerusalem.

Barag, Dan

1972 Two Roman Glass Bottles with Remnants of Oil. *Israel Exploration Journal* 22:24–26.

Barral i Altet, Xavier

1978 Mensae et repas funéraires dans la péninsule ibérique. In *Atti del IX Congresso internazionale di archeologia cristiana*. Roma, 21–27 settembre 1975, pp. 49–69. Pontificio Istituto di archeologia cristiana, Vatican City.

Basch, A.

1972 Analyses of Oil from Two Roman Glass Bottles. *Israel Exploration Journal* 22:27–32.

Ben-Nachum, Chaya

2007 Tombs of the Roman Period and Building Remains of the Byzantine and Early Islamic Periods at Kafr Kama. *'Atiqot* 56:105–112 (Hebrew; English summary 82*–83*).

Biers, William R., Klaus O. Gerhardt, and Rebecca A. Braniff

1994 *Lost Scents: Investigation of Corinthian "Plastic" Vases by Gas Chromatography–Mass Spectrometry*. MASCA Research Papers in Science and Archaeology, Vol. 11. University of Pennsylvania Museum of Archaeology and Anthropology, Philadelphia.

Bille, Mikkel, and Tim F. Sørensen

2007 An Anthropology of Luminosity: The Agency of Light. *Journal of Material Culture* 12:263–284.

Bouras, Laskarina, and Maria G. Parani

2006 *Lighting in Early Byzantium*. Dumbarton Oaks Byzantine Collection Publications, Vol. 11. Dumbarton Oaks Research Library and Collection, Washington, D.C.

Camilli, Andrea

1999 *Ampullae. Balsamari ceramici di età ellenistica e romana*. Fratelli Palombi Editori, Rome.

Classen, Constance, David Howes, and Anthony Synnott

1994 *Aroma: The Cultural History of Smell*. Routledge, London.

Covello-Paran, Karen, and Dina Avshalom-Gorni

2008 Pottery Production at Ḥorbat Rodem near Bet She'an. *'Atiqot* 58:37–46.

De Grummond, Nancy T.

2002 Review: Etruscan Mirrors Now. *American Journal of Archaeology* 106:307–311.

Ellis, Simon P.

2000 *Roman Housing*. Duckworth, London.

Fleming, Stuart J.

1997 *Roman Glass: Reflections of Everyday Life*. University of Pennsylvania Museum of Archaeology and Anthropology, Philadelphia.

1999 *Roman Glass: Reflections on Cultural Change*. University of Pennsylvania Museum of Archaeology and Anthropology, Philadelphia.

Foucault, Michel

1986 Of Other Spaces. *Diacritics: A Review of Contemporary Criticism* 16:22–27.

Gauckler, Paul

1915 *Nécropoles puniques de Carthage*. A. Picard, Paris.

Gee, Regina

2008 From Corpse to Ancestor: The Role of Tombside Dining in the Transformation of the Body in Ancient Rome. In *The Materiality of Death: Bodies, Burials, Beliefs*, edited by Fredrik Fahlander and Terje Oestigaard, pp. 59–68. BAR International Series 1768, Archaeopress, Oxford.

Giuntella, Anna Maria, Giuseppina Borghetti, and Daniela Stiaffini

1985 *Mensae e riti funerari in Sardegna. La testimonianza di Cornus*. Mediterraneo Tardoantico e Medievale: Scavi e Ricerche, Vol. 1. Editrice Scorpione, Taranto.

Green, Deborah

2008 Sweet Spices in the Tomb: An Initial Study on the Use of Perfume in Jewish

Burials. In *Commemorating the Dead: Texts and Artifacts in Context. Studies of Roman, Jewish, and Christian Burials*, edited by Laurie Brink, O.P., and Deborah Green, pp. 145–173. Walter de Gruyter, Berlin.

Greenewalt, Crawford H., Donald G. Sullivan, Christopher Ratté, and Thomas N. Howe

1985 The Sardis Campaigns of 1981 and 1982. *Bulletin of the American Schools of Oriental Research, Supplementary Studies* 23:53–92.

Hachlili, Rachel, and Ann Killebrew

1983 Jewish Funerary Customs during the Second Temple Period, in the Light of the Excavations at the Jericho Necropolis. *Palestine Exploration Quarterly* 115:109–139.

1999 *Jericho: The Jewish Cemetery of the Second Temple Period*. IAA Reports, Vol. 7. Israel Antiquities Authority, Jerusalem.

Hadad, Shulamit

1998 Glass Lamps from the Byzantine through Mamluk Periods at Bet Shean, Israel. *Journal of Glass Studies* 40:63–77.

Haddad, Elie

2007 A Burial Cave from the First–Second Centuries C.E. and Double-Arcosolia Tombs from the Fourth–Fifth Centuries C.E. on the Fringes of Ḥorbat Zikhrin. *'Atiqot* 56:25–57 (Hebrew, English summary 74*–75*).

Hamilakis, Yannis

2002 The Past as Oral History: Towards an Archaeology of the Senses. In *Thinking through the Body: Archaeologies of Corporeality*, edited by Yannis Hamilakis, Mark Pluciennik, and Sarah Tarlow, pp. 121–136. Kluwer Academic/Plenum, London.

Hamilton, Robert, and S. A. S. Husseini

1935 Shaft Tombs on the Nablus Road, Jerusalem. *Quarterly of the Department of Antiquities in Palestine* 4:170–174.

Hayes, John W.

1972 *Late Roman Pottery*. The British School at Rome, London.

1975 *Roman and Pre-Roman Glass in the Royal Ontario Museum: A Catalogue*. Royal Ontario Museum, Toronto.

1985 Sigillate orientali. In *Atlante delle forme ceramiche II. Ceramica fina romana nel Bacino Mediterraneo (tardo ellenismo e primo impero)*, pp. 1–96. Istituto della Enciclopedia Italiana, Rome.

Hirschfeld, Yizhar

1995 *The Palestinian Dwelling in the Roman-Byzantine Period*. Studium Biblicum Franciscanum, Collectio Minor, Vol. 34. Franciscan Printing Press/Israel Exploration Society, Jerusalem.

Howes, David

1991 Olfaction and Transition. In *The Varieties of Sensory Experience: A Sourcebook in the Anthropology of the Senses*, edited by David Howes, pp. 128–147. University of Toronto Press, Toronto.

Isings, Clasina

1957 *Roman Glass from Dated Finds*. J. B. Wolters, Groningen.

Jensen, Robin M.

2008 Dining with the Dead: From the Mensa to the Altar in Christian Late Antiquity. In *Commemorating the Dead: Texts and Artifacts in Context. Studies of Roman, Jewish, and Christian Burials*, edited by Laurie Brink, O.P., and Deborah Green, pp. 107–143. Walter de Gruyter, Berlin.

Johnson, Barbara L.

1988 The Pottery. In *Excavations at Jalame: Site of a Glass Factory in Late Roman Palestine*, edited by G. Davidson Weinberg, pp. 137–226. University of Missouri Press, Columbia.

2006 The Hellenistic to Early Islamic Period Pottery. In *Excavations at Tel Beth-Shean 1989–1996*. Vol. I. *From the Late Bronze Age to the Medieval Period*, edited by Amihai Mazar, pp. 523–589. Institute of Archaeology, The Hebrew University of Jerusalem, Jerusalem.

Landgraf, John

1980 Keisan's Byzantine Pottery. In *Tell Keisan (1971–1976): une cité phénicienne en Galilée*, edited by Jacques Briend and Jean-Baptiste Humbert, pp. 51–99, pl. 141. Éditions Universitaires, Fribourg.

Lawson, John C.

1910 *Modern Greek Folklore and Ancient Greek Religion: A Study in Survivals*. Cambridge University Press, Cambridge.

Lindsay, Hugh

1998 Eating with the Dead: The Roman Funerary Banquet. In *Meals in a Social Context: Aspects of the Communal Meal in the Hellenistic and Roman World*, edited by Inge Nielsen and Hanne Sigismund Nielsen, pp. 67–80. Aarhus Studies in Mediterranean Antiquity, Vol. 1. Aarhus University Press, Aarhus and Oakville, Connecticut.

Loffreda, Stanislao

2008 *Cafarnao VI: Tipologie e contesti stratigrafici della ceramica (1968–2003)*. Edizioni Terra Santa, Jerusalem.

Macalister, Robert A. S.

1912 *The Excavation of Gezer, 1902–1905 and 1907–1909*. 3 vols. J. Murray for the Committee of the Palestine Exploration Fund, London.

McNicoll, Anthony, Robert H. Smith, and Basil Hennessy

1982 *Pella in Jordan 1: An Interim Report on the Joint University of Sydney and the College of Wooster Excavations at Pella 1979–1981*. Australian National Gallery, Canberra.

Magness, Jodi

1993 *Jerusalem Ceramic Chronology circa 200–800 C.E.* JSOT / ASOR Monograph Series, Vol. 9. JSOT Press, Sheffield.

Oren, Eliezer D.

1973 *The Northern Cemetery of Beth Shan*. Brill, Leiden.

Oren, Eliezer D., and Uriel Rappaport

1984 The Necropolis of Maresha-Beth Govrin. *Israel Exploration Journal* 34:114–153.

Peleg, Michal

2004 A Late Roman-Byzantine Bathhouse at Beth She'an. *'Atiqot* 46:55–81.

Rahmani, Levi Yitzhak

1964 Mirror-Plaques from a Fifth-Century A.D. Tomb. *Israel Exploration Journal* 14:50–60.

1981a Ancient Jerusalem's Funerary Customs and Tombs: Part One. *Biblical Archaeologist* 44:171–177.

1981b Ancient Jerusalem's Funerary Customs and Tombs: Part Two. *Biblical Archaeologist* 44:229–235.

1982a Ancient Jerusalem's Funerary Customs and Tombs: Part Three. *Biblical Archaeologist* 45:43–53.

1982b Ancient Jerusalem's Funerary Customs and Tombs: Part Four. *Biblical Archaeologist* 45:109–119.

Rebillard, Éric

2009 *The Care of the Dead in Late Antiquity*. Cornell University Press, Ithaca.

Richmond, E. T.

1931 A Rock-Cut Tomb at Nazareth. *Quarterly of the Department of Antiquities in Palestine* 1:53–54, pl. XXXIII–XXXIV.

Rowe, Alan

1927 The Discoveries at Beth Shean during the 1926 Season. *Museum Journal* 18:9–45.

1930 *The Topography and History of Beth-Shan, with Details of the Egyptian and Other Inscriptions Found on the Site.* University Press, University of Pennsylvania Museum, Philadelphia.

Samellas, Antigone

2002 *Death in the Eastern Mediterranean (A.D. 50–600): The Christianization of the East. An Interpretation.* Studien und Texte zur Antike Christentum, Vol. 12. Mohr Sieback, Tübingen.

Scobie, Alex

1986 Slums, Sanitation, and Mortality in the Roman World. *Klio* 68:399–433.

Seyrig, Henri A.

1951 Le repas des morts et le 'banquet funèbre" à Palmyre. *Annales Archéologiques de Syrie* 1:1–11.

Slane, Kathleen W., and Mary E. H. Walbank

2006 Anoiting [*sic*] and Commemorating the Dead: Funerary Rituals of Roman Corinthians. In *Old Pottery in a New Century: Innovating Perspectives on Roman Pottery Studies.* Atti del Convegno Internazionale di Studi, Catania, 22–24 April 2004, edited by Daniele Malfitana, Jerven Poblome, and John Lund, pp. 377–387. Monografie dell'Istituto per I beni archeologici e monumentali, Vol. 1. IBAM, Catania.

Smith, Robert H.

1973 *Pella of the Decapolis,* Vol. I. *The 1967 Season of the College of Wooster Expedition to Pella.* The College of Wooster, Wooster, Ohio.

Smith, Robert H., and Leslie P. Day

1989 *Pella of the Decapolis,* Vol. 2. *Final Report on the College of Wooster Excavations in Area IX, the Civic Complex, 1979–1985.* The College of Wooster, Wooster, Ohio.

Synnott, Anthony

1988 Physical, Mystical, and Spiritual: The Body in Christian Thought. *Santé, Culture, Health* 5:267–289.

1991 Puzzling over the Senses: From Plato to Marx. In *The Varieties of Sensory Experience: A Sourcebook in the Anthropology of the Senses,* edited by David Howes, pp. 61–76. University of Toronto Press, Toronto.

Toynbee, Jocelyn M. C.

1971 *Death and Burial in the Roman World.* Cornell University Press, Ithaca.

Tsafrir, Yoram, and Gideon Foerster

1997 Urbanism at Scythopolis-Bet Shean in the Fourth to Seventh Centuries. *Dumbarton Oaks Papers* 51:85–146.

Vessberg, Olof

1952 Roman Glass in Cyprus. *Opuscula Archaeologica* 7:109–165.

Wallace-Hadrill, Andrew

2008 Housing the Dead: The Tomb as House in Roman Italy. In *Commemorating the Dead: Texts and Artifacts in Context. Studies of Roman, Jewish, and Christian Burials,* edited by Laurie Brink, O.P., and Deborah Green, pp. 39–77. Walter de Gruyter, Berlin.

Waterhouse, S. Douglas

1998 *The Necropolis of Hesban: A Typology of Tombs.* Andrews University Press, Berrien Springs, Michigan.

# 14. Imagined Aromas and Artificial Flowers in Minoan Society

*Jo Day*

*Abstract:* The floral world is a popular theme across a wide range of material culture from Minoan Crete. However, the ongoing difficulties encountered by scholarship in identifying many of these species and understanding their significance is suggested here to indicate that the visual appeal of these artifacts was not of primary importance. Using the concept of synesthetic material culture, examples of stone blossom bowls and Kamares-ware ceramics with relief flowers and petals are examined. As both types of vessel provide the appearance of consuming out of artificial flowers, I suggest that these vessels were deliberately intended to enhance real aromas and provoke metaphorical and mnemonic olfactory responses. The multiple social roles of olfaction are discussed in relation to palatial Crete, and it is shown how a sensorially informed approach can lead to new interpretations of well-known material.

## Senseless Archaeology

Sensory and emotional responses to objects have been omitted from the majority of traditional archaeological studies, despite the fact that such factors are "integral to the relationships between people and the material world" (Boivin 2008:113). Although as archaeologists we may enjoy the smooth feel of highly burnished pottery or form emotional connections with "our" material, we tend to dismiss these reactions as unworthy of scholarly mention.[1] In this manner, both in our own contemporary responses to archaeological material as well as in our expectations of human responses in the past, the two-way interaction between people and things as mediated through the human body usually is

*Making Senses of the Past: Toward a Sensory Archaeology,* edited by Jo Day. Center for Archaeological Investigations, Occasional Paper No. 40.  ISBN 978-0-8093-3287-8.

ignored. In the light of archaeology's recent engagement with the concepts of materiality and the agency of objects (e.g., Boivin 2008; Gosden 2005; Knappett 2005; Meskell 2005), such a statement may seem out of place. Yet even as the multiple affective connections between humans and "stuff" (Miller 2009) are explored, the cursory mentions that sensory responses are given is not sufficient. The ongoing "Sensual Revolution" (Howes 2005) in the humanities and social sciences has brought to light crucial twin realizations that archaeology would do well to consider: We must not superimpose our own culture-specific sensorium onto past cultures, and artifacts can be involved in multisensory practices and meanings that are inconceivable when analysis is based only on visual appreciation. As a way of further exploring these issues, this chapter draws on the concept of synesthetic material culture as developed by Houston and Taube (2000), using case studies from Bronze Age Crete.

## The Eastern Mediterranean: A Scented World

The Minoan civilization that flourished on the island of Crete (Figure 14-1) during the Bronze Age (c. 3300–1200 B.C.E.) gained a reputation among academics and the general public as being peaceful and "flower-loving."[2] This attitude was primarily due to the richness of the iconography of the natural world as found on frescoes, ceramics, sealstones, rings, and stone vessels, among other remains. Such material comes especially from the complexes that have been identified as "palaces" by archaeologists, following the precedent set by Sir Arthur Evans, whose early twentieth-century work at Knossos was hugely influential on later interpretations of Minoan society (Hamilakis 2002a). Current understanding of these palatial sites, however, sees them as much more than mere royal residences, providing loci for rituals, feasting, craft activity, administration, and storage (e.g., Driessen, Schoep, and Laffineur 2002; Hägg and Marinatos 1987).

Scholarly interpretation of the florally inspired material culture has preferred to see it as mainly symbolic, although there is little agreement over what exactly either the individual flowers or general landscape scenes symbolized (see Chapin 2004 for a useful summary of the main approaches to landscape frescoes and Day 2011 on one specific motif). It is argued here that this mode of interpretation often fails to consider the materiality of the artifacts themselves, preferring to see them as representations of immaterial concepts that can never be securely identified. Adopting a multisensory approach to the same body of material allows the artifacts to be reconceptualized as things that both act on and are acted on by the human body. Following this logic, suggestions about their functions are driven by these bodily interactions. To illustrate this approach, case studies of stone and ceramic vessels with floral imagery are discussed below, with particular attention paid to the real and metaphorical olfactory responses generated by these objects.

Smells themselves and the physical process of smelling are complex phenomena; odors cannot be easily classified or controlled, seen or touched, measured or discussed. We lack an explicit olfactory vocabulary, noting that smells are "like" their source—the smell of coffee, the smell of a rose, although each

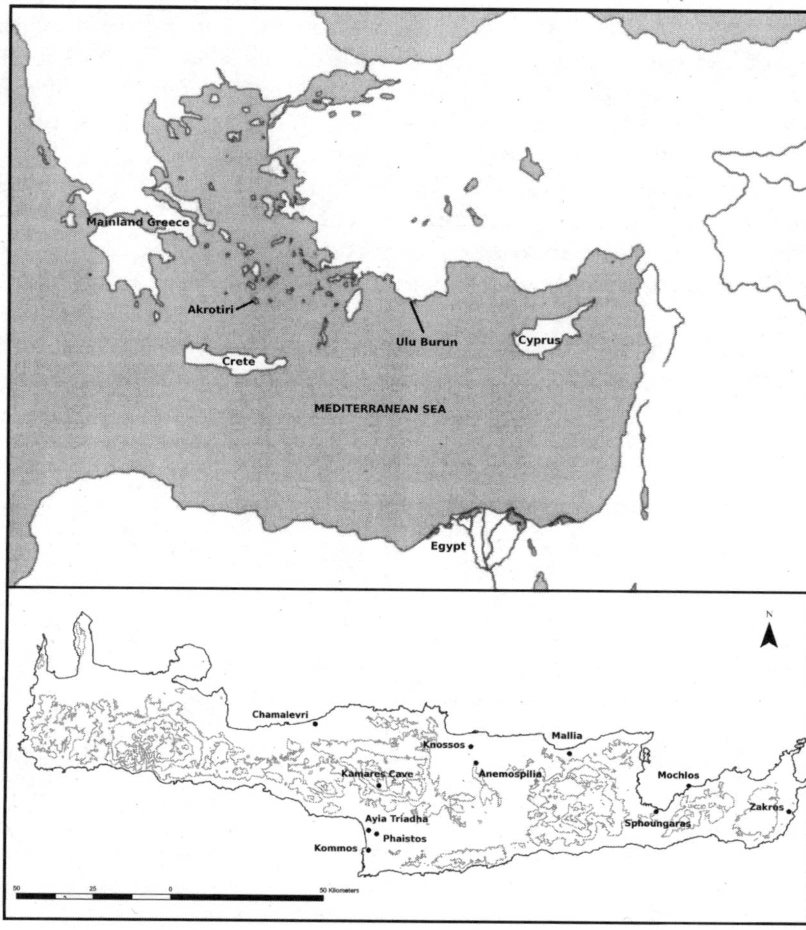


**Figure 14-1.** *Maps of the eastern Mediterranean* (top) *and Crete* (bottom), *showing locations mentioned in text.*

of these smells is actually a combination of many molecular compounds (Wilson and Stevenson 2006:6). Such olfactory muteness is not shared by all societies however. The denigration of this so-called lower sense in Western life contrasts with practices in some other cultures wherein their world is governed by osmologies, accompanied by rich olfactory vocabularies (Classen, Howes, and Synnott 1994:95–122). Like all sensory reactions, therefore, olfactory responses happen within a specific cultural sensorium that creates and reinforces the preferences and moral associations of scents.

Within this overarching social context, individual experiences of smell will also occur, with personal likes and dislikes shaping daily existence. Smells share a very personal aspect with the sense of taste too, as both require the incorporation of stimuli into the body, in contrast to touch, hearing, and sight, senses that perceive at a range of distance, from close contact to miles away. Yet, unlike taste, olfaction happens constantly and often involuntarily, leaving us with little choice about what we smell at any given time. The physiological workings of the olfactory system have been summed up by Murphy (this volume) (see also Engen 1982; Wilson and Stevenson 2006), and of particular significance is the close link between smell and emotion, facilitated by the direct access of the olfactory bulb to the brain. As odors gain their meaning through context, through the experience associated with smelling that specific smell, the emotions connected to the experience likewise become deeply embedded. It is through this link between smell, experience, and emotion that ephemeral scents become powerful social agents.

The overall use of scent and scented products on Crete during Minoan times has not, to date, received much scholarly attention (Georgiou 1974 is an exception). Yet when all the evidence is surveyed, aromatics seem to have been of not inconsiderable importance, whether for perfuming cloth, people, or places and for ritual, commensal, cosmetic, or medicinal uses. Evidence of perfumed-oil manufacturing has been found at Late Minoan Mochlos (Koh 2008) and Middle Minoan Chamalevri (Tzedakis and Martlew 1999:44–55) and also suggested at Zakros, Mallia, and Ayia Triadha (D'Agata 1997:90–92, 94–95), demonstrating that the well-known Mycenaean perfume industry (Murphy this volume; Shelmerdine 1985) had Cretan antecedents. The ceramic objects known as fireboxes have been linked to the perfume-manufacturing process (Georgiou 1980), while a variety of incense burners attest to the practice of burning fragranced substances in both tomb and settlement contexts (Georgiou 1979). The fresco known as *The Priestess* from the West House, Akrotiri, appears to show one such burner in use, as it depicts a girl sprinkling some sort of potentially aromatic substance onto hot coals (Doumas 1992:Figure 24).

This interest in scented products extended beyond the immediate Aegean region too. The site of Pyrgos-Mavroraki on Cyprus appears to have been producing perfume around 2000 B.C.E., while in New Kingdom Egypt (roughly contemporary with the Late Bronze Age on Crete), scented oils, unguents, and incense were offered to divinities and rulers, used in funerary practices, and were essential elements at banquets (Manniche 1999). Perfumed oils were also important in the Near East during the Late Bronze Age, where they were used to anoint those involved in ritual activity, often as a prelude to a feast (Fappas 2008). Late Bronze Age trade in aromatic substances was of an international character: For example, a late fourteenth century B.C.E. vessel sank at Ulu Burun, off the coast of modern Turkey, with around 120 Canaanite jars filled with a ton of fragrant terebinth resin among its cargo (Haldane 1993:352–353). This type of jar was also reported at Minoan Kommos, a port on the south coast of Crete (D'Agata 1997:85–87), suggesting the import of similar raw materials, while Mycenaean stirrup jars that contained fragranced oils are found all around the eastern Mediterranean. Royal archives of diplomatic letters and other texts (e.g., from Amarna and Mari) show that scented products, including fragrant woods as well as oils, formed important elements in elite gift exchange across the region (Knapp 1991). It is within this wider context of fragranced activity that a Minoan "smellscape," to borrow Porteous's (2006) term, and its associated material culture must be located.

## Blossom Bowls

Stone vessels first occur on Crete in contexts dating to before the rise of palatial society, such as at the EM II–MM I tholoi of the Mesara, where it is believed they played a role in funerary ritual (Warren 1969:166). It was during the Protopalatial period (c. 1900–1700 B.C.E.) that they became a more pervasive feature of life on the island however (Bevan 2007:115), and a range of stone shapes emerged, such as bird's nest bowls, alabastrons, cups, and lamps. One particular class of vessel is of interest here: a Neopalatial (c. 1700–1450 B.C.E.) type known to scholarship as the blossom bowl (Figure 14-2). Over 150 examples of blossom bowls have been recovered from Crete and farther afield, coming from both funerary and settlement contexts (Bevan 2007:130). Blossom bowls are very distinctive—they are made exclusively from serpentine and always have six petals, each with a midrib, incised on their exterior. While not every example has been found with a lid, there is evidence enough to suggest that at least some of them could have been sealed in this manner. Interestingly, ceramic imitations of blossom bowls have also been recorded, albeit relatively rarely and usually at sites beyond the reaches of direct palatial influence (Bevan 2007:130; Bevan et al. 2002:Figure 13.8; Warren 1969:169–170).

The purpose of these containers remains unclear: They are considered too fine for everyday domestic use, for example, as a mortar for grinding grain or other food substances, a function perhaps also mitigated against by the tomb findspots. One suggestion, by Peter Warren, is that they could have been used for storing valuable ointments, perfumes, or spices (1969:166). This makes sense considering their small size and the lack of traces of grinding, pounding, or other rougher uses, which would not be evident if they contained valuable organics. Indeed, the fact that blossom bowls were exported from Crete (Warren 1969:15) may support this interpretation, and they could be seen as part of the widespread trade in and use of aromatic substances around the eastern Mediterranean during the Late Bronze Age. If the contents of these vessels were indeed fragrance bearing, the link with the exterior "packaging" should be considered an intrinsic element of the overall product. Their very specific morphology allows the vessels to be more than containers and to become actual flowers.

The concept of stone vessels as flowers is not unique to Minoan Crete, and examples can be found in contemporary Egypt also. It is clear that the Egyptian stone-vessel industry influenced that on Crete to some extent, as indicated early in the Bronze Age by evidence of imported Egyptian vessels as well as Minoan imitations of Egyptian types (Bevan 2004). The blossom bowl itself may even be influenced by Egyptian designs (Hood 1994:140). Of particular relevance for this chapter are the vessels known as lotiform chalices (Figure 14-3), large faience and alabaster cups in the shape of the water-lily flower that were produced during the Eighteenth Dynasty (c. 1550–1292 B.C.E.). Nearly all the lotus vessels are in the form of *Nymphaea caerulea*, or blue lotus, although royal drinking vessels of the Amarna period (1353–1336 B.C.E.) were made in the form of the white lotus, or *Nymphaea lotus* (Tait 1963:97). This imitation of a specific species is deliberate: To the ancient Egyptians, the lotus was replete with symbolism because the sun

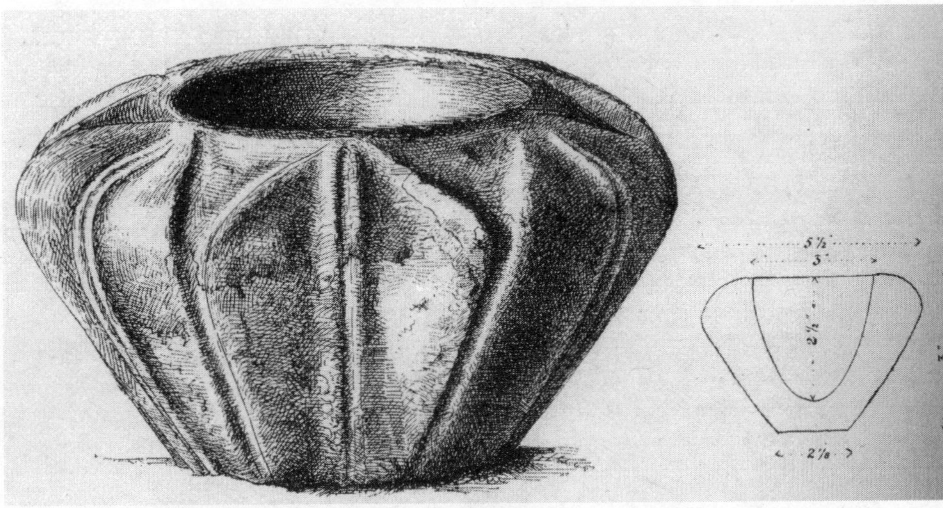

**Figure 14-2.** *Stone blossom bowl, Milatos (Evans 1895:Figure 123).*

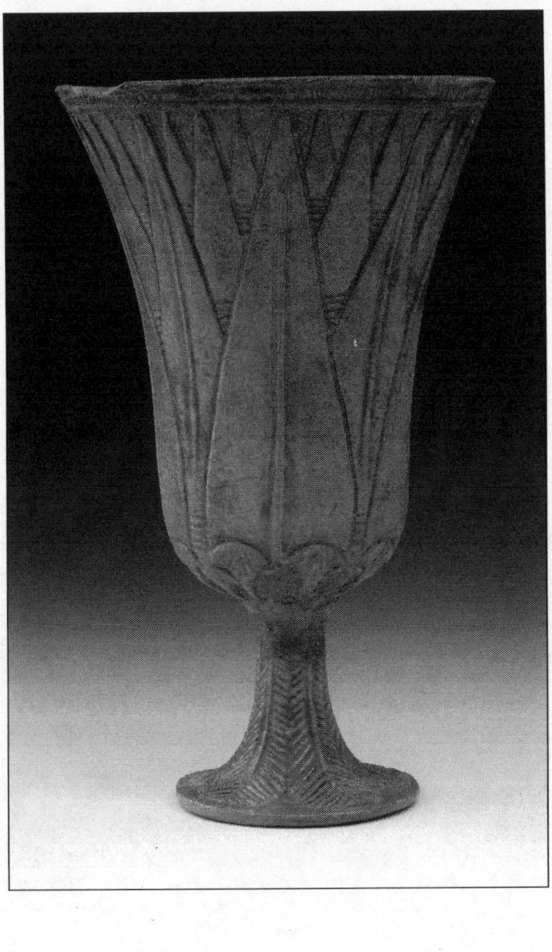

**Figure 14-3.** *Egyptian lotiform chalice. (British Museum no. 26226. © Trustees of the British Museum.)*

god, Ra, was born from this flower. Lotus imagery proliferated across dynasties and the plant became the symbol of Upper Egypt. Unlike the Amarna vessels, the *caerulea* chalices appear to have been used only in funerary contexts (Tait 1963:99). A key aspect of the blue lotus is its strong scent, and the flower is often depicted in Egyptian banquet scenes being held below guests' noses, presumably to facilitate inhalation of the sweet fragrance. This emphasis on fragrant atmospheres in life may well have continued in death, with the stone replica of the lotus ensuring eternal blossoms and a way of providing everlasting sweet smells to the dead.

Both the lotiform chalices and the Minoan blossom bowls may be seen, therefore, as examples of sensory signposting or reinforcement in which shape is neither purely functional nor purely symbolic but rather acts in an intersensorial fashion on the user.[3] Certainly the tactility of the vessels, the smooth feel of serpentine or alabaster, and the skillful use of raw materials to create a visually appealing item must not be discounted. However, it is the appeal both types of vessel make to the sense of smell that is key to their interpretation. The blue lotus chalices contained fragrant libations for funerary rituals and released metaphorical eternal scent for the dead. Similarly, the expectation of pleasant aromas emerging from a flower was confirmed when the lid was lifted from the unguents or spices contained within the Minoan blossom bowls. Considering the tomb findspots of many examples of this vessel, these too may have had a role in funerary ceremonies, and again, the stone flowers perhaps provided perpetual olfactory offerings long after the original contents had been used or decomposed.

## Artificial Flowers in Kamares Ware

Blossom bowls are a rather straightforward example of synesthetic objects, the visible artifact enhanced by metaphorical and real scents. But Minoan vessels that may have enhanced olfactory experiences are not limited to those of stone, and the ceramics of the Protopalatial period provide further food for thought. One of the most distinctive types of pottery from this first palace era is Kamares ware, with its characteristic red, black, white, and orange decoration. This rich polychrome pottery is in stark contrast to other contemporary ceramics as well as its predecessors, and the arresting visual impact should not be underestimated. Motifs are hugely varied and encompass swirls, circles, dots, spirals, and rosettes, although very few examples of what could be termed representational imagery can be identified: a fish, some trees and flowers, and a range of rather oddly shaped people are the main examples (Walberg [1987] terms these "pictorialized" and "pictorial" motifs). Much of this imagery has an overall organic air, as the motifs intertwine and curl around the vessels, often enhancing their shape, and no two vessels are the same.

The majority of Kamares ware is wheel-thrown, and some examples have such thin walls that they are known as egg-shell ware. The finest Kamares vessels are associated with the palatial sites of Knossos and Phaistos, the latter located in the fertile Mesara region just south of the eponymous Kamares cave. Indeed, while Kamares ware does occur at other nonpalatial sites (Walberg 1983), its use appears to have been restricted mainly to locations of an elite nature. The shapes of the majority of Kamares vessels—cups, jugs, bridge-spouted jars, and pedestaled bowls of varying heights—suggest that they were used for drinking, serving liquids, and perhaps displaying foodstuffs. Indeed, it is thought that sets of Kamares pottery played a part at conspicuous-consumption events, perhaps the feasts that have been suggested by some to have been a key element in the forging of alliances and status negotiations that are believed to have accompanied the emergence of palatial centers (Day and Wilson 1998; Hamilakis 2002b).

### *Relief Flowers*

A number of Kamares-ware vessels exhibit relief decoration known as barbotine work, in which surface texture is created through manipulating slip, in some instances producing an effect suggestive of rocks or barnacles (e.g., Evans 1921–1935:IV:100–106). This finish certainly adds a greater tactile dimension to the vessels, perhaps even dictating how the user consumes from or otherwise interacts with the vessel. Another relief technique is to attach mold-made or modeled motifs. These attachments typically include human figures, animals, and marine life, but also flowers, which are the focus of this chapter. Interestingly, while ceramic relief was used in the wider eastern Mediterranean during the Bronze Age (Foster 1982:123–142), floral-relief elements are limited primarily to Crete in MM II–MM III (c. 1800–1600 B.C.E.). One of the earliest examples of this technique is a bridge-spouted jar, from Quartier Gamma at Mallia, with attached rosettes (Demargne and Gallet de Santerre 1953:Plate xiv), a three-dimensional version of the common painted rosette motif (Figure 14-4). Indeed, applied rosettes remain a feature of Minoan ceramics throughout the Protopalatial period, such as those on the bull jar from Anemospilia (Sakellarakis and Sapouna-Sakellaraki 1997:548–562) or on the bridge-spouted jar from Phaistos (Levi 1976:Plate lxxviii). Other unattached molded flowers have been recovered, presumably either broken off vessels or not yet applied, for example at Kommos (Betancourt 1990:Plate 71:1341, Plate 72:1379) and Knossos (Evans 1921–1935:IV.1:Plate xxixc).

More extravagant attached flowers have also been recovered, most famously on the so-called Phaistos krater (Levi 1976:101, Plate xxviia) (Figure 14-5). This large vessel, almost half a meter tall, has received harsh treatment at the hands of some scholars and has been called an "aberration" and "perhaps the most vulgar object of Minoan workmanship so far known" (Higgins 1974:29). It is painted with a checkered pattern around the lower part of the bowl, while the vessel stem and upper part of the bowl feature red thorns or coral. It is the attached flowers, four on the bowl and three on the stem, with white petals—featuring an incised central line—and red centers, that are especially impressive. A matching jug, featuring the same checkered pattern and red coral, presumably formed part of a set with the krater, although only a broken attachment remains to indicate where the relief flower once sprouted (Levi 1976:101, Plate xxviib). These two vessels were found together, along with other ceramics, in the pottery storage area of Room LV of the Protopalatial remains at Phaistos.

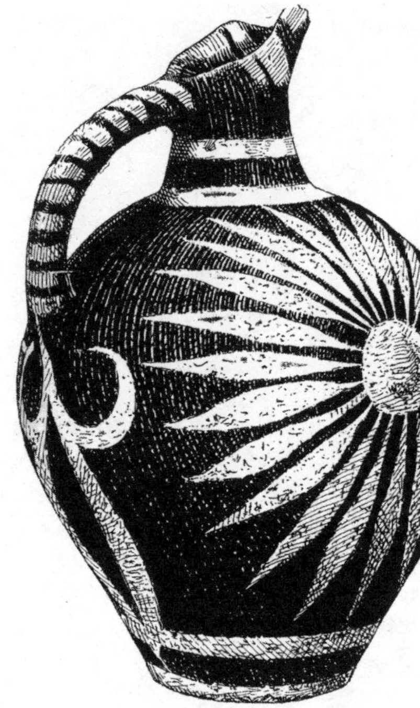

**Figure 14-4.** *Kamares-ware jug with painted rosette, Phaistos (Evans 1921–1935:I:Figure 198).*

Numerous other examples of similar attached ceramic flowers can be found.[4] An early Middle Minoan bowl (Figure 14-6) from Sphoungaras in east Crete features a pedestal topped with a red and white flower rising from its center, thus giving the impression of a lone blossom floating on the surface when the vessel was filled (Day 2007:214; Hall 1912:56–57;). Pedestaled flowers also occur on an animal-headed jug from Phaistos, rising from either side of the spout (Pernier 1935:Plate xxix), and on a globular vase from the same site (Levi 1976:Plate xlii). A similarly shaped vessel from Ayia Triadha displays twelve vertical ribs, of which six are topped with a white flower, although it probably should be assumed that all twelve were originally alike (La Rosa 1994–1996:Plate 10a-b). A Cretan export (or maybe a locally produced copy of Kamares ware) found at Qubbet el-Hawa in Egypt displays the most elaborate of this type of floral relief with five large petals flanking the vessel's mouth, thus forming a flower, and five more whole blossoms attached around the vessel's shoulder (Kemp and Merrillees 1980:Figure 60). As with the simpler rosettes, detached fragments of these higher relief flowers have also turned up in excavations at Mallia (Detournay et al. 1980:Figure 185) and Phaistos (Levi 1976:Figure 586).

### *Relief and Painted Petals*

A second type of relief floral decoration must also be included in this analysis: petal bands. Like the relief flowers, petal bands occur on Kamares-ware vessels, again especially those found at Phaistos. The Phaistos krater features one such indented relief band around its base, which is white with incised lines in the

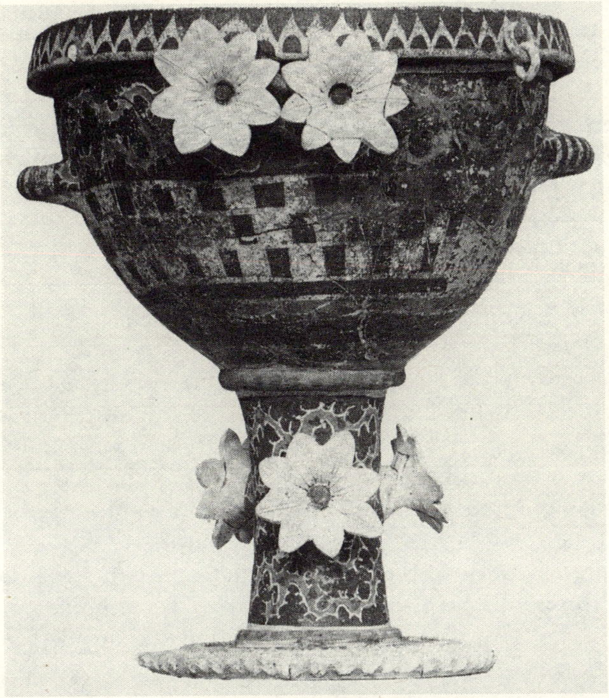

**Figure 14-5.** *Krater with floral relief, Phaistos (F1031) (Levi 1976:Plate XXVII). Used with permission of Scuola Archeologica Italiana di Atene.*

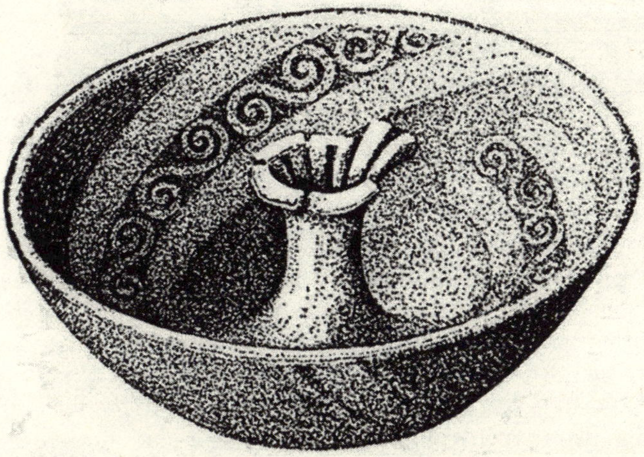

**Figure 14-6.** *Bowl with "floating" flower, Sphoungaras (Hall 1912:Figure 29).*

center of each protrusion or petal (see Figure 14-5). These central incisions link the petal bands to the relief flowers, which also display this feature, and maybe even to the later blossom bowls with their very obvious raised midribs. Identical white petals are attached to the rims of a fruitstand and two bowls, all of which are also from Phaistos (Levi 1976:Plates 62, xxviic 184e, xlib). A small piriform rhyton, again painted with the red coral motif, also has white petals around its mouth, although in this instance the petals feature a central spiral rather than a groove (Levi 1976:Plate xlvb). Further fragments of similar creamy-white petal bands come from Knossos (Evans 1921–1935:IV.1:Plate xxixa-b; MacGillivray 1998:Plates 63, 91) and Kommos (Betancourt 1990:Plate 72:1367). Perhaps the most intriguing example is the tall hollow pedestal or stand from Phaistos (Figure 14-7), which features a petal band, not only around the rim, but also one around the base and another two-thirds of the way up the vessel (Levi 1976:214, Plate lxxiv).

Less elaborate versions of this petal rim also exist, with the decoration painted instead of attached in clay. The Phaistos krater displays small white triangles running around the rim. Such bands can also be found on a variety of other shapes, such as bridge-spouted jars (Levi 1976:Plate xxa), but it is especially common on cups. On numerous examples of cups, the petals extend upward from the base, rather than down from the rim, another similarity to blossom bowls (Levi 1976:Plates 81f, 125g-k, 133k) (Figure 14-8). Evans noted this phenomenon, although it has been little remarked on since then (Evans 1921–1935:I:241, 1921–1935:II.2:697). Importantly, these painted petals are not to be confused with the fluted skeuomorphs of metal vessels that also occur (e.g., Knappett 2005:144–146). While the cups that apparently derived their inspiration from metal vessels are only fluted on the sides, the petals on the florally inspired vessels usually extend from the base upward. The term *skeuomorph* could equally be applied in this case, but here it refers to taking the form of flowers rather than that of vessels in other materials.

### *Suggested Functions of Relief and Painted Petals*

One possible explanation for the relief decoration is that the attached petals and flowers should be seen as indicators of the vessels' contents, in the same way that plastic tomatoes are filled with ketchup today (Day 2006:34–35). This is not just modern marketing practice; examples can be found among prehistoric societies in which vessels' contents may be signaled either via the shape of the vessel itself or the iconography—or even the text—on it. For example, poppy-shaped Cypriot Base Ring juglets contained opium (Bisset et al. 1996; Merrillees 1962), while certain Maya vessels displayed glyphs indicating their use for cacao consumption (Hall et al. 1990). Unsurprisingly, various attempts have been made to find a corresponding real flower with white, grooved petals and a red center, although none are wholly satisfactory. They are often assumed to be lilies, presumably because the white lily is a recurring motif in later Neopalatial frescoes and ceramics, although the actual morphological similarities to the relief flowers are limited. In other instances (e.g., Foster 1982:96; Levi 1976:72), they have been identified as marguerites—members of the daisy family—although this is an exceptionally large species group and thus not a very specific or helpful identification. In fact, it is useful to remember that the Minoans could produce recognizable models of plants, such as the faience crocuses from Knossos (Evans 1921–1935:I:Figure 358) or the relief lilies on jars from Mochlos (Brogan 2004). Therefore, the difficulties inherent in identifying a precise species for the relief flowers suggest that perhaps

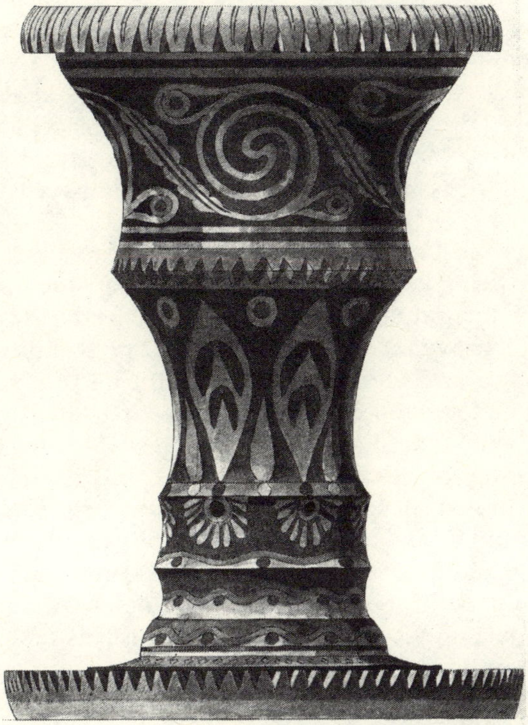

**Figure 14-7.** *Pedestal with relief petals, Phaistos (F1053) (Levi 1976:Plate LXXIV). Used with permission of Scuola Archeologica Italiana di Atene.*

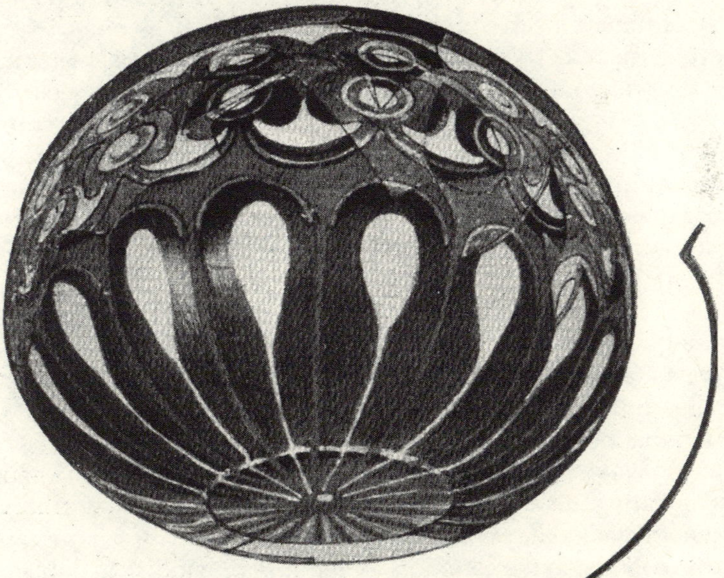

**Figure 14-8.** *Calyx cup, Knossos (Evans 1921–1935:I:Figure 181).*

no one species was intended and that thinking beyond the visual toward multisensory interpretations may be a more productive avenue.

It seems safe to assume that these elaborate vessels, both with relief petals and with attached flowers, were used at elite feasts or drinking events, whatever the exact nature of these occasions. Many of the vessels are large ones for communal use (e.g., krater, fruitstand, pedestal) and presumably would have remained on display for the duration of the event, obvious signs of access to skilled craftsmanship. Jugs, jars, and bowls would have played a more mobile role, perhaps passing from hand to hand or being controlled by hosts or other servers. The painted cups, in contrast, were for individual use, and certainly the lack of relief petals on these vessels would have made them easier to handle and to drink from. However, the fact that petals still featured as part of the decorative repertoire suggests an important role for floral decoration in feasting sets. Interestingly, Rutter (2004) has tentatively identified Late Minoan ceramic sets at Kommos, consisting of matching florally painted cups, bowls, jugs, and jars. He sees this usage of a distinctively decorated set of drinking and eating vessels as having the potential to distinguish individuals or even social groups through their material culture (Rutter 2004:79). Similarly, Knappett has discussed the vessel hierarchy evident within a ceramic deposit at Protopalatial Knossos (Knappett 2005:147–148, 2008:125; MacDonald and Knappett 2007:161–165). This same concept can be applied to the discrete group of Protopalatial relief vessels under discussion here also, a type perhaps associated in particular with Phaistos. It should be stressed that the majority of Protopalatial cups and jugs are much plainer, and any use of Kamares ware, let alone that resplendent with relief floral elements, would have been extremely noticeable.

But even if such sets were used to create or reinforce social hierarchies, the nature of the decoration itself demands further consideration. On closer inspection, it can be said that the majority of the relief-petal decoration is concentrated on the vessel rims. This serves to turn the vessels into flowers, with the aromas released by the contents wafting out of the vessel's mouth, much as a flower releases its scents. As for what these contents were, archaeological evidence shows that wine was certainly consumed on Minoan Crete (Hamilakis 1996; McGovern 2009; McGovern et al. 1996). Whether this was watered down prior to consumption, as in later Classical Greece, remains unknown. Organic residue analysis has suggested that extra flavorings, such as spices, honey, and pine resin, may have been added to Minoan beverages, although no analysis has been carried out on the elaborate vessels in question here (Tzedakis and Martlew 1999; Tzedakis et al. 2008). It could even be suggested that petals of real flowers might have been included (such as in the Caucasian drink *ovshala,* which uses rose petals), thus contributing another flavor and complementing the artificial petals on the vessel exterior. Furthermore, these drinks did not have to be served cold, and the provision of handles on Kamares-ware cups, in contrast to the common contemporary handleless goblets, facilitates holding hot liquids (although see Knappett 2005:141–142 for an opposing view). Heating whatever drink was served in the vessels would have acted not only to blend the flavors and increase fragrance, but the steam rising from the vessels may have also been perceived as making scent visible. The individual cups allowed those present to partake in this scented experience at a personal level. Moreover, when the cup is lifted to the drinker's mouth and the painted calyx becomes visible to others, it produces the appearance of consuming out of a flower, thus adding another layer of metaphorical scent to the activity.

## Aromas, Real and Imagined

The significance of vessels deliberately designed to create the effect of consuming from fragrant flowers requires further discussion, and it is here that an intersensorial explanation can help. Stephen Houston and Karl Taube, in their work on Mesoamerican senses, developed the concept of synesthetic material culture, whereby something seen by the eye conveys sensations experienced by other sensory organs like the ear or the nose (Houston and Taube 2000:263). Although ceramic or stone floral vessels do not actually exude aromas by themselves, a combination of their contents and their form reinforces the olfactory experience. The crucial fact that aromas can affect emotions and social processes was briefly introduced above, and it is in these bodily and emotional effects of scents that an explanation for such floral vessels should be sought.

The feasting events of Protopalatial Crete, and indeed other periods in the Aegean Bronze Age, have come to prominence in recent years as archaeologists explore the multiple social dramas played out over the sharing of food and drink (e.g., Halstead and Barrett 2004; Wright 2004; more generally, Dietler and Hayden 2001). In general, the multisensory nature of these events has been overlooked in favor of debate about feast typology and function (e.g., Girella 2008), although there have been some exceptions (Fox 2008; Hamilakis 2008). In the context of this chapter and indeed this volume, however, it is important to foreground the physical, sensory experience of the feast. The tastes and aromas of the beverages served in the floral Kamares-ware vessels would not have been the only olfactory stimulation. We should also bear in mind the smell of the accompanying food, including perhaps that of the actual cooking process; of aromatics smoking in ceramic burners; of the scented oils that the participants had applied to their bodies and clothes; of oil or beeswax lamps; of dogs or other animals; of a hearth; of flowers or plants in pots; and the natural smells of human bodies and waste.[5] Such atmospheres would have been accompanied by the consumption of alcoholic drinks or, indeed, other psychotropic substances, both of which bring altered states of perception. Therefore, the combination of inebriation with the many different aromas and the synesthetic floral vessels, as well as perhaps music, singing, and dancing, created a very specific shared bodily experience.

At one level, such an experience is simply pleasurable, and fun should not be written out of prehistory. But smells are never meaningless, even if their meanings often remain at a subconscious level and change over time. The selection of a perfume or an aftershave today is not a random event (unless received as an unwelcome gift!) but rather is carefully chosen not just for its smell but also for the associated values expressed through wearing that particular scent as opposed to any other.[6] For example, Christian Dior's Poison bottled the 1980s' mood of luxury and exotic seduction, in contrast to Calvin Klein's 1994 CK One, a scent that supposedly captured the disaffected, androgynous youth of Generation X (Wilson 2007). Apart from such zeitgeisty references, the link between smell and identity is also borne out by numerous anthropological studies showing how odor is important in group definition. Perhaps the most well-known example is that of the Dassanetch of East Africa, for whom it has been reported that the pastoralists view the fishermen as socially inferior, justified by a complex system of olfactory semiotics (Almagor 1987). In fact, throughout history accusations of "smelling bad" have served to reinforce and vindicate the alterity of races, religions, and classes, by thrusting a negative moral identity upon a particular population (Classen 1992; Synnott 1991:449).

To return to the Aegean Bronze Age then, the scented feasts envisaged above are not just about having a good time or displaying social status but rather about the presentation of a certain identity. As Murphy (this volume) comments regarding the distinction between persons who received perfume from the wanax (ruler) at Mycenaean Pylos and those who were not privy to such gatherings, similar experiences must be considered for inhabitants of Minoan Crete. Sharing in a fragrance creates unity with others at that moment, serving to de-individualize the participants to some extent (Borthwick 2000:132–133; Kenna 2005:58). At a time when social hierarchies were forming within and between polities on the island, sharing in such events would have helped to form strong social bonds based on bodily mnemonics. The use and reuse of such distinctive sets of drinking equipment at certain events would have produced a series of intertwined memories in which pots, people, smells, and tastes merged (an "affective field" in the phrase coined by Harris and Sørensen [2010]). Subsequent to the communal event, memories of it and of the solidarity with others could be triggered by inhaling the same smells or encountering other reminders of the sensory experience. Moreover, gatherings like this not only formed a cohesive bond between attendees but also created distance from those not present; this disparity was enhanced by the differing olfactory experiences.

We certainly should not imagine that it was only the Minoan elite who fragranced themselves and their environment. The Cretan landscape is filled with plants with aromatic properties, such as cistus (mainly *Cistus creticus*) and sages (*Salvia* sp.), which anyone could have gathered. Instead, the distinction would have been between those who had access to rarer scented products imported from overseas (like the cinnamon and myrrh referred to in the Linear B tablets from LM IIIB Knossos [Sarpaki 2001]), or at least from other regions on the island, and those who had to content themselves with locally sourced scents. These more exotic smells would have clung to the bodies and clothes of those present even after the event itself, a silent message of conspicuous inaccessibility to everyone else (following Knappett 2008:126).

The assumption of the purely secular nature of these feasts should be queried, and Hamilakis (2008:7–10) has pointed out the close ties between feasting and ritual apparent in the Aegean Bronze Age. Here, too, smell has an important role to play. Scents and scented products are often associated with deities, spirits, or other worlds, perhaps due to the somewhat ethereal nature of a smell. These nonhuman beings can sometimes receive sustenance from smells. In classical Greece, the gods feasted on the aromatic smoke produced by the meat burning on the sacrificial fire (Zaidman and Pantel 1992:36). In the Flower World spiritual complex of Mesoamerica and the American Southwest, spirits consumed smells, whether of food, flowers, incense, or blood (Taube 2004:73). In this belief system, which is just one example of the many societies in which the concepts of smell, spirit, wind, breath, and life are closely intertwined (Parkin 2007:40), fragrant blossoms were associated with life force and breath (Hays-Gilpin and Hill 1999; Taube 2010:146–147). As well as nourishing nonhuman beings with smells, the act of proffering fragrances is a medium for communication between different worlds. The visible smoke or vapor that rises upward is often conceptualized as making its way to other worlds, carrying human messages with it. This message can be a plea for the spirit or god to appear in the human world—for example, to carry out healing or bestow blessings—or an offering of thanks. To the Egyptians, incense was depicted as the sweat of the gods, and inhaling it was a way for humans to be in contact with the divine (Meskell and Joyce 2003:20). Deities and spirits can also have their own aromas, allowing humans to recognize when they are in the presence of divinity. Classical Greek gods anointed themselves with the magical fragrant substance ambrosia, which also had the benefit of preventing them from aging (Clay 1981–1982). The concept of the "odor of sanctity" pervaded early Christianity, a smell that indicated the exemplary holiness and divine favor enjoyed by the odor's producer (Classen et al. 1994:52–54; see also Ashbrook Harvey 2006).

It should also be considered, therefore, whether the use of aromatic substances at Minoan feasts, and indeed in other settings for ritual, was to feed the spirits or gods or to communicate with them in some way, perhaps even invoking their presence.[7] Creation of a scented atmosphere may have been thought to produce an environment suited to a divine visit. The choice of aromatics in such instances is deliberate, with different results attributed to different substances (e.g., Gell 1977:26; Parkin 2007:43, 46–47). Unsurprisingly, access to divinities in this manner would have contributed to the prestige of those who apparently could communicate with them. In this way, smells contribute to a specific temporality, marking a place and time as special. Howes has drawn attention to the roles of smell in moments or periods of transition, describing it as "the liminal sense *par excellence*" (1987:401). Citing a wide variety of examples, he demonstrates how there is a close connection between smell and cognitive transformations at logical, psychological, and sociological levels (Howes 1987:410). Therefore, it is to be expected that fragrances at Minoan communal events functioned on many levels also. The real scents from the drinks, food, or fragrant offerings combined with the imagined aromas of the floral vessels to create a distinct, sensory experience in which the social bonds or gulfs created between humans and the sacred bonds formed with gods or spirits became embedded in bodily memory.

## Conclusions

In a Bronze Age eastern Mediterranean world where scented substances were prevalent, the role of aromatics in Minoan Crete deserves a closer look. This chapter has adopted the methodology of synesthetic material culture to discuss how artifacts and aromatics combined together to create specific sensory experiences. The singling out of olfaction for treatment here is not intended to suggest that other senses were unimportant to the Minoans, but rather it is done to draw attention to a little-studied aspect of that society. Both the blossom bowls and the Kamares ware discussed in this chapter certainly had striking visual and tactile appeal too. However, the links between smell and emotion and memory make olfaction a particularly powerful sense; indeed, odor is "above all a statement of who one is" (Synnott 1991:438). In the context of Protopalatial feasts, olfactory stimulation contributed to the moral construction of the self or the group and the other, that is, those persons participating and those being excluded. The vessels of Kamares ware with floral or petal reliefs added an extra layer of sensory experience to an already intense event. Such events are understood to have been essential in the creation and maintenance of hierarchies on Crete, a distinction perhaps further emphasized by ritual elements in the proceedings. Smells have the power to transcend boundaries and as such are the perfect medium to feed or contact spirits, gods, or the dead. Communicating with these other beings at feasts via fragrant offerings may have lent the hosts or attendees a certain religious authority. The use of Minoan blossom bowls, as well as Egyptian lotus chalices, in funerary ritual may well be linked to this transcendent aspect of smells too. The scent of the vessel contents is important at the time of the ceremonies while the metaphorical scent released by the stone flowers left in the tomb provides sweet smells for eternity.

As a final note, some preliminary suggestions about further connections between olfaction and Minoan material culture are proposed here. As the choice in this chapter of floral artifacts from both the Protopalatial and Neopalatial periods demonstrates, the Minoans had a long-standing tradition of vibrant floral iconography in a range of media. The contextual sensory analysis adopted here has pointed toward new ways to interpret this body of material. Moving beyond the search for the meanings of individual plant motifs and specific florally decorated artifacts, it could be suggested that the Minoans may have had some kind of overall spiritual or cultural tradition centered on the floral world. In this regard, an interesting analogy can be made with the Flower World complex of Mesoamerica and the American Southwest, where floral iconography is a manifestation of an intricate system of beliefs (Hays-Gilpin and Hill 1999). Ornate carving on building facades symbolized exhalations of fragrant floral breath (Taube 2004:84–86), and ceramics with petal rims became portals to the Flower World (Mathiowetz 2010; Taube 2010:166, Figures 18–19). These artifacts were perceived to have an olfactory dimension and visual analysis alone is not sufficient to understand their significance. Attention has also been drawn to the way Mesoamerican societies could represent odor in iconography (Houston and Taube 2000), a fascinating idea but one unremarkable within the Maya or Aztec sensorium. In a similar fashion,

Egyptians may also have had an iconographic device for making the invisible visible. Depictions of banquets show what have been described as "incense cones" atop the participants' heads. Previously thought to be an actual cone of scented fat that would have melted into the wearer's wig and so released pleasant smells during a feast, it has more recently, and perhaps more plausibly, been proposed to symbolize aroma and indicate a scented environment (Meskell and Joyce 2003:56).

In the light of all these possibilities, one wonders whether more of the Minoan material might also have held olfactory meanings. For example, could the landscape frescoes of the Minoan Neopalatial era have been perceived in a synesthetic fashion, their constantly open flowers offering year-round scent to gods and spirits, as well as providing a metaphorical scented backdrop for whatever activities occured in their vicinities? Might we even consider actual scented frescoes, with aromatic substances applied to the painted images, somewhat similar to the mixing of musk with mortar to fragrance certain mosques in Persia (Green and Taylor 1986)? Only an archaeology that is open to acknowledging the full sensory and synesthetic potential of material culture can explore such previously inconceivable ideas.

## Acknowledgments

Thanks to Peter Warren for his assistance with my queries about stone vessels and to Mike Mathiowetz, whose paper at the SAA meeting in St. Louis in 2010 brought the iconography of the Flower World of Mesoamerica and the American Southwest to my attention; he also provided helpful references. William Megarry aided with map production. Thanks, too, to the other participants at the CAI conference for their comments and questions, and to Christine Morris for her thoughts on an earlier draft.

## Notes

1. For example, a recent article on emotions and material culture (Harris and Sørenson 2010) does not consider the emotions of the archaeologist at all, despite striving to incorporate them into an interpretation of past behavior.

2. Absolute dates for Minoan chronology are still debated; this article follows those used by Dickinson (1994: Figures 1.2, 1.3). Standard abbreviations for Minoan eras are used here: EM - Early Minoan, MM - Middle Minoan, and LM - Late Minoan.

3. On iconographic reinforcement, see Morris 1995.

4. See Day 2007, chapter six, for greater detail and a catalog of these vessels.

5. These suggestions are drawn from the archaeological material, with some chronological leeway within the Bronze Age. On incense burners, see Georgiou 1979; on perfumed oils, see Murphy this volume and Shelmerdine 1985; on Minoan lamps, Evershed et al. 1999; on dogs in frescoes and on seals, Marinatos and Morgan 2005; on hearths, Muhly 1984; for pot plants, see Platon 1987.

6. Much as consumers like to claim indifference to the power of branding, there is little doubt that almost every purchasing choice is a complex negotiation between perceived self-identity, aspirations, and brand values.

7. Following to its logical conclusion the idea that Minoans may have offered aromatics to spirits, gods, or the dead, it could be suggested that this implies a belief that these beings had human-type senses, that is, they could actually smell and appreciate the scented offerings.

## References


Almagor, Uri

1987 The Cycle and Stagnation of Smells: Pastoralists-Fishermen Relationships in an East African Society. *Res: Anthropology and Aesthetics* 13:106–121.

Ashbrook Harvey, Susan

2006 *Scenting Salvation: Ancient Christianity and the Olfactory Imagination*. University of California Press, Berkeley.

Betancourt, Philip P.

1990 *Kommos II. The Final Neolithic through Middle Minoan III Pottery*. Princeton University Press, Oxford.

Bevan, Andrew

2004 Emerging Civilized Values? The Consumption and Imitation of Egyptian Stone Vessels in EM II–MM I Crete and Its Wider Eastern Mediterranean Context. In *The Emergence of Civilisation Revisited*, edited by John C. Barrett and Paul Halstead, pp. 107–126. Oxbow, Oxford.

2007 *Stone Vessels and Values in the Bronze Age Mediterranean*. Cambridge University Press, Cambridge.

Bevan, Andrew, Evangelia Kiriatzi, Carl Knappett, Evangelia Kappa, and Sophia Papachristou

2002 Excavation of Neopalatial Deposits at Tholos (Kastri), Kythera. *Annual of the British School at Athens* 97:55–96.

Bisset, Norman G., Jan G. Bruhn, and Meinhart H. Zenk

1996 The Presence of Opium in a 3,500 Year Old Cypriote Base-Ring Juglet. *Ägypten und Levante* 6:203–204.

Boivin, Nicole

2008 *Material Cultures, Material Minds*. Cambridge University Press, Cambridge.

Borthwick, Fiona

2000 Olfaction and Taste: Invasive Odours and Disappearing Objects. *Australian Journal of Anthropology* 11:127–140.

Brogan, Thomas M.

2004 The Incised and Relief Lily Jars from Mochlos. In *Crete beyond the Palaces: Proceedings of the Crete 2000 Conference*, edited by Leslie P. Day, Margaret S. Mook, and James D. Muhly, pp. 29–41. INSTAP Academic Press, Philadelphia.

Chapin, Anne P.

2004 Power, Privilege, and Landscape in Minoan Art. In ΧΑΡΙΣ: *Essays in Honor of Sara A. Immerwahr*, edited by Anne P. Chapin, pp. 47–64. Hesperia Supplement 33. American School of Classical Studies at Athens, Princeton, New Jersey.

Classen, Constance

1992 The Odor of the Other: Olfactory Symbolism and Cultural Categories. *Ethos* 20:133–166.

Classen, Constance, David Howes, and Anthony Synnott
1994 *Aroma: The Cultural History of Smell*. Routledge, London.
Clay, Jenny S.
1981–1982 Immortal and Ageless Forever. *Classical Journal* 77:112–117.
D'Agata, Anna Lucia
1997 Incense and Perfumes in the Late Bronze Age Aegean. In *Profumi D'Arabia. Atti del Convegno*, edited by Alessandra Avanzini, pp. 85–99. L'Erma di Bretschneider, Rome.
Day, Jo
2006 Making 'Scents' of Flowery Pots. Considering Minoan Ceramic Vessels with Botanical Relief. In *SOMA 2004. Symposium on Mediterranean Archaeology*, edited by Jo Day, Cybelle Greenlaw, Heinrich Hall, Amanda Kelly, Lidia Matassa, Killian McAleese, Emma Saunders, and Deirdre Stritch, pp. 33–37. BAR International Series 1514. Archaeopress, Oxford.
2011 Crocuses in Context. A Diachronic Survey of the Crocus Motif in the Aegean Bronze Age. *Hesperia* 80:337–379.
Day, Joanna C.
2007 An Exploration of the Social Roles of Plants in the Bronze Age Aegean. Unpublished Ph.D. dissertation, Department of Classics, Trinity College, Dublin.
Day, Peter M., and David E. Wilson
1998 Consuming Power: Kamares Ware in Protopalatial Knossos. *Antiquity* 72:350–358.
Demargne, Pierre, and Hubert Gallet de Santerre
1953 Fouilles Exécutées à Mallia. Exploration des Maisons et Quartiers d'Habitation (1921–1948). *Études Crétoises* IX. Paul Geuthner, Paris.
Detournay, Béatrice, Jean-Claude Poursat, and Frieda Vandenabeele
1980 Fouilles Exécutées à Mallia: Le Quartier Mu II. *Études Crétoises* XXVI. Paul Geuthner, Paris.
Dickinson, Oliver T. P.
1994 *The Aegean Bronze Age*. Cambridge University Press, Cambridge.
Dietler, Michael, and Brian D. Hayden (editors)
2001 *Feasts: Archaeological and Ethnographic Perspectives on Food, Politics, and Power.* Smithsonian Institution Press, Washington, D.C.
Doumas, Christos
1992 *The Wall Paintings of Thera*. The Thera Foundation, Athens.
Driessen, Jan, Ilse Schoep, and Robert Laffineur (editors)
2002 *Monuments of Minos: Rethinking the Minoan Palaces*. Aegaeum 23. Université de Liège, Liège.
Engen, Trygg
1982 *The Perception of Odors*. Academic Press, New York.
Evans, Arthur, J.
1895 *Cretan Pictographs and Prae-Phoenician Script, with an Account of a Sepulchral Deposit at Hagios Onuphrios Near Phaestos in Its Relation to Primitive Aegean Culture*. Bernard Quaritch, London.
1921–1935 *The Palace of Minos at Knossos*. 4 vols. Macmillan, London.
Evershed, Richard P., Sarah J. Vaughan, Stephanie N. Dudd, and Jeffrey S. Soles
1999 Organic Residue, Petrographic and Typological Analyses of Late Minoan Lamps and Conical Cups from Excavations at Mochlos in East Crete, Greece. In *Palaeodiet in the Aegean*, edited by Sarah J. Vaughan and William D. E. Coulson, pp. 37–54. Oxbow, Oxford.

Fappas, Ioannis
2008 The Use of Perfumed Oils during Feasting Activities: A Comparison of Mycenaean and Near Eastern Written Sources. In *DAIS: The Aegean Feast*, edited by Louise A. Hitchcock, Robert Laffineur, and Janice Crowley, pp. 367–377. Aegaeum 29. Université de Liège, Liège.

Foster, Karen P.
1982 *Minoan Ceramic Relief*. Paul Åströms Förlag, Göteborg.

Fox, Rachel
2008 Tastes, Smells, and Spaces: Sensory Perceptions and Mycenaean Palatial Feasting. In *DAIS: The Aegean Feast*, edited by Louise A. Hitchcock, Robert Laffineur, and Janice Crowley, pp. 133–141. Aegaeum 29. Université de Liège, Liège.

Gell, Alfred
1977 Magic, Perfume, Dream. In *Symbols and Sentiments: Cross-Cultural Studies in Symbolism*, edited by Ioan M. Lewis, pp. 25–38. Academic Press, London.

Georgiou, Hara S.
1974 Aromatics in Antiquity and in Minoan Crete: A Review and Assessment. *Kretika Chronika* 25:441–456.
1979 Late Minoan Incense Burners. *American Journal of Archaeology* 83:427–435.
1980 Minoan Fireboxes: A Study of Form and Function. *Studi Micenei ed Egeo-Anatolici* 21:123–192.

Girella, Luca
2008 Feasts in 'Transition'? An Overview of Feasting Practices during MM III in Crete. In *DAIS: The Aegean Feast*, edited by Louise A. Hitchcock, Robert Laffineur, and Janice Crowley, pp. 3–19. Aegaeum 29. Université de Liège, Liège.

Gosden, Chris
2005 What Do Objects Want? *Journal of Archaeological Method and Theory* 12:193–211.

Green, Michael J. B., and Richard Taylor
1986 The Musk Connection. *New Scientist* 110(1514):56–58.

Hägg, Robin, and Nanno Marinatos (editors)
1987 *The Function of the Minoan Palaces*. Swedish Institute in Athens, Paul Åströms Förlag, Stockholm.

Haldane, Cheryl W.
1993 Direct Evidence for Organic Cargoes in the Late Bronze Age. *World Archaeology* 24:348–360.

Hall, Edith H.
1912 *Excavations in Eastern Crete: Sphoungaras*. University Museum, Philadelphia.

Hall, Grant D., Stanley M. Tarka, W. Jeffrey Hurst, David Stuart, and Richard E. W. Adams
1990 Cacao Residues in Ancient Maya Vessels from Rio Azul, Guatemala. *American Antiquity* 55:138–143.

Halstead, Paul, and John C. Barrett (editors)
2004 *Food, Cuisine and Society in Prehistoric Greece*. Oxbow, Oxford.

Hamilakis, Yannis
1996 Wine, Oil and the Dialectics of Power in Bronze Age Crete: A Review of the Evidence. *Oxford Journal of Archaeology* 15:1–32.
2002a What Future for the 'Minoan' Past? Re-thinking Minoan Archaeology. In *Labyrinth Revisited: Rethinking Minoan Archaeology*, edited by Yannis Hamilakis, pp. 2–28. Oxbow, Oxford.
2002b Too Many Chiefs? Factional Competition in Neopalatial Crete. In *Monuments of Minos: Rethinking the Minoan Palaces*, edited by Jan Driessen, Ilse Schoep, and Robert Laffineur, pp. 179–199. Aegaeum 23. Université de Liège, Liège.

2008 Time, Performance, and the Production of a Mnemonic Record: From Feasting to an Archaeology of Eating and Drinking. In *DAIS: The Aegean Feast*, edited by Louise A. Hitchcock, Robert Laffineur, and Janice Crowley, pp. 3–19. Aegaeum 29. Université de Liège, Liège.

Harris, Oliver J. T., and Tim Flohr Sørenson

2010 Rethinking Emotion and Material Culture. *Archaeological Dialogues* 17:145–163.

Hays-Gilpin, Kelley, and Jane H. Hill

1999 The Flower World in Material Culture: An Iconographic Complex in the Southwest and Mesoamerica. *Journal of Anthropological Research* 55:1–37.

Higgins, Reynold

1974 [1967] *Minoan and Mycenaean Art*. Thames and Hudson, London.

Hood, Sinclair

1994 *The Arts in Prehistoric Greece*. Yale University Press, New Haven.

Houston, Stephen D., and Karl A. Taube

2000 An Archaeology of the Senses: Perception and Cultural Expression in Mesoamerica. *Cambridge Archaeological Journal* 10:261–294.

Howes, David

1987 Olfaction and Transition: An Essay on the Ritual Uses of Smell. *Canadian Review of Sociology and Anthropology* 24:398–416.

2005 Introduction: Empires of the Senses. In *Empire of the Senses: The Sensual Culture Reader*, edited by David Howes, pp. 1–17. Berg, Oxford.

Kemp, Barry J., and Robert S. Merrillees

1980 *Minoan Pottery in Second Millennium Egypt*. Philipp von Zabern, Mainz am Rhein.

Kenna, Margaret E.

2005 Why Does Incense Smell Religious? Greek Orthodoxy and the Anthropology of Smell. *Journal of Mediterranean Studies* 15:51–70.

Knapp, A. Bernard

1991 Spice, Drugs, Grain, and Grog: Organic Goods in Bronze Age East Mediterranean Trade. In *Bronze Age Trade in the Mediterranean*, edited by Noel H. Gale, pp. 19–66. SIMA 90. Paul Åströms Förlag, Göteborg.

Knappett, Carl

2005 *Thinking through Material Culture: An Interdisciplinary Perspective*. University of Pennsylvania Press, Philadelphia.

2008 Protopalatial Crete: The Material Culture. In *The Cambridge Companion to the Aegean Bronze Age*, edited by Cynthia W. Shelmerdine, pp. 121–139. Cambridge University Press, Cambridge.

Koh, Andrew

2008 *Wreathed in a Fragrant Cloud: Reconstructing a Late Bronze Age Aegean Workshop of Aromata*. VDM Verlag Dr. Müller, Saärbrucken.

La Rosa, Vincenzo

1994–1996 Αγ ία Τριάδα. Κρητικι Εστια 5:326–332.

Levi, Doro

1976 *Festós e la civiltá minoica*. Incunabula Graeca 40. Edizioni dell'Ateneo, Rome.

MacDonald, Colin F., and Carl Knappett

2007 *Knossos Protopalatial Deposits in Early Magazine A and the South-West Houses*. BSA Supp. Vol. 41. British School at Athens, London.

MacGillivray, J. Alexander

1998 *Knossos: Pottery Groups of the Old Palace Period*. BSA Studies 5. British School at Athens, London.

McGovern, Patrick E.
2009 *Uncorking the Past: The Quest for Wine, Beer, and Other Alcoholic Beverages.* University of California Press, Berkeley.
McGovern, Patrick E., Stuart J. Fleming, and Solomon H. Katz (editors)
1996 *The Origins and Ancient History of Wine.* Gordon and Breach, Amsterdam.
Manniche, Lise
1999 *Sacred Luxuries: Fragrance, Aromatherapy, and Cosmetics in Ancient Egypt.* Cornell University Press, Ithaca.
Marinatos, Nanno, and Lyvia Morgan
2005 The Dog Pursuit Scenes from Tell el Dab'a and Kea. In *Aegean Wall Painting: A Tribute to Mark Cameron,* edited by Lyvia Morgan, pp. 119–122. BSA Studies 13. British School at Athens, London.
Mathiowetz, Michael
2010 The Aroma and Nectar of Flowers: Floral Symbolism in the Art and Ritual of the Aztatlán Tradition of Ancient West Mexico. Paper presented at the 75th Meeting of the Society for American Archaeology, St. Louis.
Merrillees, Robert S.
1962 Opium Trade in the Bronze Age Levant. *Antiquity* 36:287–292.
Meskell, Lynn M. (editor)
2005 *Archaeologies of Materiality.* Blackwell, Oxford.
Meskell, Lynn M., and Rosemary A. Joyce
2003 *Embodied Lives: Figuring Ancient Maya and Egyptian Experience.* Routledge, London.
Miller, Daniel
2009 *Stuff.* Polity Press, Cambridge, United Kingdom.
Morris, Christine E.
1995 Fishy Tales from Knossos: A Minoan Larnax and Vase-Painter. In *KLADOS Essays in Honour of J. N. Coldstream,* edited by Christine E. Morris, pp. 185–193. BICS Supp. 63. Institute of Classical Studies, London.
Muhly, Polymnia M.
1984 Minoan Hearths. *American Journal of Archaeology* 88:107–122.
Parkin, David
2007 Wafting on the Wind: Smell and the Cycle of Spirit and Matter. *Journal of the Royal Anthropological Institute,* n.s. 13, S1:S39–S53.
Pernier, Luigi
1935 *Il Palazzo Minoico di Festós.* Vol. I. Libreria dello Stato, Rome.
Platon, Maria
1987 Γλαστρεζ και ανθοδοχεια στο Μινωικο κοσμο. Ειλαπινη. Τομοζ Τιμητικοζ για τον Καθηγητη Νικολοα Πλατωνα. Βικελαια Δημοτικη Βιβλιοθηκη, Ηρακλειον Κρητηζ.
Porteous, J. Douglas
2006 Smellscape. In *The Smell Culture Reader,* edited by Jim Drobnick, pp. 89–106. Berg, Oxford.
Rutter, Jeremy
2004 Ceramic Sets in Context: One Dimension of Food Preparation and Consumption in a Minoan Palatial Setting. In *Food, Cuisine and Society in Prehistoric Greece,* edited by Paul Halstead and John C. Barrett, pp. 63–89. Oxbow, Oxford.
Sakellarakis, Yannis, and Efi Sapouna-Sakellaraki
1997 *Archanes: Minoan Crete in a New Light.* Ammos Publications, Athens.
Sarpaki, Anaya

2001 Condiments, Perfume, and Dye Plants in Linear B: A Look at the Textual and Archaeobotanical Evidence. In *Manufacture and Measurement: Counting, Measuring, and Recording Craft Items in Early Aegean Societies*, edited by Anna Michailidou, pp. 197–265. Meletemata 33. Research Centre for Greek and Roman Antiquity and National Hellenic Research Foundation, Athens.

Shelmerdine, Cynthia W.

1985 *The Perfume Industry of Mycenaean Pylos*. Paul Åströms Förlag, Göteborg.

Synnott, Anthony

1991 A Sociology of Smell. *Canadian Review of Sociology and Anthropology* 28:437–459.

Tait, G. A. D.

1963 The Egyptian Relief Chalice. *Journal of Egyptian Archaeology* 49:93–139.

Taube, Karl A.

2004 Flower Mountain: Concepts of Life, Beauty, and Paradise among the Classic Maya. *Res: Anthropology and Aesthetics* 45:69–98.

2010 At Dawn's Edge: Tulún, Santa Rita, and Floral Symbolism in the International Style of Late Postclassic Mesoamerica. In *Astronomers, Scribes, and Priests: Intellectual Interchange between the Northern Maya Lowlands and Highland Mexico in the Late Postclassic Period*, edited by Gabrielle Vail and Christine Hernandez, pp. 145–191. Dumbarton Oaks, Washington, D.C.

Tzedakis, Yannis, and Holly Martlew (editors)

1999 *Minoans and Mycenaeans: Flavours of Their Time*. Greek Ministry of Culture, Athens.

Tzedakis, Yannis, Holly Martlew, and Martin K. Jones (editors)

2008 *Archaeology Meets Science: Biomolecular Investigations in Bronze Age Greece*. Oxbow, Oxford.

Walberg, Gisela

1983 *Provincial Middle Minoan Pottery*. Philipp von Zabern, Mainz am Rhein.

1987 *Kamares: A Study of the Character of Palatial Middle Minoan Pottery*. Paul Åström, Göteborg.

Warren, Peter M.

1969 *Minoan Stone Vases*. Cambridge University Press, Cambridge.

Wilson, Donald A., and Richard J. Stevenson

2006 *Learning to Smell: Olfactory Perception from Neurobiology to Behaviour*. John Hopkins University Press, Baltimore.

Wilson, Eric

2007 How to Bottle a Generation. *New York Times* 8 March. Electronic document, http://www.nytimes.com/2007/03/08/fashion/08CALVIN.html, accessed March 28, 2012.

Wright, James C. (editor)

2004 *The Mycenaean Feast*. American School of Classical Studies at Athens, Princeton, New Jersey.

Zaidman, Louise B., and Pauline S. Pantel

1992 [1989] *Religion in the Ancient Greek City*. Translated by Paul Cartledge. Cambridge University Press, Cambridge.

# 15. Craft and Sensory Play in Late Bronze Age Boeotia

*Anastasia Dakouri-Hild*

*Abstract:* This paper deals with an assemblage of mostly unfinished, failed, and partially recycled artifacts, as well as roughouts, scraps, and raw materials, excavated from the destruction fill of a large palatial building at the center of the citadel of Thebes. More specifically, I discuss the complex biographies and materialities of these objects in both visual and nonvisual terms. Based on this analysis, I entertain the somatic engagement of Theban minds with things and the agentive force of sensed matter. Finally, I consider cultural classifications and likely sensorial conflicts illuminated through this unique assemblage.

The study of craftsmanship is intertwined with the anthropology of technology, as well as with cognitive approaches to material culture and the theorized body and senses. Scholarly interest in craft and technology is represented by complementary approaches, ranging from traditional studies focusing on the identification of tools and technique how-tos to techno-psychological and linguistic models and operational sequences (e.g., Gibson and Ingold 1993; Lemonnier 1992, 1993; Renfrew and Zubrow 1994). From a social and multisensory perspective, on the other hand, craft and technology do not merely produce things but are regarded as a means of asserting and contesting social relations and values through the sensuous experience of working with matter (e.g., Dobres 2000; Dobres and Hoffman 1999; Knappett 2005).

In this chapter, I explore the latter direction, aiming to bring craft and the theorized senses closer together. In particular, I discuss the mutable material "careers" of certain workshop-derived objects from Late Bronze Age Thebes in

*Making Senses of the Past: Toward a Sensory Archaeology*, edited by Jo Day. Center for Archaeological Investigations, Occasional Paper No. 40.  ISBN 978-0-8093-3287-8.

Greece, specifically looking at the complex materialities of unfinished, flawed, and/or recycled agate artifacts.

Taking into account the socioeconomic context of these artifacts (an elite-controlled system of production), their location within a palatial complex, and their archaeological (hoarding) context, I explore the non-linear aspects of Theban workmanship beyond the predictable operational sequence: the drama and playful experimentation entailed by an inherently risky craft and a challenging yet intriguing material; the visual and tactile affordances of agate that were creatively and uniquely grappled with, sometimes to the point of captivation and against the logic of functionality; and the mutual intercalibration of matter and ideas through the somatic and sensorial experiences of Late Bronze Age minds.

Moreover, I attempt to discern emic determinations of "failure" on the basis of the archaeological context of the assemblage and discuss possible sensorial clashes between the craftspeople and the palatial patrons who commissioned, organized, and exclusively controlled the manufacture of the artifacts in question.

## Biographical Things

Tracking down the lives of artifacts, understood as sequences of both human behavior and natural processes, is key to archaeology. From the procurement of raw materials to the preservation of completed artifacts in the archaeological record, things are gradually transformed to become archaeological finds. Teasing apart the historical, social, and economic trajectories of things as a means to reconstruct and understand the past is indeed what archaeology is about. In addition to this general biographical orientation of the field, two biographical approaches aiming to document the social lives or deaths of artifacts specifically have taken hold in the last decade, largely thanks to Arjun Appadurai's seminal volume *The Social Life of Things* (1984).

First, there is an emphasis on the *material lives of people*. Things are regarded as integral to human action, inextricably linked to personhood and identity. Of particular interest in this approach is the investment of human biographies and memories in significant artifacts such as trophies, framed diplomas, collections, and family heirlooms (e.g., Herva and Nurmi 2009; Hoskins 1998; Weiner 1992). There is a parallel focus on the intersubjective fame of artifacts or monuments obtained by their cumulative association with people—their "aura" (e.g., Hamilakis 2007; Shanks 1998:19–20)—or the fame that people can derive by means of association with particular things (e.g., Whitley 2002). From this perspective, material culture becomes inalienable from persons or social groups and can define human relationships. Alfred Gell's (1998) "distributed mind" or Marilyn Strathern's (1988) "partible person" encapsulate this inalienability and stress the idea that humans are divisible into material things because they tend to form object identities (see also Hoskins 2006:76).

Other studies have focused on the active nature of material culture and the *social lives of things*, especially their changing semiotic and functional status in different contexts (e.g., Holtorf 2002; Langdon 2001; Shanks 1998). According to the latter viewpoint, artifacts cannot be reduced simply to the kind of things that they were intended to be but must also be regarded as the things that they become in social praxis. The biography of a find does not end with deposition but encompasses all sumptuary episodes in its life span, including for instance excavation, interpretation, installation in a museum, and physical or ideological appropriation by a social group. All episodes in their lives need to be taken into account, including their diversion from predetermined paths in social performance: for instance, the radical and sometimes rapid transformation of utilitarian objects into museum art, artworks into commodities, masterpieces into fakes, heirlooms into trash or *Antiques Roadshow* national treasures.

In a nutshell, biographical approaches to material culture are aimed at blurring the ontological line and binary distinction between people and things, predicating that these are intermingled, and simultaneously and mutually constructed in social life (Gosden and Marshall 1999; Kopytoff 1984:90).

## Material Lives

The biographical approaches mentioned above relate more to the "culture" part of material culture, that is, the mutability of meaning and/or function, which are always situational and culturally specific. Can materiality itself be construed as a mutable quality, rather than as a static and unchangeable property of things? The material identities of things seem, at first sight, static, unchangeable, and permanently crystallized in their given forms through manufacture or industrial production. Marcel Duchamp's famous porcelain urinal has been relabeled a "fountain" and set up as an exhibit in an art museum, evoking water and possibly acting as a metaphor for artistic inspiration. It may at once allude to and mock sculpture, challenging traditional concepts of art, and assert the aesthetic value of ready-made art; yet its materiality stubbornly continues to evoke its original function (Risatti 2007:141).

It is difficult to envisage multiple material lives for a single object that are distinguishable from each other. However, works in progress, repaired and recycled objects fit comfortably in this domain. The life cycles of unfinished and incomplete artifacts, especially handcrafted ones—the physical changes, processes, and multiple transformations that they undergo—can be seen as attributes of their biographies as well. In a similar vein, artifacts can be reworked and given "new life." Fixing them necessitates regular maintenance and intervention programs (Shanks 1998:16–17, 19), but their wear and repair can contribute to their perceived cumulative patination or "aura" (Herva and Nurmi 2009:175; see also Pye 1995:36, 65). Such special things become even more special by their treatment as repair worthy, and their extended social lives can be informed by their previous material lives, provided the modifications or repairs are obvious.

Alternatively, artifacts can be recycled and treated as raw material without any consideration for their previous function or form. Such treatment implies indifference or even hostility to the original artifacts, as for instance in the case of monument and statue usurpation and recycling as a performance of memory

(Crawford 2007:34–38; see also Feldman 2009; Kinney 1997). Recycling can also emerge as a final option ensuing a series of unsuccessful repair attempts. Conceivably the full range of the unfinished, repaired, recycled states can be attested on a single artifact, for instance in a workshop context. To sum up, the notion of biography is not only applicable to the meaning or function of things. Rather, their materialities are also potentially mutable and multifaceted (Holtorf 2002:49).

## Thebes

Mycenaean Thebes is one of four known palatial centers on the Late Bronze Age Greek mainland (Figure 15-1). As the seat of palatial authority and administration in the state of East Boeotia from the fourteenth to the twelfth century B.C.E., the site commanded substantial territory that appears to have reached beyond the geographical confines of Boeotia and enjoyed a prominent political and economic role in the eastern Mediterranean (Dakouri-Hild 2005:208). Excavations since the early twentieth century on the citadel, or Kadmeia, have produced a wealth of evidence regarding the arrangement and functions of the palatial complex, the fortified town with which it seems to have been interwoven, and the nearby cemeteries.

Thebes appears to have been a major center for the ornamental industries, especially lapidary, ivory, and gold work. A number of workshops on the citadel have produced evidence for the manufacture of appliqués, inlays, finials, and moldings for furniture pieces (Dakouri-Hild 2010a:701–702 and Figure 52.2 for other sites; Symeonoglou 1973), paralleled by the elaborate furnishings described in the Pylian Linear B documents (Ta series, Ventris and Chadwick 1973:332) and actual finds from other Mycenaean sites (e.g., Poursat 1977:Plates I, XVI; Tournavitou 1995:Frontispiece, Plate 22; Xenaki-Sakellariou 1985:Plates 20, 25, 27, 96). The local production of jewelry, cloth attachments, grooming accessories, equestrian ornaments, and decorative weapon parts is also attested archaeologically at Thebes (Dakouri-Hild 2004, 2005), with parallels (in agate and other materials) from other Theban (Demakopoulou and Konsola 1981:Plates 18–19, 23; Platon and Touloupa 1965:Plate 276; Spyropoulos and Chadwick 1975: 38; Symeonoglou 1973:Figure 272) and mainland sites (e.g., Blegen 1937:Plates 85–286; Blegen and Rawson 1966:Plates 266, 273; Krzyszkowska 2007:Plate 6; Persson 1931:Plates XX, XXV; Rahmstorf 2008:Taf. 58).

The goods produced tend to be associated with the elite body. They are frequently iconographic, composite, and materially complex: They are made using numerous parts from various imported materials. Their manufacture entailed multiple transformations: from raw materials to individual parts to dazzling, complex artifacts. The palace allocated raw materials to the workshops with the expectation that unused raw materials, or scraps thereof, and unfinished or completed objects were returned to the palatial depots for long-term hoarding or temporary storage while awaiting further work (e.g., Krzyszkowska 1996:101). These ornamental industries involved virtuoso craftspeople and their apprentices, who were fully supported by and worked exclusively for the palace within the palatial complex

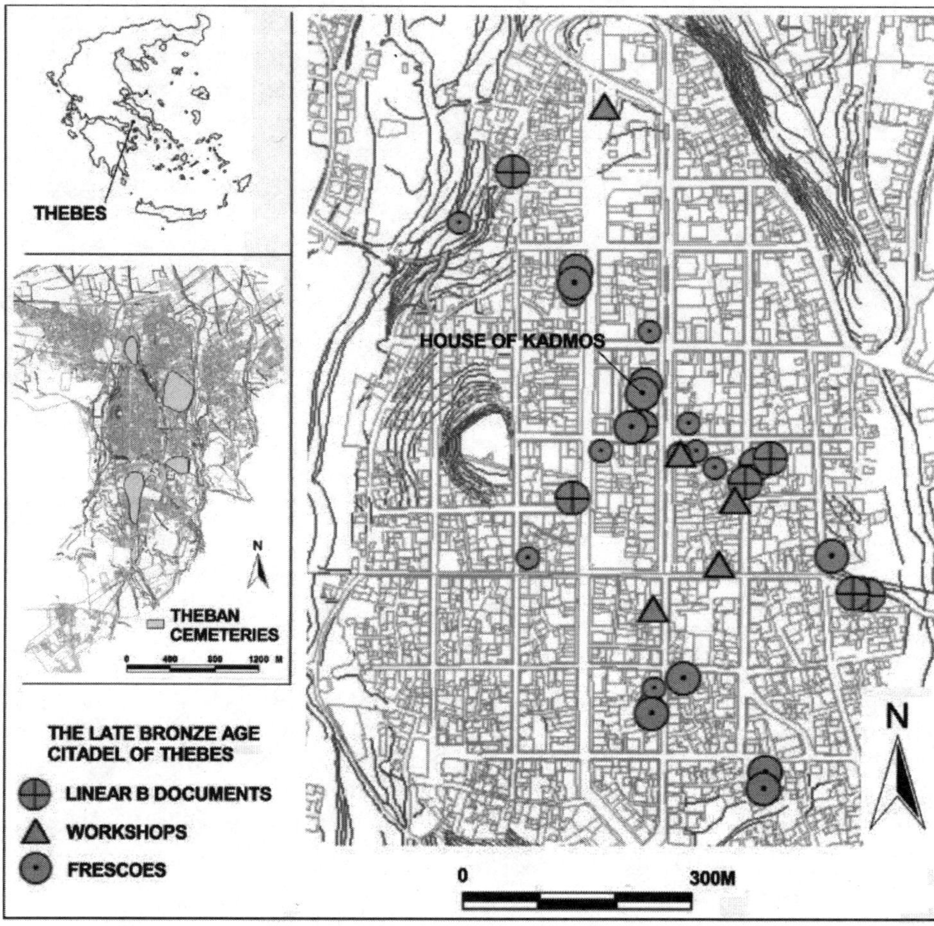


**Figure 15-1.** *The citadel of Thebes with surrounding cemeteries and distribution of workshops. (Drawing © Anastasia Dakouri-Hild.)*

itself (Halstead 1992; Killen 1988). The exclusivity of such goods is reflected in the sumptuary realm as well (Dakouri-Hild 2004:184–185).

Artifacts produced under these conditions required more than just the expenditure of energy or the use of exotic materials. They necessitated the convergence of skill, talent, authenticity, equipment, material resources, distant knowledge and connections; an elite taste and lifestyle; and the symbolic and performative amalgamation of the above through liminal processes at the heart of the kingdom (Dakouri-Hild 2005:210). Artifacts brought about in this way necessitated a practical and ideological momentum that could only have been gained by the palatial center. They bear the undeniable stamp of the authoritative, symbolically charged palatial townscape that was Thebes.

The assemblage discussed in this paper originates from the so-called House of Kadmos, or Old Palace of Thebes (Figures 15-1 and 15-2). This is a monumental, and at one point frescoed, building at the center of the citadel. It served a

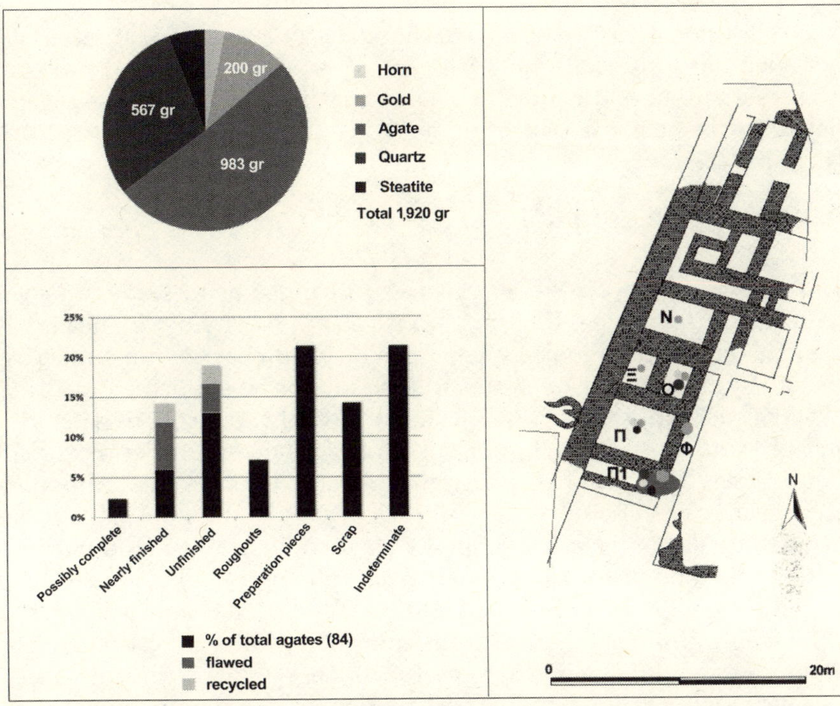


**Figure 15-2.** *The House of Kadmos with the distribution* (right) *and absolute quantities of workshop-related finds* (top left)*, and the production stages and states represented by the agate material* (bottom left)*. (Drawing © Anastasia Dakouri-Hild.)*

variety of functions associated with palatial administration: storage for bulk liquid commodities (wine and/or oil); storage for mostly plain but otherwise fine ceramic vessels suitable for ceremonial banqueting; the production of pottery at a nearby workshop with a kiln; and the safe-keeping of prestige artifacts made from various metals, stones, organic materials, and glass paste.

The workshop material, in particular (Dakouri-Hild 2006, 2010b, 2010c), consists mostly of stone objects. Other than the agate artifacts, which are the focus of this paper, there are quartz pieces (raw nuclei, leftovers, and shattered fragments in areas O and Π1) and black steatite and ofite objects (areas Π, Π1). Scrap gold and preprocessed gold in the form of spooled wire of various thicknesses and sections as well as semiprocessed boar tusks and horns (cores, slices) have also been found (areas N, Ξ, O, Π, Π1). The overlapping distribution of these different kinds of materials and object types over several rooms in the south-west part of the building (Figure 15-2), coupled with the recent discovery of additional gold wire spools (Dakouri-Hild 2010b) in the fused limestone elevation of a basement wall (area Π1), suggest that the objects originally derive from a single context in the upper story of the House of Kadmos.

The building was destroyed by a violent fire in the transition from the fourteenth to the thirteenth century B.C.E. (Dakouri-Hild 2001:100–101). The collapsed and fused elevation debris sealed off the habitation deposit and protected it from the post-Mycenaean habitation in the area. Thus, the destruction has brought about a rare snapshot of the functional use of the building and the associated assemblages shortly before it was abandoned.

## Artifacts of Many Lives

About half of the 84 objects made of banded agate represent a variety of recognizable artifact types (Figure 15-3). There are jewelry pieces (beads of various shapes, blank seal-like objects, pendants), weapon parts ("mushroom" pommels, knobs, handle or hilt covers), and furniture or box attachments drilled or scored at the back (appliqués, inlays, inserts). Notably, some of the latter are zoomorphic or skeuomorphic (a lion or lioness head, bucranium, griffin or sphinx wing, miniature half-columns) and were probably intended as components of larger pictorial compositions.

The agates also represent a variety of stages and states of manufacture (see Figure 15-2). Roughouts are understood as morphologically incomplete artifacts that would have required substantial additional work in order to enter the consumption realm. Unfinished artifacts are morphologically complete objects that are missing perforations and other key functional details. Nearly finished artifacts are morphologically complete and perforated but may have required additional detailing. Possibly complete artifacts are fully formed objects, though the context argues against the idea that they were simply hoarded at the site. Notably, the fact that many such artifacts find parallels in consumption contexts at Thebes and other Mycenaean sites (see previous section) makes them easily recognizable in functional terms and enables an emic determination of "roughout," "nearly finished," or "complete." In addition to the recognizable artifact types, there are many nondescript objects (by-products, leftovers, and a bark slice) that were probably kept for reuse (see Figure 15-2).

Since no debitage or tools were found at the site, it is unlikely that the objects derive from a workshop context per se. The mixed nature of the agate material, found alongside scraps of gold, wire, raw quartz, and steatite nuclei, suggests that the House of Kadmos functioned in part as a collection hub, where artifacts in various stages of manufacture, raw materials, leftovers, and mistakes were kept temporarily before they were released to the workshops for further work (Dakouri-Hild 2006:181–185). However, similarities in the veined patterns, which act as fingerprints for identifying the original stock material used for different objects (Dakouri-Hild 2010c), suggest that some artifacts derive from the same nuclei and possibly from a single workshop.

Salvaging failed objects and reworking them into forms different from the ones originally intended can lead to the "continual coming into being" of artifacts (Herva and Nurmi 2009:175), the protean material biographies of which are hard to decipher and distinguish. The various stages of, and intentions represented by, such complex biographies may or may not leave archaeologically detectible traces behind, depending on whether the objects were completed or not in the

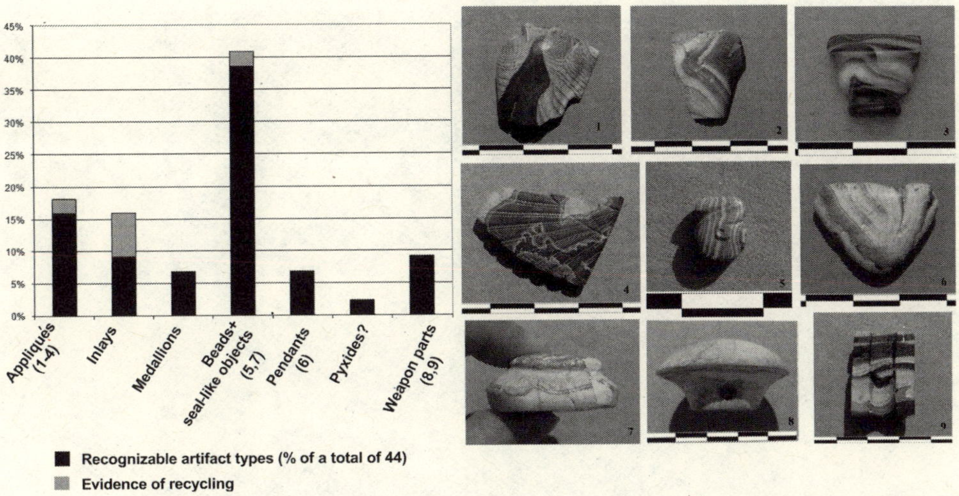


**Figure 15-3.** *Types of recognizable artifacts represented by the agate assemblage. (Photograph © Anastasia Dakouri-Hild.)*

end. Finishing processes (abrasion of tool marks, polishing, etc.) will generally eliminate clues regarding the prior material identities of reworked things. On the other hand, the work episodes leading to the incipient lives of artifacts can be teased apart if the work was never completed.

If the potential for failure is part and parcel of design, the concept of failure in itself is not necessarily self-evident. After all "failure" and "success" are value judgments regarding what is acceptable, proper, ready, and what is not. An actor's choices and implicit beliefs can be comprehended better through what she rejects rather than what she keeps: "the word changed, the sentence deleted, and other alterations that may be traced through successive drafts' failures to contribute to the end worked towards" (Petroski 1992:75, 77). Thus, artifacts classified as failures from an emic perspective can facilitate an understanding of the constellations of knowledge that guide decisions and present a range of conceivable choices; they are a part of the social, ideological, and technological narratives that organize existence materially and mentally in a society (Lipartito 2003:54, 57).

Interestingly, several unfinished agates from the House of Kadmos have been used as a source of raw material, and in some cases it can be established with certainty that the objects were flawed in functional terms: For example, their perforations failed, they were redrilled in a manner that rendered them unusable, or they broke as a result of perforation work (Figure 15-4). A striking example is a cylindrical bead failed during perforation work, which was subsequently sliced across its diameter, recycled into a pictorial appliqué (a griffin or sphinx leg, see Tournavitou 1995:Frontispiece), and left unfinished (Figure 15-5).

Some of the agates, then, appear to have biographies of a different kind than expected: not careers of mutable meanings and sumptuary uses, but rather different material trajectories within the domain of production that are partially preserved in the composite, abandoned forms of objects. They were made using

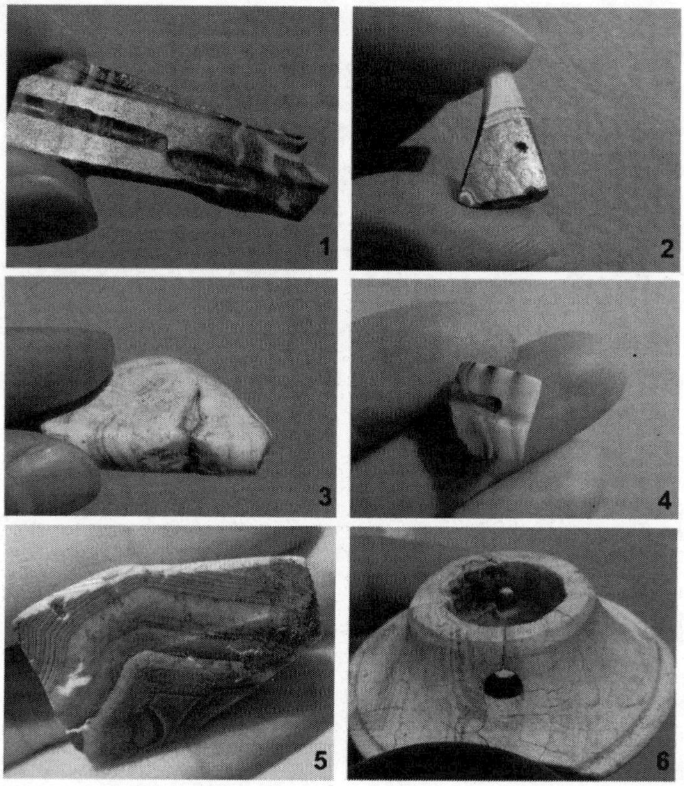


**Figure 15-4.** *Failed artifacts among the agate finds, some showing attempts at repair (3, 6), others recycled (1, 4). (Photograph © Anastasia Dakouri-Hild.)*

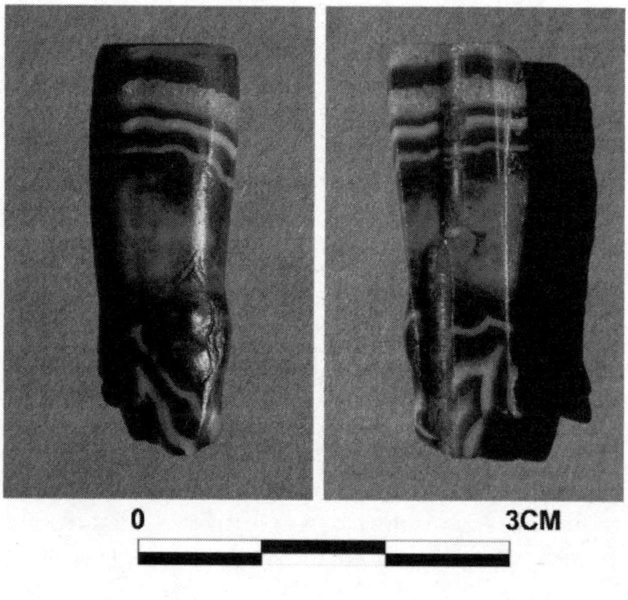


**Figure 15-5.** *The multiple lives of an agate object: a cylindrical bead that failed during perforation, recycled into a griffin leg appliqué and subsequently left unfinished. (Photograph © Anastasia Dakouri-Hild.)*

other, recycled things as a source of raw material, and their transformations and renewals have brought along threads of previously intended material lives; these artifactual identities have been preserved to some extent (cf. Dipert 1993:123–124). At the same time, their "lives" were never lived socially even as the objects were recycled and re-recycled.

## Beyond *Chaînes*

I turn now to the interrelationship between matter and ideas as it emerges through a sensory approach. In a different study (Dakouri-Hild 2010c), I employed a *chaîne opératoire* approach to reconstruct a stratigraphy, as it were, of actions that brought about these artifacts. Since operational sequences are not just the outcome of material and technical constraints but are also due to culture-specific choices, I was able to catch a glimpse of the cultured, doing mind in action, understood not as an essentialistic, deep-seated "Mycenaean mind" but rather as a workmanship style in this specific context. Although there are no complete sequences for each artifact type represented and, in some cases, a single object represents several attempts at making different types of goods, it has been possible to reconstruct a standard operational sequence relating to all types of artifacts (roughing out, polishing, carving, perforating) and another that relates to the initial process by which raw material was broken down based on the anticipated volume of artifacts. These observations betray some planning and foresight, at least in the original stages of such work, and a systematic approach possibly aided by workshop guidelines.

However, this study revealed the drawbacks of a traditional *chaîne opératoire* approach, in which it is assumed that manufacture is a linear process, from raw material to finished product, and that the actions entailed are planned and executed from start to finish without a glitch. The Theban artisans who handled this material seem to have employed tactics, not grand strategies, in their work. Their goals seem to have been articulated dynamically; that is, in the process of doing, they sometimes overrode the original objective due to breakage and so on. A second problem is that this method works best for things produced en masse and that conform to very standardized kinds of artifacts, like stone tools. Some types of artifacts attested here are served well by such an analysis because they are predictable and well known from consumption contexts. Others, however, do not conform to functional or formal stereotypes and their uniqueness cannot be accounted for through this approach.

## Mind, Body, Matter

This leads me to a third, more fundamental problem. From a *chaîne* perspective things tend to be regarded as passive, inert, blank media on which mental templates are stamped. The very term *medium* implies this mentalistic approach, in which the manipulation of materials is understood to take a backseat to thought processes. In recent years, scholarship has moved away from the Cartesian divide between mind and matter, mind and body, subject and object; pure materialist and mentalist approaches have been tempered with a more complex understanding of the dynamic feedback between cognition and material culture.

With the advent of embodied cognition in the 1990s, materiality has ceased to be regarded as a passive repository for the download of preconceived mental schemata (Boivin 2004a:63; Knappett 2005). Neurophenomenological analysis of the experiential structure of visualization has also cast doubt on the existence of mental images in the brain stricto sensu (Thompson 2007:10–11, 302; cf. Kosslyn 2006). In what has also been called the situated, or distributed, cognition model, the mind is not simply a computational device and filing cabinet for external stimuli and representational structures (Malafouris 2004:54). Ideas and matter are considered to be codependent and coemergent (Knappett 2005:43; Renfrew 2004:23; see also Knappett and Malafouris 2008; Malafouris and Renfrew 2010): Thought and manufacture, visualization and execution, *theoria* and *praxis* are interwoven. Ideas lead to the transformation of materials and materials prime ideas; therefore, cognition is a blend of interactions between an embodied mind and the world (Kirsh 2009:278; Risatti 2007:169; Ullrich 2004:208). Thus, while certain ideas must predate action—for instance, abstract knowledge on how to deal with stone, how to use tools, what the patron expects, what the workshop guidelines are—others are more ambiguous and articulated in the process of creatively and somatically grappling with matter (cf. Clark 2008:170).

Meaning is bestowed on things by working through materiality, not against it. The physicality of objects is not a tabula rasa for the inscription of meaning: It is strongly agentive in itself, resisting some options while permitting others (Boivin 2004a:64). This view lends support to the notion that not all meaning resides outside an object; indeed, some things have an indissoluble reality in matter (Renfrew 2004:25; Risatti 2007:255). Also critical to the process by which "brains make up their minds" and bodies and matter interact is socialized action. It takes a *doing* mind to shift through the affordances and potentialities of materiality. This is the case with crafted objects as well as paintings. The physical description of paint will not capture the nuance of the medium as a painter uses it: It "is something that only is what it is through being used' (Wentworth 2004:34). Meaning emerges not only between matter and the embodied mind but also socially, between different minds (Johnson 2007:151; Knappett 2005:46–49; Malafouris 2004:58–59).

Some of the House of Kadmos agates show that the material is neither just a constraint—a problem to be dealt with—nor a blank medium on which preconceived ideas are downloaded. For example, in the lion's head (Figure 15-6.1) the natural patterns of the stone are framed to enhance form, plasticity, volume, and details—such as the eye socket and the muzzle; in the case of the griffin or sphinx wing (Figure 15-6.4), form is worked around the natural round patterns of the stone to suggest elaborate plumage; in a likely figure-eight shield appliqué (Figure 15-6.2), the pattern of the stone could suggest a dappled skin hide. There are also many examples of artifacts the shape of which has been adapted to the natural veins of the material (e.g., Figure 15-6.3). The feedback between idea and

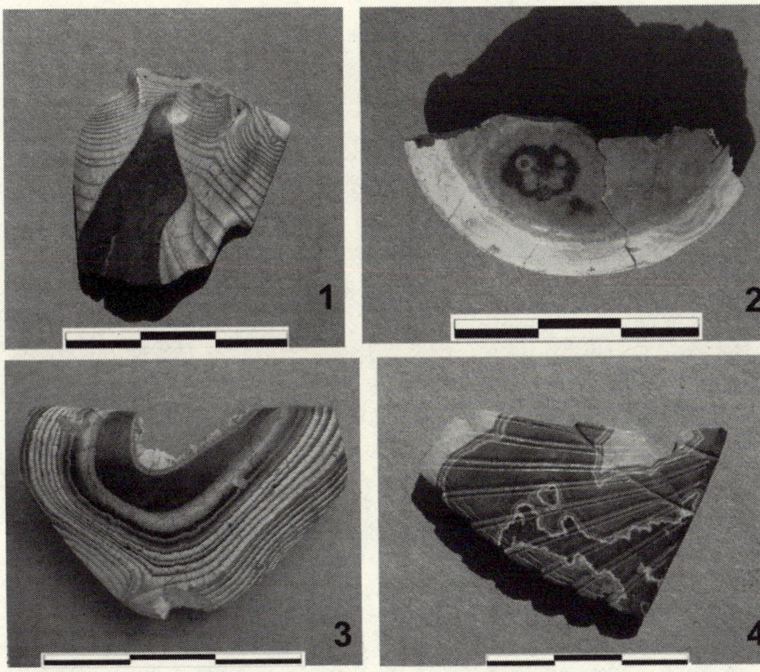


**Figure 15-6.** *Affordances of agate in action. (Photograph © Anastasia Dakouri-Hild.)*

matter, as witnessed here, has been described by Alfred Gell (1998) as "tuning," that is, framing an idea against a suitable portion of the material and articulating an idea in the process of working the material. But what is seen is invisible until seeing is done in a particular way (Hutchins 2010:43).

An understanding of perception, and by extension artistic production, as a blend between the body and the world "out there," engaging sensory and intellectual capacities alike, seems particularly apposite here. In these crafted objects, thought and matter interface in a dynamic way, and we catch a rare glimpse of prehistoric artisans thinking on their feet, or rather with their hands and eyes.

## Prehistoric Eyes and Hands

Western culture has long favored vision as a more rational, disembodied, and therefore, objective means to perceive and experience the world compared to the other senses (Edwards et al. 2006:7; MacGregor 1999:264). According to this model, non-Western, non-literate, or prehistoric societies emerge as largely aural, tactile, olfactory, and gustatory, whereas Western, literate, or modern societies are understood to be primarily visual. Although some things invite visual scrutiny, having been purposefully configured as signs within a specific semiotic system (Risatti 2007:127), a sharp binary distinction between cultures and historical times centered either on visuality or tactility does not necessarily correspond to historical reality. Despite their rhetorical value, such sensory stereotypes tend to "other" the cultures or social groups under study (Smith 2007:11–12) and must be tempered by taking into account the complex, cross-modal synergies of the senses.

Although different aspects of perception appear to rely on discrete areas of the brain, each sense does not constitute an independent perceptual system but rather relies on others for the synergistic compilation of correlated information (Spence 2007:45–46). Experimental studies, for instance, have demonstrated the close interaction of vision and touch in the evaluation of objects. Skin mechanoreceptors on the hands are employed for the determination of microgeometry (texture) and thermal conductivity relative to the body; muscle mechanoreceptors are used for perceiving weight, hardness, stiffness, and volume. Yet vision is just as important for the assessment of macrogeometry (size, shape, pattern) (Spence 2007:48; Wing et al. 2007:31–32). Even the determination of texture itself is a multisensory task, involving haptics, vision, and audition: Reflectance and sound further help evaluate the degree of friction presented to the hand by an object (Lederman and Klatzky 2004:107–110); in turn, seeing texture invites tactility (Kreitler and Kreitler 1972:205).

Handcrafted objects, specifically, demand an "active reading" that engages several senses because their creation necessitates and encodes a somatic, kinesthetic, multisensorial approach (Risatti 2007:147). Such objects are—in their shape, size, texture, or function—sympathetic to the human hand as they are "made by the body for the body." Indeed, the hand can be seen as a measure for judging the appeal of "handsome" things (Risatti 2007:108–110). Tools involved in manufacture are also phenomenologically involved in the creative dialectic and frequently manifest themselves on the end product (Wentworth 2004:32). The crafting hand-cum-tool is not just about effort, skill, technique, and the purposeful manipulation of raw material. It enables a mind's thinking through matter, it is a means of expressing one's being in the world, and it helps place objects in human perspective (Risatti 2007:196, 202–205). With the House of Kadmos agate assemblage, the mutual feedback between mind and matter is not just visual but also tactile—it is about the look as well as the feel of shiny, smooth, intricately patterned stone.

The natural properties of agate are worth discussing in more detail here, as they inform its "affordances" (see O'Connor and Cooney 2009:xxii) and uses in the hands of the Theban artisans. The origin of agate, which occurs in nature in the form of dull-looking rocks, is unknown. Sources can be found on Crete and in the Near East; the ancient Greek author Theophrastus mentioned a Sicilian source (Katerinopoulos 1993:27). Agate, a type of chalcedony, is rigid and hard enough to scratch glass (Mohs 6.5–7) but fractures and chips easily (Pabian et al. 2006:19–23), properties that make it a material difficult to work with. The level of difficulty experienced by the craftspeople is hinted at by the variety and nature of tools necessary for its processing, ranging from saws to tube-drills and chisels, and also by their sheer impatience, documented by examples of snapped–off, incomplete cuts. Agate is not a very dense stone (2.66 $g/cm^3$), though its compactness can vary, and has low thermal conductivity, which makes it feel cool and light in the hand.

Many of the House of Kadmos agates are polished to a very smooth, almost soapy surface, with outlines and contours likewise finely abraded to form gentle curves soft to the touch. Such surfaces, despite their opacity, are quite luminous and release an eye-catching sheen through their high polish (Figure 15-7). Looking at these artifacts, we are reminded of Nicholas Saunders's (1999) "biographies of brilliance" and his discussion of the symbolic significance of dazzling or iridescent materials in Amerindian material culture. Whether the luminosity and shine of these objects, or indeed their geological origins and mineral journeys and biographies (e.g., Boivin 2004b:4–14; see also Saunders 2004), were invested with cosmological meaning in Theban society is hard to know in the absence of Mycenaean literature, but it does appear to be one of their most striking and surely deliberate attributes. As David Pye (1995:91) remarked, polishing in itself suggests special attention lavished on an object, almost lovingly: "It glitters. It catches the eye. It has an element of excitement. It is not dull." This property of chalcedony is so potent it was noted by the Renaissance artist Lorenzo Ghiberti to compete with carved decoration under certain light conditions (Gage 1999:100).

Some materials create special sensory effects that contribute to their aesthetic diversity (Daston 1998:239; Pye 1995:36) and affect the ways the artifacts from which they are made are incorporated into symbolic schemes (Boivin 2004a:65; Owoc 2004:221). The multiple, variegated colors of agate—black, brown, taupe, beige, white—further enhance the look and feel of surface and form. Color is not a trivial adjunct to design and form; rather, it is a highly agentive expressive force, capable of effecting transformations in perception. Color relationships can contribute to or shape form in things. Moreover, in combination, they can create captivating effects, "fetishizing and bringing things alive" (Young 2006:181–182). I return to this captivation effect subsequently, as it is directly linked to the notion of material agency.

Pattern, formed by means of color contrasts, is another striking property of the House of Kadmos agates. Certain materials, especially grained or veined ones, lend themselves to certain shapes; not only is it impossible to deny their patterns but these also can be exploited to enhance an artifact (Pye 1995:86, 88). Some colors, in this case black and white, are "stickier" than others and lend themselves more easily to patterning, creating a dazzling effect (Young 2006:176). Pattern has an active, structuring ability. It can create spatial structures, intricate topographies, symmetries, rhythmic repetitions, and juxtapositions on objects (Figure 15-8). Some patterns induce suggestibility of the mind by carrying, to use Dario Gamboni's term (2002), "potential images." Such images lurk somewhere between perception and imagination; they are interpretations of mental derivation but also motivated by things and rely on the beholder for their realization. Gamboni understands the interpretation of such potential images as an ambiguous, oscillating, open process in which new possibilities are constantly perceived. Roger Callois (1985) has also explored the potentiality of certain materials. Commenting on the natural fantasy and "graphic madness of contrasting and merging colors" of agate specifically, he has gone on to recognize the mesmerizing, almost meditative quality of the material.

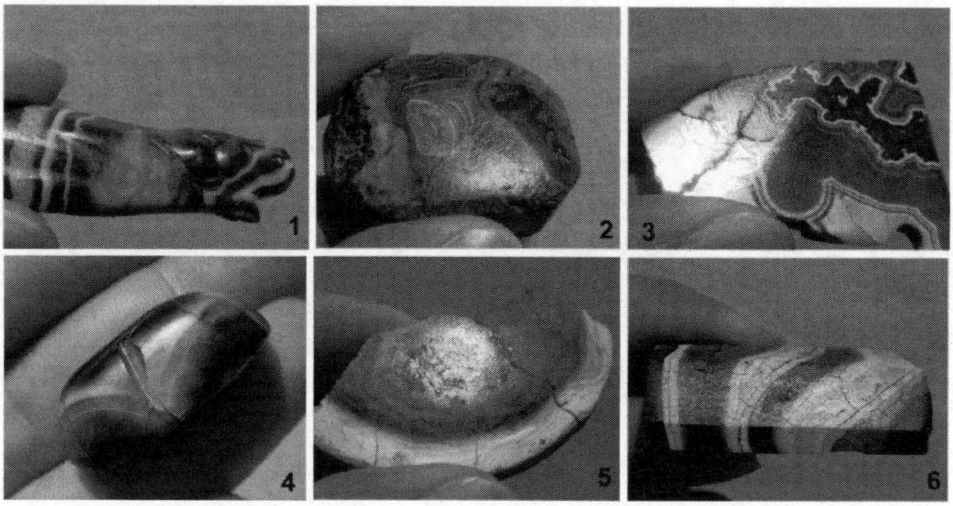

**Figure 15-7.** *Shiny things. (Photograph © Anastasia Dakouri-Hild.)*

Such natural patterns are not semiotic but are, nevertheless, potentially evocative. Their elusive suggestiveness can be clarified through imagination and creativity, for instance by framing an appropriate area of a natural pattern and working form around it.

## Risk and Failure

From an engineering perspective, failure is an unavoidable but also useful aspect of design in that it encourages improvement (e.g., Petroski 1992:82). In industrial production, lessons learned from failure contribute to a rational and linear redesign process; the choices are clear, and the outcomes are to a large extent predictable. Yet, in nonlinear systems of production, the available choices are not as clearly articulated, the outcomes are not easily predictable, and as a result, the overall process is more ambiguous and opaque (Lipartito 2003:55–56). However, the increased potential of risk might contribute to the aesthetic value of produced goods. As Shanks (1998:19) has remarked, handcrafted artifacts are denials of pure repetition; their value resides, at least partly, in their very unpredictability. In a similar vein, in David Pye's "workmanship of risk," the quality of the result is highly unpredictable and depends on the judgment, dexterity, and care of the maker. The work is continually at risk, as it can be ruined at any moment during the manufacturing process. The "tension and drama" entailed (Risatti 2007:165) enhances the performative, experimental, ludic flavor of work undertaken under such conditions. Unsurprisingly, although more prone to failure, the workmanship of risk is responsible for most unique and artistic work. By contrast, in the "workmanship of certainty," associated with mass production, the quality of the result is predetermined. Hybrid forms of production—for instance, craft-based industries—may be characterized both by the workmanship

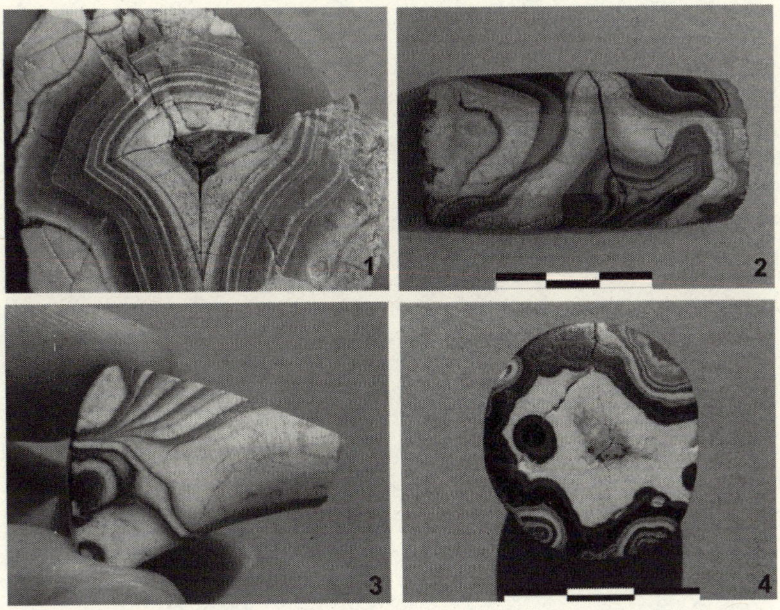


**Figure 15-8.** *Pattern and contrasts in the agate finds. (Photograph © Anastasia Dakouri-Hild.)*

of certainty and of risk, at different phases of the production process (Pye 1995:20, 22–23).

While the workmanship of risk is closely associated with visual appeal, not all such workmanship is necessarily good, since the outcome depends heavily on the performance and talent of the maker. Quality, according to Pye, is not brought about simply through precise execution. While imprecision stemming from a lack of time, knowledge, patience, or dexterity can certainly destroy a project, roughness is deemed as necessary for the workmanship of risk as a sketch is to a Rembrandt painting (Pye 1995:30, 32–33). In some cases, even accidental modification can be of value in the workmanship of risk, for example if it augments a design by introducing "diversity" previously lacking (Pye 1995:66). Such high-risk work, seconds Polly Ullrich (2004:206–207), can be especially revealing of "the sense of life and the moment-by-moment human decisions" recorded in the process of making an artifact. The narratives of revision encapsulated by things with multiple material lives, in particular, cast light on the workings of the mind as it meanders and experiences matter through the senses.

Some of the House of Kadmos agates are unparalleled things that defy the structural logic and stylistic vocabulary of Mycenaean ornaments, having been adapted from the natural shape of the stone's outline or its patterns. David Pye has made a useful distinction between "regulated work" on one hand, in which disparities between idea/design and execution/performance is minimal and the result is formulaic, predictable, and nearly flawless by means of sheer dexterity, and "moderately free" or "free-style" work on the other, which is characterized by slight to major, intentional disparities (Pye 1995:34, 63). The free-style agate objects from the House of Kadmos have no apparent flaws but are unfinished. They are unique, apparently unusable things that were never completed even if some surfaces were perfectly smoothed to a high polish (Figure 15-9). The material actually inspires the artifact: It is the concept that is formulated based on the material, not the other way round. To use a culinary example, the cook is not simply adjusting food to taste but improvising using textures, flavors, and smells. Sometimes it works, and sometimes it does not. But the cook is willing to take that risk, and potentially fail, in the process of creative action.

## Agency and Sensoria

Putting their multiple semantic, functional, or formal lives aside, artifacts can be understood to hold an active role in social life: Upon their materialities converge minerals, metals, ideas, tools, craftspeople, patrons, traders, designs, style, the body, deities, workshops, palaces and graves, and human relations across time and geographical space. Such convergences act on humans in very real ways, with artifact trajectories engendering aspirations, ambitions, and desires both in the past and in the present (Shanks 1998:24).

Artifacts are made to purposefully act on their social environment. They tend to be compatible with certain usages and "reject" others (Hoskins 2006:75, 81; Robb 2004:133). They demand and structure human responses figuratively and literally: "A heavy-looking object stimulates a firmer grip, a light or fragile-looking object a gingerly touch. . . . How we sit in a massive chair differs from how we sit in a delicate one—we may plop in one but not the other" (Risatti 2007:114; see also Edwards et al. 2006:12). Moreover, the iconographies, visual metaphors, and metonymies exhibited by artifacts stimulate cognition (D'Alleva 2001:82) and profoundly affect perception and interpretation. Yet it is not only through function, representation, and symbolism that artifacts affect the mind. The complex materialities of things are inseparable from their semiotic attributes, such as form and iconicity.

Alfred Gell posited that art is a form of instrumental action intended to act on people and that it is agentive when it has the ability to captivate the viewer. By extension, the virtuosity and "technologies of enchantment" that artful things entail can mesmerize (Gell 1999; see also Campbell 2001). Thus, even if they lack consciousness, self-government, and volition, artifacts exert a secondary agency that mediates and stands for the primary agency of people. Paradoxically, such secondary agency ultimately springs from the very habitus of those whom it affects; that is, it stems from the structured beliefs and values that surround material culture in a society (Gell 1998:21; Robb 2004:131–133, 137). Thus, human values and agency constitute a sine quibus non for material agency.

The theory of material engagement goes hand in hand with the theorized senses, as the latter enable the intercalibration of cognition and materiality. Recent scholarship has explored the individual, cultural, and political dimensions of the senses, beyond their role as physiological apparatus for interfacing with the world. The age, sex, genes, and expertise of the person sensing and the duration

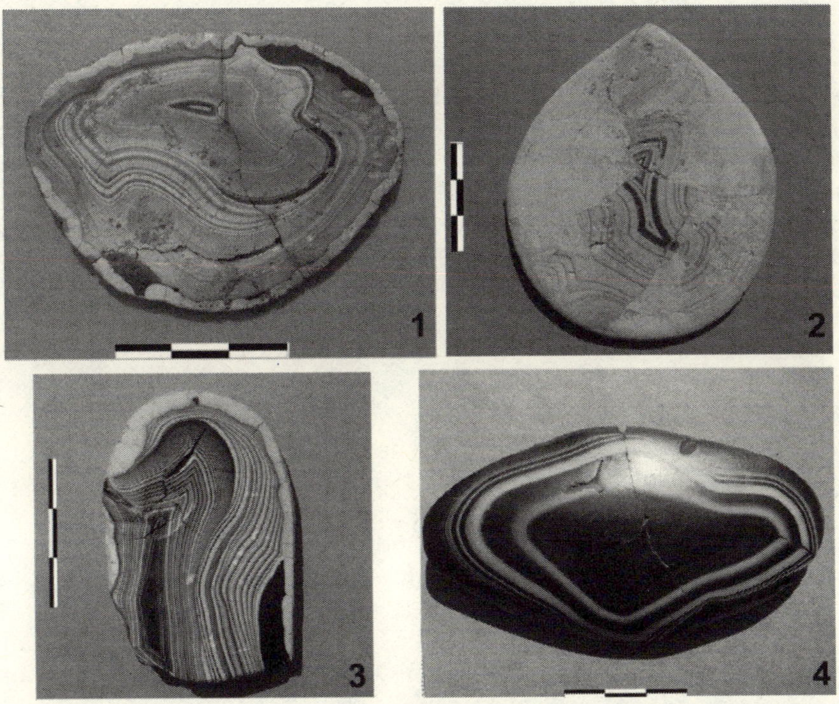


**Figure 15-9.** *Free-style agate objects. (Photograph © Anastasia Dakouri-Hild.)*

and nature of the encounter with specific sensed objects can bring about marked differences in perceptual abilities and effects, leading to individualistic sensory styles or "sensotypes" (Spence 2007:54). Furthermore, the senses are not passive devices deployed in cross-culturally and transhistorically similar ways but are the product of education and filtered through culture. Sensory categories are unstable and may differ across time and space; the range of sensory concepts and appropriate responses in a society bespeak the beliefs and values of those who uphold them (Edwards et al. 2006:5, 8; Gosden 2001:163; Smith 2007:3).

It follows from these observations that the archaeological sensorium itself is culturally and temporally specific and as such must be consciously reflected on and critiqued. Innocently "stepping into someone else's shoes" and ignoring the sensorial habitus under study runs the risk of interpretivist naivete (Gosden 2001:166; Renfrew 2004:24).

A further point to be made is that the senses and the discourses pertaining to them cannot be taken at face value. The senses are political, as they can be employed to advance normative constructions of the world that strategically contradict others. The articulation of sensoria and indigenous aesthetics actively shape social relations and engender hierarchical distinctions (Edwards et al. 2006:3, 24; Gosden 2001:163, 165). Since any given sensorium is intrinsically suspect, as Smith (2007:15, 17) has remarked, not only do we need to contextualize the senses but we must also explore the multiple sensory discourses within a given society.

If the House of Kadmos agates highlight the captivating allure of materiality, to what extent do they illuminate differing sensoria in Theban society circa 1400 B.C.E.? Archaeological finds from other palatial sites in the Aegean and, in part, epigraphic documents from associated archives indicate that the production of elaborate artifacts was highly regulated. Craftspeople specializing in the ornamental industries worked exclusively for the palaces as full-time employees. Exotic and rare raw materials were procured by the palaces through international exchange networks inaccessible to most. The materials were allocated to artisans and processed in workshops within confined, performative spaces, such as fortified citadels, while the inputs and outputs were closely monitored and safeguarded.

There seems to be little leeway for experimentation, sensory play, and artisan agency within such a framework of production. However, agency is intrinsic in craftsmanship: Materials and designs have promise that can only be brought about by the performance of craft (Pye 1995:18). On the other hand, the patron does not necessarily have full control over the outcome of the creative process, as good workmanship cannot be commanded by the terms of a contract: "If the work is not what he had in mind, he can only say 'do it again' and if it's bad a second time his resources are at an end" (Pye 1995:51).

There is no doubt that many of the artifacts discussed here are failures in functional terms. Others are not "damaged goods," however. They are just unique and somewhat strange compared with the typical repertoire of Mycenaean ornaments, which would indeed suggest some space for artistic experimentation on behalf of the Theban artisans. Nevertheless, judging from the context in which failed and strange objects alike were found—unfinished pieces, scraps, unworked raw materials—it seems that they were treated as substandard by elite authority. That is to say, the objects are rejects in emic terms: Their material biographies were "killed," terminated prematurely by those who commissioned them.

If we agree that sensoria, or sensory habitus, are in part social and cultural constructs, engendered by cognition as well as an education of the senses, we might ask, based on these findings, whether certain types of sensory responses in Late Bronze Age Thebes were deemed less important, or even inappropriate, and if so, why.

The study of this assemblage reveals cultural responses not only to functional errors but also to certain kinds of aesthetic experiments. Stripped of their functional and artistic value and potential, such experiments were good to keep only as recyclable material. Can the removal of substandard works from circulation be regarded as a sensory "pruning" of sorts, on behalf of the palatial patrons? Or does it even betray "sensory clashes," to use Yannis Hamilakis's term (this volume)? Such experiments presuppose free sensory play, which mobilizes pattern in unconventional ways and privileges a more intimate, somatic connection with matter through haptics. On the other hand, the formulaic repertoire of Mycenaean ornaments reveals a lesser interest in the tactile properties of things, combined with an emphasis on visuality, in particular symmetry, structure, uniformity, and specificity of form tied to the function and display of objects within the elite ambit. While this assemblage shows that the "workmanship of risk" was possible, its outcomes were not necessarily appreciated and were subject to filtering and adjustment by the commissioning patrons. Chris Gosden (2001:164–165) has stressed the power that materiality has as "prosthetic extension" of the self, in creating or subverting values attached to human relations. It would not be surprising, then, to find that the senses, which mediate materiality, also mediate the politics of identity.

## Acknowledgments

I would like to thank V. Aravantinos for allowing me to study the material from the House of Kadmos and J. Day for the invitation to participate in the conference and the resulting publication. I am also grateful to the faculty of the Lindner Center for Art History at the University of Virginia, especially P. Barolsky, M. Bell, and T. J. Smith, for useful comments and bibliographical suggestions on an earlier version of the paper presented as a departmental seminar (2007); and to D. Sutton and Y. Hamilakis for feedback during the conference. A special thanks goes to M. Bonanno-Aravantinos, whose casual comment on the House of Kadmos agates, in the summer of 2001 ("Look how they *shine*!") sparked an interest in their exuberant materialities.

## References

Blegen, Carl W.
1937 *Prosymna: The Helladic Settlement Preceding the Argive Heraeum*, Vol. II (plates). Cambridge University Press, Cambridge.

Blegen, Carl W., and Marion Rawson
1966 *The Palace of Nestor at Pylos in Western Messenia*, Vol. II (plates). Princeton University Press, Princeton.

Boivin, Nicole
2004a Mind over Matter? Collapsing the Mind-Matter Dichotomy in Material Culture Studies. In *Rethinking Materiality: The Engagement of the Mind with the Material World*, edited by Elizabeth DeMarrais, Chris Gosden, and A. Colin Renfrew, pp. 63–71. Cambridge University Press, Cambridge.
2004b From Veneration to Exploitation: Human Engagement with the Mineral World. In *Soils, Stones, and Symbols: Cultural Perceptions of the Mineral World*, edited by Nicole Boivin and Mary A. Owoc, pp. 1–29. UCL Press, London.

Callois, Roger
1985 *The Writing of Stones*. University Press of Virginia, Charlottesville.

Campbell, Shirley
2001 The Captivating Agency of Art: Many Ways of Seeing. In *Beyond Aesthetics: Art and the Technology of Enchantment*, edited by Christopher Pinney and Nicholas Thomas, pp. 117–134. Berg, New York.

Clark, Andy
2008 *Supersizing the Mind: Embodiment, Action, and the Cognitive Extension*. Oxford University Press, Oxford.

Crawford, Catherine L.
2007 Collecting, Defacing, Reinscribing (and Otherwise Performing) Memory in the Ancient World. In *Negotiating the Past in the Past: Identity, Memory, and Landscape in Archaeological Research*, edited by Norman Yoffee, pp. 10–42. University of Arizona Press, Tucson.

Dakouri-Hild, Anastasia
2001 The House of Kadmos in Mycenaean Thebes Reconsidered: Architecture, Chronology, and Context. *Annual of the British School of Archaeology* 96:81–122.
2004 Value and Values in a Mycenaean Society: Production and Consumption of Commodities in Late Bronze Age East Boeotia. Unpublished Ph.D. dissertation, Faculty of Classics, University of Cambridge.
2005 Breaking the Mould? Production and Economy in the Theban State. In *Autochthon: Papers Presented to O.T.P.K. Dickinson on the Occasion of His Retirement*, edited by Anastasia Dakouri-Hild and Sue Sherratt, pp. 207–224. Archaeopress, Oxford.
2006 Something Old, Something New: Current Research on the 'Old Kadmeion' of Thebes. *Bulletin of the Institute of Classical Studies* 48:173–186.
2010a Thebes. In *The Oxford Handbook of the Bronze Age Aegean*, edited by Eric H. Cline, pp. 690–711. Oxford University Press, Oxford.
2010b An Update on the House of Kadmos: The Latest Study Campaigns. In *Proceedings of the 5th International Conference on Boeotian Studies*, edited by Vassilis Aravantinos, pp. 203–218. Society of Boeotian Studies, Athens.
2010c Lives in Chains: Artifact Biographies in LBA Thebes. AIA 110th Annual Meeting Abstracts, Vol. 32. Archaeological Institute of America, Philadelphia.

D'Alleva, Anne
2001 Captivation, Representation, and the Limits of Cognition: Interpreting Metaphor and Metonymy in Tahitian Tamau. In *Beyond Aesthetics: Art and the Technology of Enchantment*, edited by Christopher Pinney and Nicholas Thomas, pp. 79–96. Berg, Oxford.

Daston, Lorraine
1998 Nature by Design. In *Picturing Science, Producing Art*, edited by Caroline A. Jones and Peter Galison, with Amy Slaton, pp. 232–253. Routledge, New York.

Demakopoulou, Katie, and Dora Konsola
1981 *Archaeological Museum of Thebes*. Greek Ministry of Culture, Athens.

Dipert, Randall R.
1993 *Artifacts, Art Works, and Agency*. Temple University Press, Philadelphia.

Dobres, Marcia-Anne
2000 *Technology and Social Agency: Outlining a Practice Framework for Archaeology*. Blackwell, New York.

Dobres, Marcia-Anne, and Christopher R. Hoffman
1999 *The Social Dynamics of Technology: Practice, Politics, and World Views*. Smithsonian Institution Press, Washington, D.C.

Edwards, Elizabeth, Chris Gosden, and Ruth Phillips
2006 Introduction. In *Sensible Objects: Colonialism, Museums, and Material Culture*, edited by Elizabeth Edwards, Chris Gosden, and Ruth Phillips, pp. 1–31. Berg, Oxford.

Feldman, Marian H.
2009 Knowledge as Cultural Biography: Lives of Mesopotamian Monuments. In *Dialogues in Art History, from Mesopotamian to Modern: Readings for a New Century*, edited by Elizabeth Cropper, pp. 41–55. National Gallery of Art, Center for Advanced Study in the Visual Arts and Yale University Press, New Haven.

Gage, John
1999 *Color and Meaning: Art, Science, and Symbolism*. University of California Press, Berkeley.
Gamboni, Dario
2002 *Potential Images: Ambiguity and Indeterminacy in Modern Art*. Reaktion, London.
Gell, Alfred
1998 *Art and Agency: An Anthropological Theory*. Oxford University Press, Oxford.
1999 The Technology of Enchantment and the Enchantment of Technology. In *The Art of Anthropology: Essays and Diagrams*, edited by Eric Hirsch, pp. 159–186. Athlone, London.
Gibson, Kathleen R., and Tim Ingold (editors)
1993 *Tools, Language, and Cognition in Human Evolution*. Cambridge University Press, Cambridge.
Gosden, Chris
2001 Making Sense: Archaeology and Aesthetics. *World Archaeology* 33:163–167.
Gosden, Chris, and Yvonne Marshall
1999 The Cultural Biography of Things. *World Archaeology* 31:169–178.
Halstead, Paul
1992 The Mycenaean Palatial Economy: Making the Most of the Gaps in the Evidence. *Proceedings of the Cambridge Philological Society* 38:57–86.
Hamilakis, Yannis
2007 *The Nation and Its Ruins*. Oxford University Press, Oxford.
Herva, Vesa-Pekka, and Risto Nurmi
2009 Beyond Consumption: Functionality, Artifact Biography, and Early Modernity in a European Periphery. *International Journal of Historical Archaeology* 13:158–182.
Holtorf, Cornelius
2002 Notes on the Life History of a Pot Sherd. *Journal of Material Culture* 7:49–71.
Hoskins, Janet
1998 *Biographical Objects: How Things Tell the Stories of People's Lives*. Routledge, New York.
2006 Agency, Biography, and Objects. In *Handbook of Material Culture*, edited by Christopher Tilley, Webb Keane, Susanne Küchler-Fogden, Mike Rowlands, and Patricia Spyer, pp. 74–84. Sage, London.
Hutchins, Edwin
2010 Enaction, Imagination, and Insight. In *Enaction: Toward a New Paradigm for Cognitive Science*, edited by John Stewart, Oliver Gapenne, and Ezequiel A. Di Paolo, pp. 425–450. MIT Press, Cambridge, Massachusetts.
Johnson, Mark
2007 *The Meaning of the Body: Aesthetics of Human Understanding*. University of Chicago Press, Chicago.
Katerinopoulos, Athanasios
1993 *Theofrastou Peri Lithon*. Society for Greek Mineral and Fossil Collectors, Athens.
Killen, John T.
1988 The Linear B Tablets and the Mycenaean Economy. In *Linear B: A Survey*, edited by Anna Morpurgo Davies and Yves Duhoux, pp. 241–305. Peeters, Louvain-la-Neuve.
Kinney, Dale
1997 Spolia: Damnatio and Renovatio Memoriae. *Memoirs of the American Academy in Rome* 42:117–148.

Kirsh, David
2009 Problem Solving and Situated Cognition. In *The Cambridge Handbook of Situated Cognition*, edited by Philip Robbins and Murat Aydede, pp. 264–306. Cambridge University Press, Cambridge.
Knappett, Carl
2005 *Thinking through Material Culture: An Interdisciplinary Perspective*. University of Pennsylvania Press, Philadelphia.
Knappett, Carl, and Lambros Malafouris
2008 *Material Agency: Towards a Non-Anthropocentric Approach*. Springer, Berlin.
Kopytoff, Igor
1984 The Cultural Biography of Things: Commoditization as Process. In *The Social Life of Things: Commodities in Cultural Perspective*, edited by Arjun Appadurai, pp. 64–91. Cambridge University Press, Cambridge.
Kosslyn, Stephen M.
2006 Mental Image. In *Sensorium: Embodied Experience, Technology, and Contemporary Art*, edited by Caroline A. Jones, pp. 169–170. MIT Press, Cambridge, Massachusetts.
Kreitler, Hans, and Shulamith Kreitler
1972 *Psychology of the Arts*. Duke University Press, Durham, North Carolina.
Krzyszkowska, Olga H.
1996 Furniture in the Aegean Bronze Age. In *The Furniture of Western Asia, Ancient and Traditional. Papers of the Conference Held at the Institute of Archaeology, University College London (28–30 June 1993)*, edited by Georgina Herrmann, pp. 85–103. Von Zabern, Mainz am Rhein.
2007 *Well Built Mycenae, Fascicule 24: The Ivories and Objects of Bone, Antler, and Boar's Tusk*. Oxbow Books, Oxford.
Langdon, Susan
2001 Beyond the Grave: Biographies from Early Greece. *American Journal of Archaeology* 105:579–606.
Lederman, Susan J., and Roberta L. Klatzky
2004 Multisensory Texture Perception. In *The Handbook of Multisensory Processes*, edited by Gemma Calvert, Charles Spence, and Barry E. Stein, pp. 107–122. MIT Press, Cambridge, Massachusetts.
Lemonnier, Pierre
1992 *Elements for an Anthropology of Technology*. University of Michigan, Ann Arbor.
Lemonnier, Pierre (editor)
1993 *Technological Choices: Transformation in Material Cultures since the Neolithic*. Routledge, London.
Lipartito, Kenneth
2003 Picturephone and the Information Age: The Social Meaning of Failure. *Technology and Culture* 44:50–81.
MacGregor, Gavin
1999 Making Sense of the Past in the Present: A Sensory Analysis of Carved Stone Balls. *World Archaeology* 31:258–271.
Malafouris, Lambros
2004 The Cognitive Basis of Material Engagement: Where Brain, Body, and Culture Conflate. In *Rethinking Materiality: The Engagement of the Mind with the Material World*, edited by Elizabeth DeMarrais, Chris Gosden, and Colin Renfrew, pp. 53–62. Cambridge University Press, Cambridge.

Malafouris, Lambros, and Colin Renfrew
2010 *The Cognitive Life of Things: Recasting the Boundaries of the Mind*. McDonald Institute for Archaeological Research, Cambridge.
O'Connor, Blaze, and Gabriel Cooney
2009 Introduction: Materialitas and the Significance of Stone. In *Materialitas: Working Stone, Carving Identity*, edited by Blaze O'Connor, Gabriel Cooney, and John Chapman, pp. xxi–xxv. Oxbow, Oxford.
Owoc, Mary A.
2004 Epilogue: Humans in a Mineral World. In *Soils, Stones, and Symbols: Cultural Perceptions of the Mineral World*, edited by Nicole Boivin and Mary A. Owoc, pp. 217–225. UCL Press, London.
Pabian, Roger, Brian Jackson, Peter Tandy, and John Cromartie
2006 *Agates: Treasures of the Earth*. Firefly, London.
Persson, Axel W.
1931 *The Royal Tombs at Dendra Near Midea*. Gleerup, Lund.
Petroski, Henry
1992 *To Engineer Is Human: The Role of Failure in Successful Design*. Vintage, New York.
Platon, Nikolaos, and Evi Touloupa
1965 Kadmeion. Oikopedon A. kai S. Tzortzi (Pindarou kai Antigonis). *Archaiologikon Deltion* 20 B2, pp. 231–232.
Poursat, Jean-Claude
1977 *Catalogue des ivoires mycéniens du musée national d'Athènes*. Diffusion de Boccard, Paris.
Pye, David
1995 *The Nature and Art of Workmanship*. Herbert, London.
Rahmstorf, Lorenz
2008 *Tiryns XVI. Kleinfunde Aus Tiryns: Terrakotta, Stein, Bein und Glas/Fayence vornehmlich aus der Spätbronzezeit*. Reichert, Wiesbaden.
Renfrew, A. Colin
2004 Towards a Theory of Material Engagement. In *Rethinking Materiality: The Engagement of the Mind with the Material World*, edited by Elizabeth DeMarrais, Chris Gosden, and A. Colin Renfrew, pp. 23–31. Cambridge University Press, Cambridge.
Renfrew, A. Colin, and Ezra B. W. Zubrow
1994 *The Ancient Mind: Elements of Cognitive Archaeology*. Cambridge University Press, Cambridge.
Risatti, Howard A.
2007 *A Theory of Craft: Function and Aesthetic Expression*. University of North Carolina Press, Chapel Hill.
Robb, John
2004 The Extended Artefact and the Monumental Economy: A Methodology for Material Agency. In *Rethinking Materiality: The Engagement of the Mind with the Material World*, edited by Elizabeth DeMarrais, Chris Gosden, and A. Colin Renfrew, pp. 131–139. Cambridge University Press, Cambridge.
Saunders, Nicholas
1999 Biographies of Brilliance: Pearls, Transformations of Matter, and Being, c. A.D. 1492. *World Archaeology* 31:243–257.
2004 The Cosmic Earth: Materiality and Mineralogy in the Americas. In *Soils, Stones, and Symbols: Cultural Perceptions of the Mineral World*, edited by Nicole Boivin and Mary A. Owoc, pp. 123–141. UCL Press, London.

Shanks, Michael

1998 The Life of an Artifact in an Interpretive Archaeology. *Fennoscandia Archeologica* XV:15–30.

Smith, Mark M.

2007 *Sensing the Past: Seeing, Hearing, Smelling, Tasting, and Touching in History*. University of California Press, Berkeley.

Spence, Charles

2007 Making Sense of Touch: A Multisensory Approach to the Perception of Objects. In *The Power of Touch: Handling Objects in Museum and Heritage Contexts*, edited by Elizabeth Pye, pp. 45–61. Left Coast, Walnut Creek, California.

Spyropoulos, Theodore, and John Chadwick

1975 *Thebes Tablets II*. Ediciones Universidad Salamanca, Salamanca.

Strathern, Marilyn

1988 *The Gender of the Gift: Problems with Women and Problems with Society in Melanesia*. Studies in Melanesian Anthropology, University of California Press, Berkeley.

Symeonoglou, Sarantis

1973 *Kadmeia I: Mycenaean Finds from Thebes, Greece. Excavation at 14 Oedipus Street.* Paul Åström, Göteborg.

Thompson, Evan

2007 *Mind in Life: Biology, Phenomenology, and the Sciences of the Mind*. Harvard University Press, Cambridge, Massachusetts.

Tournavitou, Iphiyenia

1995 *The 'Ivory Houses' at Mycenae*. British School at Athens, London.

Ullrich, Polly

2004 Workmanship: The Hand and Body as Perceptual Tools. In *Objects and Meaning: New Perspectives on Art and Craft*, edited by M. Anna Fariello and Paula Owen, pp. 198–214. Scarecrow, Lanham, Maryland.

Ventris, Michael, and John Chadwick

1973 *Documents in Mycenaean Greek*. 2nd edition. Cambridge University Press, Cambridge.

Weiner, Annette B.

1992 *Inalienable Possessions: The Paradox of Keeping While Giving*. University of California Press, Berkeley.

Wentworth, Nigel

2004 *The Phenomenology of Painting*. Cambridge University Press, Cambridge.

Whitley, James

2002 Objects with Attitude: Biographical Facts and Fallacies in the Study of Late Bronze Age and Early Iron Age Warrior Graves. *Cambridge Archaeological Journal* 12:217–232.

Wing, Alan, Christos Giachritsis, and Roberta Roberts

2007 Weighing Up the Value of Touch. In *The Power of Touch: Handling Objects in Museum and Heritage Contexts*, edited by Elizabeth Pye, pp. 31–43. Left Coast, Walnut Creek, California.

Young, Diana

2006 The Colours of Things. In *Handbook of Material Culture*, edited by Christopher Tilley, Webb Keane, Susanne Küchler-Fogden, Mike Rowlands, and Patricia Spyer, pp. 173–183. Sage, London.

Xenaki-Sakellariou, Agne

1985 *Oi Thalamotoi Tafoi ton Mykenon Anaskafis Chr. Tsounta (1887–1898)*. Diffusion de Boccard, Paris.

# 16. Scents and Sensibilities: The Phenomenology of Late Neolithic Iberian Slate Plaque Production

*Jonathan T. Thomas*

*Abstract:* The engraved slate plaques of Late Neolithic (3500–2500 B.C.E.) Iberia are some of the most enigmatic expressions of prehistoric European art, capturing the imagination of the public and archaeologists alike during the past century. Thousands of these hand-size, perforated plaques have been found in Neolithic collective burials, and they are thought to have served as mnemonic, prestigious, or ritual objects, perhaps for specific individuals. Large numbers of plaques were initially experimentally replicated to answer questions related to the *chaîne opératoire* of their production. These experiments, however, also yielded valuable phenomenological information about the sensory—the haptic, olfactory, auditory, visual, and even gustatory—experience of plaque making. Some of the results of this research allow us to actually identify individual plaque makers in the archaeological record in certain cases and to better understand the emergence of organized craft production in early complex societies.

We and the people of the past share carnal bodies.

—Christopher Tilley (2004:201)

Following the immensely ambitious and productive period associated with the New Archaeology, a number of archaeologists began to voice epistemological concerns with the discipline's embrace of empirical positivism, questioning not only the interpretation of archaeological evidence but also the types of archaeological knowledge considered valid within orthodox scientific frameworks.

*Making Senses of the Past: Toward a Sensory Archaeology,* edited by Jo Day. Center for Archaeological Investigations, Occasional Paper No. 40.  ISBN 978-0-8093-3287-8.

One emblematic and now rather well-known response to what was seen as an increasingly mechanistic, impersonal view of people's lives in the past was the question, "Why have archaeologists produced a prehistory of genderless, faceless blobs?" (Tringham 1991:97).

This desire for a thick—or at least thick*er*—description of individuals in prehistory resonated with a great number of archaeologists. In a few instances, the discipline had actually done a fairly good job of fleshing out a limited number of (typically androcentric) "types." However, although we found it fairly easy to envision the faces of the chiefs, the shamans, and the other prehistoric movers and shakers, the "blob problem" remained. Out of frustration with this perceived one-dimensional understanding of people in the past, an interest in phenomenology, or the nature of individual embodied experience in various environments (sensu Brück 2005), began to gain currency.

While many archaeologists often associate phenomenology with the influence of postmodernism on British landscape archaeologists such as Christopher Tilley or Julian Thomas, the use of individual physical and perceptual experience as a heuristic tool or means of descriptive analogy has arguably been a core element of anthropology since its inception and is certainly one of the advantages of anthropology over closely related disciplines. Clearly archaeologists should not make the mistake of using modern embodied experiences as *direct* analogies to those of people in the past or in other cultures, but we certainly can—and should—use phenomenological information to generate both heuristic and testable ideas that aid in the interpretation of archaeological data. In keeping with this, this chapter presents information related to the southern Iberian Late Neolithic engraved slate burial plaques and to the sensory experiences of modern slate-plaque makers. This information, unobtainable through historical research, contributes to our understanding of the *chaîne opératoire* of archaeological plaque production and to our knowledge of the emergence and organization of prestige-goods production in early complex societies.

## The Late Neolithic of Southwestern Iberia

The experimental replication of the southwestern Iberian Late Neolithic engraved slate plaques was initially designed to clarify aspects of archaeological plaque production related to engraver skill and engraving-tool technology. The resulting phenomenological information about the sensory experience of plaque making was initially an unintended by-product of these experiments. Before describing these replication experiments, however, a brief introduction to the Iberian Late Neolithic and to the engraved burial plaques is necessary.

In southwestern Iberia, the Late Neolithic is generally considered a period of social and political transformation often associated with a new emphasis on agriculture (Gonçalves 1999), social differentiation, and the cyclical integration and fission of groups responsible for the construction of large, fortified settlements (e.g., Zambujal, Vila Nova de São Pedro, Leceia) and elaborate, labor-intensive collective tombs (Fohrenbaher 1999). This region has long been known as a core area of prehistoric population aggregation and is particularly rich in terms of Late Neolithic archaeological sites and materials (Cardoso 2000; Kunst and Trindade 1990). Although incipient elites may have been emerging in southern Iberia during the Late Neolithic, the evidence of institutionalized class division, differential access to productive resources, political centralization, or rigid hierarchical systems is scarce (Chapman 2003). Most evidence indicates that Late Neolithic groups were not highly stratified, but it is generally agreed that some social differentiation existed and that this differentiation generally increased over time (Díaz-del-Río 2006; Forenbaher 1999; Gilman 1987; Jorge 1990; Jorge 1995; Kunst 1995; Lillios 1995). Large Late Neolithic and Copper Age craft production centers such as Zambujal in southwestern Portugal appear to be contemporary with and roughly equivalent (in terms of cultural complexity) to those in southeastern Spain such as Los Millares. However, it must be reiterated that evidence of craft production in southern Iberia during this period is highly variable, both from site to site and through time.

Similar to people from elsewhere in Atlantic Europe, Late Neolithic groups in southwestern Iberia typically buried their dead in collective tombs: megaliths (dolmens, passage graves, or corbel vaulted tombs), caves, rock shelters, or rock-cut tombs. Collective burials were used and reused for extensive periods of time (Jorge and Jorge 1997), and newer megalithic structures were often constructed upon or annexed to older ones. While the specific sequence of interment and subsequent manipulation of skeletal remains or secondary burial is generally unknown, the commingling of bones at these locations suggests that as part of the funerary process some human remains from previous burials were moved and reconfigured. Burial goods such as bifacial flint tools; bone tools and ornaments; ceramic vessels and "loom weights"; ground stone axes, adzes, chisels, and hammers; and decorated ritual objects typically referred to as "idols"—made from limestone and bone—were commonly deposited in these burials (Thomas 2009). In addition to these, perforated beads and pendants similar to the slate plaques but made from a variety of materials are common.

The engraved slate burial plaques are some of the more enigmatic types of material culture found in the Late Neolithic collective burials (Figure 16-1). Several thousand engraved slate plaques have been recovered from over 200 burials in southwestern Iberia (Lillios 2008). While some of the largest Late Neolithic tombs contain hundreds of these objects (e.g., Escoural, Olival da Pega, Ante Grande do Zambujeiro), in most collective burials, plaques are typically found one at a time or in small groups. With the exception of Águas Frias (Alandroal), where the entire *chaîne opératoire* of plaque production is attested to (Gonçalves and Calado 2006), plaque workshops are absent from the archaeological record. Thus, a single modality for plaque making is unlikely. It appears that a spectrum of plaque making existed across different production contexts, perhaps culminating in their ritual production at the largest megalithic tombs by the end of the Late Neolithic.

In the past, plaques have been interpreted as depictions of the European Mother Goddess (e.g., Almagro Gorbea 1973; Gimbutas 1991; Gonçalves 1992, 1999; Rodrigues 1986a, 1986b), as heraldry (Lillios 2008; Lisboa 1985), or as ethnic

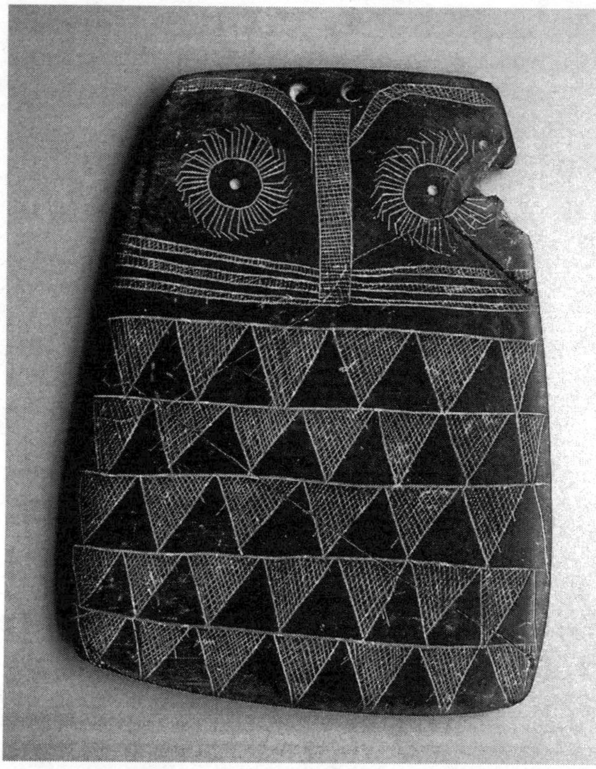

**Figure 16-1.** *Enigmatic engraved slate plaque from Valencina de la Concepción (Seville, Spain) featuring a common cross-hatched triangle pattern underneath more rarely occurring ocular imagery. (Photograph © Jonathan T. Thomas; used with permission of Museo Arqueológico de Sevilla.)*

identifiers (Bueno Ramírez 1992). Based on an analysis of over 1,300 plaques, Lillios has suggested that the majority of them functioned as mnemonic or genealogical markers (2008). When found with an articulated individual, engraved plaques were thought to have been placed on the chest of, or next to, the skeleton (Gonçalves 1999:87). Because the minimum number of individuals (MNI) in a tomb is always higher than the number of plaques recovered (Silva 1999:356–357; Spindler 1981:224), it is clear that not everyone in the Late Neolithic was interred with a plaque. This suggests that they might have been ritual or prestige objects or restricted in some other sense.

With a few exceptions, Late Neolithic plaques are made from slate from the Iberian interior. They are hand sized (~15 cm high) and perforated with several holes at the top, ostensibly for cordage. Most are thin (~.5 cm), trapezoidal, and engraved on one side, although some plaques are partially or completely engraved on both sides. Typically, these engravings conform to a fairly specific design grammar: zigzags, triangles, chevrons, checkerboards, herringbones, and occasionally zoomorphic or anthropomorphic imagery (Lillios 2008). This decorative imagery is found on other types of Late Neolithic material culture, such as megalithic art, limestone figurines, and ceramics, as well as on later Bell Beaker ceramics (Bradley 1997:2002; Bueno Ramírez 1992; Bueno Ramírez and Balbín Behrmann 1992). Though the engraved plaques represent a coherent element of a larger corpus of Iberian visual imagery that existed prior to and following the Late Neolithic, relatively little is known about plaque production or who plaque makers were. While archaeologists have contested the meaning of plaque imagery, it typically evokes imagery found on other Late Neolithic material culture such as stone axes, dolmen orthostats and capstones, ceramics, basketry, textiles, and other woven materials (Lillios and Thomas 2010). Thus, although the plaques are contextually associated with death, their form and imagery simultaneously reference aspects of Late Neolithic life.

In earlier work with the engraved slate plaques, Katina Lillios and I briefly described some of the phenomenological information that can be derived from their design and shape. The relatively small size of the plaques (ranging roughly from 10 to 20 cm) encourages individuals to be in close proximity in order to see their designs and, at the same time, restricts the number of people who are able to effectively view them at any one time. In addition to this, many of the plaques have anthropomorphic or zoomorphic designs dominated by ocular motifs. These "eyed individuals" in some ways act as what Alfred Gell (1996) refers to as "Secondary Agents." In this capacity, they command the focus of the viewer, drawing direct attention to their imagery, in essence trapping our gaze and in some ways our imagination. Because the emphasis has largely been placed on the visual qualities of the plaques, little or no work has focused on the other sensory stimuli they evoke, a problem common to phenomenological research (see Brück 2005 for a more extensive discussion).

## Plaque Replication Experiments

As a raw material, slate lends itself to experimental analysis. Slate is a durable but easily worked material: It is malleable and highly responsive to engraving tools of varying hardnesses. Incisions made on slate tend to be resistant to taphonomy and to some degree even record the directionality and force of the motion that created them. Against the dark luster of slate, engraved lines appear much brighter and are easily analyzed visually, without optical aids or with microscopy.

In initial plaque replication experiments, replica plaques were created and worn by volunteers around their necks (using different cordage materials) each day for over a month to determine if archaeological plaques showed signs of use wear, either within the perforation or on the surface (Woods and Lillios 2006). The results show that slate, when worn in daily contexts, absorbs oils that quickly obscure lighter-colored engraving lines. The perforations on this set of experimental plaques were then analyzed in order to determine if the archaeological plaques were worn by living, moving individuals prior to their deposition in burials. The use-wear experiment on the replica plaques demonstrated that different types of cordage leave very distinct evidence of wear, which was not present on the archaeological plaques. Because archaeological plaques have little if any use wear within their perforations, it was concluded that the plaques were likely placed on the dead upon interment rather than worn on a regular basis. The fact that the engraving lines on archaeological plaques are still quite bright even today also suggests that the plaques were likely worn by the dead upon interment rather than in day-to-day life.

Starting in 2005, I began to conduct another series of replication experiments designed to answer questions about the degree of skill and labor involved in plaque production. In these experiments, groups of volunteer plaque makers were asked to engrave copies of a single archaeological plaque repeatedly. The goal of producing a large number of facsimiles of a single plaque was to hold constant as many aspects of variation—material, functional, technological, and decorative—as possible in order to better interpret variation in archaeological assemblages. The results of these experiments demonstrated that variation related to fine-motor skills was greater between individual engravers than within the work of a single engraver, allowing the work of more skilled engravers to be consistently and accurately identified. The traits distinguishing experimental plaque makers were applied to several sets of archaeological plaques, in which a number of distinct plaque making "experts" were identified at several sites (Thomas et al. 2009). A third series of plaques were experimentally replicated to analyze technological variation in terms of engraving tools (lithic, bone, copper, etc.). The results of microscopic use-wear analysis on the third set of replica plaques indicated that stone tools work as well as if not better than copper tools to engrave plaques. While copper tools existed at the end of the Late Neolithic, they would have been relatively rare and difficult to obtain.

The production of the replica plaques was based on the methods employed by Woods and Lillios (2006). Because we know next to nothing about the actual *chaîne opératoire* of plaque production, we intentionally kept our technology as simple as possible and variability to a minimum. With the assistance of volunteers, I typically began by breaking apart large compositionally homogenous slate chalkboards. In contrast, Neolithic Iberians were likely quarrying large blocks of slate and reducing them to blanks or preforms (Gonçalves and Calado 2006), such as can be found at Águas Frias (Alandroal) (Figure 16-2). Subsequent experiments in reducing and engraving larger chunks of several types of quarried slate demonstrate that it is a much more laborious process than was initially thought.

After examining a number of unfinished or unengraved Late Neolithic plaques, we began making plaque preforms by breaking and grinding pieces of slate into trapezoidal shapes of roughly the desired size (Figure 16-3). A large stock of standardized blank slate plaques was produced. After individual preforms were broken into trapezoidal shapes, their edges were ground to the desired size on concrete (approximately 15 cm tall by 7.5 cm wide). Although it is certain that archaeological plaques were not ground on a cement sidewalk or pavement, Late Neolithic Iberians would have had a variety of slates, limestones, sandstones, granites, and other types of coarse stones on which to grind their own plaques. These replica plaques were then perforated with a flint burin, polished with a piece of leather to bring out the natural dark luster of slate,

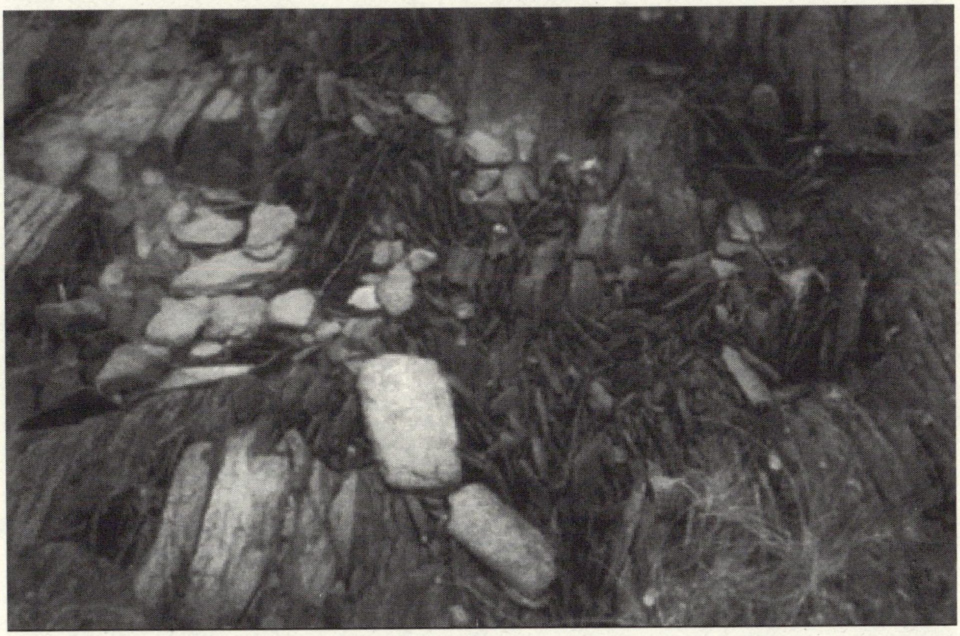

**Figure 16-2.** *The only known plaque production site at Águas Frias (northern Portugal), where the entire* chaîne opératoire *of plaque making from quarrying to finished, perforated plaques is evident. (Photograph © Rafael Henriques; used with permission.)*

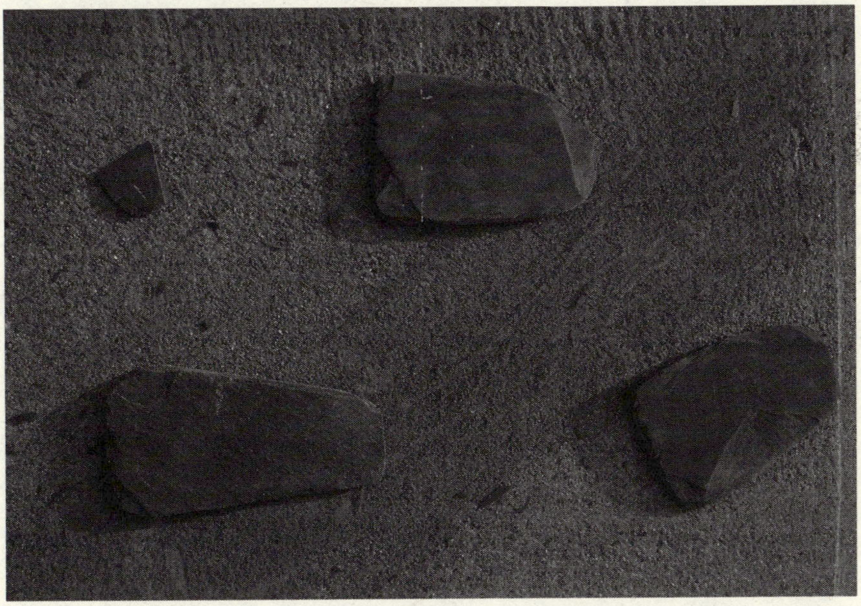

**Figure 16-3.** *Experimental slate plaque preforms in the process of being ground into trapezoidal shapes on the pavement. (Photograph © Jonathan T. Thomas.)*

and engraved with flint, quartz, or copper tools. After beveling the edges of the replica plaques, a sanding pad was used to smooth the engraving face, and then a piece of leather was used to bring out the luster of the slate's surface. The surfaces of the replica plaques are, to the eye, indistinguishable from their Neolithic counterparts (although distinct surface-wear and trace elements left by engraving tools are detectable using SEM-EDX microscopy). It took approximately two hours to prepare a blank, unengraved plaque from blackboard slate; quarried slate requires two to three times as long to reduce to preforms.

In each replication experiment, volunteers were given a photograph of an archaeological plaque from Pedra Branca (Figure 16-4) and asked to engrave a copy of it as closely as possible. Thus, the resulting 20 plaques were engraved with an identical design motif, although executed with individual styles. The archaeological plaque selected for replication represents one of the most common types and is decorated with one of the most commonly found geometric motifs: the triangle. Triangular shapes also tend to be relatively easy to engrave in comparison to some of the more complicated anthropomorphic or zoomorphic plaque motifs. After a few engraving sessions, it became clear that our student plaque makers were primarily proceeding from their mental template of the design. While they occasionally referred to the photographs, each plaque maker spent a majority of his or her time concentrating on engraving and only occasionally consulted the photograph for landmarks and visual verification. The engraving sessions lasted approximately 30–60 minutes and were followed by extensive exit interviews.

The sensory information that resulted from these replication experiments was largely the result of these exit interviews. While I attempted to design questions that would elucidate the degree of skill involved, plaque makers consistently seemed to want to convey their ideas about the sensory aspects of plaque making. After grinding the slate on the concrete, plaque makers vociferously noted the burning, pungent smell of the slate particles, which not only fill the nose but also end up in the mouth, forming an acrid-tasting, moisture-absorbent, chalky dust necessitating the use of masks. This dust is not only unpleasant to breathe or taste, but it also occasionally produces a slight burning sensation in the eyes that causes them to tear. When slate is worked on the ground it also becomes very hot to the touch. Yet, at the same time as the slate is hot and smooth to the touch, it also has jagged edges that lacerate the palms and fingers, occasionally causing small cuts on the hands of plaque makers. All plaque makers consistently commented on the wear and tear plaque making causes on the hands and described soreness and pain associated with their weekly endeavors turning jagged, unworked, abrasive slate into finished, polished plaques. Thus, the experience of plaque making for Late Neolithic plaque makers might not have been an entirely pleasant one. Pain and discomfort, while not an essential part of plaque making, may have come to be associated with it. In addition, this would have added to the process a mnemonic component, in which the sensory experience of making a plaque recalled the difficulties of earlier episodes of plaque making.

Plaque makers reported that different engraving tools each had a unique feel, and they often developed specific preferences for tools they felt were easier

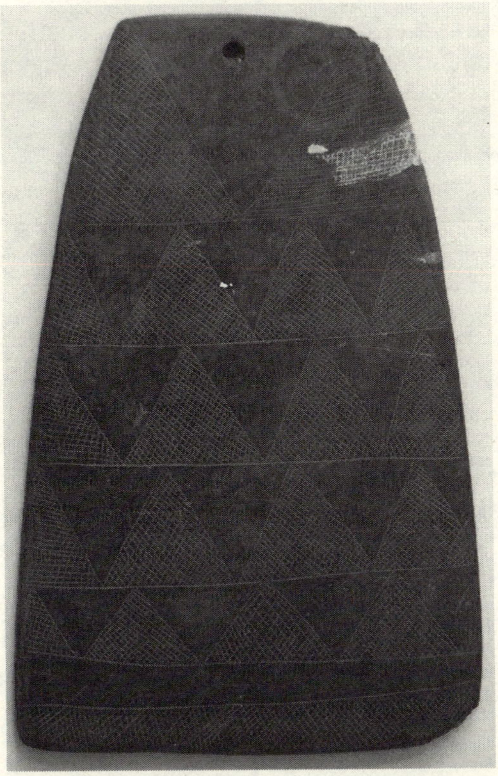

**Figure 16-4.** *The engraved slate plaque from Pedra Branca that was used as a template for modern experimental plaque makers. It was chosen for the regularity of its incised shapes and overall simplicity of design. (Photograph © Jonathan T. Thomas; used with permission of Museu Geológico de Lisboa.)*

or more comfortable to work with. Different engraving tools also created a variety of different sounds: the engraving sessions were often brought to a halt with groans and some good-natured laughing when an engraver's tool resulted in a loud, screeching noise identical to the sound of chalk or fingernails running down a slate blackboard. Engraving slate resulted in a unique and quickly recognizable set of sounds that soon became familiar.

Plaque makers repeatedly expressed their appreciation of the tactile properties of slate, which—in addition to being visually attractive—is soft, smooth, and quickly becomes warm to the touch. Slate was described as an inviting material to hold in one's hand or otherwise pleasurable to touch and look at. Despite this, plaques proved to be cumbersome objects to wear, and often went from a chalky-grey to a dark, glossy black after absorbing the oils from people's clothing, skin, and hair.

In terms of skill, plaque makers repeatedly noted the period in which they felt their engraving skills were improving and the point at which they felt their skills had essentially plateaued. In general, however, most plaque makers reported being increasingly satisfied with their engraving abilities and the outcome of their work over time. They developed, in the words of one volunteer, a sense of "plaqueness"—that is, a sensibility about when plaques were finished, the amount of acceptable error, and what conventions could or could not be broken in terms of a plaque's acceptability. Plaque makers reiterated that any pain or physical stress incurred during the process, an important part of the tactile-kinesthetic component of phenomenological experience, was outweighed by the positive parts of the experience and the final result.

Most important, I recorded numerous examples of culturally coded cross-modal synesthesia. As described by Houston and Taube (2000), cross-modal synesthesia is similar to physiological synesthesia, in which the brain interprets a particular sensation using a sense that would not normally be used (e.g., hearing or tasting a color; seeing an odor). Culturally coded synesthesia occurs when a sensory input triggers parallel sensations in other senses or when one type of sensory experience triggers the memory of other types of sensory experience that are not immediate. Often, plaque makers would enter the laboratory and upon smelling the somewhat burnt scent of ground slate begin to speak of their own experiences with plaque production. Loud noises produced during the engraving process would elicit discussions of particular problems or similar experiences in the past. While it is of course difficult to demonstrate this type of sensory-memory effect among the original Late Neolithic plaque makers, it is clear that plaque making had a sensory component as well a mnemonic one and reasonable to assume that these components were somehow interrelated. Thus, different sensory inputs—the sights, sounds, and scents of plaque making—affected plaque makers' sensibilities about the process and their memories of it afterward.

Much like my experimental plaque makers, Late Neolithic plaque makers certainly must have had a sense of their own work, their own plaque-making style. This sense of individual style was not something that I was initially aware of when I began to explore technological variation among the plaques; only after collecting the exit interviews about plaque engravers' experiences did I realize that it might be possible to quantitatively examine the variation related to an individual plaque maker's fine-motor skills. This is an encouraging example of how phenomenological approaches can provide testable hypotheses and generate new answers to archaeological questions.

## Discussion

Because an archaeology of the senses is closely related to phenomenological approaches, a brief discussion of the development of phenomenological archaeology is warranted. During the past twenty years, anthropologists have increasingly added phenomenological approaches to the conceptual tools they have had at their disposal (e.g., Tilley 1994, 2004), emphasizing the subjective aspects of personal experience within our broader understanding of patterns in human culture. Because corporeal experience is highly variable for physical (age, sex, and health related), biological, and cultural reasons, the replicability and epistemological validity of phenomenological knowledge claims about the past have been hotly contested. In spite of this, most archaeologists would be hard pressed to deny that, at some level, the human body is a valid link between the past and the present (Sanders 1990).

One way in which phenomenology has been used—and the manner in which it is employed here—is as a hermeneutic tool for interpreting material culture and describing "the character of human experience, specifically the ways in which we apprehend the material world through directed intervention in our surroundings" (Brück 2005:46). The use of phenomenology within archaeology has by far had the most impact on archaeological theory in Britain, where scholars such as Christopher Tilley have argued that individuals do not experience the world in terms of two-dimensional abstract space but rather through the sensuous world in which the human body is embedded. Thus, the world as humans actually perceive it is experienced as a sensuous, three-dimensional (or four-dimensional, if we count time) space and an embodied engagement with the landscape and the entirety of the material world is central to human experience (Tilley 2004:10–12). Simply put, as archaeologists, our encounters with archaeological landscapes and objects provide valuable insights into the ways in which prehistoric individuals experienced and understood the world. Because our experience is mediated through the human body, modern ideas and perceptions of the landscape may share many elements with and serve as analogues to those of people in the past (Tilley 1994, 2004:201–202). Theoretically, phenomenology privileges subjective, lived understandings of the world over objective or scientific understandings of it and is more broadly an assault on Cartesian positivism (Brück 2005:45).

In many ways, the development of an archaeology of the senses is an outgrowth, or perhaps a elaboration, of the phenomenological interest in landscapes and architecture that coalesced into an interest in the realm of material culture. Research on the individual experience of landscapes has broadened into an interest in smellscapes, soundscapes, tastescapes, and touchscapes. As with my research on the Late Neolithic engraved slate plaques, many of the chapters in this volume focus on the sensory impact of a restricted type of material object or a particular sensory experience within a delineated space. As an archaeology of the senses moves forward, I have little doubt that we will see more in-depth work that zeros in on highly specific sensory experiences. However, as I have discovered in my own foray into phenomenological archaeology, an archaeology of the senses deals not only with an individual's immediate sensory experience but also with the effect of that sensory experience on meaning and memory.

## Obstacles for an Archaeology of the Senses

It is also important to address some of the obstacles brought to light specifically by this project that archaeologists who use phenomenological approaches face. One common critique of phenomenological approaches to archaeology is that we risk creating for ourselves a series of imaginative just-so stories about human life in the past. While I think this concern is completely warranted, I do not think that just-so stories are strictly the purview of phenomenological approaches. One need only open any volume on Mother Goddesses, shamans, or Neandertals to realize that many approaches, even those based on hard science, can lead to anthropological just-so stories. As I have tried to demonstrate in this chapter, testable ideas can come from anywhere, including from our own admittedly subjective sensory experience of the world.

As noted by several contributors to this volume, phenomenological questions and the reconstruction of ephemeral past experiences can be difficult to address via material culture. Many critics of phenomenology have pointed out that the representation of a "universal human body" or a "universal sensuous experience" is highly problematic for several reasons (Hamilakis et al. 2002:9; Hodder 1999; Meskell 1996). For biological and physical reasons related to—among other things—age, health, and sex, sensory experience of the physical world is a highly variable, complex phenomenon, from which the singular sensory experience is irreducible.

Similarly, individual experience of the physical world is highly variable for cultural reasons as well. The human body and the range of its potential experience is clearly socially and culturally constructed. According to Brück, the body "forms a locus for the construction of identity and the mediation of the relationship between individual and society. As such, it is a site of contested meanings" (2005:55). Thus, even given identical material conditions, individual physical experience is highly variable both within and between cultures. Because of this, archaeologists' encounters with landscapes and material culture may not serve as appropriate analogues to those of people in the past. By focusing on own our experience of the sensuous world without critically reflecting on the implications of phenomenology as a heuristic tool, we run the risk of adopting a process of interpretation that is so idiosyncratic that it is likely to be of little value to anyone other than ourselves. Nonetheless, although a sense of "individual experience" connected to sensory perception of the physical world is no doubt culturally constructed, biologically contingent, and quite different from that of people in the past, it can still be used as a productive method of indirect analogy. I would have never investigated whether or not Late Neolithic plaque makers could be identified stylistically had not one of my modern-day plaque makers begun to sense the development of his own unique plaque-making style.

## Conclusion

We are still working on giving faces to the "faceless blobs" in prehistory. To avoid doing so is to do violence to the people of the past and to perpetuate a dehumanized, unreflexive anthropology that the discipline has been attempting to escape from for the past three decades. An archaeology of the senses has the potential for being a powerful avenue for such research.

What is the value of my own experiences with making plaques and that of my plaque makers in terms of understanding the archaeological record and, more generally, life in the Late Neolithic? The jury is still out on this one. While a great deal of phenomenological information was gleaned through the process of plaque making, my interest in the sights, sounds, smells, and other sensations of plaque making was perhaps more hypersensitive than someone not ruminating on such sensory qualities. I have no way of knowing if the smell of making plaques went unnoticed by prehistoric plaque makers or if it was intimately linked to the creation of memory associated with plaque making nor of knowing if the pain involved was a crucial (i.e., "ritual") or simply an epiphenomenal part of plaque making. It is possible that the burning sensation in the eyes mimicked or was associated with the tearful mourning for those about to be buried with a freshly made plaque, but this idea is beyond my own capability to test. Was my plaque makers' sense of "plaqueness" similar or even relatable to that of the ancient Iberians? While this is not difficult to imagine, it is certainly difficult to prove beyond a reasonable doubt.

In my case, the potential narratives of plaque making are highly dependent on who plaque makers were and who witnessed plaque production. Certainly, the visual qualities of the plaques had great power, as attested to by their uniform shape and design and their long life as funerary phenomena. However, the potential narrative of the individual perspective of plaque making differs according to the relationship of the plaque maker to both the deceased and the community. Mnemonic qualities related to the sensory aspects of plaque making are clearly different if close family members were responsible for making plaques. In this case, the sights, sounds, smells, and tastes involved in plaque making might be associated with mourning or with religious experience. However, if plaques were produced by extralocal specialists with no connection to the dead, then the sensory experiences and resulting potential narratives of plaque making are something altogether different. We can also envision a combination of these scenarios that would result in an experience that was variable in terms of meaning, emotion, memory, and sensory stimulus. Similarly, the sensory experience of making a single plaque (or even a few initial plaques) is drastically different from a lifetime spent making them.

This project has also led to me to the realization that archaeologists need to engage more with the phenomenological experience of producing the material culture that they study. Critics of experimental archaeology have largely missed the boat, often criticizing the highly specific information produced by experimental archaeology (e.g., how many kilocalories it takes to chop down a tree with a groundstone axe). While this information can be valuable, on the one hand it is perhaps too specific and contingent to have been of realistic concern to people in the past and on the other completely ignores the sensory experience of making and handling an object. In many ways, archaeologists have always used phenomenologically derived knowledge (although they may not have referred to it as such) in order to generate ideas from which to form the bases of testable hypotheses; the onus is now on us to develop methodologies to test these ideas. In this case, sensory archaeology allowed me to begin to distinguish individual plaque makers in the archaeological record and to better understand their role in the organization of prestige-goods production during the Late Neolithic. As I see it, experimental archaeology and phenomenology, as exemplars of processual and postprocessual research paradigms, are not mutually exclusive but rather quite complementary; it is only the epistemological blinders that we so often wear that have kept us from this realization.

## References


Almagro Gorbea, Martín J.
1973 *Los Idolos del Bronce I Hispano*. Consejo Superior de Investigaciones Científicas, Madrid.
Bradley, Richard
1997 *Rock Art and the Prehistory of Atlantic Europe*. Routledge, London.
2002 Access, Style, and Imagery: The Audience for Prehistoric Rock Art in Atlantic Spain and Portugal, 4000–2000 B.C. *Oxford Journal of Archaeology* 21:231–247.
Brück, Joanna M.
2005 Experiencing the Past? The Development of a Phenomenological Archaeology in British Prehistory. *Archaeological Dialogues* 121:45–72.
Bueno Ramírez, Primitiva
1992 Les plaques décorées Alentéjaines: Approche de leur étude et analyse. *L'Anthropologie* 96:573–604.
Bueno Ramírez, Primitiva, and Rodrigo de Balbín Behrmann
1992 L'art mégalithique dans la Péninsule Ibérique: Une vue d'ensemble. *L'Anthropologie* 96:499–572.
Cardoso, João Luís
2000 The Fortified Site of Leceia (Oeiras) in the Context of the Chalcolithic in Portuguese Estremadura. *Oxford Journal of Archaeology* 19:37–55.
Chapman, Robert W.
2003 *Archaeologies of Complexity*. Routledge, London.
Díaz-del-Río, Pedro
2006 An Appraisal of Social Inequalities in Central Iberia (c. 5300–1600 cal B.C.). In *Social Inequality in Iberian Late Prehistory*, edited by Pedro Díaz-del-Río and Leonardo García Sanjuán, pp. 67–77. BAR International Series 1525. British Archaeological Reports, Oxford.
Forenbaher, Staso
1999 *Production and Exchange of Bifacial Flaked Stone Artifacts during the Portuguese Chalcolithic*. BAR Series 756. British Archaeological Reports, Oxford.
Gell, Alfred F.
1996 Vogel's Net: Traps as Artworks and Artworks as Traps. *Journal of Material Culture* 1:15–38.
Gilman, Antonio
1987 Unequal Development in Copper Age Iberia. In *Specialization, Exchange, and Complex Societies*, edited by Elizabeth M. Brumfiel and Timothy Earle, pp. 22–29. Cambridge University Press, Cambridge.
Gimbutas, Maria A.
1991 *The Civilization of the Goddess*. Harper, San Francisco.
Gonçalves, Victor S.
1992 *Revendo as Antas de Reguengos de Monsaraz*. Instituto Nacional de Investigação Cientifica, Lisbon.
1999 *Reguengos de Monsaraz: Territórios Megalíticos*. Câmara Municipal de Reguengos de Monsaraz, Lisbon.
Gonçalves, Victor S., and Manuel Calado
2006 Working at Home (and Abroad): The Atelier of Engraved Schist Plaques of Águas Frias (Alandroal). *Abstracts of the UISPP XV Congress*. UISPP, Lisbon.
Hamilakis, Yannis, Mark Pluciennik, and Sarah Tarlow
2002 Introduction. In *Thinking through the Body: Archaeologies of Corporeality*, edited

by Yannis Hamilakis, Mark Pluciennik, and Sarah Tarlow, pp. 1–21. Springer, New York.

Hodder, Ian
1999 *The Archaeological Process. An Introduction*. Blackwell, Oxford.

Houston, Stephen, and Karl Taube
2000 An Archaeology of the Senses: Perception and Cultural Expression in Ancient Mesoamerica. *Cambridge Archaeological Journal* 10:261–294.

Jorge, Susana O.
1990 Desenvolvimento da hierarquizacao social e da metalurgia. In *Nova Historia de Portugal, Vol. 1: Portugal das Origens a Romanizacao*, edited by Jorge de Alarcão, pp. 184–185. Editorial Presença, Lisbon.

Jorge, Susana O., and Victor O. Jorge
1997 The Neolithic/Chalcolithic Transition in Portugal. In *The Archaeology of Iberia: The Dynamics of Change*, edited by Margarita Díaz-Andreu and Simon Keay, pp. 128–142. Routledge, London.

Jorge, Victor
1995 Late Prehistoric Funerary Mounds in Northern Portugal as Indicators of Social Complexity. In *The Origins of Complex Societies in Late Prehistoric Iberia*, edited by Katina T. Lillios, pp. 140–152. University of Michigan Press, Ann Arbor.

Kunst, Michael
1995 Central Places and Social Complexity in the Iberian Copper Age. In *The Origins of Complex Societies in Late Prehistoric Iberia*, edited by Katina T. Lillios, pp. 32–43. University of Michigan Press, Ann Arbor.

Kunst, Michael, and Leonel Trindade
1990 Zur besiedlungesgeschicte des Sizandrotals: Ergebnisse aus der küstenforshung. *Madrider Mitteilungen* 31:34–83.

Lillios, Katina T.
2008 *Heraldry for the Dead: Memory, Identity, and the Engraved Stone Plaques of Neolithic Iberia*. University of Texas Press, Austin.

Lillios, Katina T. (editor)
1995 *The Origins of Complex Societies in Late Prehistoric Iberia*. University of Michigan Press, Ann Arbor.

Lillios, Katina T., and Jonathan T. Thomas
2010 Speaking of Stone, Speaking through Stone: An Exegesis of an Engraved Slate Plaque from Late Neolithic Iberia. In *Materialitas: Working Stone, Carving Identity*, edited by John Chapman, Gabriel Cooney, and Blaze O'Conner, pp. 138–146. Oxbow, Oxford.

Lisboa, I. M. G.
1985 Meaning and Messages: Mapping Style in the Iberian Chalcolithic. *Archaeological Review from Cambridge* 4(2):181–196.

Meskell, Lynn
1996 The Somatisation of Archaeology. Institutions, Discourses, Corporeality. *Norwegian Archaeological Review* 29:1–16.

Rodrigues, María da Conceição Monteiro
1986a *Código Para a Análise das Placas de Xisto Gravadas do Alto Altentejo—Nova Estratégia Para o Tratamento de Dados em Arqueologia*, Vol. I. Câmara Municipal de Castelo de Vide, Castelo de Vide, Portugal.
1986b *Estudo Ideológico-Simbólico das Placas de Xisto Gravadas—Alto Alentejo*, Vol. II. Câmara Municipal de Castelo de Vide, Castelo de Vide, Portugal.

Sanders, Donald H.
1990 Behavioral Conventions and Archaeology: Methods for the Analysis of Ancient

Architecture. In *Domestic Architecture and the Use of Space: An Interdisciplinary Cross-Cultural Study*, edited by Susan Kent, pp. 43–72. Cambridge University Press, Cambridge.

Silva, Ana Maria

1999 A Nécropole Neolitica do Cabeço da Arruda (Torres Vedras, Portugal): Os Dados Oaleobiológicos. In *Sagvntvm (Actes del II Congrés del Neolitic a la Peninsula Ibérica), Valencia, Espanha, 7–9 April*, pp. 355–360. Departament de Prehistòria i d'Arqueologia, Universidade de Valencia, Valencia.

Spindler, Konrad

1981 *Cova da Moura: Die Besiedlung des Atlantischen Küstengebietes Mittelportugals vom Neolithikum bis an das Ende der Bronzezeit*. Von Zabern, Mainz am Rhein.

Thomas, Jonathan T.

2009 Approaching Specialization: Craft Production in Late Neolithic/Copper Age Iberia. *Papers from the Institute of Archaeology*, Vol. 19, pp. 67–84. University College London, London.

Thomas, Jonathan T., Grant McCall, and Katina T. Tobias

2009 Revisiting the Individual in Prehistory: Idiosyncratic Engraving Variation and the Neolithic Slate Plaques of the Iberian Peninsula. *Cambridge Archaeological Journal* 19:53–72.

Tilley, Christopher Y.

1994 *A Phenomenology of Landscape: Places, Paths, and Monuments*. Berg, Oxford.

2004 Round Barrows and Dykes as Landscape Metaphors. *Cambridge Archaeological Journal* 14:185–203.

Tringham, Ruth E.

1991 Households with Faces: The Challenge of Gender in Prehistoric Architectural Remains. In *Engendering Archaeology: Women and Prehistory*, edited by Joan M. Gero and Margaret W. Conkey, pp. 93–131. Blackwell, Oxford.

Woods, Alexander D., and Katina T. Lillios

2006 Wearing Stone: Experimental Use-Wear Analysis of the Iberian Engraved Slate Plaques. In *Actas do IV Congresso de Arqueologia Peninsular (Faro 2004)*, edited by Nuno Bicho, pp. 29–37. Centro de Estudos de Património, Faro, Portugal.

# 17. The Production Process as Sensory Experience: Making and Seeing Iron in Colonial New England

*Krysta Ryzewski*

*Abstract:* Making objects, whether by wrought or mechanized techniques, is now and was in the past a multisensory affair, but a challenge exists as to how to identify and interpret these sensory acts of production in archaeological materials. Using examples from colonial-period iron production sites in New England, this discussion demonstrates how archaeological assemblages may be uniquely suited to address the social, material, and sensory complexities of craft production. Written documentation of metal (and other) production processes is often limited in its description of craft operations, which were largely guided by tactile engagements, sensory cues, and experience. Differential access to and command over these bodies of practice by those who participated in and observed iron manufacture resulted in concomitantly differential multisensory experiences and understandings of the production process. Three points of consideration—the cooperation of the senses, material properties, and performance—are raised here as the basis for questioning how archaeologists might use archaeological materials to access these practice-oriented elements of production. Using a suite of methods drawn from archaeology and materials science, the following examples demonstrate how technological tools allow archaeologists to read evidence of the sensory production process from metals—which act as documents that contain otherwise inaccessible information about the traditions of and engagements with craft technologies.

Technique and technology, art and craft, material and social agency, science and the humanities—these relations are often set apart from each other at the outset of archaeological studies of production and technology. The following

*Making Senses of the Past: Toward a Sensory Archaeology,* edited by Jo Day. Center for Archaeological Investigations, Occasional Paper No. 40.  ISBN 978-0-8093-3287-8.

discussion considers sensory engagements and experiences in relation to acts and enactments of the production process, with specific examples from three iron-production sites in New England (see Dobres 2000; Ingold 2000; Shanks and McGuire 1996). The questions and examples that follow are a brief introduction to thinking about how, by operating beyond these sometimes polarizing distinctions, archaeologists might recognize and learn from the generative movements and highly experiential and sensory processes that were involved in the making of materials that we excavate and study.

## Colonial Iron Production: Traditions and Innovations

Archaeological assemblages are uniquely suited to address the inseparable social and material complexities and textilities of craft techniques, technologies, and associated things (Ingold 2010; Webmoor and Witmore 2008). In considering the relationships between sensory experience and production, this discussion draws on objects excavated and studied from three sites (Figure 17-1) of colonial-period iron production associated with the Greene family from Warwick, Rhode Island: Greene Farm (ca. 1730–1781 C.E.), Potowomut (ca. 1690–1820 C.E.), and Coventry (1742–ca.1800 C.E.). According to historical accounts, no iron-production operations of consequence existed in Rhode Island during the colonial period (Bining 1933). Archaeological excavations and subsequent archival research, however, point to the existence of a thriving iron industry during this period, one that was intentionally omitted from official record keeping (Ryzewski 2008). Iron production in the American colonies was outlawed by the British in 1750 because, like other manufacturers and raw-material processors, the many small industries gradually increased in quantity and output to the point where, by midcentury, the amount of iron that England consumed from North America was notably greater than it produced (Bridenbaugh 1950). The successes of these small-scale and often domestic-based production operations were seen as a threat to the British colonial system because they demonstrated the American colonists' potential to gain material independence.

During the eighteenth century, the British worried that the establishment of home-based manufacturing industries like the Greene iron operations would reduce the colonists' reliance on British-supplied iron objects. And they did. Although the Iron Act of 1750 did allow colonists to produce bar iron, it stipulated that the raw bar, or pig iron, they produced was to be shipped to England where British forges would produce finished objects to sell back to the colonists at a profit. These objects—farming implements, household utensils, weaponry, anchors, and tools—were basic and utilitarian necessities for the colonists' survival and everyday affairs in New England. The long turnaround time and the higher cost of obtaining these finished objects from England encouraged many Rhode Island colonists to illegally produce their own objects. Surviving historical accounts and excavated remains of iron smelting and smithing confirm that the three Greene iron operations spanned the colonial period and, in fact, expanded considerably in output and influence after 1750 (Greene and Co. Papers, Providence, Rhode Island; Greene and Greene Papers, Providence, Rhode Island;

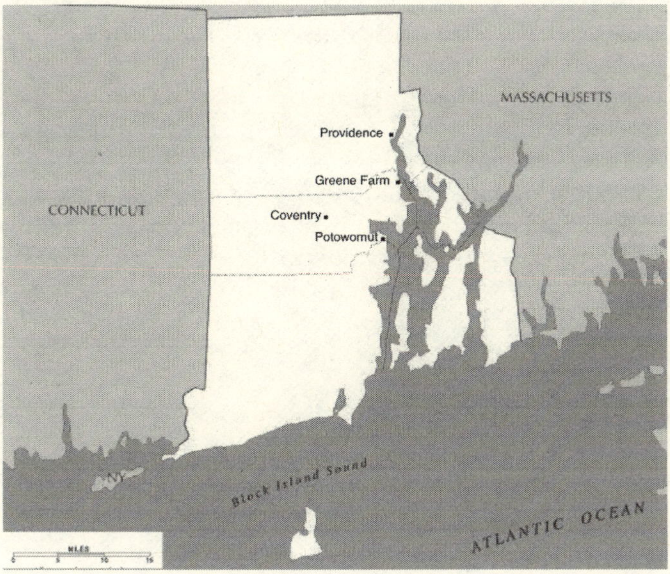


**Figure 17-1.** *Map of Rhode Island with Greene Farm, Potowomut, and Coventry—the Greene family iron-production sites—labeled. (Adapted from U.S. Department of Interior, National Atlas, 2010.)*

Ryzewski 2008). This increase could be interpreted in part as acts of defiance or resistance against colonial rule, but it also speaks to the continuity of a largely undocumented traditional craft industry that was established based on a mixture of European, African, and North American traditions and had been growing steadily since the mid-seventeenth-century arrival of European settlers to Rhode Island.[1] While documentary evidence of how these operations worked is sparse, the traditions of production from the three Greene sites can be addressed from the associated historical and archaeological evidence. Emerging from these assemblages is a series of questions that are of particular interest when considering the involvement of sensory engagements during the production process:

- How did the Greene family ironmasters, who were descended from generations of English metalworking specialists, adapt their industries and skilled traditions of iron production and working to the very different, unfamiliar environmental and demographic situation of New England?
- How was iron produced and worked in New England?
- How did the craftspeople involved in Greene iron production transfer what was primarily tactile, nonverbal, and experiential knowledge about these processes to other groups of craftspeople, apprentices, and associated laborers?
- How did the consumers of the production experience who were *not* specialists or producers engage with and understand the production process through sensory mediations?

The roles that sensory, experiential, and embodied actions play in these processes of making and transmission underlie the remainder of this discussion.

## Craft Production and Sensory Experiences

In the process of smelting and forging, iron takes many forms and textures depending on the stage of production. Success during each step of the process results from the craftsperson's ability to understand and adjust to the continuously variable signals emitted by the furnace and materials by the negotiation of nonverbal, sensory clues, identifiable based on the individual's intuition, experience, and empirically derived knowledge.

This interplay raises several avenues for further attention in archaeological studies of production. Here, the intent is to briefly introduce and explore three aspects of production as they relate to sensory experience:

- Metal production as achieved by the successful cooperation of the senses
- Human-material interrelationships as seen and felt in materials' properties *and* in microscopic views
- Production as performance, from the stance of the ironworker-actor and of the witness-audience subjected to a diversity of sensory consumption

### *Metal Production and Cooperating Senses*

From the linguistic and spiritual importance of ancient Chinese bronzes to the insatiable appetites for gold and silver of the early Spanish explorers in South America, the worldwide appeal of metals is rooted in varying circumstances and cultural contexts but they are recurrently valued across space and time for their aesthetic qualities, rarity, mystifying production process, acoustic properties, unique textures, and durability (Killick 2004; Saunders 2003; Schmidt 2009). Here the focus is on iron: specifically, on the producers and processes of making and working wrought iron, which, depending on the stage of the process, involves converting ore to metal or working red-hot masses of spongy blooms into finished objects.

Just as archaeological sites of production leave ephemeral traces on the landscape, so too do the steps and conditions of manufacture in documentary records and the sensory components of the experience in either material or written forms. Those descriptions of iron production or other craft processes that do survive often take the form of step-by-step explanations of an externally observed *chaîne opératoire*, but when we consider the craft process itself, and the fact that, historically, many craftspeople were not the authors of these descriptions,[2] it is perhaps frustratingly evident that there are no recipes for (material) success that archaeologists can distill into a linear process, bounded description, or reliable, replicable formula. Instead, as numerous ethnoarchaeological and ethnohistorical studies illustrate, producing wrought iron involves the culmination and flow of carefully orchestrated combinations of tacit negotiation, experience, memory, and skill by the craftsperson, embodied in performed technique and bodily interactions with materials (Keller 2001; Knappett and Malafouris 2008; Lechtman 1977, 1999; van der Leeuw 2008).

Consider as an archaeological example the bloomery furnace in which iron at Greene Farm was smelted from combinations of local mineral and bog ores

(Ryzewski 2008). What were the sensory clues that ironworkers engaged with in order to extract iron from the bloomery? What traces, if any, do these leave archaeologically? As Robert Gordon and David Killick (1993:246) emphasize, in processes of iron smelting, sensory clues and timing were vital to the successful operation of a bloomery. The color of the flame indicated the temperature and reducing or oxidizing atmosphere within the furnace. The smelter used tongs to feel how spongy the nonmolten bloom was in order to determine whether silica and flux impurities were being removed from the proto-iron. The viscosity of slag running from the bloomery also communicated the temperature and the course of the smelt. The sounds and smells emanating from within the furnace were physical, acoustic, and olfactory components of the generative process of material transformation. In the process of witnessing and negotiating these clues, the ironworkers knew that if the bloomery was working below the 1200°C temperature necessary to remove slag from the iron bloom, poorly performing metal would result. In the surviving microstructure of these metals, large slag inclusions and other impurities would be visible. The smiths' ability to gauge furnace temperature in this case was the first step in a multisensory process of adjustments, which involved any combination of alterations and embodied acts, including the addition of more fuel, increasing the force applied to the bellows, or changing the speed of airflow.

The process of iron production and subsequent ironworking by hammering variably hot, cold, and reheated iron at the forge demanded the coordination and cooperation of multiple senses into the performance of a repeated, rhythmic series of gestures (Figure 17-2). Until very recently, thermometers, automatic controls, and other standardizing devices were not involved in ironworking; sensory cues were the gauges by which craftspeople determined whether materials were ready or needed adjustment. Ancient and historical processes of making iron were fundamentally multisensory coordinations of time, temperature, atmosphere, gesture, technique, and material. The emergent iron object was a testimony to the craftsperson's skillful negotiation of the clues and conditions of a furnace and the flow of materials: It was a victory over unquantifiable, intangible conditions. Ancient Greek texts and modern studies of African bloomery smelting alike demonstrate how this victory often inspired awe, attributed status, associated elements of the supernatural, and invited ritual benefaction to the producers and the process (Killick 2004; Schmidt 2009; van der Merwe and Avery 1987; Wisseman and Wendell 1994).[3] As the next section details, archaeological remains of these objects preserve, in their microstructures, details of these intangible conditions and skillful negotiations.

In the case of the Greene iron-production operations, craftspeople combined deep-rooted skill, practice, and coordinated sensory information with the involvement of new materials and environments. The enactment of these embodied, habitual gestures is particularly interesting given that the ores used in these operations were compositionally different from the European counterparts (Greene Family Papers, Providence, Rhode Island). As the furnace heated these ores, and as the smiths forged the resulting iron, associated sounds, smells, colors, and temperature indicated various states of material readiness. The Greene craftsperson's ability to understand these properties demanded sensory awareness and

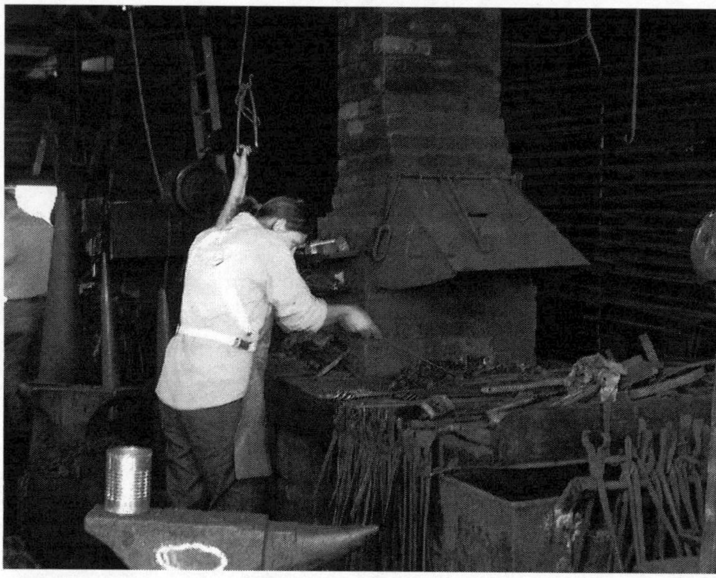

**Figure 17-2.** *The cooperation of multiple senses of the smith is involved in iron forging at Mystic Seaport Museum in Connecticut. (Photograph © Krysta Ryzewski.)*

expertise that was difficult, if not impossible, to communicate verbally. In considering, as Pfaffenberger (1992:508) notes, "the portion of technical knowledge that people can verbalize represents only the tip of the iceberg," the question of how this sensory knowledge passed between craftspeople across time and place is especially intriguing. Nevertheless, the successful production of iron and iron objects is testimony that the Greene ironworkers, using accepted and improvised gestures, successfully translated and incorporated new sensory enactments, nonverbal clues, and unfamiliar material properties into an established tradition of ironworking, which they identified with a specific and proven realm of possible choices and alternatives (see Bourdieu 1977; Chilton 1998; Dietler and Herbich 1998; Killick 2004). These situations of cooperative sensory negotiation and adaptation are, however, just a starting point; they are especially beneficial in orienting sensory-production studies back to the archaeological assemblages, specifically toward materials' properties, a focus that is the physical basis for archaeologically examining sensory interactions and coexistence.

### *Material Properties and Microscopic Views*

It is in combining these ideas about multisensory engagements with information about artifacts' material properties that we can pursue more detailed, empirically and contextually rich discussions about object making.

Today, engineers can identify and explain precisely why properties of materials interact in specific and predictable ways when subjected to variables like heat, force, water, and chemicals. The tools of twenty-first-century science allow researchers to quantify and see these interactions on atomic, and even nano, scales. Novel as these understandings may seem, these properties and their interactions are not the discovery of modern scientists; for millennia craftspeople measured, identified, and predicted materials' properties through a combination of sensory mediations—sight and color, sound, weight, temperature, texture. While ancient craftspeople could not see or understand how these phenomena worked at the microscale, they certainly would have had a sensual awareness of materials' properties and their behavior under certain conditions (Figure 17-3). For example, following his visit to what were probably metals workshops, Aristotle identified and described 18 different properties that craftspeople followed and used to their advantage in working metal (*Meteorologica* 378.ii.26ff). These properties, which included crystallization, viscosity, plasticity, tension, color changes, and various states of oxidation, are some of the foundational material relationships and terminologies that materials scientists study today (see Smith 1981:114). The engagement of craftspeople with materials' properties raises questions about how, in the past, people understood and mastered these properties through sensory perceptions. Traces of these sensory perceptions, I argue, are visible archaeologically, preserved in the microstructural remains of crafted iron (and other) objects.

In iron production, touch, sight, hearing, and smell have material correlates and consequences that affect a furnace's operating temperature, the metal's texture, and the material's consistency, purity, and performance. The new types of mineral and bog ore—cumberlandite and local limonite—that the Greene family incorporated in their smelting operations (Figure 17-4) were uncharacteristically high in titanium, a chemical that required a higher furnace temperature to extract iron from the ore and that caused resulting iron objects to be structurally unstable (Ryzewski 2008; Urban, Ryzewski, and Hermance 2010). Of course, the ironworkers did not know that the cumberlandite ore performed differently because of the elemental presence of titanium, but they would have recognized that the ore's composition had different properties and performance characteristics as they used it at Greene Farm and Potowomut, and importantly, despite the difficulties posed by the ores' properties, the Greene ironworkers chose to continue working with it. The reason the ironworkers made this decision strikes at some of the most pressing debates in the anthropology of technology and production studies about how and where to locate motivations for technological choice making. Trends vary from technologically and materially focused explanations to interpretations rooted in social phenomena. The role of archaeological objects and materials' properties in these discussions, and the complexities of arguably inseparable human-material relationships, can be neglected in these conversations.

The literature on the archaeology and anthropology of technology is rich with discussions of the roles that technical choices, techniques, and embodied or social actions and other phenomena play in the making of things (Ingold 2000; Lechtman 1977; Lemonnier 1992, 1993; Schiffer 2001). How close these approaches come to articulating the complexity of sensory involvement in the production process—especially in regard to materials' properties and human-material

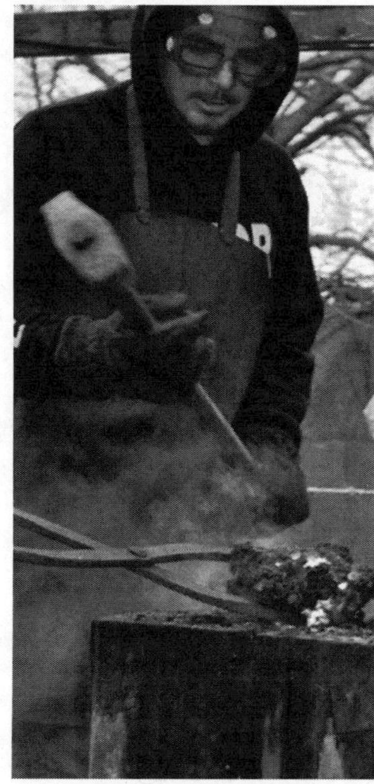

**Figure 17-3.** *The craftsperson judges the appropriate force and duration for hammering an iron bloom based on the iron's material and sensory properties. (Photograph © K. Ryzewski.)*

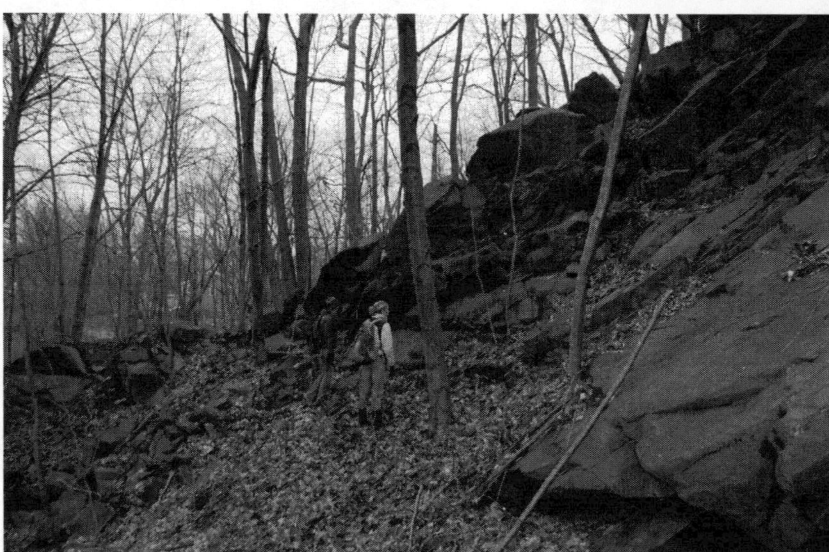

**Figure 17-4.** *One of the last remaining outcrops of cumberlandite ore, which was mined by the Greene family and other iron producers between the seventeenth and nineteenth centuries in Cumberland, Rhode Island. (Photograph © Krysta Ryzewski.)*

interrelationships—varies, however, and in some cases is challenged by basic questions about the very process of production. For example, what happens to conventional models of the *chaîne opératoire* (Leroi-Gourhan 1964) of forging an iron tool when the archaeologist is asked to account for concurrent sensory variables? Or, how do we locate and explain the reasons why the smith corrects an object's shape when a step in the production sequence fails?

When considering the sensory experience of production, and working from the material properties of archaeological objects, different perspectives on human-material interaction emerge. Human-material relationships are fundamentally important for thinking about the sensory realm of production and for considering how materials' properties might act back at or act with the craftspeople and with each other during the production process. Current approaches that recognize the importance of bodily experience in production activities tend to situate agency and traces of interactions with materials within the realm of the subject and associated social phenomena. In her discussions of object making and sensual material practice, Marcia-Anne Dobres notes that the craftsperson's body was "a sensual, socially constituted and gendered being making sense of the world and themselves as they made and used material culture during the mundane routines of everyday practice" (2010:108; see also 2000). Though the importance of bodily experience is undeniably integral to the sensory craft process, attention here remains primarily focused on the subject as the agent of change rather than the interaction between materials, people and materials, and subsequent material traces of the craftsperson's embodied gestures in the making of the object.

While the relationships between techniques of production and social phenomena have been convincingly demonstrated in contextual discussions of ritual knowledge, symbolism, practice theory, and technical choice making (Bourdieu 1977; Killick 2004; Lemonnier 1992; Schmidt 2009; Van der Leeuw 2008), in considering the sensory aspects of production, however, it is perhaps not necessary (or timely) to shift questions of agency and influence entirely away from the object in order to address these social or intangible aspects of production. Such a shift would be detrimental to considering production and the sensory experience, primarily because the interrelationships between materials' properties and many of the perceived "social" dimensions remain entangled and have been only preliminarily explored by archaeologists.

An alternative perspective and encouraging influence for examining human-material interrelationships as they relate to production studies is Tim Ingold's recent notion of the "textility of making" (2010:91). In his discussion, Ingold reflects on how craftspeople, in their work with wood (a varied and heterogeneous material), are guided by tactile and sensuous knowledge of line and surface. Although he does not specifically refer to properties of materials in the sense that they are understood in the field of materials science, Ingold speaks of a similar notion of sensual engagement with materials during processes of production. During these processes, materials are mixed together, the craftsperson weaves and moves through and with them, based on his or her understanding of specific properties (e.g., the grain of the wood, the malleability of iron, how the hammer sounds when it strikes warm metal). As is the case with the Greene ironworking practices, these understandings are critically important in working with materials that, because of their specific properties, are neither predisposed to form into the desired shape nor to remain permanently in that shape once the object-making process is completed (Ingold 2010:93; Ingold and Hallam 2007:3–4).

How material properties are harnessed by the ironworker and made to interact in the process of making—as the iron is exposed to heat, to repeated blows from the hammer, and to flux and as decisions are made by the experienced craftsperson—exemplifies the relations between material properties, sensory clues, and the reading of these clues by the craftsperson. All of these decisions must mix with each other effectively in the generative process of making an iron object successfully. As Ingold notes, borrowing from Deleuze and Guattari (2004:377), the relations that emerge from the mixture of these materials (human and nonhuman) in the making of things is a very different way of understanding how and why things are made, especially because they invite the incorporation of sensual elements into consideration. This generative view acts against a hylomorphic model of production, in which form is imposed by an agent on matter that is understood as being passive and inert (Ingold 2010). This emphasizes the importance of considering the mixture between people and things in views about technology. As a consequence, the process of formation is viewed as one that operates against a final product—where the flows and transformations of materials are against states of matter (Ingold 2010:92). Rather than viewing the final object, or form, as the grounds for working backward from thing to thought or along a linear, reconstructive *chaîne opératoire*, they encourage us to work forward by following the materials and how they intervene with each other and the world as they vary during the process of production (see Deleuze and Guattari [2004:451] on matter-flow).

Returning to the questions posed at the outset of this discussion, the power of sensory perception in lending specific and masterful understanding of materials' properties to the Greenes and to other ironworkers in historical metalworking contexts is documented in the presence of lasting industries, the generations of kin-based production units, and the reputable objects that they produced (Figure 17-5).[4] The ephemeral traces of sensory experiences associated with iron production cannot be reexperienced in movement, at least not from the external surface of objects. We can, however, see *traces* of these movements archaeologically by examining objects' microstructure in relation to the process of production, using various instruments, including optical, scanning electron, and focused ion beam microscopes, tools beyond the standard archaeological tool kit but common to materials scientists. A recent trend in sensory archaeology may be to move away from touch and sight in favor of new and experimental directions (see also Classen 2005; Howes 1991, 2005). In the discussion of craft technologies, however, these senses of touch and sight become quite complicated when considered in light of materials' production; much more exploration of the interplay between these senses during the process of making remains ahead.

One opportunity to see and think about sensory archaeology in relation to production is through images of iron objects' microstructures, which preserve traces of gesture and negotiation, material constituents, and other details about

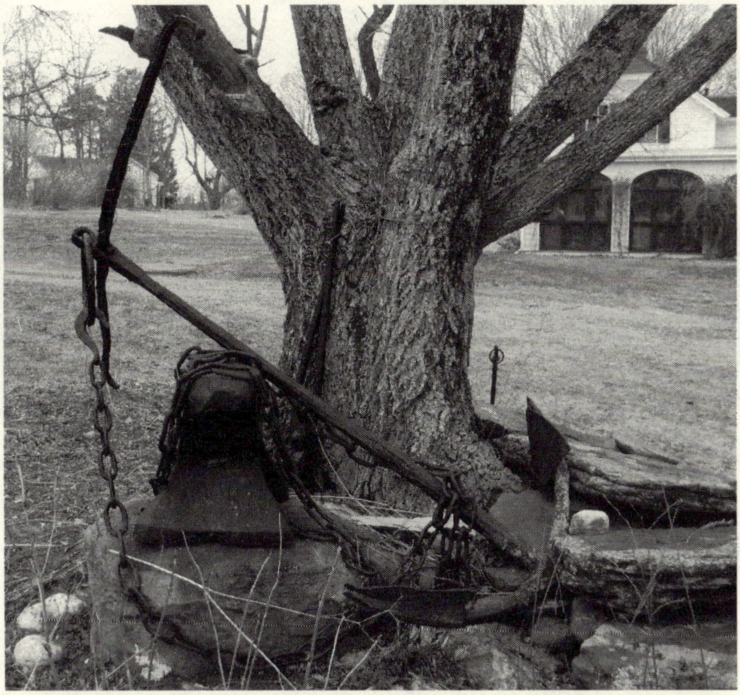

**Figure 17-5.** *At Potowomut, the lawn in front of the main house is presently decorated with an anvil from the eighteenth-century Greene family forge and an anchor produced there. (Photograph © Krysta Ryzewski.)*

the process of object making from start to finish. In the following micrographs, the microstructures of iron objects from the Greene production operations show, in vivid detail, the properties of these materials for archaeologists to experience and interpret. To read them, one must incorporate technical knowledge from materials science, metallurgy, and engineering, as well as knowledge of the choices and production processes available to the makers of these objects (see Ryzewski and Gordon 2008). Three examples illustrate differences in visibility and how the type of information that can be read from these material documents relates directly and indirectly to sensory aspects of the production process.

Figures 17-6 and 17-7 are micrographs of the ferrite grains of two iron nails produced at the Greene Farm and Potowomut iron-production sites. Visible in both microscopic images are the striations between the ferrite grains, the textured appearance caused by phosphorous impurities, and the inclusions of slag that were not successfully removed by the ironworkers during production. These traces are micro-artifacts of sensory clues, of gestures, and of experiential knowledge that relate to the resulting production of wrought objects of mediocre quality and performance.

Figure 17-8 is a low-magnification image of a wrought nail. In this micrograph, the black lines are inclusions of slag that were not successfully removed during smelting or smithing. Though a sign of what might be considered (at best)

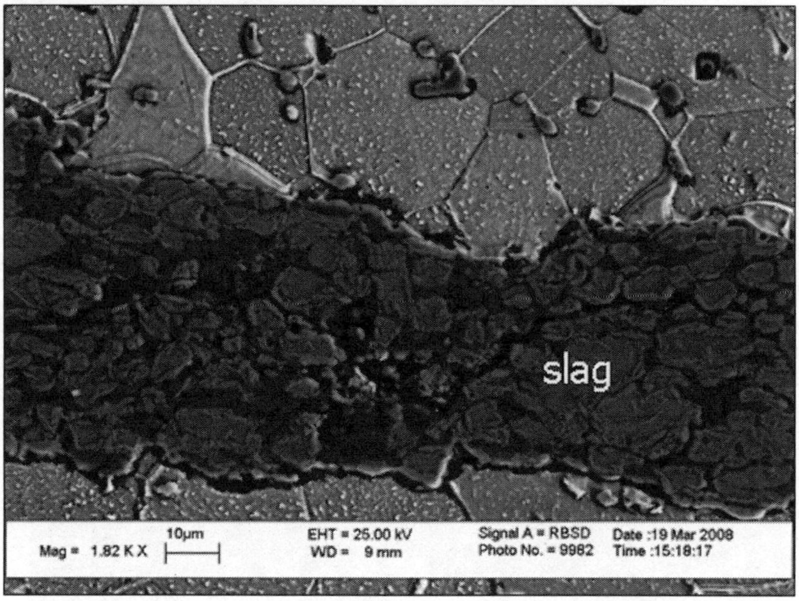


**Figure 17-6.** *Electron microscope image (1.82Kx) of slag structures in a wrought-iron tool from Greene Farm.*

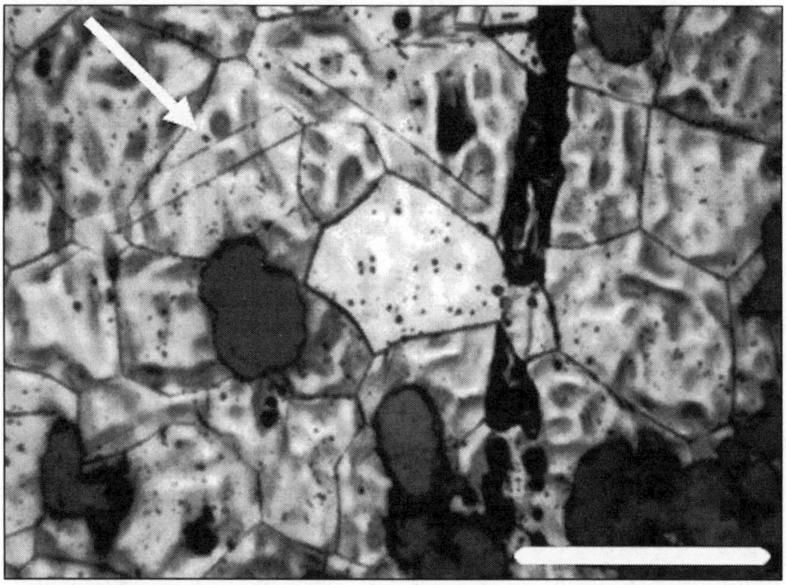

**Figure 17-7.** *Optical microscope image of a nail sample from Greene Farm in which high phosphorus content (textured surface) and Neuman bands (arrow) are visible, evidence of the cold-working stage in an iron artifact (210x, scale bar = 2 mm).*

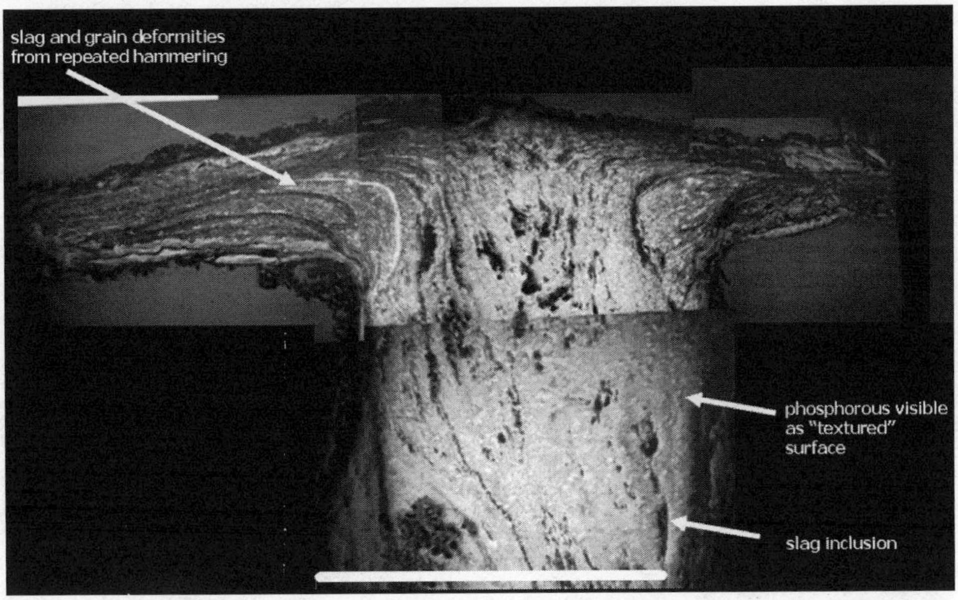


**Figure 17-8.** *Photomosaic of the cross section of a wrought nail from the Greene Farm iron-production site. Features of working are visible in the nail's microstructure, even at low magnification (4x, scale bar = 1 cm).*

moderately skilled iron production, these failures preserve, in their curvature and compact alignments along the nail's head, the repeated hammering gestures and rhythms of the smith, which became part of the material's structure as he struck and shaped the nail head with enough force to cause dislocations among strongly bonded atomic structures within the object.

Figure 17-9 is a micrograph of an iron tool from Greene Farm. This image is a biography: It documents the production process of the tool and the stages of reheating and reworking that the smith performed. The smaller ferrite grains around the edges document that the object was at one point reintroduced into the fire; the object would have been reheated to more than 650°C in order for grain recrystallization to have occurred. In reheating the object, the smith gauged when it was hot enough to work and how he wanted to follow the material in working it. These decisions were influenced by sensory clues as felt and heard indirectly through his hammer and by sight—the ductility and texture of the metal and its color. The smith did not necessarily have to reheat the iron to this temperature; it is possible to "cold work" iron at a temperature below the recrystallization phase. In this case, however, a desire to work with properties of the iron at this temperature informed the choice he made; this choice was perhaps based on his past experience or expectations for the finished object. In a final step of the process, the small grains on the edge formed because the iron, after it was worked, was cooled rapidly—possibly by being submerged in cool water or placed outdoors.

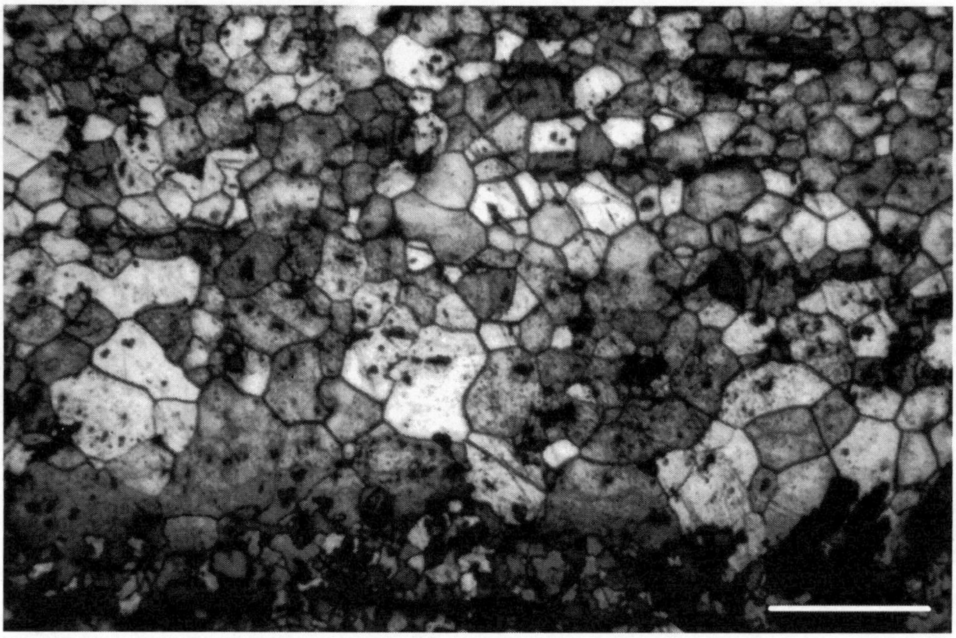

**Figure 17-9.** *Optical microscopy image of an iron tool from Potowomut showing variable ferrite grain size, moderate phosphorus content, and recrystallization along top edge and bottom (278x, scale bar = 2 mm).*

In all of these micrographs, we see traces of the synergies between tools, gestures, relations with materials, and traditions of crafting preserved in the microstructural details of iron artifacts (Ingold 2000; Lemonnier 1992; Leroi-Gourhan 1964). The phosphorus is diagnostic of locally available bog ore, which tells us that the craftspeople were extracting local resources for production. The properties of this high-phosphorus ore would have adversely affected the strength of the objects in which it occurred. Similarly, the presence of excess slag communicates that the furnace temperature was either not hot enough or not regulated enough to remove it from the iron bloom during smelting. The interrelationships of these variables alone convey the complexity of the production process as multisensory and difficult, if not impossible, to understand through a step-by-step reconstruction of the production's operational sequence. To understand how these materials, their properties, and their makers interacted in the textility of making, these microstructural images should be viewed as movements through the material-making process and this movement considered as it related to sensory and embodied experiences, skilled knowledge and practice, and various other conditions of the production process. Accordingly, to understand how the craftsperson followed materials in his or her work, so too must those who study that work also study the material. In other words, as the archaeologist joins and follows forces and flows of material that bring the form of work into being through countless sensory mediations, the micrograph, in this case, invites the viewer to join the craftsperson in the experience of crafting. With the relevant technical know-how, one can follow the process as it unfolds through multiple relations and socio-material interactions (see Ingold 2010:97).

### *Craft Production as Performance and Sensory Consumption*

The final point of interest in examining multisensory aspects of production archaeologically moves beyond the realm of the craft specialist and the microstructure of iron objects to reflect on the diversity of sensory participation and perception that was involved in the process of iron production. Following Tristan Carter (2007), production is also understood to be a performative process, where the making of things is a well-orchestrated activity involving multiple groups of people, ranging from master craftsperson to laborer and from unaffiliated audiences of consumers to more distant witnesses of the production operation. Despite the fact that the Greene iron-production facilities were illegal according to British law, all three were long-standing, conspicuous operations, prominently placed on the properties' landscapes alongside major thoroughfares, where they were visible to all who passed by. Given their locations, the size of their labor force, and their output—which supplied many local merchants, farmers, and other consumers—the Greene ironworks were spectacles offering differing degrees of sensory experiences and inclusion to those who interacted with or benefited from them (Figure 17-10).

In the course of smelting and forging iron at the Greene operations, a successful production performance would have resulted in appreciation and reputation for the producers because certain sensory and other elements of the process were made inaccessible (both intentionally and unintentionally) to the general public. Ironworkers, including the Greene family, often operated in tight-knit kin-based groups who carefully guarded the intricate details of production. These trade secrets were bodies of knowledge and practice rooted in generations of experiential learning and sensory mastery that effectively shrouded the process of metalworking in mystery and awe for those outside the group (see Bourdieu 1977; Brandt 1980; Hendon 2006). The result was a division along lines of accessibility to specialized knowledge and experience between the skilled, or at least active, craftspeople and those with decreased access to such information. This inequality casts the production process as an experience that displayed producers and the production operations to a wider audience of affiliated and unaffiliated people who consumed the production experience through witnessing its activities and consequences.

In the Greene operations, where iron production was the backbone of a family dynasty for a century and a half, this type of experiential knowledge was certainly communicated across generations and across cultures, as the Greenes trained their family members, as well as enslaved and itinerant Native American and African laborers—all of whom came to the stage with culturally and technologically diverse understandings of raw materials, iron production, and sensory engagements.

In addition to cultural diversity among Greene ironworkers, a stark contrast in sensory awareness and experience existed between those who crafted the iron and those who did not.

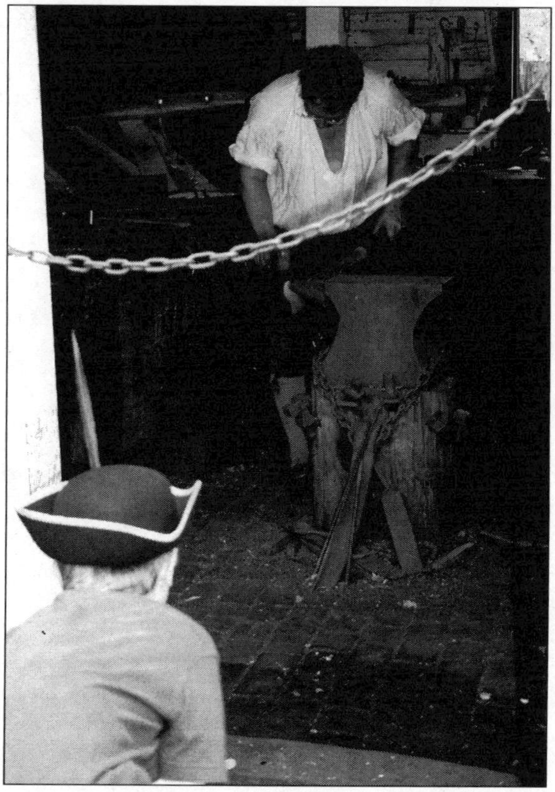

**Figure 17-10.** *The smith at the Colonial Williamsburg blacksmith shop and his audience: a scene that communicates the different sensory experiences of and witnesses to the production process. (Photograph © Krysta Ryzewski.)*

The unequal access to knowledge and experience shaped how sensory elements of the production process were received and embodied. For both performers and audience, the process of production was also one of differential sensory consumption and translation. In some non-Western contexts, necessary or everyday production activities of forge workers were revered by outsiders and perceived to be acts of magic or ritual (Schmidt 2009). This was not the case in Rhode Island, where outsiders' perceptions were more negative, providing a basis for casting judgment on producers, sometimes using sensory perceptions as the means for bolstering critique. Surviving records and complaints from colonial period Rhode Island townspeople, the audience of the Greene iron-production operations, refer to iron-production as noisy, onerous, and polluting, activities responsible for clogging waterways and disrupting landscapes (Greene Family Papers, Providence, Rhode Island; Greene and Co. Papers, Providence, Rhode Island). The ironworkers affiliated with these operations were similarly cast as pollutants of the moral fabric of local society and were chastised for their loud, rowdy, and drunken behavior (Greene Family Papers, Providence, Rhode Island; Greene and Co. Papers, Providence, Rhode Island). As these examples illustrate, in examining how sensory differences develop and unfold among those engaged with the production process, sensually based or sensually driven interactions should be approached as fluid, accumulative, and diverse processes that involve many groups of participants with varying degrees of inclusivity.

## Concluding Thoughts: Making Sense of Craft Production

The sensory-driven practice and performance of production is a topic that demands multidisciplinary orientations capable of identifying the interrelationships between people, materials, and modes of engagement in the making of material culture. As the Greene-produced iron objects demonstrate, these mixtures are present even in the generation and enactment of seemingly sensible, everyday things. These examples, and the instrumental, archaeological, and documentary tools they enlist, are an introduction to seeing the multisensory aspects of production archaeologically. As highlighted in these discussions, the three specific avenues along which the multisensory aspects of the production process can be approached are examples for considering the many faces of production studies, including those individuals who understood the intricate details of the craft process, those who witnessed the making of objects, and by those who now study them. Such diversity of experience and multiplicity of actors underscore the need for careful attention to how the participants in craft activities operated with varying degrees of technical understanding or investment and, therefore, with equivalently different experiences of sensory participation and awareness.

## Acknowledgments

Many thanks to Jo Day for the invitation to participate in the Carbondale conference, to Karen Holmberg for her willingness to present the original version of this paper in my absence, and to Rod Campbell for additional insights into archaeological production contexts. Any omissions or shortcomings are my own.

## Notes

1. In 1771, the American colonies produced 30,000 tons of iron, only 7,000 tons of which was shipped to Britain (Lewis 1979:11).

2. In many cases, craftspeople were illiterate (see Smith 1981).

3. For example, a poem about kiln conditions in Pseudo-Herodotus's *Life of Homer* (second or third century C.E.) describes the demons associated with the critical firing process. The firing demons' names are the equivalent of sounds and sensual conditions for breaking: "Smasher," "Cracker," "Shake-to-pieces." These names evoke sounds that related to other sensual components of temperature, atmosphere, time, heating and cooling speed, all critically important parts of the

process of successful pottery production (adapted from Noble 1988; also quoted in Wisseman and Wendell 1994:23).

4. This is a reminder that archaeologists have much to learn about how these craftspeople negotiated such complicated behavioral properties of materials that they could not possibly (but also, did not necessarily need to) understand from modern scientific perspectives.

## References

Aristotle

1952 *Meteorologica*. Translated by Sir Henry Desmond Pritchard Lee. Loeb Classical Library. Heinemann, London.

Bining, Arthur Cecil

1933 *British Regulation of the Colonial Iron Industry*. University of Pennsylvania Press, Philadephia.

Bourdieu, Pierre

1977 *Outline of a Theory of Practice*. Cambridge University Press, Cambridge.

Brandt, Elizabeth

1980 On Secrecy and the Control of Knowledge: Taos Pueblo. In *Secrecy: A Cross-Cultural Perspective*, edited by Stanton K. Tefft, pp. 123–146. Human Sciences Press, New York.

Bridenbaugh, Carl

1950 *The Colonial Craftsman*. New York University Press, New York.

Carter, Tristan

2007 The Theatrics of Technology: Consuming Obsidian in the Early Cycladic Burial Arena. In *Rethinking Craft Specialization in Complex Societies: Archaeological Analyses of the Social Meaning of Production*, edited by Zachary X. Hruby and Rowan K. Flad, pp. 88–107. Archeology Papers of the American Anthropological Association, No. 17, Washington, D.C.

Chilton, Elizabeth

1998 The Cultural Origins of Technical Choice: Unraveling Algonquian and Iroquois CeramicTraditions in the Northeast. In *The Archaeology of Social Boundaries*, edited by Miriam T. Stark, pp. 132–160. Smithsonian Institution Press, Washington, D.C.

Classen, Constance (editor)

2005 *The Book of Touch*. Berg, Oxford.

Deleuze, Gilles, and Felix Guattari

2004 *A Thousand Plateaus*. Translated by Brian Massumi. Continuum, London.

Dietler, Michael, and Ingrid Herbich

1998 Habitus, Techniques, Style: An Integrated Approach to the Social Understanding of Material Culture and Boundaries. In *The Archaeology of Social Boundaries*, edited by Miriam T. Stark, pp. 232–263. Smithsonian Institution Press, Washington, D.C.

Dobres, Marcia-Anne

2000 *Technology and Social Agency: Outlining a Practice Framework for Archaeology*. Blackwell, Oxford.

2010 Archaeologies of Technology. *Cambridge Journal of Economics* 34:103–114.

Gordon, Robert B., and David J. Killick

1993 Adaptation of Technology to Culture and Environment: Bloomery Iron Smelting in America and Africa. *Technology and Culture* 34:243–270.

Greene, Elihu, and Christopher Greene
1786–1830 Papers. Mss 459, Rhode Island Historical Society Manuscript Collections, Providence.
Greene Family
1783–1853 Papers. Mss 1043, Rhode Island Historical Society Manuscript Collections, Providence.
Greene, James, and Co.
1786–1830 Papers. Mss 459, Elihu and Christopher Greene Records, Rhode Island Historical Society Manuscript Collections, Providence.
Howes, David (editor)
1991 *The Varieties of Sensory Experience.* University of Toronto Press, Toronto.
2005 *Empire of the Senses: The Sensual Culture Reader.* Berg, Oxford.
Ingold, Timothy
2000 *The Perception of the Environment: Essays in Livelihood, Dwelling, and Skill.* Routledge, London.
2010 The Textility of Making. *Cambridge Journal of Economics* 34:91–102.
Ingold, Timothy, and Elizabeth Hallam (editors)
2007 *Creativity and Cultural Improvisation*. Berg, Oxford.
Iron Act
1750 Parliamentary Statute 23 Geo. 2, c. 23
Keller, Charles M.
2001 Thoughts and Production: Insights of a Practitioner. In *Anthropological Perspectives on Technology*, edited by Michael Schiffer, pp. 33–45. University of New Mexico Press, Albuquerque.
Killick, David
2004 Social Constructionist Approaches to the Study of Technology. *World Archaeology* 34:571–578.
Knappett, Carl, and Lambros Malafouris (editors)
2008 *Material Agency: Towards a Non-anthropocentric Approach.* Springer, New York.
Lechtman, Heather
1977 Style in Technology: Some Early Thoughts. In *Material Culture: Styles, Organization, and Dynamics of Technology,* edited by Heather Lechtman and Robert Merrill, pp. 3–20. American Ethnological Society, St. Paul, Minnesota.
1999 Afterword. In *The Social Dynamics of Technology: Practice, Politics, and World Views,* edited by Marcia-Anne Dobres and Christopher R. Hoffman, pp. 223–232. Smithsonian Institution Press, Washington, D.C.
Lemonnier, Pierre
1992 *Elements for an Anthropology of Technology.* University of Michigan, Ann Arbor.
Lemonnier, Pierre (editor)
1993 *Technological Choices: Transformation in Material Cultures since the Neolithic.* Routledge, London.
Leroi-Gourhan, André
1964 *La Geste et la Parole: Technique et Language.* Albim Michel, Paris.
Lewis, Ronald L.
1979 *Coal, Iron, and Slaves: Industrial Slavery in Maryland and Virginia, 1715–1865.* Greenwood Press, Westport, Connecticut.
Noble, Joseph V.
1988 *The Techniques of Painted Attic Pottery.* Thames and Hudson, London.
Pfaffenberger, Bryan
1992 Social Anthropology of Technology. *Annual Review of Anthropology* 21:419–516.

Ryzewski, Krysta
2008 *Archaeology of a Colonial Industry: Domestic Ironworking and Industrial Evolution in Rhode Island, 1642–1800.* Master's thesis, Brown University, Providence. University Microfilms, Ann Arbor.
Ryzewski, Krysta, and Robert B. Gordon
2008 Historical Nail-Making Techniques Revealed in Metal Structure. *Historical Metallurgy* 42:50–64.
Saunders, Nicholas J.
2003 "Catching the Light": Technologies of Power and Enchantment in Pre-Columbian Goldworking. In *Gold and Power in Ancient Costa Rica, Panama, and Colombia,* edited by Jeffrey Quilter and John W. Hoopes, pp. 15–48. Dumbarton Oaks, Washington, D.C.
Schiffer, Michael (editor)
2001 *Anthropological Perspectives on Technology.* University of New Mexico Press, Albuquerque.
Schmidt, Peter
2009 Tropes, Materiality, and Ritual Embodiment of African Iron Smelting Furnaces as Human Figures. *Journal of Archaeological Method and Theory* 16:262–282.
Shanks, Michael, and Randall McGuire
1996 The Craft of Archaeology. *American Antiquity* 61:75–88.
Smith, Cyril S.
1981 *Search for Structure: Selected Essays on Science, Art, and History*. MIT Press, Cambridge, Massachusetts.
Urban, Thomas, Krysta Ryzewski, and John Hermance
2010 Cumberlandite: Using Residual Gravity to Delineate an Historically Important Ore Body. Paper presented at the 75th Annual Meeting of the Society for American Archaeology, St. Louis.
van der Leeuw, Sander
2008 Agency, Networks, Past and Future. In *Material Agency: Towards a Non-anthropocentric Approach,* edited by Carl Knappett and Lambros Malafouris, pp. 217–247. Springer, New York.
van der Merwe, Nikolaas J., and Donald H. Avery
1987 Science and Magic in African Technology: Traditional Iron Smelting in Malawi. *Africa* 57:143–172.
Webmoor, Timothy, and Christopher Witmore
2008 Things Are Us! A Commentary on Human/Things Relations under the Banner of a 'Social' Archaeology. *Norwegian Archaeological Review* 41:53–70.
Wisseman, Susan, and Wendell Williams (editors)
1994 *Ancient Technologies and Archaeological Materials.* Routledge, London.

# 18. Beyond the Display Case: Creating a Multisensory Museum Experience

*Catherine P. Foster*

*Abstract:* Museums play a critical role in the development and dissemination of sensory archaeological research. To accomplish this, they must go beyond their visual presentation of material culture to encourage the stimulation of all senses—a shift that would coincidently bring these institutions back to their organizational roots. Drawing from collaborative exhibitions sponsored by the Badè Museum and the Doug Adams Gallery, this paper shows how a sensory exploration of ancient Israelite society can be exhibited through innovative use of archaeological materials. This study extends to include modern artistic interpretation of prehistoric artifacts as a meditation on measurement, a challenge to our sensory perceptions, and an example of the power of contemporary art and artists to deepen our understanding of ancient cultures.

Since the early nineteenth century, the evolution of modern Western ethnographic and archaeological museums has largely supported a single-sensory visitor experience, one based on sight, in which museumgoers or "viewers" can only look at displays. This visual presentation of material culture has dominated to the detriment of the other, "lesser" senses of touch, smell, taste, and hearing, which at one time figured prominently within the larger museum sensescape (Classen and Howes 2006; see also Classen 2007). A static picture has been drawn inside this stale environment of past and present cultures—their art and objects locked away behind cases that serve as both a physical and a psychological barrier. How can museums break free of this ocular framework to embrace a truly sensory narrative of the cultures their visual and material collections represent?

*Making Senses of the Past: Toward a Sensory Archaeology,* edited by Jo Day. Center for Archaeological Investigations, Occasional Paper No. 40.  ISBN 978-0-8093-3287-8.

In this chapter, I explore the dissemination of sensuous pasts and presents in museum space through the use of art and objects at the Badè Museum of Biblical Archaeology and the Doug Adams Gallery, both located on the campus of the Pacific School of Religion in Berkeley, California. Using dual collaborative exhibitions from 2010 as case studies, I provide examples of how a sensory exploration of ancient Israelite society can be exhibited through innovative use of archaeological materials. My study extends to contemporary artistic interpretations of prehistoric artifacts both as a meditation on measurement and as a challenge to visitors' perceptions about lived experience in the past.

I contend that, despite traditional practices, museums are suitable venues for presenting sensuous pasts and can offer unique settings for the proliferation of sensory archaeological research. Likewise, history and visual culture museums have the ability to further develop sensory approaches and bring about tactile experiences through a marriage of contemporary art and archaeology. Only when museums and their curators look beyond the display case will a truly holistic narrative of the human experience in both the past and the present be understood, acknowledged, and shared.

## Museums: Shaping History and the Modern Corporeal Experience

In the rubric of current museum best practice, where the pursuit of lifelong learning is mediated by a responsibility to protect and preserve, it seems inconceivable that exhibitions of material and visual culture could lend themselves to fully tactile and exploratory experiences. Yet this is the exact environment in which the museum, as we know it today, developed. The private collections of the sixteenth- and seventeenth-century aristocracy served as the earliest templates. Their libraries and studies were a cornucopia of art pieces, historic artifacts, and biological specimens (Alexander and Alexander 2008; Impey and MacGregor 2001). Ethnographic objects were also of interest both for their strangeness in the context of European or North American upper society and for what they represented: a material symbol of colonial conquest over the collected objects' former owners and places of origin (Classen and Howes 2006:209). These "cabinets of curiosity" contained no artificial divisions between scholarly fields such as we see today in our museums of art, archaeology, and natural sciences. They were also the privileged arena of usually small, discrete groups of people, even when the first public museums like the Ashmolean Museum of Art and Archaeology in Oxford and the British Museum in London opened in the late seventeenth and mid-eighteenth centuries.

Perhaps surprising to us, with our modern sensibilities about museum etiquette, at that time visitors to both public and private galleries could physically interact with objects: They were allowed to hear, touch, and even taste items on display. Many travel accounts describe the smell of scented woods and taxidermic animals or the pleasing tones produced by historical musical instruments (von Uffenbach 1934:83). Religious relics were especially prone to tactile engagements.

In an extreme case, Samuel Pepys notes his opportunity to kiss the corpse of Queen Katherine, wife of Henry V, during his tour of Westminster Abbey in 1669 (Pepys, *Diary* IX:457, as cited in Classen 2007). More mundane tactile inspection, however, appears to have been the normal practice. On her 1694 visit to the Ashmolean Museum, the proficient traveler Celia Fiennes (1949:33) describes a certain "cane [on display] which looks like a solid heavy thing but if you take it in your hands it's as light as a feather."

Fiennes's appraisal of this cane by physically holding the object underscores one of the foundational measures of these early museums, many of which were curated by scientists for the purpose of serious academic study. Tactile access to artifacts provided an essential means of acquiring knowledge that outweighed the potential risks of wear, breakage, or theft (Classen and Howes 2006:201). As Classen (2007:901) notes in her examination of the sensory life of things, "a hands-on approach to exhibits enabled visitors to acquire an embodied understanding of the nature of the display." It is also apparent through these travel stories that physical interaction with objects, especially those of great antiquity, contributed to feelings of a special bond between modern visitors and ancient peoples. A wonderful example comes from Sophie de la Roche in which she ponders a collection of Roman mirrors from Herculaneum on display in the British Museum. She imagines that "maybe chance has preserved amongst these remains some part of the dust from the fine eyes of a Greek or Roman lady, who so many centuries ago surveyed herself in this mirror" (de la Roche 1933:107–108).

These sensory experiences, of course, do not relate to the lived experience of the people who created and used these objects. Instead, these examples show the level of personal engagement with objects that was once commonplace for and expected by museum visitors. These examples also highlight what is perhaps a very innate requirement for learning on the part of many people: direct interaction with objects.

By the nineteenth century, shifts in scientific practice, aesthetic appreciation, and sociopolitical frameworks led to changes in museum display and how visitors interacted with exhibits. An increased concern for the preservation and conservation of museum objects necessarily limited the level of physical engagement by the public. In the wake of European colonialism, sight was favored as the appropriate sense for aesthetic appreciation by "civilized" persons, relegating the "lower" senses of smell, taste, touch, and hearing to the non-Western "savages" (Classen and Howes 2006:207).

The development of modern public museums in the mid-nineteenth century also coincided with a reformation of governmental structures. Cultural institutions like museums, libraries, and parks were quickly appropriated as vehicles for the exercise of new forms of power (Bennett 1995:19). Museums in particular acquired three new roles. First, they became social spaces detached from their prior exclusive forms as private collections. A broader section of the public was allowed, and sometimes even encouraged, to patronize these spaces and marvel at exotic objects brought back as part of the imperial project. Second, museums were wielded as organizational tools to represent and arrange the natural and cultural orders of the world, preferably in line with Western sentiments. Third, galleries transformed into spaces of both observation and regulation. Within this politicized space, the visitor body could be molded according to newly emerging social norms in terms of public conduct. Museums thus became the "passionless reformers" (Goode 1895:71) to ebb the tide of public drunkenness and debauchery frequently associated with places of popular assembly. This was accomplished by implementing underlying rules of engagement enforced through strict dress codes, restrictions on eating and drinking in the galleries, and prohibitions on touching exhibits.

This development, from full tactile engagement with material culture to hands off, naturally puts archaeological and ethnographic museums currently at odds with presenting a sensory narrative of the past. Many (though not all; see Owen 1999) modern archaeological museums use video or film to overcome this divide and "flesh out" exhibitions. This practice, however, preserves the primacy of vision while once more putting the visitor in the position of passive learner with little or no participation. An issue also lies in the division between art and sciences in both displays and, more often, museum institutions, which not only furthers the decontextualization of objects but also detracts from the mutually beneficial relationship that can exist between the two fields. How then can curators reinsert a sensory visitor experience that not only allows more personal engagement with objects but also creates the possibility for imaginings of lived experience for both present and past civilizations through this tactile encounter?

## Coming to Our Archaeological Senses

The exhibitions at the Badè Museum and the Doug Adams Gallery supply only a few of the many ways museums can engage the visitor with a multisensory experience. This involves looking beyond scientific objectivity as the sole means of understanding the function and meaning of things—the goal of modern archaeological enterprises—and considering how these objects constituted a real lived experience by ancient and historic peoples. For example, can we hold a small ceramic lamp and consider not only its particular form or utility but also imagine how warm it would feel in the palm of the hand when lit? How slowly we would have to walk when holding it so as not to spill the olive oil that serves as the fuel? Or how the dim light would barely illuminate our footsteps? In other words, can we move beyond a rigid, scientific approach to understand how life was truly experienced in the ancient past? Several pioneering museums have made this move, including the Sensory Museum Project of Concordia University (Classen 2007; Classen and Howes 2006), the 2005 *Touch Me* exhibition at the Victoria and Albert Museum in London, and the 2010 *Touchstone* exhibition at the Salisbury Museum.

My exhibition, *Lived Experience in Ancient Judah,* at the Badè Museum represents a further meditation on this sensory approach. It was based on artifacts excavated at the ancient town of Mizpah (modern Tell en-Nasbeh), a 2,500-year-old settlement located in the hill country of modern Israel north of Jerusalem, in an area known in biblical times as Judah. The town was excavated between 1926 and 1935 by William F. Badè, a professor at Pacific School of Religion (McCown

1947; Wampler 1947; Zorn 1993). This exhibition, both physically and conceptually, was based on two primary concerns: (1) the juxtaposition between traditional scientific methods and embodied approaches to archaeological material and (2) the greater depth of understanding to be gained by a sensory approach to the ancient past.

The exhibition space was designed around a traditional wood and plexiglass vitrine; a potent symbol for a stale, senseless archaeology (Figure 18-1). Inside were the tools of scientific archaeological endeavors most studiously used by Dr. Badè at Tell en-Nasbeh: metal calipers, measuring stand, pottery drawing, photograph, camera, and a reconstructed cook pot. But behind this central case, "sensory envelopes" (Frieman and Gillings 2007) based on discrete contexts for visitor exploration (discussed below) became the backdrop to enable a more dynamic, enlivened approach. In this space, the cook pot was no longer simply a utilitarian object to be measured and recorded, but rather it became a prop in the larger theater of lived experience at ancient Mizpah.

To ground the exhibition, I chose three dynamic points of interest based on archaeological contexts from Tell en-Nasbeh: a house, the town gateway, and a family tomb.[1] The organization of the exhibition based on these particular locations derived from both practical and philosophical concerns. Discrete contexts helped visitors channel their intellectual attentions to specific places in space and time, lessening the effects of sensory overload that might occur in simulated immersive environments or in the presentation of site- or culture-wide sensory perceptions.[2] By focusing on contexts and not individual senses, I was also able to simultaneously preserve the holistic nature of sensory perception (i.e., that our senses are not isolated but work together) and undermine the rigid Western categorization of the five senses that is not represented cross-culturally (Day, this volume; Hamilakis 2002; Howes and Classen 1991; Stewart 1999).

Each section of this fully tactile exhibition included a combination of artifact replicas, interactive models, visual imagery, and traditional museum pieces inside display cases. Visitors held ceramic bowls, smelled fragrant spices like cinnamon and cumin, and felt the cold touch of rough-hewn limestone common to tombs at Mizpah. Visitors were also encouraged to test the coarseness of mud bricks akin to those from Mizpah houses and shake (and listen to!) rattles modeled on ancient examples in the Badè collection.

To further approach the concept of lived experience, formal text labels featured exclusively a first-person narrative alongside traditional object labels. This technique of micronarrative has been previously used in the presentation and performance of archaeological storytelling to great effect (e.g., Edmonds 1999; Shanks 1992; Spector 1993; Tringham 1991, 1994; Van Dyke, this volume; see summary in McCarthy 2003), though its exclusive use in museum display I have yet to encounter. In *Lived Experience*, visitors were introduced to Hannah, a (fictitious) teenage girl living in a middle-class household at Mizpah. They journeyed with her as she moved about and experienced life in the town, from her daily chores to her excitement at the harvest festival staged in the town gateway.

The use of narrative allows for a personal connection with museumgoers that is not possible with dry factual labels. This was especially indicated by visitors

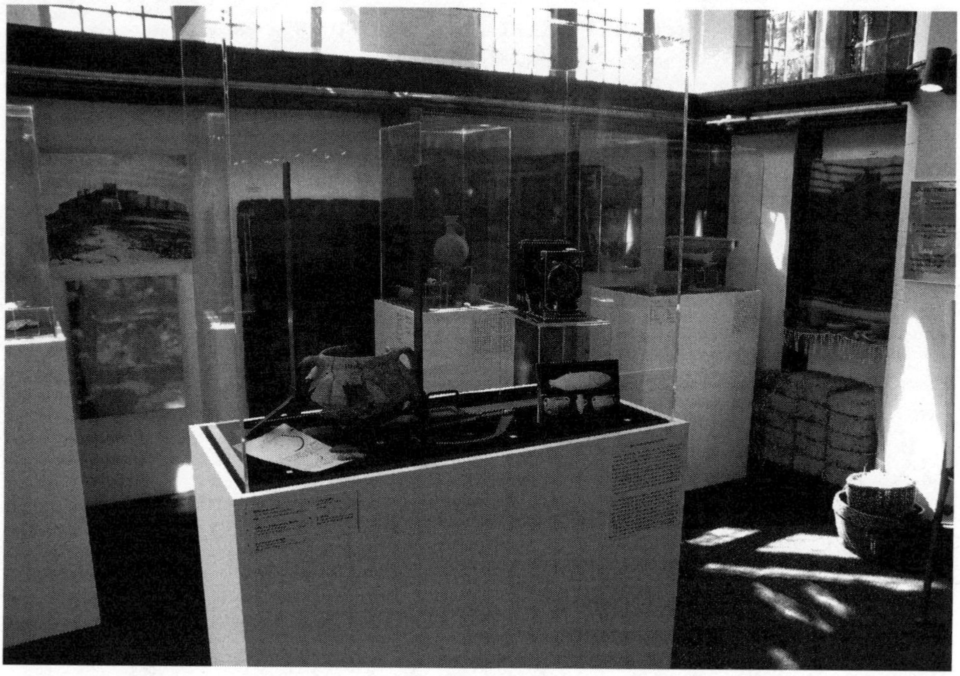

**Figure 18-1.** Lived Experience in Ancient Judah *exhibition at the Badè Museum of Biblical Archaeology, Berkeley, California. (Photograph © Catherine P. Foster.)*

to the exhibition who noted in both written and verbal comments how the story of Hannah provided contextualization for the objects on display while simultaneously transporting them back in time. For this exhibition, the history of Mizpah was thus no longer a recitation of occupation levels and ceramic styles, but a story told by an "eyewitness" whose thoughts, emotions, and actions were woven throughout the narrative. For example, in this label Hannah describes a visit to her family's tomb where she brings offerings to a deceased loved one:

> Outside the town walls to the west, my brothers help me move the stone door of our family tomb and I gingerly walk down the rough steps to enter the dark, cool crypt. The tiny lamp in my hand barely illuminates my footsteps and in its flickering, the shadows seem to dance before me as I move deeper inside. The smell of stale incense and rotting flesh mingle with the sweetness of the pomegranates and figs in my hand. I set them gently upon the stone bench next to my grandfather's body, now reduced to dry bones that will one day turn to dust, as we all do. (Foster 2010)

By using a first-person narrative approach, curators are able to connect visitors on a personal level and transcend the impersonal expression of an ancient past by blending imaginative renderings with ethnographic and archaeological evidence.

It is important to stress that Hannah's story, like other iterations of interpretive narrative archaeology (McCarthy 2003), developed from both scientific and creative sources. Her situations and surroundings were founded on a study of the archaeological materials from ancient Mizpah, ethnoarchaeological research, biblical texts, and scholarly treatments of everyday life in ancient Israel that have begun, in some small ways, to envision a truly embodied past (see especially King and Stager 2001:8–12). Hannah's emotions, reactions, and internal thoughts derived from my historical imaginings as both an archaeologist and a curator. In turn, such imaginings can give museum visitors permission and encouragement to create their own stories about this or other exhibitions—a practice that can only strengthen interest in ancient materials in general. Indeed, visitor feedback reinforced how this narrative presentation promoted appreciation and "mental visualizations" of the objects on display as being created, used, and discarded by persons in the past.

While storytelling as a museum device has the power to "bring history alive," it can also be limiting if we stop to consider whose history, exactly, we are portraying. In *Lived Experience*, Hannah and her adolescent perceptions dictate the story and, thus, what visitors learn about daily life in ancient Mizpah. To preserve clarity, the plurality of dynamic human experiences is lost while a distinct curatorial voice remains foregrounded.[3] In an effort to overcome this, prominent text panels embedded within the exhibition space prompted visitors to consider several questions. These included: "Is it possible to truly understand the lived experiences of ancient peoples? How are your modern experiences similar to those experienced in the past? How are they different?" Beyond prompting discussions by visitors, these panels underscored a level of curatorial transparency by raising questions that could potentially undermine some messages of the exhibition. The panels also acknowledged the diversity of personal experiences in the present as well as in the past.

## Sensory Art and Archaeological Interpretation

Archaeological exhibitions that present the entire sensorium through storytelling and interactive displays are only one way to disseminate and encourage sensory research. Contemporary art can also enrich sensory scholarship and provide a stimulus for archaeological imagining, all while encouraging an embodied experience in display space. In fact, there is a long history of interaction between contemporary art and archaeology with increasingly dynamic relationships being developed by practitioners of both fields (see Russell 2008 for a succinct discussion of this history). But while there is a definitive trend of contemporary artists being inspired by both ethnographic and archaeological artifacts (Picasso and Braque, for example), many have gone well beyond this "art source" approach. Artists like Mark Dion, Paul Nash, Simon Callery, Daniel Spoerri, Andy Goldsworthy, and Antony Gormley have all explored aspects of the archaeological process as well as the politics of display. For example, Colin Renfrew (2003:39) has noted that the environmental pieces of Richard Long, like *A Line Made by Walking* (1965), demand a personal experience. This physical interaction with the art and landscape both heightens our modern sensory perceptions and makes the viewer (no, the participant!) ponder experiences of ancient peoples in this same space. My point (shared by Bailey 2008; Noble 1991; Renfrew et al. 2004) is that contemporary art can make archaeologists conceptualize material culture in new and different ways. Art is not just an illustrative tool to relate archaeological information (Jameson 2003; Lippard 1983; Pate 2003), but rather it is a medium that challenges, shapes, and alters our archaeological perceptions. Artists and archaeologists also share similar processes of interaction and interpretation of the physical environment. Through this tactile engagement with the material world, creative processes are nurtured, and past and present realities are constructed (Renfrew 2003:138).

The use of art and artists to elicit embodied understandings of the past has been widely embraced in the arenas of landscape art (Tilley et al. 2000), aesthetics of excavation and process (Vilches 2007), urban environments (Rendell 2007), and even theatrical performance (Pearson and Shanks 2001). For museums, pioneering examples include the Art of Archaeology Initiative (Owen 2002) and the 2008 *Abhar agus Meon* exhibition series at University College Dublin (Russell 2008). These recent efforts undercut temporal divisions between contemporary and heritage spaces and infuse emotional sensibilities to objects normally overshadowed by the need for scientific objectivity. They also raise awareness that, by performing archaeology as a scientific discipline, we are constructing a "fourth wall" between humans and things, one that is physically materialized as the museum display case (Russell 2008:89).

Viewed within this analytical framework, the impact of contemporary artist Pamela Blotner's fully tactile exhibition at the Doug Adams Gallery, located in the Badè Museum, becomes apparent. Her pieces featured in *An Archaeology of the Senses* (curated by Carin Jacobs) represent her personal exploration of archaeological discovery, sensory perceptions, and spirituality (the "sixth sense"). As artist-in-residence,[4] Blotner relished the rather daunting opportunity to mine the collection of the Badè Museum, which holds "many beautiful and mysterious objects, whose both obvious and presumed functions provide the viewer—artist and archaeologist alike—a world of real and conceptual roads to travel" (Pamela Blotner, personal communication 2010). For Blotner, a noted San Francisco Bay Area artist for over 15 years, these roads traversed dynamic landscapes of archaeological process and interpretation, as well as the human experience of daily living in both a spiritual and profane sense.

Blotner's work acknowledges that the act of constructing history and meaning from the fragmentary evidence is itself based on some speculation (in her words, "an act of faith"), despite modern archaeological science and extensive scholarship of the Near East. Take, for example, her sculptural piece *What Remains*, based on footed bowls and incense burners in the Badè collection (Figure 18-2). The single ceramic sherd ensconced within a steel structure resembling a computer-generated 3-D wire frame is the artist's reaction to the fragmented and reconstructed vessels commonplace in archaeological collections. Both the artistic and scientific fields, it seems, are fascinated by absence and what it implies. In this situation, the missing parts and the fillings of these ancient objects speak both to archaeology in part as an act of conjecture and to the ongoing richness of the human imagination.

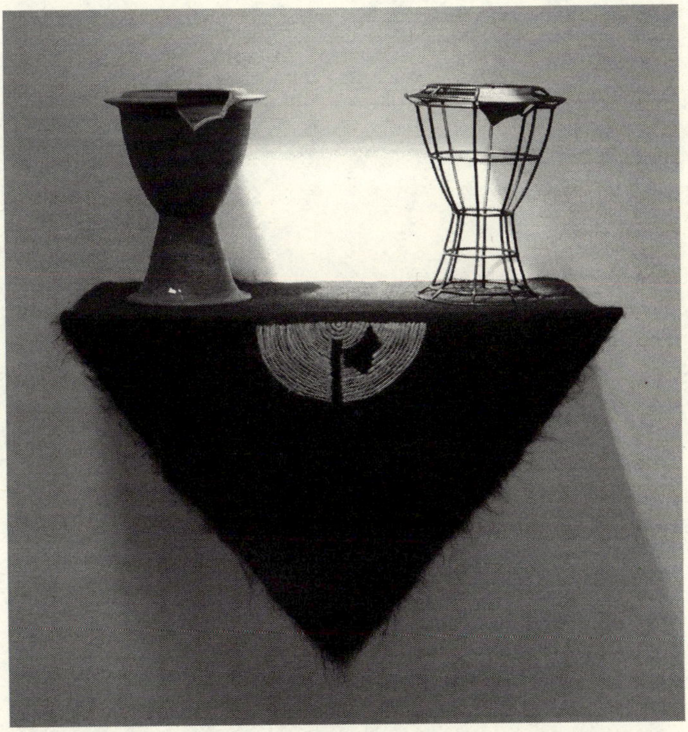

**Figure 18-2.** *Archaeology as faith:* What Remains, *2010, by Pamela Blotner. (Photograph © Pamela Blotner; used with permission.)*

A direct contemplation on the quantification of senses is also explored in *Six Visions*, a composite piece of felted wool and alpaca that visitors were encouraged to both touch and view (Figure 18-3). Drawn from the iconic multilimbed Hindu gods, the bent arms are emblematic of powers and sensuous experiences encapsulated within our visual perceptions. Each of the six hands uses, what is for many, an instantly recognizable gesture: pointing, cradling, waving, indicating "stop," indicating "all right," and praying (Pamela Blotner, personal communication 2010). This final gesture is in many ways representative of our "inner vision" embodied by the sixth and most cognitive sense of intuition, emotions, or spirituality. This is further reinforced by wool tendrils strung with wooden "worry beads": a contemporary play on ancient ceramic and glass beads from the Near East that feature an "evil-eye" decoration and were believed to ward off malignant spirits.

Finally, in Blotner's piece *Day by Day* we are reminded that sound-making elements encompass the realms of both music and noise (Figure 18-4). For example, the shape of the artwork resembles a stringed instrument with a pair of female musicians drumming along to the psalm carved into the crossbeam.[5] But suspended below, ceramic rattles, metal bells, obsidian blades, and potsherds act as unusual strings. The combination of these seemingly unrelated objects reconceptualizes how everyday items when in use (and in this case, when being strummed

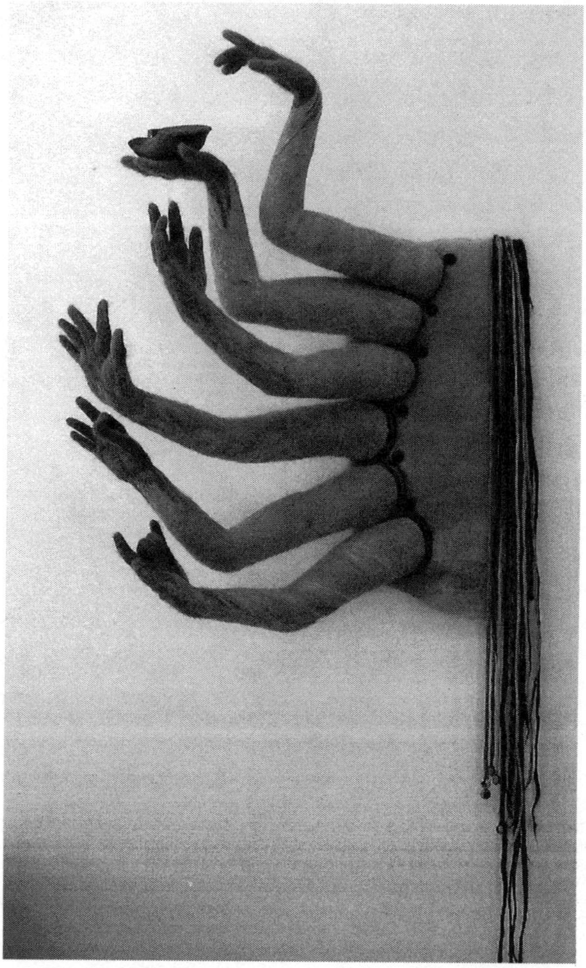

**Figure 18-3.** *The quantification of senses:* Six Visions, *2010, by Pamela Blotner. (Photograph © Pamela Blotner; used with permission.)*

by visitors) make unique noises that produce a sort of daily music or, in grander terms, daily rhythm of life. Seen in this light, the piece looks less like an instrument and is more reminiscent of a vertical loom, its warp threads being held taut by the bell "weights" that knock together as the weaver works.

Blotner's visceral reaction and subsequent presentation in *An Archaeology of the Senses* are both complementary and divergent from *Lived Experience*. Many of the archaeological objects on display—four-handled krater, loom weights, beads—were mirrored in Blotner's show, where they were treated as more than artistic inspiration but also as contemporary interpretation. But while my conscious curatorial decision involved a holistic conceptualization of sensory experiences, Blotner chose to display her work divided by individual senses. The artist believed this particular format of installation helped pace the visitor so that the essence of the works would have an accumulative weight (Pamela Blotner, personal communication 2010). This contrast in presentation of the senses between the two

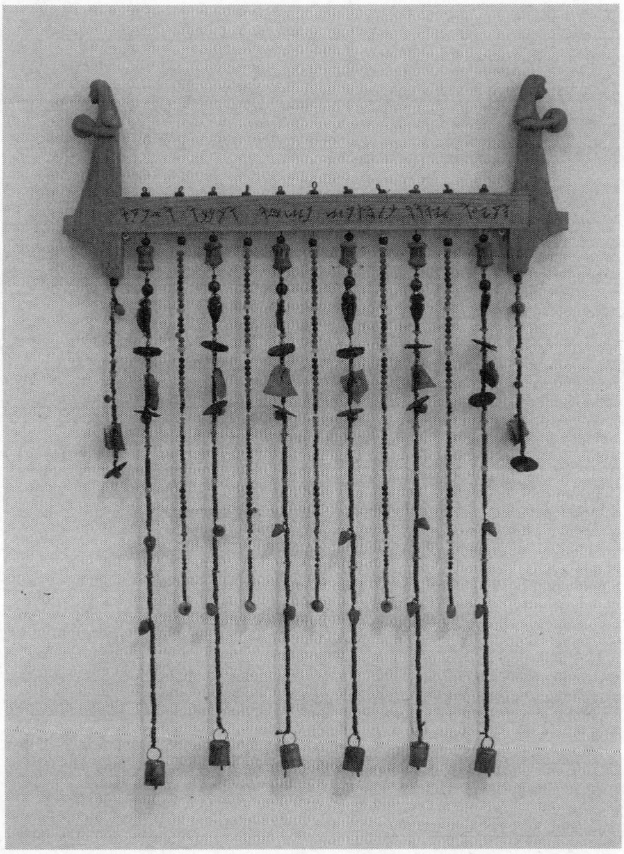

**Figure 18-4.** *Musical rhythms of daily life:* Day by Day, *2010, by Pamela Blotner. (Photograph © Pamela Blotner; used with permission.)*

exhibitions poses an interesting question for curators, artists, and sensory scholars about how best to present our information. Is a holistic sensory approach that envelops visitors most engaging or is a gradual layering of senses a more dramatic experience? Further experimentation and collaboration between these vested groups will, it is hoped, shed light on this question.

## Beyond the Display Case

The exhibitions at the Badè Museum and the Doug Adams Gallery call attention to the great potential museums have in presenting sensory narratives. More important, sensory-based narratives and interactive displays that encourage "surprise encounters" with objects, senses, and emotions are able to connect archaeology with a nonspecialist audience. This is no small concern considering the future of museums rests on their relevance to the broader public.

The two exhibitions presented here also underscore the rich dialog that exists between contemporary art and archaeology that is only now being realized.[6] It is a strongly reciprocal relationship. Artists have long drawn inspiration from the art, architecture, and cultural materials of ancient and historic civilizations brought to light by the archaeological community. But just as objects become "art sources" for artists, so too do these objects regain some of the centrality they had in the past as functional, artistic, and material objects (Paternosto 2006:167; see also Gosden 2001). As the modern divide between "high art" and craft is rendered invisible, the true multiplicity of object meanings can be highlighted and celebrated. The somewhat stifling mold of "artist-archaeologist" is also being broken by the work of Christopher Tilley, Barbara Bender, Sue Hamilton (Bender et al. 2008; Tilley et al. 2000) and others who do not simply view contemporary art as a convenient tool set for progressive archaeological interpretations but who foresee a fusion of the two fields to create an entirely new way of envisioning and presenting the past (Bailey 2008).

Not only can contemporary artists help represent history, but their work also "can be the expression in the material world of a concept" (Renfrew 2003:99). Art can give shape to the unknown and convey emotion that we cannot simply dig up in archaeological sites. Especially fruitful for sensory studies is the fact that visual art also insists on personal interaction. In *Archaeology of the Senses*, all pieces were on a human scale, challenging the visitor's own physical relationship with them and relying on a tactile encounter. This physical relationship naturally goes beyond the visual—all of Blotner's artworks were available for touching, smelling, hearing, and viewing.

Finally, these contemporary artistic imaginings can portray those things not normally preserved in the archaeological record of the Near East, like wooden implements or basketry. Art can fill the conceptual gaps many archaeologists struggle with in portraying a holistic picture of ancient life. Artists may thus make associations that archaeologists may have disregarded or never envisioned. In essence, they recontextualize ancient objects and can demand a nonlinear understanding of and deeper experience with these objects.

This kind of recontextualized engagement is mandated in particular by Blotner's *Gathering*, a composite sculpture of wood and ceramic inspired by a large four-handled krater from ancient Mizpah (Figure 18-5). Harkening back to Diane Ackerman's (1991:127) notion that taste may be our most social sense, the large communal vessel and carved wooden spoons, or ladles, attest to and become symbolic of community. Taste and smell are also linked through the application of spruce oil to the table and cumin and clove oils in the fired clay of the krater. The number of ladles furthers this contemplation with both the various foods depicted on each and also the number of diners. How many sat around this vessel to feast together? Who was included and why? Who was excluded? How did the meal change based on the company, season, or location? These are only a few of the questions considered by visitors as they engaged in their own musings and interpretations of what these objects mean outside the display cases and in real life.

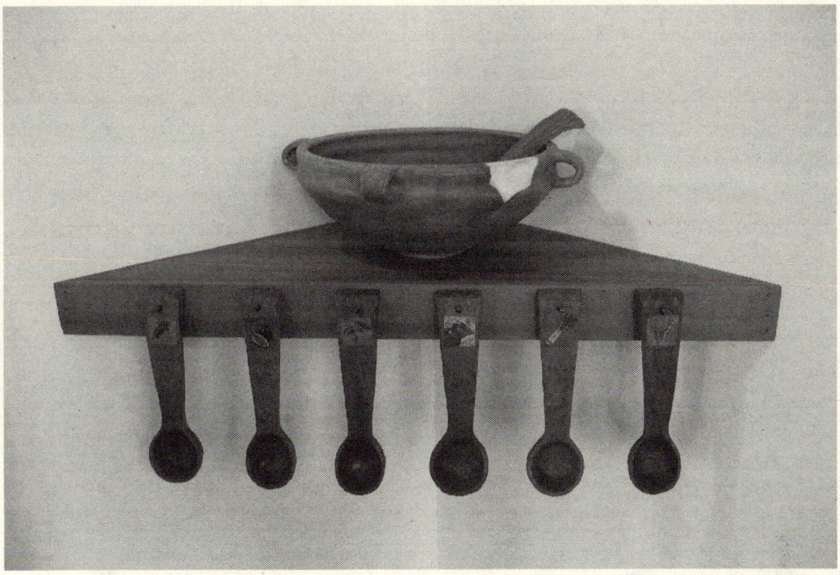

**Figure 18-5.** *The social sense of community:* Gathering, *2010, by Pamela Blotner. (Photograph © Pamela Blotner; used with permission.)*

## Conclusion

This chapter has been a meditation on various ways museums, archaeologists, and contemporary artists can work together to promote sensory archaeological research and create truly engaging presentations to the public that rely on a multisensory experience. Museums were founded on principles of physical encounters with objects to facilitate learning. In the case of historical, ethnographic, and archaeological museums, this tactile approach encouraged real connections with peoples of long ago or from halfway across the globe. Coincidently, this same focus on physicality, embodiment, and human interaction with the material world is shared by archaeologists and contemporary artists. This distinct relationship could be explored and promoted further in a museum setting. The two sensory archaeology exhibitions at the Badè Museum and the Doug Adams Gallery were founded on this concept of open dialog to not only bridge the gap between the two fields but to also use the great tools and strengths of each to explore concepts of lived experience in ancient Judah and our current lives.

*Lived Experience in Ancient Judah* and *An Archaeology of the Senses* represent only a pair of examples of multisensory exhibitions as a starting point for what I hope will develop into larger museum practice. There is much to be incorporated into these types of exhibitions that was not utilized in the Badè Museum and the Doug Adams Gallery shows due to budgetary and space issues. One example would be combined exhibitions that feature contemporary art and archaeological objects melded within the same display space.[7] Another example could be the continued lessening of the curatorial voice and greater encouragement of museum visitors to offer their own interpretations. This approach supports much of sensory archaeological research that reinforces the multivocality involved with understanding, interpreting, and presenting embodied experiences of the past. Sensory perceptions are indeed personal and dictated by social relations and cultural values (Brück 2005), underscoring the necessity for plurality. The re-creation of a singular "true" narrative should not be the goal.

A third example of how exhibitors and curators could further grasp the sensuous exploration of ancient pasts through tactile exhibitions would be a larger use of sensory perceptions not normally found within gallery settings, including smells, tastes and sounds. While Owen (1999:180) has already remarked that hands-on activities are becoming more commonplace in the permanent galleries of archaeological and historical museums, I would emphasize that these types of learning experiences focus only on touch and sight. Even when offered the opportunity of these activities, in many cases it is difficult for visitors to overcome their learned museum actions. I observed on several occasions the reluctance and refusal of several visitors to touch, smell, and listen to display pieces in *Lived Experience* and *Archaeology of the Senses*, despite the addition of prominent "Please Touch Gently" signs.

I believe our hard wiring for traditional museum etiquette can be overcome by focusing on other senses and sensory research. The inclusion of sounds in exhibition spaces would impart both the study and presentation of ambient noise, sound cutouts, and copresence zones (Mongelluzzo, this volume; Williams, this volume). It is impossible to evoke smell using language or vision (Day, this volume; Weddle, this volume), making the use of scent within gallery spaces essential. Sound and scent also circumvent our learned gallery behaviors; unlike touch, we cannot simply choose to stop hearing and smelling inside the exhibition. Though the idea of edible exhibitions seems unfeasible, the re-creation of ancient dishes in museum cafeterias might be a more logical extension of a unique visitor experience. In the end, however, curators must be careful that these sensuous representations do not purposefully or inadvertently support sensory stereotypes.[8] The Western five-sense schema may be a starting point for some, but it should not be the final conceptualization.

Referring to the priority most museums place on preservation of objects for future generations, Elizabeth Pye (2007:26) has remarked that "the obligation to preserve is so future-oriented that it is preventing access to collections now." So what is the future of multisensory museum exhibits in the face of preservation responsibilities? I believe it involves a delicate balancing act between curators and conservators who want to maintain the structural integrity of their collections on the one hand and the interested public who are starved for tactile engagement on the other.

While the option of virtual touch based on 3-D renderings may be satisfactory for remote interaction via the Internet, this method still removes objects from their culturally significant and tactile environments, essentially substituting a digital case for a glass one. Truly sensory appreciation of the lived experiences of past peoples relies on a full engagement of the senses in contexts that, although re-created, stimulate engagement with material artifacts, both real and replicated. Visitors should be challenged to consider and perhaps reconceptualize their own beliefs about past and present lifeways through tactile engagement with art and objects. More so than traditional books, films, or even television shows, I am confident that museums stand ready to support and promote a sensory exploration of the past while still maintaining established practices of preservation and stewardship. We have only to look—touch, taste, smell, and hear—beyond the display case.

## Acknowledgments

This chapter is based on research and exhibitions generously supported by the Badè Museum of Biblical Archaeology, Doug Adams Gallery, Pacific School of Religion, and Center for Arts, Religion and Education (CARE) at the Graduate Theological Union. I am indebted to Dr. Aaron Brody, director of the Badè Museum; Carin Jacobs, director of the Doug Adams Gallery and CARE; and Pamela Blotner, who was coauthor on the original conference paper and artistic collaborator for this project. I also wish to extend my thanks to Dr. Brian A. Brown and Dr. Jo Day for their insightful comments.

## Notes

1. Skeates (2008) took a similar approach in his analysis of sensory stimuli and full-bodied experiences on prehistoric Malta by referencing three dynamic place types (houses, caves, and temples).

2. This sentiment is echoed by Classen and Howes (2006:218–219), who are against total sensory immersion and argue that objects of simulated reality should not have to vie for authenticity with actual cultural materials.

3. A similar problem was noted by Piccini (1999:170) who found open-air reconstructions of ancient sites to be static, one-dimensional, and capable of offering only a general picture of the society being represented.

4. Blotner served as the Doug Adams Gallery's inaugural (2009–2010) artist-in-residence, an annual program organized by Carin Jacobs and sponsored by the Center for Arts, Religion, and Education (CARE) at the Graduate Theological Union.

5. Written in Paleo–Hebrew based on letterforms found on other inscribed objects from Tell en-Nasbeh, the verse reads, "Make a joyful noise unto the Lord, all the earth; make a loud noise and rejoice, and sing praise" (Psalms 98:4).

6. A 2009 conference in Paris hosted by the Institut National d'Histoire de l'Art (INHA) addressed this very subject.

7. A wonderful example is the Oakland Museum of California where objects from California's history intermingle with contemporary art and specimens from the natural world that share similar thematic or material elements. This multidisciplinary approach is a future phase of the Badè Museum and the Doug Adams

Gallery, which currently occupy the same large display space but do not as yet stage fully integrated exhibitions.

8. As is the case with many nonsensory museum displays and public installations that, for example, reinforce the inferiority of Africans because of their role in human origins (Scott 2005) or maintain a hyperrealistic image of modern Egyptian society as idyllic and unchanged since pharaonic times (Meskell 2003).

## References

Ackerman, Diane
1991 *A Natural History of the Senses*. 4th ed. Vintage, New York.
Alexander, Edward P., and Mary Alexander
2008 *Museums in Motion: An Introduction to the History and Function of Museums*. 2nd ed. Altamira, Walnut Creek.
Bailey, Douglass
2008 Art to Archaeology to Archaeology to Art. In *Archaeologies of Art: Papers from the Sixth World Archaeological Congress*, edited by Ian Russell, UCDscholarcast. Electronic document, http://www.ucd.ie/scholarcast/transcripts/Art_to_Archaeology.pdf, accessed July 8, 2010.
Bender, Barbara, Sue Hamilton, and Christopher Tilley
2008 *Stone Worlds: Narrative and Reflexivity in Landscape Archaeology*. Left Coast, Walnut Creek.
Bennett, Tony
1995 *The Birth of the Museum: History, Theory, Politics*. Routledge, New York.
Brück, Joanna
2005 Experiencing the Past? The Development of a Phenomenological Archaeology in British Prehistory. *Archaeological Dialogues* 12:45–72.
Classen, Constance
2007 Museum Manners: The Sensory Life of the Early Museum. *Journal of Social History* 40:895–914.
Classen, Constance, and David Howes
2006 The Museum as Sensescape: Western Sensibilities and Indigenous Artifacts. In *Sensible Objects: Colonialism, Museums and Material Culture*, edited by Elizabeth Edwards, Chris Gosden, and Ruth B. Phillips, pp. 199–222. Berg, Oxford.
Edmonds, Mark
1999 *Ancestral Geographies of the Neolithic: Landscape, Monuments and Memory*. Routledge, London.
Fiennes, Celia
1949 *The Journeys of Celia Fiennes*. Cresset, London.
Foster, Catherine P.
2010 "Lived Experience in Ancient Judah." Badè Museum of Biblical Archaeology, Berkeley, California.
Frieman, Catherine, and Mark Gillings
2007 Seeing Is Perceiving? *World Archaeology* 39:4–16.
Goode, George Brown
1895 The Principles of Museum Administration. *Annual Report of the Museums Association*, pp. 69–148.

Gosden, Chris
2001 Making Sense: Archaeology and Aesthetics. *World Archaeology* 33:163–167.
Hamilakis, Yannis
2002 The Past as Oral History: Towards an Archaeology of the Senses. In *Thinking through the Body: Archaeologies of Corporeality*, edited by Yannis Hamilakis, Mark Pluciennik, and Sarah Tarlow, pp. 121–136. Kluwer Academic/Plenum, New York.
Howes, David, and Constance Classen
1991 Sounding Sensory Profiles. In *Varieties of Sensory Experience*, edited by David Howes, pp. 257–288. University of Toronto Press, Toronto.
Impey, Oliver, and Arthur MacGregor
2001 *The Origins of Museums: The Cabinet of Curiosities in Sixteenth- and Seventeenth-Century Europe*. House of Stratus, London.
Jameson, John H., Jr.
2003 Art and Imagery as Tools for Public Interpretation and Education in Archaeology. In *Ancient Muses: Archaeology and the Arts*, edited by John H. Jameson Jr., John E. Ehrenhard, and Christine A. Finn, pp. 57–64. University of Alabama Press, Tuscaloosa.
King, Philip J., and Lawrence E. Stager
2001 *Life in Biblical Israel*. Westminster John Knox, Louisville.
Lippard, Lucy
1983 *Overlay: Contemporary Art and the Art of Prehistory*. New Press, New York.
McCarthy, John P.
2003 More than Just "Telling the Story": Interpretive Narrative Archaeology. In *Ancient Muses: Archaeology and the Arts*, edited by John H. Jameson Jr., John E. Ehrenhard, and Christine A. Finn, pp. 15–24. University of Alabama Press, Tuscaloosa.
McCown, Chester C.
1947 *Tell En-Nasbeh I: Archaeological and Historical Results*. Palestine Institute, Pacific School of Religion and American Schools of Oriental Research, Berkeley, California.
Meskell, Lynn
2003 Pharaonic Legacies: Postcolonialism, Heritage and Hyperreality. In *The Politics of Archaeology and Identity in a Global Context*, edited by Susan Kane, pp. 149–171. Archaeological Institute of America, Boston.
Noble, Alexandra (editor)
1991 *From Art to Archaeology*. South Bank Centre, London.
Owen, Janet
1999 Interaction or Tokenism? The Role of 'Hands-On Activities' in Museum Archaeology Displays. In *Making Early Histories in Museums*, edited by Nick Merriman, pp. 173–189. Leicester University Press, London.
2002 *Society of Museum Archaeologists Art of Archaeology Initiative: Summary Report*. Electronic document, http://www.socmusarch.org.uk/artofarch.pdf, accessed July 8, 2010.
Pate, Martin
2003 Archaeology in Two Dimensions: The Artist's Perspective. In *Ancient Muses: Archaeology and the Arts*, edited by John H. Jameson Jr., John E. Ehrenhard, and Christine A. Finn, pp. 49–56. University of Alabama Press, Tuscaloosa.
Paternosto, Cesar
2006 No Borders: The Ancient American Roots of Abstraction. In *Contemporary Art and Anthropology*, edited by Arnd Schneider and Christopher Wright, pp. 157–168. Berg, Oxford.

Pearson, Mike, and Michael Shanks
2001 *Theatre/Archaeology*. Routledge, London.
Piccini, Angela
1999 Wargames and Wendy Houses: Open-Air Reconstructions of Prehistoric Life. In *Making Early Histories in Museums*, edited by Nick Merriman, pp. 151–172. Leicester University Press, London.
Pye, Elizabeth
2007 Introduction: The Power of Touch. In *The Power of Touch: Handling Objects in Museums and Heritage Contexts*, edited by Elizabeth Pye, pp. 13–30. Left Coast, Walnut Creek.
Rendell, Jane
2007 Not Yet . . . Art and Archaeology in the Context of Urban Renewal. In *Situations*. Electronic document, http://www.situations.org.uk/_uploaded_pdfs/JaneRendell_000.pdf, accessed July 15, 2010.
Renfrew, Colin
2003 *Figuring It Out: What Are We? Where Do We Come From? The Parallel Vision of Artists and Archaeologists*. Thames and Hudson, New York.
Renfrew, Colin, Chris Gosden, and Elizabeth DeMarrais (editors)
2004 *Substance, Memory, Display: Archaeology and Art*. McDonald Institute for Archaeological Research, University of Cambridge.
de la Roche, Sophie
1933 *Sophie in London*. London: Jonathan Cape.
Russell, Ian
2008 Art, Archaeology and the Contemporary: The Abhar Agus Meon Exhibitions. *Museum Ireland* 18:85–105.
Scott, Monique
2005 "We Grew Up and Moved On": Visitors to British Museums Consider Their "Cradle of Mankind." In *Envisioning the Past: Archaeology and the Image*, edited by Sam Smiles and Stephanie Moser, pp. 29–50. Blackwell, Malden, Massachusetts.
Shanks, Michael
1992 *Experiencing the Past*. Routledge, London.
Skeates, Robin
2008 Making Sense of the Maltese Temple Period: An Archaeology of Sensory Experience and Perception. *Time and Mind: The Journal of Archaeology, Consciousness and Culture* 1:207–238.
Spector, Janet D.
1993 *What This Awl Means: Feminist Archaeology at a Wahpeton Dakota Village*. Minnesota Historical Society, St. Paul.
Stewart, Susan
1999 Prologue: From the Museum of Touch. In *Material Memories: Design and Evocation*, edited by Marius Kwint, Christopher Breward, and Jeremy Aynsley, pp. 17–36. Berg, Oxford.
Tilley, Christopher, Sue Hamilton, and Barbara Bender
2000 Art and the Re-Presentation of the Past. *Journal of the Royal Anthropological Institute* 6:35–62.
Tringham, Ruth
1991 Households with Faces: The Challenge of Gender in Prehistoric Architectural Remains. In *Engendering Archaeology: Women and Prehistory*, edited by Joan M. Gero and Margaret H. Conkey, pp. 93–131. Blackwell, Oxford.
1994 Engendered Places in Prehistory. *Gender, Place and Culture* 1:169–203.

Vilches, Flora
2007 The Art of Archaeology: Mark Dion and His Dig Projects. *Journal of Social Archaeology* 7:199–223.
von Uffenbach, Zacharias Conrad
1934 *London in 1710*. Translated by W. H. Quarrel and Margaret Mare. Faber and Faber, London.
Wampler, Joseph C.
1947 *Tell En-Nasbeh II: The Pottery*. Palestine Institute, Pacific School of Religion and American Schools of Oriental Research, Berkeley, California.
Zorn, Jeffery R.
1993 Tell En-Nasbeh: A Re-Evaluation of the Architecture and Stratigraphy of the Early Bronze Age, Iron Age and Later Periods. Unpublished Ph.D. dissertation, Department of Near Eastern Studies, University of California, Berkeley.

# 19. Imagined Narratives: Sensory Lives in the Chacoan Southwest

*Ruth M. Van Dyke*

*Abstract:* In this chapter, I use the Chacoan archaeology of the Southwest United States to illustrate the power of imagined narratives to take us out of the two-dimensional world of data and interpretation and into the three-dimensional world of sensory lives. Imagined narratives are essentially creative nonfiction—the use of archaeological information to construct imagined lives in the past. Narratives must resonate coherently with, and be grounded in, archaeological evidence. Imagined narratives can give voice to multiple perspectives, emphasizing the interplay among past peoples' experiences, roles, genders, ages, statuses, ethnicities, and occupations. Imagined narratives can be analytical tools that provide us with alternative ways of thinking about, not just representing, the past. As I try to imagine a series of events in ancient Chaco from the point of view of a particular individual, not only does the past become closer, more personal, and more humanized, but the effort brings into relief the many things I do not know and the questions I have not yet thought to ask.

It's early summer in 1050 C.E. The corn is just beginning to stretch green shoots upward from the dry fields planted along Coyote Wash, amidst the beige-brown cliffs and the sandstone hoodoos of the western San Juan basin, in a place today they call New Mexico. At Chaco Canyon, soon it will be time for the summer solstice ceremonies. I imagine that I am a 10-year-old girl living in the Whirlwind outlier community, about 35 km southwest of Chaco. This is the first summer I am old enough to join my grandmother and older sister on the journey to Chaco for the solstice ceremonies. We travel together across the rugged terrain, the desert gravels crunching in time with our footsteps. My early morning excitement dissipates gradually into fatigue, because it's a long walk, and it's very hot during the day, and I have short legs. My sister runs ahead of me, gossiping with the other girls her age. We walk along

*Making Senses of the Past: Toward a Sensory Archaeology*, edited by Jo Day. Center for Archaeological Investigations, Occasional Paper No. 40.  ISBN 978-0-8093-3287-8.

the paths that connect the outliers, from our home at Whirlwind, north to the community at Escalon, then east along the Chaco Wash to Lake Valley, and then farther east to Casa del Rio. The paths are broad, straight, and well trampled—many people have passed this way. Along the way, prominent, odd-looking landforms such as Bennett Peak and White Rock shift into and out of view. My grandmother tells me stories about things that happened to the ancestors at those peaks long ago. And she tells me stories about other journeys she has made to Chaco, as a young mother and as a girl like me. One time a man was bitten by a rattler, and another time the special offering jars were left behind, and another time they met strange traders on the road who carried bracelets carved of white shell.

It takes us four days to make the journey. We stop each night at a different community, visiting the homes of relatives and cousins. My sister and grandmother catch up on the news and gossip; I play with my cousins and the other children. Some people are joining us on the journey; others are not. We share shelled corn and savory deer jerky that we have brought, and people feed us and give us things to take to Chaco for them—offerings such as red dog shale pendants, or Narbona Pass chert, or pieces of special pottery. There are so many new experiences that each day seems to last a week. Each morning I wonder, who will we meet today? What will we eat? Where will we sleep tonight? We sing traveling songs as we walk. More and more people join us each day as we go—some come from distant communities to the north or south. Some speak with strange accents, and some we cannot understand at all.

On the fourth day of our journey, we walk east up the Chaco Wash from the great house of Casa del Rio toward West Mesa. In the distance, I see a row of watchers standing atop the mesa edge, silhouetted against the sky . . . but as we move nearer I can see that these are not people, but shrines. My heart pounds with excitement. Chaco, at last! We round the edge of the mesa and enter the canyon, and suddenly we are assaulted by a cacophony of drumming and singing, barking dogs, and babbling voices. We climb the short staircase up the cliff to the great house of Peñasco Blanco, where we will stay with our relatives for the week of the ceremonies. The building resembles our great house at home at Whirlwind, but it is so much bigger! As we approach, we smell venison roasting, and we see people running to and fro along the third-story rooftops. Someone calls and waves to my grandmother, and we have arrived.

## From Chaco Canyon to Phenomenology

A millennium ago, Chaco Canyon in northwest New Mexico (Figure 19-1) was the center of a polity held together by ritual (e.g., authors in Lekson 2006; Lekson 1999, 2008; Sebastian 1992; Van Dyke 2007). Canyon builders constructed monumental architecture in the form of great houses, great kivas, earthworks, and road segments (Figure 19-2). Thousands of people from an area within a 150 km radius of Chaco traveled to the canyon for major ceremonial events that probably coincided with astronomical phenomena. These events were presided over by an elite group of Chacoan residents. Although most Chaco scholars see periodic ritual gatherings in the canyon as central to social and political organization, it is difficult to reconstruct the specific nature of Chacoan ceremonialism.

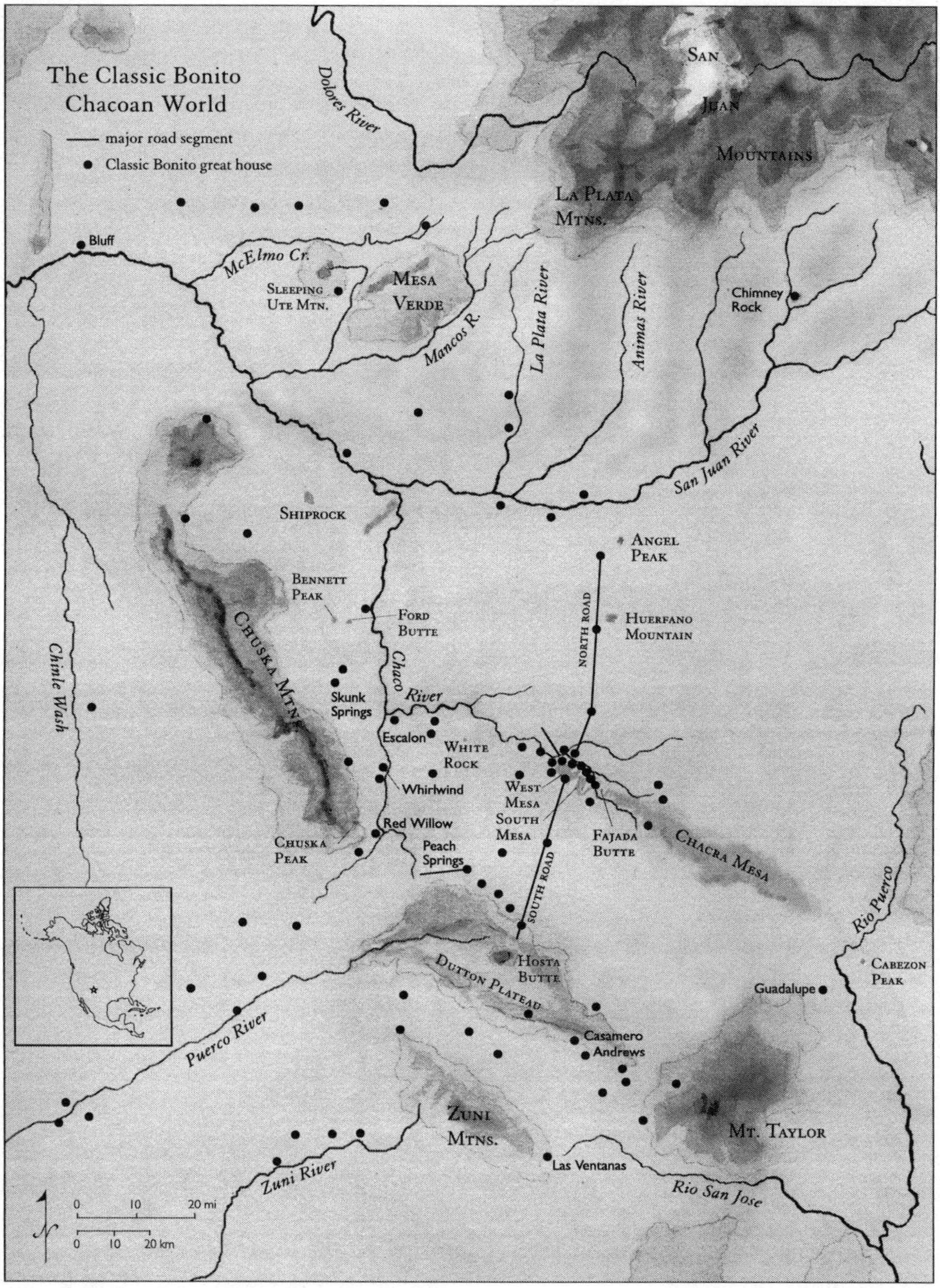


**Figure 19-1.** *The San Juan basin (northwest New Mexico and surrounding areas) showing Chaco Canyon, outlier great houses, and other landscape features circa 1020–1100* C.E. *(Map by Molly O'Halloran, with modifications by Ruth M. Van Dyke.)*

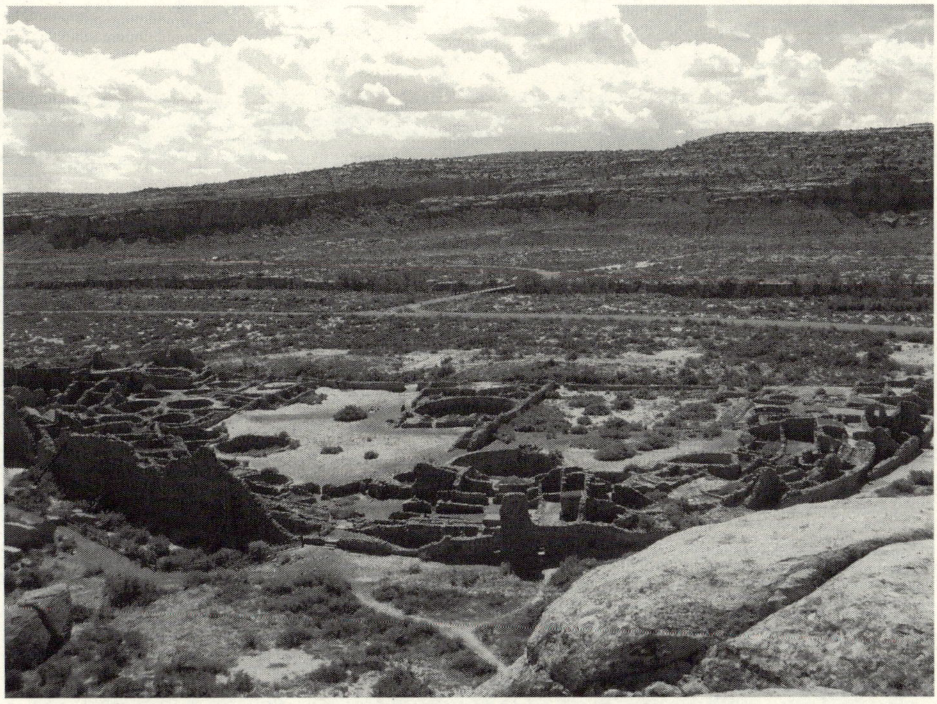

**Figure 19-2.** *The great house of Pueblo Bonito, looking south from the north rim of Chaco Canyon. (Photograph © Ruth M. Van Dyke.)*

The material evidence for ritual at Chaco consists of the public architecture, rock art, portable objects, and unusual depositional events. Clues to Chacoan cosmology are contained in the orientations, positions, and other aspects of great houses, great kivas, road segments, earthworks, and shrines. Landscape and architecture embodied ideas—such as center place—that were important to the Chacoans, and this constructed environment encouraged particular kinds of bodily experiences that supported a Chacoan ideology (Van Dyke 2007). Archaeo-astronomical alignments and rock art tell us that the Chacoan ritual cycle probably incorporated solstices, equinoxes, and lunar standstills (Malville 2004; Sofaer 2007). Archaeological signatures of feasting include unusual food remains, cooking vessels, cooking facilities, and special trash middens (Toll 1985, 2001; Windes 1987). Ritual paraphernalia from Chacoan great houses include carved and painted wooden altar furniture (Vivian et al. 1978), cylinder jars that held cacao (Crown and Hurst 2009), decorated baskets, cornhusk containers, feather and reed items, and rush bundles (Webster 2011). Chacoans interred turquoise, shell, and lignite beads, pendants, and other materials with burials, in sealed niches, and under roof-support columns (Judd 1954:338–339; Pepper 1909, 1920; Vivian and Reiter 1960). The caching of these inalienable objects (Mills 2004, 2008), the repeated obliteration and redecoration of cylinder vessels (Crown and Wills 2003), and the frequent remodeling of great houses and great kivas (Van

Dyke 2004, 2007) suggest a concern with inscribed and embodied social memory (Connerton 1989).

How are we to approach the sensory, human experiences behind these collections of artifacts, features, and ideas? For empirical as well as epistemic reasons, archaeologists are well situated to think about generalizing processes and large-scale social transformations over long spans of time. In the American Southwest, we have a long tradition of relying heavily on the direct historical approach, even though we know that Pueblo society and ritual could not have been the same in 1050 C.E. as it was during the ethnohistoric past (Lekson and Cameron 1995; Plog and Solometo 1997; Van Dyke 2012). Ethnographic analogies, while useful in many respects, create the illusion of a past that is temporally flat and populated by generalities. As Ruth Tringham famously avowed, all too often we think of past peoples as "faceless blobs" (Tringham 1991:94).

Whether one studies the emergence of the state or household craft production, our interest in the past has ultimately to do with the human experience. A past with faces is a past filled with sensory experience, emotion, and meaning. The burgeoning of archaeological interest in agency over the past decade (e.g., Dobres and Robb 2000; Dornan 2002; Varien and Potter 2008) might be seen in part as an attempt to recolonize archaeological interpretations with actual people. Although peoples in the past probably did not view themselves as "individuals" in the Western, modern sense of bounded, isolated entities (Bernbeck 2003), "it is at the human scale that contradictions and conflicts are worked out, lived through, and resolved" (Hodder 2000:26). We need creative ways to evoke the sensory experiences of the past peoples we study.

There has recently been a great deal of phenomenological interest in evoking the sights, sounds, smells, tastes, and textures of the past (e.g., Cummings et al. 2002; Cummings and Whittle 2003; Hamilakis 2002; Hamilton and Whitehouse 2006; Ryzewski 2009; Tilley 1994, 2004, 2008). Phenomenology posits the human body as the point of dialectical mediation between consciousness and the physical world (Casey 1996; De Certeau 1984; Heidegger 1962; Merleau-Ponty 1962; Thomas 1996). As we move through archaeological spaces, we can learn about how ancient builders intended their world to be perceived. Correspondingly, I have spent a good deal of time walking, with video camera and notebook in hand, across the Chacoan landscape (Van Dyke 2007, 2011).

However, archaeological phenomenology is problematic in many respects (Barrett and Ko 2009; Brück 2005; Fleming 1999, 2005, 2006). Interpretations tend to rely on universalisms. Phenomenological work often privileges the visual (Day, this volume). But what of the other senses? Acoustic, haptic, olfactory, and savory somatic experiences are just as integral to human life. And phenomenological accounts are often written from the perspective of the solitary walker encountering the past for the first time—but past meanings were created and negotiated across repeated, multiple encounters with places (Figure 19-3). My phenomenological experiments have not gotten me much closer to Chacoan sensory experiences, as I tend to end up with unsatisfying lists of things that I could see, or could not see, on a given pedestrian route. It is all too easy to generalize and universalize past

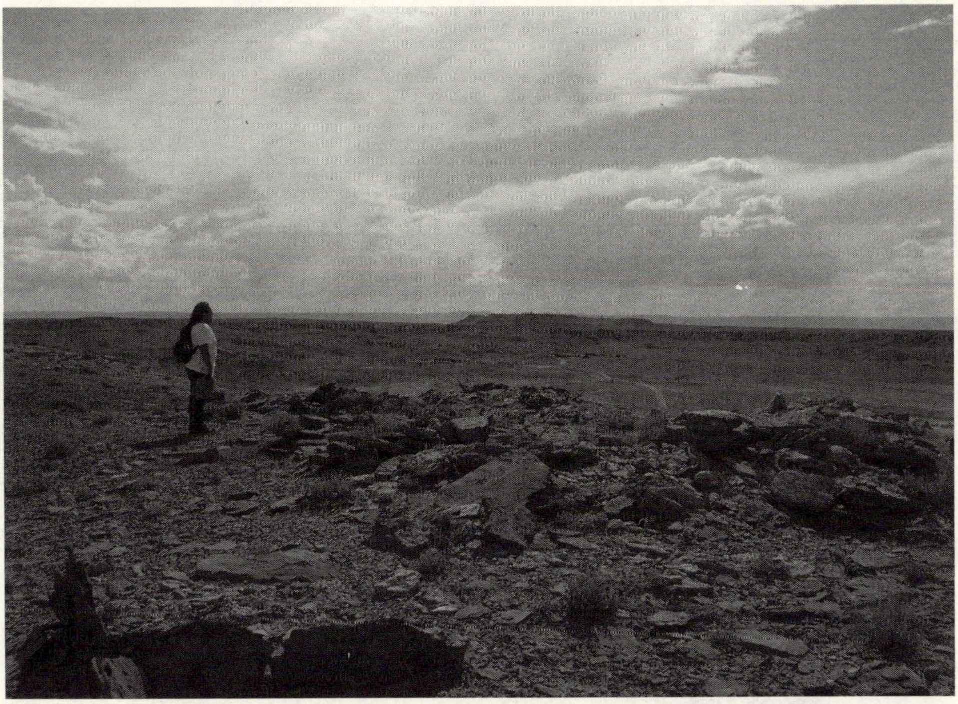

**Figure 19-3.** *Navajo archaeologist Davina Two Bears contemplates a tenth-century enclosure at the Willow Canyon complex south of the Chaco Wash, along the route described in the imagined narratives. (Photograph © Ruth M. Van Dyke.)*

bodies, but experiences would have been different for individuals depending on age, gender, and social standing (Figure 19-4).

And so I have begun to explore imagined narratives, such as the one presented above. Imagined narratives bring memory, meaning, and emotion into archaeological interpretations while circumventing some of the problems inherent in phenomenological approaches. They provide a means to more vividly engage the senses in archaeological interpretation.

## Imagined Narratives as Archaeological Interpretation and Analysis

I conceive of imagined narratives as creative nonfiction—the use of archaeological information to construct imagined lives. This is not the same thing as archaeological fiction. I am not attempting to write a story, complete with plot and character development, nor am I attempting to use archaeological knowledge as a jumping-off point for the creation of a fictional world. I ground my narratives in empirical data (McCarthy 2003). I draw on the notion of coherence

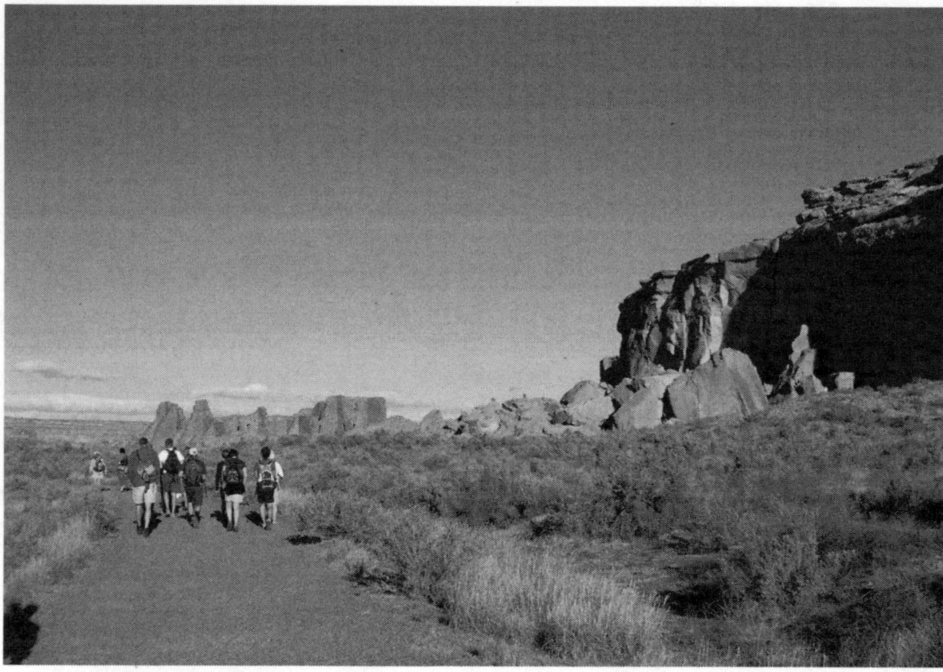

**Figure 19-4.** *A group of Colorado College students approaches Pueblo Bonito from the east, along the modern park-service trail. (Photograph © Ruth M. Van Dyke.)*

(Bradley 1914; Davidson 1986; Hodder 1991:60–61) to construct interpretations that resonate with multiple strands of archaeological evidence—interpretations that encompass rather than ignore the interstices among archaeological data, linking these data into a coherent and plausible whole.

Creative, interpretive methods are not new in archaeology. Over the past decade, quite a few archaeologists have engaged in artistic representation as one means for transcending the limitations of traditional prose formats (e.g., Avikunthak 2001; Cochrane and Russell 2008; Pearson and Shanks 2001; Renfrew 2003; Vilches 2007; Witmore 2005). The categorical separation of "art"—as something to be passively, aesthetically appreciated—from "science"—as a systematic mode of enquiry into the nature of the world—is a Cartesian, modern Western ontology (Thomas 2004). Archaeologists have inseparable engagements with intuitive and analytical, emotional and rational sensibilities as we seek to understand the past. Even the most rigorous processual archaeologist does not approach her research devoid of emotional attachments and creative inspirations.

Many archaeologists have incorporated imaginary or fictional vignettes into their work (e.g., Deetz 1977, 1993; Edmonds 1999; Joyce and Tringham 2007; Joyce et al. 2000; Lopiparo and Joyce 2003; Praetzellis 1998; see also Praetzellis et al. 1997; Spector 1991, 1993; Tringham 1991); some have engaged in the construction of complete novels (e.g., Bandelier 1971 [1916]; Nelson 1999, 2004). Artistic approaches have been embraced in Americanist historical archaeology, where scholars have created or sponsored paintings, plays, fiction, and even an opera based on archaeological research (Bullard and Bryant 1999; Gibb 1998, 1999; authors in Jameson et al. 2003; Praetzellis 1998; Praetzellis et al. 1997; Yamin 1998, 2008).

Much of this creative work has sprung from a laudable desire to do a better job of communicating with the public (McCarthy 2003; Masson and Guillot 1994). Indeed, first-person narratives and stories tend to be perceived as legitimate scholarly contributions to museum exhibits, whose primary purpose is popular education. Of course, this raises all sorts of ontological and political issues about the presumed appetite of the predominantly white, middle-class museumgoer for truths about the past as presented by authoritative specialists (Leone et al. 1995). But in a world saturated with nonspecialist, popular representations of the past (e.g., Auel 1980; Diamond 2005; Gibson 2008; Spielberg 1981), archaeologists who want to present their views to audiences beyond the scholarly and the professional must find creative ways to leap into the fray.

However, imagined narratives are not simply appealing tools for conveying archaeological knowledge to the public. There are compelling political and intellectual reasons for us to stretch ourselves beyond the familiar rhetorical constructions of technical, expository writing. Many archaeologists who have attempted fictional or interpretive narratives have done so explicitly to humanize the past, to sensualize the past, to facilitate multivocality, and to expose the constructed nature of archaeological knowledge. Following the lead of James Gibb (2000), I would add to these aims another reason to write imagined narratives: They can serve as analytical tools that enable archaeologists to think differently about the pasts we study.

### *Multivocality and the Grandmother's Narrative*

One of the great strengths of imagined narratives, and indeed of many experimental forms that push beyond the objective expository text, is that these forms facilitate archaeologists' representation of diverse voices. Often these are voices that are otherwise silent. Imagined narratives can be a way to give voice to subaltern peoples, such as slaves, and women. It is no coincidence that there is a burgeoning archaeological literature in feminist interpretive writing (e.g., Joyce et al. 2000; Joyce and Tringham 2007; Spector 1991, 1993; Tringham 1991).

Yet many archaeologists may feel an inherent reticence in speaking for past peoples. If we imagine voices for subjects in other times and places, are we not actually silencing them by placing our own words in their mouths (Bakhtin 1990:27–36)? Experimental writers in historic archaeology sometimes sidestep this problem by juxtaposing their own words with the words of their subjects, taken from journals, letters, or other literary sources (e.g., Beaudry 1998; Spector 1991, 1993; Yamin 1998), but as these authors are well aware, literary sources speak only for the literate. Reinhard Bernbeck (n.d.) suggests that archaeologists working in ahistoric contexts might do well to emulate Robbe-Grillet's (1957) *nouveau roman*, in which repetitive descriptions of objects reveal the emotions and motivations of unnamed characters. But I would counter the "inappropriate appropriation" critique by arguing that we are already speaking for past peoples when we engage in any form of archaeological representation. Because an imagined first-person narrative is overtly constructed, it actually represents a more transparent authorial hand than does an oblique, ostensibly subjectless narrative.

Archaeological texts are inherently multivocal, whether we acknowledge this fact or not. Employing concepts derived from Bakhtin (1981; Todorov 1984:49–56), Joyce (2002:8–10) suggests that there are at least three voices present in an archaeological (or any) text—those of the speaker/writer, the listener/reader, and the dialogic others who have used the words in the past, thereby imbuing them with meanings that both speakers and listeners can understand. The construction of archaeological texts thus entails dialogue not only between writer and reader but also between writer and other archaeologists past and present, as well as with diverse peoples in the past (e.g., Praetzellis and Praetzellis 1998).

These multivocal, reflexive, nonlinear qualitities are explicit in the work of archaeologists who have created multidimensional Web sites, hypertext through which viewers/readers browse in free play, charting their own pathways through interrelated concepts and voices (e.g., Joyce and Tringham 2007; Lopiparo and Joyce 2003; Metamedia 2010; Shanks 2011; Webmoor 2005). For example, Joyce et al.'s (2000) nonlinear, Web-published *Sister Stories* incorporates Nahuatl voices through the writings of Bernardino de Sahagún, a sixteenth-century Spanish cleric who created the Florentine Codex by compiling the words of male elites at Tenochtitlán.

I chose to initiate the narrative presented above from the perspective of a 10-year-old girl from the Whirlwind outlier because, like my archaeological self, this imaginary girl would have been a relative outsider at Chaco, old enough to undertake the pilgrimage but young enough to have only a naive and partial understanding of the events she witnessed. But it is possible—indeed, desirable—to attempt narratives from a host of different perspectives. In the process, it is possible to think through the gendered, identity-specific experiences of a panoply of players at Chaco. For example, an imagined narrative from the grandmother's perspective might sound something like this:

> So I said to my daughter, I said, why not let me take the girls to Chaco this summer if you don't feel you are up to it, with such a new young baby? The other girls are all old enough to make the journey and they will be good company for me. That is how we came to walk the solstice road together. My footsteps along the path weave my life together with this place, as they echo alongside all the other footsteps from all the other times we passed this way. But how many more times will these legs carry me to Chaco, I wonder? The sand hills seem steeper every year. Eh, but the sun feels good on my bones, and there's a nice breeze keeping the gnats away. Here is the rock overhang where my sister and I were sitting in the shade long ago, in our new reed sandals, snacking on sweet pinyon nuts, when the shell jewelry man passed by. Eh, but he was a beautiful man, almost as beautiful as the bracelets he carried. I wish I knew where that bracelet of mine has got to. It must have broken off my wrist that time I was carrying a water jar over to Red Willow Wash. My mother used to say to me, she'd say, don't wear that bracelet out into the fields, but I sure didn't listen. My sister, of course, she always listened, and she was buried with hers. I sure wish your

> aunty were here now to see all of you girls, so grown up, traveling to Chaco together. Chaco is a grand place, girls—there is great power there, and we must treat it with respect. Not everyone gets to witness the high priests of the center place calling upon the cloud beings and making the rain. I wonder if I will be able to exchange these red dog shale pendants your father made at the fair after the ceremonies—maybe trade them for some turquoise beads, if the turquoise traders come this year. Eh, child, leave that rattlesnake alone—he's not bothering you! He is following his own path across the earth, just as we are. We will stop awhile at the shrine on top of the first bluff along the Chaco Wash, up there at the old village. There's nobody living there now but ancestors, but it is important for us to honor the old ones. Do you have those black-on-white sherds I gave you to carry? When the baby knocked over my best water jar, I said to your mother, I said, we'll keep those pieces. I spent hours with my yucca brush decorating that pot with fine black hachure, and it fired so nice and hard. Those pieces will make a good offering for the old ones, along with a little yellow corn pollen. The ancestors are pleased when they are remembered. So many young people today, they don't keep to the old ways any more. I wonder if you girls will remember to leave offerings for me when I am gone?

With the grandmother's voice, I am imagining the memories, emotions, and physical sensations of an older woman who has made this journey many times over the years. I am attempting to evoke a sense of repetitive, multilayered, bodily engagement with place. This imagined voice contrasts with and complements that of the naive young girl, experiencing everything for the first time and cataloging each day's events in her mind.

### *New Analytical Directions*

Imagined narratives as thought experiments have the potential to be analytical tools that provide us with alternative ways of thinking about, not just representing, the past. I cannot write a narrative from the point of view of a settlement pattern or a potsherd; I can only write from the perspective of a person. And as I try to imagine a series of events in ancient Chaco from the vantage point of human individuals, I must make a host of decisions grounded in what I know. This effort brings into instant, sharp relief the many things I do not know, and raises questions I had not previously thought to ask—questions that can subsequently guide future empirical research.

Table 19-1 summarizes some of the narrative decision points and accompanying research issues associated with the imagined narratives in this chapter. The first column lists a number of decisions I had to make, or questions I had to answer, to construct a first-person narrative. The second column briefly outlines areas where existing archaeological research provides some insights. The third column catalogs poorly explored research topics or new questions that sprang to mind in the context of column 1 decisions. The table is not meant to be comprehensive or exhaustive. Rather, it is meant to demonstrate how constructing an imagined narrative can help nudge the archaeological writer out of learned, prescribed patterns of thought and toward new research.

**Table 19-1.** *How Narrative Decision Points Articulate with Existing Issues and Lead to New Research Questions*

| *Imagined Narrative Question* | *Existing Research Issues and Data* | *New Research Questions* |
|---|---|---|
| From whose perspective do I write? A young girl? A middle-aged man? A grandmother? | ? | How did people of different ages, genders, social standings, and ethnicities experience Chaco differently? |
| Who goes to Chaco? Why am I going? | Outlier residents gathered periodically, perhaps seasonally, in Chaco. | Does everyone in a family, or community, or ritual society go to Chaco? Why or why not? How frequently? |
| With whom do I travel? | ? | Did people travel with relatives, friends, fictive kin, strangers? |
| What items do I bring with me? | Many nonlocal materials were carried to Chaco, for practical as well as votive reasons. | Who carried these materials? |
| What specific route will I follow? | People moved along drainages and along some Chaco road segments, but these do not connect most settlements. | Can we use LIDAR, other remote sensing, and/or ground survey to identify nonroad paths on logical routes? |
| How long will it take to make the journey? Where will I spend the night? | Why are outliers spaced at 5–10 km intervals along the Chaco River? Are there way stations along roads? | Could an experimental journey on foot answer this question? |
| What relationships do I have to people I encounter along the way? | The distribution of nonlocal materials indicates a low level of interaction among outliers, as opposed to between outliers and Chaco. | Could bioarchaeological studies help identify kinship among outlier populations? |
| When I get to Chaco, where will I stay? | Roasting pits and trash deposits suggest large, periodic influxes of people at one excavated great house (Pueblo Alto). | Could remote sensing in unexcavated great house plazas shed light on this?* |
| How long do gatherings at Chaco last? | Ethnographic evidence suggests at least several days, probably longer for those participating in key roles. | Can we come up with some creative way to measure this? |
| What will I get to experience, see, hear about, and do? With whom, and why? | Ethnographic and archaeological evidence suggests hierarchical, differential access to ritual events. | What is the capacity of various potential public spaces (great house plazas, great kivas, kivas)? |

* Currently, Chaco Culture National Historical Park policies favor nondestructive, noninvasive investigations such as remote sensing; new excavations are not particularly feasible.

The nature of the social and political relationship between outliers and Chaco Canyon is a major topic of debate and likely varied considerably across time and space (Kantner 2003; Kantner and Mahoney 2000; Van Dyke 1999). Chaco scholars have no definitive answers for the question of which outlier residents made visits to the canyon and in what specific social contexts. Some of the questions raised in column 3 may not be answerable, but others could lead directly to new field projects.

My imagined narrative for the young girl's pilgrimage with her grandmother is plausible and fits with existing data, but it is not the only possible nor, indeed, the only likely experience. I can use imagined scenarios to explore multiple possibilities. For example, what if, rather than extended families of both genders and all ages, only elite male community leaders made the pilgrimage to Chaco? As I construct and consider alternative scenarios, I am refining multiple possible interpretations, and I am gaining insights into new ways to collect and utilize material information to address these questions. In these ways, imagined narratives can become a powerful tool for analysis.

## Conclusion

Imagined narratives have the power to take us out of the two-dimensional world of data and interpretation and into the three-dimensional world of sensory lives, bringing us closer to human somatic experiences in the past and allowing us to explore territory beyond the flat landscape of generalizing patterns. The writer of imagined narratives can give voice to multiple perspectives, emphasizing the interplay and differences among past peoples' experiences, roles, genders, ages, statuses, ethnicities, and occupations. And imagined narratives can be useful tools to help us recharge our analyses and interpretations.

Our choice of prose styles affects the way we think about the past (e.g., Clifford and Marcus 1986; LaTour 1986; Shanks 1997; Shanks and Tilley 1987a, 1987b). Traditionally, we archaeologists have constructed our arguments through expository texts supported with images. But relationships among ideas and representations are not limited to specific formats, nor are our choices regarding these relationships ever innocent. The third-person passive style we commonly employ obscures the role of the archaeologist in constructing knowledge, and it keeps the peoples of the past at a safe and unknowable distance (Joyce 2002; Plucienník 1999). The third-person passive denies agency to past peoples, as material remains become self-evident references to monolithic meanings and events. In the cognitive environment created by expository texts, some questions, but not others, may be legitimately raised by archaeologists.

By contrast, first-person narratives bring past peoples sharply (perhaps uncomfortably) into focus, and they expose the constructed nature of archaeological knowledge. Some scholars may be concerned that an interpretive approach of this kind decenters archaeological authority to a troubling degree. But we need not open the door for radical relativism. On the contrary, I envision imagined narratives as a realist, interpretive archaeological method. I do not suggest that we archaeologists should abandon our empirical and deductive tools and methods. Rather, I want to advocate a legitimate, scholarly space for creative, sensory engagement with the peoples who inhabit our constructed pasts.

## Acknowledgments

As I have developed this argument for imagined narratives, I have benefited from constructive criticism, encouragement, and suggestions offered by many people. I especially want to thank Robin Beck, Reinhard Bernbeck, Jo Day, Michael Heckenberger, Scott McEachern, Randy McGuire, Joanne Murphy, Tim Pauketat, Corin Pursell, Susan Pollock, John Robb, Ken Sassaman, Kath Sterling, Jonathan Thomas, Ruth Tringham, and Yannis Hamilakis. Their input has made the paper stronger, but I take full responsibility for the final product.

## References

Auel, Jean M.
1980 *The Clan of the Cave Bear*. Crown, New York.

Avikunthak, Ashish (director)
2001 *Rummaging for Pasts: Excavating Sicily, Digging Bombay*. 27 min. DVD. Available from the author at http://www.avikunthak.com.

Bakhtin, Mikhail M.
1981 *The Dialogic Imagination: Four Essays*. Translated by Caryl Emerson and Michael Holquist, edited by Michael Holmquest. University of Texas Press, Austin.
1990 *Art and Answerability: Early Philosophical Essays by M. M. Bakhtin*. Translated by Vadim Liapunov and Kenneth Brostrom, edited by Michael Holquist and Vadim Liapunov. University of Texas Press, Austin.

Bandelier, Adolf F.
1971 [1916] *The Delight Makers*. Harcourt Brace/Harvest, Orlando.

Barrett, John, and Ilhong Ko
2009 A Phenomenology of Landscape: A Crisis in British Landscape Archaeology. *Journal of Social Archaeology* 9:275–294.

Beaudry, Mary C.
1998 Farm Journal: First Person, Four Voices. *Historical Archaeology* 32:20–33.

Bernbeck, Reinhard
2003 The Ideologies of Intentionality. *Rundbrief der Arbeltsgemeinschaft Theorie en der Archäologie* 2(2):44–50.
2014 From Archaeological Knowledge to Narratives without Subjects. In *Subjects and Narratives in Archaeology*, edited by Ruth M. Van Dyke and Reinhard Bernbeck. University Press of Colorado, Boulder, in press.

Bradley, Francis H.
1914 *Essays on Truth and Reality*. Clarendon, Oxford.

Brück, Joanna
2005 Experiencing the Past? The Development of a Phenomenological Archaeology in British Prehistory. *Archaeological Dialogues* 12:45–72.

Bullard, Mary R., (librettist) and Curtis Bryant (composer)
1999 *Zabette: An Opera in Three Acts*. Performed at the Rialto Center for the Performing Arts, Atlanta, Georgia, April 29–30, 1999.

Casey, Edward S.
1996 How to Get from Space to Place in a Fairly Short Stretch of Time: Phenomenological Prolegomena. In *Senses of Place*, edited by Steven Feld and Keith H. Basso, pp. 13–52. School of American Research Press, Santa Fe.

Clifford, James, and George E. Marcus (editors)
1986 *Writing Culture: The Poetics and Politics of Ethnography*. School for American Research Press, Santa Fe.

Cochrane, Andrew, and Ian Russell
2008 Archaeoclash: Manifesting Art and Archaeology. *Archaeologies of Art: Papers from the Sixth World Archaeological Congress*. UCD Scholarcast Series 2, edited by Ian Russell. Electronic document, http://www.ucd.ie/scholarcast/transcripts/Archaeoclash.pdf, accessed December 27, 2008.

Connerton, Paul
1989 *How Societies Remember*. Cambridge University Press, Cambridge.

Crown, Patricia, and Jeffrey Hurst
2009 Evidence of Cacao Use in the Prehispanic American Southwest. *Proceedings of the National Academy of Sciences of the United States of America* 106:2110–2113.

Crown, Patricia, and Wirt H. Wills
2003 Modifying Pottery and Kivas at Chaco: Pentimento, Restoration, or Renewal? *American Antiquity* 68:511–532.

Cummings, Vicki, Andrew Jones, and Aaron Watson
2002 Divided Places: Phenomenology and Asymmetry in the Monuments of the Black Mountains, Southeast Wales. *Cambridge Archaeological Journal* 12:57–70.

Cummings, Vicki, and Alisdair Whittle
2003 *Places of Special Virtue: Megaliths in the Neolithic Landscape of Wales*. Oxbow Books, Oxford.

Davidson, Donald
1986 A Coherence Theory of Truth and Knowledge. In *Truth and Interpretation, Perspectives on the Philosophy of Donald Davidson*, edited by Ernest LePore, pp. 307–319. Basil Blackwell, Oxford.

De Certeau, Michel
1984 *The Practice of Everyday Life*. Translated by Steven Rendall. University of California Press, Berkeley.

Deetz, James
1977 *In Small Things Forgotten: The Archaeology of Early American Life*. Anchor, Garden City, New Jersey.
1993 *Flowerdew Hundred: The Archaeology of a Virginia Plantation, 1619–1864*. University Press of Virginia, Charlottesville.

Diamond, Jared
2005 *Collapse: How Societies Choose to Fail or Succeed*. Viking Penguin, New York.

Dobres, Marcia-Anne, and John Robb
2000 Agency in Archaeology: Paradigm or Platitude? In *Agency in Archaeology*, edited by Marcia-Anne Dobres and John Robb, pp. 3–17. Routledge, London.

Dornan, Jennifer L.
2002 Agency and Archaeology: Past, Present, and Future Directions. *Journal of Archaeological Method and Theory* 9:303–329.

Edmonds, Mark
1999 *Ancestral Geographies of the Neolithic: Landscape, Monuments, and Memory.* Routledge, London.
Fleming, Andrew
1999 Phenomenology and the Megaliths of Wales: A Dreaming Too Far? *Oxford Journal of Archaeology* 18:119–125.
2005 Megaliths and Post-modernism: The Case of Wales. *Antiquity* 79:921–932.
2006 Post-processual Landscape Archaeology: A Critique. *Cambridge Archaeological Journal* 16:267–280.
Gibb, James
1998 *London Shades: A Play in Three Acts.* Performed in October 1998 and October 1999 at the London Town Historic Site, Edgewater, Maryland.
1999 *Revolutionary Spirits: A Play in Two Acts.* Performed in April 1999 at the London Town Historic Site, Edgewater, Maryland.
2000 Imaginary, but by No Means Unimagineable: Storytelling, Science, and Historical Archaeology. *Historical Archaeology* 34(2):1–6.
Gibson, Mel (director)
2008 *Apocalypto.* 140 min. DVD, Touchstone Pictures, Los Angeles.
Hamilakis, Yannis
2002 The Past as Oral History: Towards an Archaeology of the Senses. In *Thinking through the Body: Archaeologies of Corporeality,* edited by Yannis Hamilakis, Mark Pluciennik, and Sarah Tarlow, pp. 121–136. Kluwer Academic/Plenum, New York.
Hamilton, Sue, and Ruth Whitehouse
2006 Phenomenology in Practice: Towards a Methodology for a "Subjective" Approach. *European Journal of Archaeology* 9:31–71.
Heidegger, Martin
1962 *Being and Time.* Translated by John Macquarrie and Edward Robinson. Blackwell, Oxford.
Hodder, Ian
1991 *Archaeological Theory in Europe: The Last Three Decades.* Routledge, London.
1999 *The Archaeological Process: An Introduction.* Blackwell, Oxford.
2000 Agency and Individuals in Long-term Processes. In *Agency in Archaeology,* edited by Marcia-Anne Dobres and John Robb, pp. 21–33. Routledge, New York.
Jameson, John H., Jr.
2003 Art and Imagery as Tools for Public Interpretation and Education in Archaeology. In *Ancient Muses: Archaeology and the Arts,* edited by John H. Jameson Jr., John E. Ehrenhard, and Christine A. Finn, pp. 57–64. University of Alabama Press, Tuscaloosa.
Jameson, John H., Jr., John E. Ehrenhard, and Christine A. Finn (editors)
2003 *Ancient Muses: Archaeology and the Arts.* University of Alabama Press, Tuscaloosa.
Joyce, Rosemary A.
2002 *The Languages of Archaeology.* Blackwell, Oxford.
Joyce, Rosemary A., Carolyn Guyer, and Michael Joyce
2000 *Sister Stories.* New York University Press, New York. Electronic document, http://www.nyupress.org/sisterstories, accessed March 14, 2010.
Joyce, Rosemary A., and Ruth Tringham
2007 Feminist Adventures in Hypertext. *Journal of Archaeological Method and Theory* 14:328–358.
Judd, Neil M.
1954 *The Material Culture of Pueblo Bonito.* Smithsonian Miscellaneous Collections 124, Smithsonian Institution, Washington, D.C.

Kantner, John (editor)
2003 The Chaco World. *Kiva* 69(2).
Kantner, John, and Nancy Mahoney (editors)
2000 *Great House Communities across the Chacoan Landscape*. Anthropological Papers of the University of Arizona 65. University of Arizona Press, Tucson.
Laneri, Nicola
2003 Is Archaeology Fiction? Some Thoughts about Experimental Ways of Communicating Archaeological Processes to the "External World." In *Ancient Muses: Archaeology and the Arts*, edited by John H. Jameson Jr., John E. Ehrenhard, and Christine A. Finn, pp.179–192. University of Alabama Press, Tuscaloosa.
LaTour, Bruno
1986 Visualization and Cognition: Thinking with Eyes and Hands. *Knowledge and Society* 6:1–40.
Lekson, Stephen H.
1999 *The Chaco Meridian: Centers of Political Power in the Ancient Southwest*. AltaMira, Walnut Creek, California.
2008 *A History of the Ancient Southwest*. School for Advanced Research Press, Santa Fe.
Lekson, Stephen H. (editor)
2006 *The Archaeology of Chaco Canyon: An Eleventh-Century Pueblo Regional Center*. School of American Research Press, Santa Fe.
Lekson, Stephen H., and Catherine Cameron
1995 The Abandonment of Chaco Canyon, the Mesa Verde Migrations, and the Reorganization of the Pueblo World. *Journal of Anthropological Archaeology* 14:184–202.
Leone, Mark
1995 Can an African American Historical Archaeology Be an Alternative Voice? With Paul Mullins, Marian C. Creveling, Laurence Hurst, Barbara Jackson-Nash, Lynn Jones, Hannah Kaiser, George Logan, and Mark Warner. In *Interpreting Archaeology: Finding Meaning in the Past*, edited by Ian Hodder, Michael Shanks, Alexandra Alexandri, Victor Buchli, John Carman, Jonathan Last, and Gavin Lucas, pp. 110–124. Routledge, London.
Lopiparo, Jeanne, and Rosemary A. Joyce
2003 Crafting Cosmos, Telling Sister Stories, and Exploring Archaeological Knowledge Graphically in Hypertext Environments. In *Ancient Muses: Archaeology and the Arts*, edited by John H. Jameson Jr., John E. Ehrenhard, and Christine A. Finn, pp. 193–203. University of Alabama Press, Tuscaloosa.
McCarthy, John P.
2003 More than Just "Telling the Story": Interpretive Narrative Archaeology. In *Ancient Muses: Archaeology and the Arts,* edited by John H. Jameson Jr., John E. Ehrenhard, and Christine A. Finn, pp. 15–24. University of Alabama Press, Tuscaloosa.
Malville, J. McKim (editor)
2004 *Chimney Rock: The Ultimate Outlier*. Lexington Books, Lanham, Maryland.
Masson, Pierre, and Hélène Guillot
1994 Archeofiction with Upper Primary-School Children, 1988–1989. In *The Presented Past: Heritage, Museums, and Education*, edited by Peter G. Stone and Brian L. Molyneaux, pp. 375–383. Routledge, London.
Merleau-Ponty, Maurice
1962 [1981] *Phenomenology of Perception*. Translated by Colin Smith. Routledge, London.
Metamedia: A Collaboratory at Stanford University
2010 Electronic document, http://metamedia.stanford.edu, accessed March 15, 2010.

Mills, Barbara J.

2004 The Establishment and Defeat of Hierarchy: Inalienable Possessions and the History of Collective Prestige Structures in the Puebloan Southwest. *American Anthropologist* 106:238–251.

2008 Remembering While Forgetting: Depositional Practices and Social Memory at Chaco. In *Memory Work: Archaeologies of Material Practices*, edited by Barbara J. Mills and William H. Walker, pp. 81–108. School of Advanced Research Press, Santa Fe.

Nelson, Sarah M.

1999 *Spirit Bird Journey*. RKLOG Press, Littleton, Colorado.

2004 *Jade Dragon*. RKLOG Press, Littleton, Colorado.

Pearson, Mike, and Michael Shanks

2001 *Theatre/Archaeology*. Routledge, London.

Pepper, George H.

1909 The Exploration of a Burial Room in Pueblo Bonito, New Mexico. In *Anthropological Essays Presented to Frederick Ward Putnam in Honor of His Seventieth Birthday*, pp. 196–252. G. E. Stechert, New York.

1920 *Pueblo Bonito*. Anthropological Papers Vol. 27. American Museum of Natural History, New York.

Plog, Stephen, and Julie P. Solometo

1997 The Never-Changing and the Ever-Changing: The Evolution of Western Pueblo Ritual. *Cambridge Archaeological Journal* 7:161–182.

Pluciennik, Mark

1999 Archaeological Narratives and Other Ways of Telling. *Current Anthropology* 40:653–678.

Praetzellis, Adrian, and Mary Praetzellis

1998 A Connecticut Merchant in Chinadom: A Play in One Act. *Historical Archaeology* 32(1):1–3.

Praetzellis, Adrian, Grace H. Ziesing, and Mary Praetzellis

1997 *Los Vaqueros Final Project Report: 5. Tales of the Vasco*. Anthropological Studies Center, Sonoma State University Foundation, Rohnert Park, California.

Praetzellis, Mary (editor)

1998 Archaeologists as Storytellers. *Historical Archaeology* 32(1).

Renfrew, Colin

2003 *Figuring It Out: What Are We? Where Do We Come From? The Parallel Visions of Artists and Archaeologists*. Thames & Hudson, London.

Robbe-Grillet, Alain

1957 *La Jalousie*. Éditions de Minuit, Paris.

Ryzewski, Krysta (editor)

2009 Experiences, Modes of Engagement, Archaeology. Theme Issue, Archaeologies. *Journal of the World Archaeological Congress* 5(3).

Sebastian, Lynne

1992 *The Chaco Anasazi: Sociopolitical Evolution in the Prehistoric Southwest*. Cambridge University Press, Cambridge.

Shanks, Michael

1997 Photography and Archaeology. In *The Cultural Life of Images: Visual Representation in Archaeology*, edited by Brian L. Molyneaux, pp. 73–107. Routledge, London.

2011 *The Archaeological Imagination*. Left Coast, Walnut Creek, California.

Shanks, Michael, and Randall H. McGuire

1996 The Craft of Archaeology. *American Antiquity* 61:75–88.

Shanks, Michael, and Christopher Tilley
1987a *Re-constructing Archaeology: Theory and Practice*. Cambridge University Press, Cambridge.
1987b *Social Theory and Archaeology*. Polity, Cambridge.
Sofaer, Anna
2007 *Chaco Astronomy: An Ancient American Cosmology*. Ocean Tree Books, Santa Fe.
Spector, Janet
1991 What This Awl Means: Toward a Feminist Archaeology. In *Engendering Archaeology*, edited by Joan M. Gero and Margaret Conkey, pp. 388–406. Blackwell, Oxford.
1993 *What This Awl Means: Feminist Archaeology at Wahpeton Dakota Village*. Minnesota Historical Society, St. Paul.
Spielberg, Steven (director)
1981 *Raiders of the Lost Ark*. 115 min. DVD, Paramount Pictures, Los Angeles.
Thomas, Julian
1996 *Time, Culture, and Identity*. Routledge, London.
2004 *Archaeology and Modernity*. Routledge, London.
Tilley, Christopher
1994 *A Phenomenology of Landscape*. Berg, Oxford.
2004 *The Materiality of Stone: Explorations in Landscape Phenomenology*. Berg, Oxford.
2008 *Body and Image: Explorations in Landscape Phenomenology 2*. Left Coast, Walnut Creek, California.
Todorov, Tzvetan
1984 *Mikhail Bakhtin: The Dialogical Principle*. Translated by Wlad Godzich. University of Minnesota Press, Minneapolis.
Toll, H. Wolcott
1985 Pottery, Production, and the Chacoan Anasazi System. Ph.D. dissertation, Department of Anthropology, University of Colorado, Boulder.
2001 Making and Breaking Pots in the Chaco World. *American Antiquity* 66:56–78.
Tringham, Ruth
1991 Households with Faces: The Challenge of Gender in Prehistoric Architectural Remains. In *Engendering Archaeology: Women and Prehistory*, edited by Joan Gero and Margaret Conkey, pp. 93–131. Blackwell, Oxford.
Van Dyke, Ruth M.
1999 The Chaco Connection: Evaluating Bonito-Style Architecture in Outlier Communities. *Journal of Anthropological Archaeology* 18:471–506.
2004 Memory, Meaning, and Masonry: The Late Bonito Chacoan Landscape. *American Antiquity* 69:413–431.
2007 *The Chaco Experience: Landscape and Ideology at the Center Place*. School for Advanced Research Press, Santa Fe.
2011 Anchoring Identities: Iconic Landforms across San Juan Time and Space. In *Changing Histories, Landscapes, and Perspectives: The Twentieth Anniversary Southwest Symposium*, edited by Margaret C. Nelson and Colleen A. Strawhacker, pp. 403–422. University Press of Colorado, Boulder.
2012 Ritual, Timelessness, and Lived Experience in the Pueblo World. In *Big Histories, Human Lives: Tackling Problems of Scale in Archaeology*, edited by John Robb and Timothy Pauketat, pp. 193–206. School of Advanced Research Press, Santa Fe.
Varien, Mark D., and James M. Potter (editors)
2008 *The Social Construction of Communities: Agency, Structure and Identity in the Prehispanic Southwest*. Altamira, Walnut Creek, California.

Vilches, Flora
2007 The Art of Archaeology: Mark Dion and His Dig Projects. *Journal of Social Archaeology* 7:199–223.
Vivian, R. Gordon, and Paul Reiter
1960 *The Great Kivas of Chaco Canyon and Their Relationships*. Monographs of the School of American Research and the Museum of New Mexico, No. 22, Santa Fe.
Vivian, R. Gwinn, Dulce N. Dodgen, and Gayle H. Hartman
1978 *Wooden Ritual Artifacts from Chaco Canyon, New Mexico*. Anthropological Papers Vol. 32. University of Arizona Press, Tucson.
Webmoor, Timothy
2005 Mediational Techniques and Conceptual Frameworks in Archaeology: A Model in "Mapwork" at Teotihuacan, Mexico. *Journal of Social Archaeology* 5:52–84.
Webster, Laurie
2011 Perishable Ritual Artifacts at the West Ruin of Aztec, New Mexico: Evidence for a Chacoan Migration. *Kiva* 77:139–172.
Windes, Thomas C.
1987 *Investigations at the Pueblo Alto Complex, Chaco Canyon, New Mexico, 1975–1979* Vols. I and II, Pts. 1 and 2. Chaco Canyon Studies, Publications in Archeology No. 18F, National Park Service, Santa Fe.
Witmore, Christopher L.
2005 Four Archaeological Engagements with Place: Mediating Bodily Experience through Peripatetic Video. *Visual Anthropology Review* 20:57–71.
Yamin, Rebecca
1998 Lurid Tales and Homely Stories of New York's Notorious Five Points. *Historical Archaeology* 32(1):74–85.
2008 *Digging in the City of Brotherly Love: Stories from Philadelphia Archaeology*. Yale University Press, New Haven.

# 20. Afterword: Eleven Theses on the Archaeology of the Senses

*Yannis Hamilakis*

## I

An archaeology of the senses is an impossible task. By this I mean that it is both unattainable and futile to attempt to produce a new subfield, in the same way that we have an archaeology of food, of death, of texts and documents, of pottery, and so on. This is not only because the senses occupy a different ontological ground in comparison with the kinds of materials and social practices and phenomena that are at the center of customary archaeological endeavor; it is also because to attach the research field of the "senses" to an accepted disciplinary category that we call "archaeology," in other words to continue practicing "archaeology" as usual following the same norms and the same ontological and epistemological principles, and to expect to derive new, more "truthful" and more valid insights into the past would be a fallacy. It would soon lead to triviality, disappointment, and abandonment of the whole endeavor; the search for novel, trendier, and perhaps seemingly more "feasible" approaches would soon commence.

## II

Archaeologies of the senses are, however, not only possible but also essential and feasible, not as representations of the past but as evocations of its materiality, contingency, and (multi)temporality, not as mimetic exercises or reconstructions but as explorations of the range of sensorial possibilities and affordances. The rich and insightful papers contained in this important volume testify to it. Sensorial experience produces place and materiality (cf. Williams, this volume) but at the same time relies on materiality in order to be set into

*Making Senses of the Past: Toward a Sensory Archaeology,* edited by Jo Day. Center for Archaeological Investigations, Occasional Paper No. 40.  ISBN 978-0-8093-3287-8.

motion. The field of archaeology, having primary access to the materiality of the world through time, is in a privileged position, thus, to explore sensoriality and to contribute to the broader discussion on bodily experience and its social-power effects. The constitution of these archaeologies of the senses, however, requires the reconfiguration of the field of archaeology as a whole. The starting point for an archaeology of the senses should be a dual genealogical inquiry: the interrogation of the researcher's personal sensory and sensuous stratigraphy, his or her sensorial education and socialization into specific modes of embodied interaction and conduct in the world; and the exploration of *ab/senses* in our own scholarly heritage, our socialization and incorporation into the apparatus of a (dis)embodied archaeology, an apparatus that was shaped by Western modernity and its dominant (but often diverse) bodily and sensorial regimes. These two genealogical projects should run in tandem, rather than as isolated exercises. Personal (as well as disciplinary) reflexivity is an essential requirement for an archaeology of the senses (cf. Holmberg, this volume). This excavation of one's sensorial stratigraphy is necessary for many reasons: For a start, in our exploration of the sensoriality of the past, our own bodies are the most important guides and research tools; to unearth and thus expose one's own sensorial education and conduct would be an important act of intellectual honesty and an opportunity for the reader or the intended audience to judge the validity and plausibility of statements. Furthermore, such an in-depth exploration of one's sensorial past could become an important process of instruction, a corporeal education on the links between bodies, senses, memories, and materials. The biographical sensorial knowledge thus gained can prove invaluable for any further attempts to evoke past sensorialities.

## III

The Western intellectuals' inherited Aristotelian heritage, which divides the senses into distinct and finite entities (sight, hearing, touch, smell, taste) and imposes a hierarchy on them (high/low, distant/close, primary/secondary, and so on), is an extremely problematic framework for any archaeology of the senses. As several anthropological studies have shown (e.g., Geurts 2002), this is a Western folk taxonomy, intricately linked to social and racial hierarchies, to logocentrism, to patriarchy, and more recently to capitalist modernity and middle-class values and norms of social engagement. Norbert Elias (1994) has eloquently demonstrated, for example, how sensorial bodily conduct, such as appropriate table manners, was a learned code and an index of upper- and middle-class respectability and distinction. Certain archaeological attempts, which implicitly adopt this Western sensorium, place one isolated sense at the center of their inquiry, often for purely heuristic purposes and for methodological convenience. Some of these efforts are successful in evoking specific sensorial experiences of the past, but their de facto emphasis on distinct and often autonomous sensorial interactions reproduces static, mechanistic, and often modernistic discourses. All sensorial experience is synesthetic; it is activated and enacted by the merging of different sensory modalities (cf. Avery; Hunter-Crawley; Day; Pursell; Ryzewski; Weddle; and others, this volume).

Michel Serres, one of the most interesting contemporary philosophers who has dealt with the senses, chose to grapple with this conundrum, the perception of the senses as distinct and finite, in an interesting and rather ironic manner: He titled his book *The Five Senses* (2008 [1985]), but then he held a surprise for the unsuspecting reader. His five chapters do not deal with the five distinct Aristotelian senses, although they do address some of them in an indirect manner. In the first chapter, "Veils," one would expect a discussion on vision, yet he discusses touch and skin and tattoos, in an attempt to evoke not a sense in the abstract but the act of reaching out, of being in contact, of relating to the world through the largest bodily organ (cf. Connor 2004). It is this centrality of fully embodied tactility that is also foregrounded by several authors in this volume, most notably by Tringham. In Serres's second chapter, "Boxes," he talks about audibility and sound ("Before making sense, language makes noise," [2008:120]), but in the third, "Tables," he offers a combined discussion on eating and drinking, on smell and taste (and of course, on memory). The fourth chapter is the one devoted to vision, but it is telling that he chose to call it "Visit" instead. With this he did not simply want to point to the etymological connection between the word for seeing and the word for going somewhere (cf. Connor 2008). More important, he wanted to reinstate vision as inseparable from movement. The five senses were exhausted with one chapter to go, hence his decision to call the final one "Joy" in order to invite us to place at our center of attention the living body but also to make space for all other sensory modalities that are not covered by the taxonomy of the Western sensorium (temperature? movement? balance? . . . ). The senses are infinite, and their isolation, taxonomic classification, and separation from the acting, moving body or, to be more precise, the multisensorial, corporeal-material experiential field are doomed to failure.

## IV

The human individual, especially as perceived and enacted in Western capitalist modernity, is not the most appropriate unit of analysis for an archaeology of the senses. This is not only because, as anthropological accounts have shown, human persons can be conceptualized and embodied in diverse ways: at times as indivisible and autonomous entities, at other times as dividuated/fractal ones, part of social collectives and constantly in motion and circulation as part of sets and networks. More important, such an analytical category is inappropriate because sensorial experience is activated at the moment of a trans-corporeal encounter; this is an encounter among human bodies, between human bodies and the bodies of other beings, and between human bodies and objects, things, and environments. Sensoriality takes place in a trans-corporeal landscape, and it is that process of trans-corporeal sensorial experience that should form the unit of analysis, not a singularized, individualized human (or other) body. This is what Michael Serres tried to evoke when he put as the subtitle of his book "A Philosophy of *Mingled* Bodies" (italics added). To put it another way (and combining theses III and IV), neither the designation of individual senses nor the analytical separation of the "body" (whether it be of a human, of an animal, or of an object) constitutes an adequate starting point for an archaeology of the senses. Rather we should proceed by defining and understanding the field of trans-corporeal sensorial relationships, a field that is produced by the materiality and agency of mingled corporeal beings, objects, things, and environments.

This has been one of the major flaws of approaches such as landscape phenomenology, as practiced in the study of British prehistory, for example (e.g., Tilley 1994, 2004). It attempted to reconstruct sensorial experience from the point of view of the singular observer-wanderer who experiences natural features or megalithic monuments. As such, not only did it project the modernist notion of personhood into prehistory, but it also operated within the Cartesian subject/object dichotomy whereby the solitary observer/subject perceives and experiences a monument or a hill/object. Even if we assume, however, that such an observer was in prehistory wandering in the landscape on his or her own (as the modern archaeologist-phenomenologist does), the corporeal contact with the land, the rocks, the monuments, other nonhuman beings, the weather, and the horizon would have produced a continuous field, a relationship, a sensorial common ground that transcended the bounded individual.

## V

Archaeologies of the senses have to confront the ocular-centricity of the discipline. They will have to point to the paradoxical situation of an intensely physical craft (one based, for example, on handling, closely observing, and drawing/photographing material things, and even tasting sediments to determine their texture and composition) that was nevertheless construed by dominant discourses and practices as an exhibitionary apparatus of Western modernity (cf. Bennett 1988; Hamilakis 2007); an apparatus that very often transforms the physicality of past objects into bloodless and soulless narratives, abstract sequences and typologies, and disembodied museum exhibits destined to be appreciated exclusively by the sense of autonomous vision. But our battle with this modernist heritage will have to point out that our enemy is not vision per se; it is, rather, the de-corporealization of vision, its divorce from all other sensory modalities. It will also have to remind that, in fact, even within the Western sensorium, vision was not autonomous and disembodied: For example, as part of the ancient Greek and medieval/Byzantine sense of extramission, it was thought that the eyes could emit as well as receive rays of light (cf. Hamilakis 2011a; Hunter-Crawley, this volume). They could touch objects, producing thus a tactile sense of vision. There are countless examples that can demonstrate the multisensorial character of what we tend to classify as primarily visual phenomena: Icons in Byzantine churches were/are not merely visual representations of saints but objects that would be/are experienced through tactile vision and through touch itself—they could be kissed—and were/are infused with incense and decorated with flowers, thus producing additional olfactory experiences. Likewise, both the figures in the icons and more so the figures in wall paintings lit by the flickering light of the candles were perceived as moving (cf. Pentcheva 2006). To cite another example, film theorists such as Michel Chion (1994) have coined the term *audio-vision* to describe the synesthetic experience of film audiences who see the moving image on the screen and at the same time phenomenologically experience sound coming out of that same screen. Our laudable desire to reinstate other sensory modalities that have been obscured by the dominance of disembodied vision should not thus lead us to produce a series of separate archaeologies of hearing, smell, touch, and so on (cf. Ingold 2000), especially since senses are infinite, but instead to demonstrate the mingled and synesthetic character of all sensorial experience. In that effort, we should recall Serres's link between seeing and movement (see above) and accept that all sensorial interaction is an *encounter in motion*, all human experience is kinesthetic, as well as synesthetic (cf. papers in Ingold and Vergunst 2008).

## VI

"Perception is never a mere contact of the mind with the object present; it is impregnated with memory-images which complete it as they interpret it," says the early phenomenologist Henri Bergson (1991:133), and elsewhere he notes that "there is no perception which is not full of memories (1991:33). The archaeologies of the senses cannot be developed separately from the archaeologies of remembering and forgetting. All archaeology is engaged in the re-collecting of fragments of materiality, and as such it is a mnemonic practice (cf. Hamilakis 2010). But the connection between the archaeologies of the senses and memory is much closer, more direct, and thus more fundamental. If remembering and forgetting are primarily collective experiences (cf. Connerton 1989; Halbwachs 1992), then these experiences are generated through trans-corporeal sensorial interactions such as commensal events (recall feasts and other convivial eating and drinking events), embodied rituals and performances, habitual synesthetic and kinesthetic routines. Memory is a collective meta-sense that activates and structures time and experience (cf. papers in Seremetakis 1994). The senses are thus the materiality's way of producing remembering and forgetting. Through sensorial experiences, "mnemonic records" are produced: Memories are generated in the bodies of the participants, creating complex and rather messy sensory stratigraphies. These memories are re-collected through repetition and citation, but every such recollection reshuffles these messy mnemonic stratigraphies; every recollection generated through sensorial experience reshapes these memories, casts them anew in a continuous and dynamic process.

If every sensorial experience carries within it the mnemonic weight of countless other experiences, then our attempt to evoke other people's sensorial experiences in the past becomes even more complicated. Phenomenological studies of landscapes by present-day researchers, for example, make the implicit assumption that what the researchers experience, often for the first time, would loosely correspond to the experiences of past people, forgetting thus that these past sensorial experiences would have been infused with people's memories, memories that would have shaped that sensorial experience. The same applies to the contemporary researcher, of course, which makes the interrogation of his or her own mnemonic biography and stratigraphy even more important.

## VII

Archaeologies of the senses are also archaeologies of affect. The transcorporeal sensorial field is at the same time an affective field, a field where emotions are generated or rather affective interactions and relationships are being produced, reiterated, and recollected. One only needs to recall the affective relationships and memories produced through eating and drinking with others or the emotional and affective impact of powerful and highly evocative works of art or reflect on the connotations of English words for tactility ("I was touched by her kindness"). A natural history of the senses is a fallacy, not only because of the socially and culturally mediated nature of sensorial experience, but also because such a natural history devoid of mnemonic and affective interactions leads to mechanistic and static narratives inscribed into the dominant Cartesian mind/body dichotomy. That is why attempts by computer scientists to replicate sensorial experiences by electronic, mechanical, and biochemical means are doomed to fail.

Take, for example, the device called the virtual cocoon, which was launched in 2009 and hailed by its inventors and by the press as a machine that could mimic "all five senses and make the virtual world as convincing as real life" (Derbyshire 2009). The inventors of this device, Alan Chalmers and Eva Zanyi, in an article entitled "Real Virtuality: Emerging Technology for Virtually Re-creating Reality" (2009), suggest that virtual reality has promised much and until now delivered relatively little, hence the need to move to the concept of real virtuality instead, which the virtual cocoon is an embodiment of. They hail this as a major step-change of immense potential. For example, in education, they claim, the applications are many: "re-creating the past, such as experiencing a full multisensory ancient Rome during history or Latin lessons" or "experiencing the world by, for example, visiting a café in France while remaining in the classroom in the UK" (Chalmers and Zanyi 2009:17). The device itself is a helmet that connects wirelessly to a computer that feeds it information on the specific locale of the real world that you wish to visit virtually or a virtual reality altogether. It features a high-definition screen and it is connected, through a tube, to a box of chemicals that are released into your nose to produce the sense of smell; a similar tube can spray flavors directly into your mouth to provide a taste sensation. The heat and humidity can be regulated using a fan and a heater and so on.

Claims such as these, of course, have been pronounced many times in the past by several inventors of mimetic devices. Apart from the science-fiction "time travel" machines, one can recall the mid late-nineteenth- and early twentieth-century excitement over the invention of the stereoscope and the stereograph. Their inventors, too, believed that through the illusion of three-dimensionality that these devices produced and the total immersion they demanded, the viewer could be transported to other places and other times, without moving from his or her living room (cf. Malin 2007). Yet the device proved short-lived and never delivered on the hype it generated. For how can we claim to mimic, through a static, isolated body, the sensorial experience of another time and another place without the affective and mnemonic weight that a lived experience of such a place and time generates on moving, mingled bodies? These mimetic exercises will, of course, produce their own distinctive mnemonic and possibly affective traces, but their relationship to the destination of the intended "sensorial travel" would be tangential, to say the least.

## VIII

The sensorial field is also a field of power, a terrain of contestations. The Foucaultian concept of biopolitics (as outlined in the first volume of his *History of Sexuality* [1998], for example) has attempted to capture the intersection between the body and the regimes of power and authority especially in Western modernity, although its emphasis on constraining and subjugating power has limited its potential. The same author has also shown, among others, the power effects of vision as surveillance, and other critics with Guy Debord (1995) as the most prominent have demonstrated the immense power inherent in the obverse side of surveillance that is the spectacle. But it is another, more recent theoretician, Jacque Rancière, who has produced some of the most interesting insights on the matter (2004). In his treatment of the field of aesthetics, not as an abstract philosophical academic specialization that it has become, but as the arena of sensorial experience (from the ancient Greek word for sense, *aesthesis*), he claims that aesthetics and politics share the same ontological ground; they are both about *the distribution of the sensible*: what is allowed to be sensed and experienced and what is not, what is deemed appropriate or permissible to be sensorially appreciated and embodied and by whom. Moreover, his distinction between *consensus*, that is, established (imposed or tacitly accepted) sensorial order, and *dissensus*, the challenge to that order by posing new and heterodox sensorial regimes, holds great potential for the archaeologies of the senses (see for example, Rancière 2004).

It is in the arena of the politics of vision, for example, that the debates around the location, exhibition logic, and character of the new Acropolis Museum in Athens are played out: the insistence by the authorities on the visual contact of the museum with the site of the Acropolis, but not with the "ugly" modern building blocks, which are blocked out with panels; the suggestion to demolish the art-deco buildings in front of the museum, which are seen as obscuring the view toward the rock, especially since their back, ugly side is visible from the museum; the emphasis on visuality and, at the same time, the prohibition for visitors to take any photos inside the museum. In other words, the authorities in charge of this institution strive to not only direct and guide sensorial experience for all visitors but to also control the dissemination of visual/sensorial traces and mnemonic objects in the form of photographs: Visitors will have to buy the official photographs (postcards, museum photo-guides) sold in the museum shop. In this case, several citizens and urban movements, through protests and court battles, challenged the orthodox, consensual regime and succeeded in rescuing the offending twentieth-century art-deco buildings from demolition, while clandestine photographing takes place inside the museum (cf. Hamilakis 2011b). Such *sensory clashes* are common today: One need only recall the constant debates on the appearance, and thus sensorial reception, of public and civic buildings, monuments, or war memorials. They would have also been common in the past (cf. Dakouri-Hild, this volume). In this volume, Weismantel has eloquently shown the political effects of directed sensoriality (vision as well as movement) through architectural arrangement and the careful positioning of features and objects at the Peruvian site of Chavín de Huantar. The distribution of the sensible in this site would have led to what she calls the "manufacture of wonder," through anticipation, lack of predictability, and surprise (cf. also Mongelluzzo, this volume). Could it be possible, however, that this consensual regime would have been undermined by the inhabitants and visitors to this site, who might have produced their own dissensual experiences?

Sensorially generated and activated bodily memory has its own political economy. Feasting events, for example, derive their immense power not only from the conspicuous generosity of the hosts but also from the intense sensorial and affective experiential effects they instill in the bodies of the participants, effects that will produce strong memories (and perhaps countermemories), which can be recalled and perhaps mobilized and deployed expediently by various aspiring authorities at a later occasion (cf. Hopwood, this volume; Hamilakis 2002). Along with the manufacture of wonder, the manufacture of sensorial remembering (which always involves selective forgetting) is a central feature of many diverse social practices and materialities, from communal eating to olfactory experience (cf. Day; Murphy, this volume), from public rituals and performances to architecture. Yet as with that other mnemonic practice, in archaeology, wherein unanticipated materials and objects can be unearthed, involuntary sensorial and embodied memories can spring up unexpectedly, as Proust so profoundly and elegantly described, and can upset the mnemonic and sensorial consensus.

## IX

The archaeologies of the senses are about presence, not representation. Yet their practitioners still agonize over the most appropriate means through which its results can be conveyed and communicated to peers and the broader publics (cf. Foster; Tringham; Van Dyke; and others, this volume). Such a task will become easier if we move from the archaeologies *of* the senses to archaeologies *with* the senses: if our task reconnects with, acknowledges, and foregrounds its inherent multisensoriality from the beginning, and practices multisensorial archaeology all along, rather than at the stage of communicating the results with others; if the language of research designs and reports, field-recording processes, and teaching practices becomes multisensorial; in other words, if our practices conjure up the presence of the material past and evoke its palpable, corporeal existence. To that effect, experimentation with materials (cf. Thomas, this volume), with all available aesthetic forms (from creative writing and poetry to photography, theater, film, and sculpture, to name but a few), and perhaps more important, the production of hybrid academic, creative media should be the way forward.

## X

The job of the archaeologies of the senses would not have been completed with the production of an evocative and rich narrative of the bodily experiences of people in a specific archaeological-historical context. The act of scholarly reflexivity should come full circle. The power of a sensorial archaeology emanates primarily from its ability to reshape the field of archaeology as a whole, to liberate it from its modernist and objectivist shackles, to reclaim it as a multisensorial-cum-mnemonic practice that can be central in helping us reconfigure our trans-corporeal experiential encounter with materiality and temporality. The theses advocated above, if taken to their logical conclusion, carry implications well beyond the archaeological. Sensoriality as the trans-corporeal mingling of bodies, materials, and environments undermines much more than the body/mind dichotomy. It also dissolves the object/subject and the self/other divides: As sensorially active bodies (as part of a trans-corporeal terrain) reach out and enact multisensorial encounters, as they incorporate food and drink substances that become integral parts of their bodies in a participatory relationship, as they exchange with others not only sensorial experiences but also organic and bodily substances (along with emotions, feelings, and memories), the distinctions between objecthood and subjecthood and between self and other become obsolete. A new ontological ground is created, an affective terrain that is produced at the moment of the sensorial encounter, a moment that can acquire duration through materiality.

As with the archaeology of memory, the archaeologies of the senses open a Pandora's box: They dislodge the foundational logic of our scholarly and broadly social endeavors. It is a daring move, but despite the anticipated challenges it is worth the risk.

## XI

Thesis Eleven is by someone else. It could have been also Thesis One (or his other Thesis Eleven): "The *forming* of the five [*sic*] senses is a labour of the entire history of the world down to the present" (Marx 1975: 302 [1844]).

## Acknowledgments

I am grateful to Jo Day and to the Center for Archaeological Investigations at Southern Illinois University Carbondale for the kind invitation to be part of the symposium on which this volume is based and for their hospitality and care; to Jo again for waiting so patiently for this contribution; and to Costas Papadopoulos (at Southampton University) for educating me on virtual realities and real virtualities.

## References

Bennett, Tony
1988 The Exhibitionary Complex. *New Formations* 4(1):73–102.
Bergson, Henri
1991 *Matter and Memory*. Translated by Nancy Margaret Paul and W. Scott Palmer. Zone, New York.
Chalmers, Alan, and Eva Zanyi
2009 *Real Virtuality: Emerging Technology for Virtually Re-creating Reality*. Becta, Coventry, United Kingdom.
Chion, Michel
1994 [1990] *Audio-Vision: Sound on Screen*. Translated by Claudia Gorbman. Columbia University Press, New York.
Connerton, Paul
1989 *How Societies Remember*. Cambridge University Press, Cambridge.
Connor, Steven
2004 *The Book of Skin*. Reaktion, London.
2008 Introduction. In *The Five Senses: A Philosophy of Mingled Bodies*, by Michel Serres, pp. 1–16. Continuum, London.
Debord, Guy
1995 [1967] *The Society of the Spectacle*. Zone, New York.
Derbyshire, David
2009 Revealed: The Headset That Will Mimic All Five Senses and Make the Virtual World as Convincing as Real Life. Electronic document, http://www.dailymail.co.uk/sciencetech/article-1159206/The-headset-mimic-senses-make-virtual-world-convincing-real-life.html, accessed 20 July 2012.
Elias, Norbert
1994 [1939] *The Civilizing Process*. Translated by Edmund Jephcott. Blackwell, Oxford.
Foucault, Michel
1998 [1976] *History of Sexuality: Volume 1, The Will to Knowledge*. Translated by Robert Hurley. Penguin, London.
Geurts, Kathryn Linn
2002 *Culture and the Senses: Bodily Ways of Knowing in an African Community*. University of California Press, Berkeley.
Halbwachs, Maurice
1992 [1952] *On Collective Memory*. Edited, translated, and with an introduction by Lewis A. Coser. Chicago University Press, Chicago.
Hamilakis, Yannis
2002 The Past as Oral History: Towards an Archaeology of the Senses. In *Thinking*

*through the Body: Archaeologies of Corporeality*, edited by Yannis Hamilakis, Mark Pluciennik, and Sarah Tarlow, pp. 121–136. Kluwer/Plenum, New York.

2007 *The Nation and Its Ruins: Antiquity, Archaeology, and National Imagination in Greece*. Oxford University Press, Oxford.

2010 Recollecting the Fragments: Archaeology as Mnemonic Practice. In *Material Mnemonics: Everyday Memory in Prehistoric Europe*, edited by Katina T. Lillios and Vasilis Tsamis, pp. 188–199. Oxbow, Oxford.

2011a Archaeologies of the Senses. In *The Oxford Handbook on the Archaeology of Ritual and Religion*, edited by Tim Insoll, pp. 208–225. Oxford University Press, Oxford.

2011b Museums of Oblivion. *Antiquity* 85:625–629.

Ingold, Tim

2000 Stop, Look and Listen! Vision, Hearing and Human Movement. In *The Perception of the Environment: Essays in Livelihood, Dwelling and Skill*, pp. 243–287. Routledge, London.

Ingold, Tim, and Jo Lee Vergunst (editors)

2008 *Ways of Walking: Ethnography and Practice on Foot*. Ashgate, Aldershot.

Malin, Brent

2007 Looking White and Middle Class: Stereoscopic Imagery and Technology in the Early Twentieth-Century United States. *Quarterly Journal of Speech* 93:403–424.

Marx, Karl

1975 [1844] Economic and Philosophical Manuscripts of 1844. In Marx, Karl and Engels, Friedrich, *Collected Works*, Vol. 3, pp. 231–246. International, New York.

Pentcheva, Bissera V.

2006 The Performative Icon. *Art Bulletin* 88:631–655.

Rancière, Jacques

2004 *The Politics of Aesthetics: The Distribution of the Sensible*. Translated by Gabriel Rockhill. Continuum, London.

Seremetakis, Nadia C. (editor)

1994 *The Senses Still: Perception and Memory as Material Culture in Modernity*. University of Chicago Press, Chicago.

Serres, Michel

2008 [1985] *The Five Senses: A Philosophy of Mingled Bodies*. Translated by Margaret Sankey and Peter Cowley. Continuum, London.

Tilley, Chris

1994 *A Phenomenology of Landscape*. Berg, Oxford.

2004 *The Materiality of Stone*. Berg, Oxford.

# Contributors

*William A. Allen* is a researcher at Heritage One, Burk's Falls, Ontario, Canada.

*Emerson Avery* is a Ph.D. candidate in the Graduate Group of the Art and Archaeology of the Mediterranean World, University of Pennsylvania, Philadelphia.

*Anastasia Dakouri-Hild* is visiting assistant professor, McIntire Department of Art, University of Virginia, Charlottesville.

*Jo Day* is a lecturer in classical archaeology and a curator in the Classical Museum, Department of Classics, University College Dublin, Ireland.

*Perry T. Fletcher* is an archaeological and a historical consultant in Taupō, New Zealand.

*Catherine P. Foster* is co-executive director of the Ancient Middle East Education and Research Institute, Oakland, California.

*Yannis Hamilakis* is professor of archaeology at the University of Southampton, United Kingdom.

*Karen Holmberg* is a lecturer at the Stanford Archaeological Center, Stanford University, Stanford, California.

*Marie Hopwood* is a visiting assistant professor at Central College, Pella, Iowa.

*Heather Hunter-Crawley* is a Ph.D. candidate in the Department of Classics and Ancient History, the University of Bristol, Bristol, United Kingdom.

*Ryan Mongelluzzo* is a lecturer in the Department of Anthropology, University of California–Riverside.

*Joanne M. A. Murphy* is an assistant professor in the Department of Classical Studies, University of North Carolina Greensboro.

*Roger Noganosh* is a Traditional/Cultural Elder of the Magnetawan First Nation in Britt, Ontario, Canada, and a coauthor.

*Gerard O'Regan* (Ngai Tahu tribe) is a Ph.D. candidate in the Anthropology Department at the University of Auckland, Auckland, New Zealand.

*Corin C. O. Pursell* is a Ph.D. candidate in the Department of Anthropology, Southern Illinois University Carbondale.

*Krysta Ryzewski* is an assistant professor in the Department of Anthropology, Wayne State University, Detroit, Michigan.

*Jonathan T. Thomas* is a Ph.D. candidate in the Department of Anthropology, University of Iowa, Iowa City.

*Ruth Tringham* is a professor of the Graduate School in the Department of Anthropology, University of California Berkeley, and the president and creative director of the Center for Digital Archaeology (CoDA).

*Ruth M. Van Dyke* is associate professor in the Department of Anthropology at Binghamton University–SUNY, Binghamton, New York.

*Candace Weddle* is assistant professor of art history at Anderson University, Anderson, South Carolina.

*Mary Weismantel* is the director of gender studies and a professor of anthropology at Northwestern University, Evanston, Illinois.

*Joe Willliams* is a Ph.D. student in the Department of Classical and Archaeological Studies, University of Kent, Canterbury, United Kingdom.

# Index

The letter *n* following a page number denotes an endnote and the letter *t*, a table.


access analysis, 200, 201, 202, 208, 209
acoustic(s), 2, 11; cut out effect and, 101–102; in iron production, 355; Maya, 96; of metal, 354; at rock art sites, 44; at Shiloh, 86. *See also* sound
affordance, 162, 173, 174, 322, 409; kinesthetic, 167; materiality and, 320; tactile, 311; visual, 311
agency, 5, 229, 287, 323, 326, 359, 394, 401, 412; and color, 73; and craftsmanship, 328; and landscape, 7
altered state of consciousness, 12, 20, 43, 299. *See also* hallucinogen; psychotropics
ambrosia, 301
ancestors, 7, 35, 42, 43, 82, 84, 128
apprenticeship, 20, 188; apprentices and, 313, 353
archaeoacoustics, 11–12. *See also* sound
archaeoastronomy, 44, 393
archaeological practice: sensory aspects of, 6, 21, 120, 178, 412, 417
archaeomusicology, 11, 197
Aristotle: and the senses, 4, 50, 51, 62, 410; and craftspeople, 357
aroma. *See* smell
aromatics, 140, 289, 299; blessing of, 276; for deities, 301; in frescoes, 303; in landscape, 300; in perfume manufacture, 251, 252; spices used as, 250, 252, 256, 277, 290, 292, 298, 375; in tombs, 273; trade in, 289, 290
art, 133n10; and archaeology, 55, 377–378, 382, 383, 396; and emotion, 414; and ruler portraits, 96, 102; sensory nature of, 2, 56
art exhibitions, 8, 56, 312, 374, 377, 378
audio-vision, 413
auditory experiences, 36, 109, 118, 138, 165, 171, 173. *See also* sound
awe, 12, 20, 118, 127, 355, 365

balance, 51, 178, 411
banquet. *See* feasting
bells, 169, 216, 379, 380
Benjamin, Walter, 18
body: bodily effects of things, 10, 286; bodily experiences, 2, 62, 128, 359, 399, 410; bodily memory, 14, 15, 300, 416; Christian idea of, 161, 166; and environment, 9, 50, 120, 126, 131, 182, 359; the living, 394, 411, 412; in museums, 374; physical aspect of the, 5, 6, 344, 345, 346; and power, 415; techniques of, 20. *See also* embodiment
burial: at Beth She'an-Scythopolis, 266–280; at Çatalhöyük, 185; cemeteries as heterotopias, 277; at Chaco, 393; Egyptian, 251; Iberian, 336, 337; Minoan, 289, 292; at Mizpah, 375, 376; Mycenaean, 243; Roman, 275; at Shiloh, 70, 82–83, 84

cave: Areni-1, 186; burial in, 337; Kamares, 292; rock art and, 39; sound in, 12, 36, 57; of the Whales, 43
ceramic(s): Aztec, 225; beads, 379; Bell Beaker, 339; at Chavín, 117; cooking vessels, 230, 231, 232, 251, 393; grave goods, 337; Kamares ware, 292; lamp, 270; Mayan, 95, 102, 104; Minoan, 287, 289, 298; mirror plaque, 270; Mississippian, 70; organic residue analysis of, 249; production, 367n3; at Pylos, 253, 254, 256; rattles, 379; relief decoration, 293–296; restricted shapes, 232; sensory interaction, sound of, 113, 237; sensory interaction, tactility of, 286, 293, 374; storage vessels, 231, 232, 233, 234, 251, 274, 278; at Thebes, 315; unguentaria, 273; use alteration, 224, 229, 237
*chaîne opératoire*, 16, 319, 336, 337, 340, 354, 359, 360
Christian: Apocryphal writings, 171; attitudes about the senses, 10, 162, 276; light and spirituality, 164–165, 170; material culture, 160–161; music, 199, 211; odor of sanctity, 301; ritual practice, 162, 168, 172, 173; theologians, 197
color, 6, 323; in craftsmanship, 355, 357, 363; dye and, 164; earth and, 70, 73, 76, 82, 83; on Kamares ware, 292; in mounds, 70, 81; in perfume, 250; symbolism of, 8, 70, 72, 73, 84–85; symbolism of, red as blood, 145; symbolism of, red paint, 57, 270; symbolism of, red in rock art, 32, 33, 37, 39, 40, 42, 45; symbolism of, red as sacred, 37; symbolism of, red stucco, 95. *See also* ochre
commensality, 13, 223, 244, 257, 413. *See also* feasting; meals
consumption: of alcohol, 299; of food, 3, 14, 173, 223–224, 225, 227, 234, 235, 237; of goods, 243, 249, 257, 258, 293, 316; sensory, 354, 365–366
cooking, 3, 237, 279; smells, 226, 235, 299; sounds, 226; vessels, 230, 231, 232, 251, 393. *See also* cuisine; food
craftsmanship, 16, 17, 298, 310, 328; of architect, 92; of artisan, 122, 321; builders and, 130; craftspeople and, 20, 311, 322, 326, 328, 353, 354, 355, 356, 357, 359, 360, 364, 365, 367n1, 368n4; and craft specialization, 243, 249; in Minoan palaces, 287
cuisine, 13, 256. *See also* cooking; food
cultural geography, 124, 178

dancing, 79, 299
Descartes, René, 4, 161; Cartesian mind-body duality, 4, 10, 50, 161, 174, 174n2, 320, 345, 396, 412, 414, 417
digital technologies, 20, 188–189; and touch, 17–18, 188–189, 384. *See also* virtual reality
discourse, 5, 161
drawing: in archaeology 6, 9, 54, 114, 120, 126, 131, 180, 375, 412
drink(ing), 183, 299, 411, 417; and memory, 14, 300, 413, 414; in museums, 374; offerings of, 275; vessels, 225, 274, 290, 293, 298

embodiment, 177, 383; and Christianity, 161, 165, 166, 168, 172; of cognition, 320; of memory, 15, 394, 416; and museums, 377, 378, 384, 412; of practice and experience, 21, 61, 188, 226, 267, 336, 345, 355, 357, 364, 410, 411, 413. *See also* body
emotion: in archaeology, 5, 244, 396, 414; and architecture, 90, 96; and art, 382; and commensality, 257; and food, 237; and material culture, 14, 21, 286, 303n1, 347, 378, 379; in narrative, 376, 377, 381, 395, 399; and smell, 15, 16, 246–248, 253, 289, 299, 302; and vision, 128
ethnography, 3, 248; analogy of, 70, 118, 276, 394; and artists, 377; and autoethnography, 142; and

fieldwork, 21; and museums, 371, 372, 374; record of in archaeology, 46, 82, 129, 182, 376, 400t
etiquette: in museums, 384; of table manners, 410
exchange: in the Eucharist, 166; of gifts, 257, 289; Locard's principle of, 180; networks and, 250, 328; Tennessee river route and, 77
experimental archaeology, 17, 347; replication and, 17, 182, 336, 339–342
extramission, 10, 162, 165, 412

feasting, 13, 223, 238, 255, 299, 413, 416; Aztec, 225; aromatics and perfume at, 244, 256, 257, 258, 259, 289, 302, 303; ceramic sets for, 298, 315; at Chaco, 393; funerary, 275, 279; and identity, 256, 300; Late Antique, 165; in Minoan palaces, 287, 293, 299, 300; and power, 237, 293; and ritual, 300–301; sacrificial banquet and, 148, 153, 301; scene of, 249, 257, 292, 303. *See also* commensality; meals
flavor, 3, 13, 227, 414
flavorings, 57, 234, 298
food, 3, 13, 165, 223, 225, 237, 299, 417; and hierarchy 256; and memory, 14, 226. *See also* cooking; cuisine; feasting
footwear, 186
Foucault, Michel, 277, 280, 415
fragrance. *See* smell

gastronomy: molecular, 3
Geertz, Clifford, 18; thick description of, 18, 336
Gell, Alfred, 311, 321, 326, 339
gender, 224, 395, 398, 401; and food, 222; and space, 214
Geographic Information Systems (GIS), 7, 124
gesture, 183, 229, 379; in craftsmanship, 355–356, 359, 361, 363, 364; ritual, 79; of supplication, 102
gold, 164, 165, 166, 249, 313, 315, 316, 354
grave goods, 272, 275, 337, 393
graves. *See* burial
gustemology, 13

*habitus* 14, 226, 326, 327, 328
Halbwachs, Maurice, 60
hallucinogen, 119, 129. *See also* altered state of consciousness; psychotropics
haptics, 10, 178, 180, 181, 182, 186, 322; digital, 17, 188–189. *See also* tactile; touch
hearing, 3, 5, 21, 50, 58, 97, 357; in museums 371, 384; zone, 201. *See also* auditory experiences; sound
Hegel, Friedrich: on art, 55–56
Heidegger, Martin, 5, 7
hierarchy: sensory, 3, 4, 9, 11, 59, 161, 162, 172, 248, 276, 277, 374, 410 (*see also* ocularcentrism); in ritual, 172; social, and aromatics and perfumes, 254, 300, 302; social, and ceramics, 298; social, and gift giving, 258; social, and feasting, 13, 256; social, in Late Neolithic Iberia, 337; social, at Pylos, 249; social, and spatial restriction, 9, 102, 103; social, Western construct of, 410
Hume, David, 4
hybrid: figures at Chavín, 117, 129; hallucinations, 119; Maya palaces as, 105; media, 417

iconography, 94, 126, 129, 130, 163, 167, 174n2, 287, 296, 302
identity: Christian, 173; and food, 222, 225, 256; and smell 15, 246, 259, 300; and things, 311
incense, 138, 140, 168, 169, 170, 172, 173, 277, 289, 301, 413; burner, 289, 299, 378; censers, 10, 169, 174n8; cone, 303
Ingold, Tim, 178, 179, 184, 186, 359, 360

interoception, 162, 172
interoceptive sensations, 3, 173
ivory, 169, 313

jade, 96
jewelry, 104, 258, 313, 316

Kant, Immanuel, 51, 63
kinesthetic: affordances, 162, 167; experiences, 8, 125, 413; memory, 14; objects, 166, 168, 322; and tactile sense, 178, 179, 184, 344
kivas, 118, 391, 393

landscape, 7, 8, 52, 62, 345, 393; aromatic, 300; art and, 287, 303, 377–378; indigenous understandings of, 7, 33; and movement, 20; sacred, 42, 46; urban, 97, 108, 109; volcanic, 50, 52, 56, 57, 59, 60, 62
landscape archaeology: and phenomenology, 5, 7, 18, 124, 177, 336, 345, 412
light, 8, 9, 33, 36, 39, 44, 45, 166, 173, 240, 270, 279, 374, 413; ambient, 97, 271; brilliance of, 166; Christ as, 171; lamps and, 169, 170, 270, 271, 279, 290, 299, 374; luminous quality of, 323; spiritual attributes and, 42, 164, 166, 167; sunlight as source of, 7, 20, 32, 33, 34, 35, 37, 41, 43, 97; from textile, 255. *See also* mirrors
lightscape, 271, 272
Locke, John, 4

McLuhan, Marshall, 4–5
magic: food as, 226; forging as, 366; fragrances, 301
magnetoreception, 21
Märtens's rule, 74
material culture, 5, 10, 60, 63, 131, 298, 312, 346, 367, 378; Christian, 160–161, 173, 174n1; and cognition, 310, 320; and emotion, 303n1; and memory, 14, 52; in museums, 371, 374; and phenomenology, 345; and social life of things, 16, 237, 311; synesthetic, 15, 287, 299, 302
materiality, 10, 162, 163, 225, 227, 287, 311, 312, 320, 326, 329; archaeology of the senses and, 409, 410, 411, 412, 413, 417
meals, 142, 198, 215, 226, 227, 234, 275, 276, 279, 382
memory, 14, 52, 55, 59, 60, 172, 178, 257, 300, 312, 344, 411; archaeology of, 417; bodily, 8, 14, 15, 301, 416; and color, 73; and craftsmanship, 354; and food, 14, 223, 225, 226, 267, 414; imagined narratives and, 395; past sensorialities and, 410; and perception, 413, 414; and smell, 3, 14, 15, 244, 246–247, 248, 249, 253, 258, 280, 302, 347; social, 50, 59, 60, 63, 394; and time, 413; and vision, 128, 189
Merleau-Ponty, Maurice, 5, 7, 114, 179
middle-range theory, 6
mirrors, 118, 270, 271, 272, 373
mnemonic(s), 14, 344, 347, 413, 414, 415, 417; devices, 169, 338; and feasting, 165, 300; and pain, 342; and smell, 244, 258; texts, 173
movement, 9, 11, 20, 73, 189, 202, 227, 411, 413, 416; through Chavín de Huantar, 122, 124, 125, 126, 128, 130, 131; in craftsmanship, 352, 360, 364; in the Eucharist, 166, 172, 173; goal oriented, 184, 185, 186; through Maya palaces, 96, 97, 98, 99, 100, 101; and sound, 107, 197, 199, 211, 214, 215; and taskscapes, 178, 179, 181, 182, 183. *See also* kinesthetic
museum, 17, 127, 312; of the Acropolis, 415–416; evolution of the, 17, 371, 372–373, 383; multisensory experiences in, 17, 20, 374, 383, 384; narrative in exhibits at, 377, 395, 397; visual emphasis of, 161–162, 371, 412
music, 11, 106, 107, 249, 299, 379; chant and, 118, 172, 199, 211; drumming and, 118, 138; futurist,

196; in monastic life, 199, 210, 211; musical instruments and, 117, 118, 132n1, 138, 140; musicians and, 96; the organ and, 199, 211, 213; in sacrifice, 138, 140, 149, 150, 152; song and, 138, 140, 216, 299, 391. *See also* archaeomusicology
myth, 8, 57, 127, 153

narrative: in archaeology, 18–19, 21, 375–376, 381, 395, 397–401
nationalism: and archaeology, 14
neurophenomenology, 320
New Archaeology, 5, 335
noise, 12, 196–197, 379; ambient, 384. *See also* sound

obsidian, 182, 183, 186, 379
ochre: red, 32, 33, 35, 37, 39, 42
ocularcentrism, 4, 11, 161, 371, 373, 374, 412
odor. *See* smell
offerings: aromatic, 138, 140, 255, 289, 292, 301, 302; ceramics and, 117; to the dead, 275; and power, 156; for protection, 41; supplication gestures and, 102; as thanks, 301; tobacco, 33; votive, 165, 400t; wine, 140. *See also* sacrifice
Oken, Lorenz, 4
olfactory system, 15, 246–247, 289. *See also* smell
Ong, Walter, 4–5
osmologies, 288

pain, 16–17, 178, 182, 342, 344, 347
perception, 3, 21, 51, 114, 129, 321, 322, 384; of color, 72, 323; control of, 70, 90–91, 105, 109; in craftsmanship, 360, 365–366; cross-modal, 15; environmental, 53, 55, 62; of flavor, 3; of landscape, 345; olfactory, 246; of place, 178; of taste, 225; visual, 74, 94, 379
performance, 20, 73, 74, 79, 83, 227, 312, 363, 413, 416; craft production as, 17, 314, 324, 325, 328, 354, 365; and the Eucharist, 172–173; space in Maya palaces, 103, 109
perfume: containers, 273, 290; divine, 173; industry, 244, 249–254, 289; and perfumers, 251, 255; scented oil as, 169–170, 250, 255, 256–257, 289, 299; unguent, 250, 251, 256, 276, 289, 292; unguentaria 273, 274, 275, 278
personhood, 4, 311, 412
phenomenology, 5, 55, 177, 336, 344–345, 394, 413; criticism of, 7, 114, 339, 345, 346, 394, 412; in experimental archaeology, 17, 55, 347; in landscape archaeology, 7, 18, 124, 336, 413–414
pilgrimage, 114, 117, 120, 127, 128, 130, 167, 209, 398, 401
postprocessual archaeology, 5, 55, 347
pottery. *See* ceramics
power, 8, 102, 130, 132, 255, 258, 373, 415; and color, 73, 82; and feasting, 237, 416; and food, 238; of God, 168; royal/elite, 77, 81, 83, 84, 90, 92, 95, 99, 104, 106, 109, 257; and sacrifice, 156; and smell, 244, 255, 258; and sound, 12, 106, 107
prestige goods, 253, 255, 258, 315, 336, 338, 347
processual archaeology, 5, 13, 347, 396
Proust, Marcel, 246, 416; madeleine and, 52; Proustian moment, 14
proxemics, 103, 201
psychotropics, 118, 119, 129, 130, 299; opium, 296. *See also* hallucinogen

quartz, 315, 316, 342
quiet. See *silence*

race: and the senses, 4, 300, 373, 410
replicas, 18, 19, 20, 189, 292, 340, 375
residue analysis, 181, 183, 249, 273, 298
rhythm, 11, 183, 184, 187, 216, 323, 363, 380

ritual, 74, 96, 128, 138, 139, 153, 255, 393, 413, 416; and color, 85, 86; coming-of-age, 128; construction, 73, 77, 82; of the Eucharist, 163, 165, 168, 169, 172; funerary, 72, 267, 275, 290, 292, 337, 347; of Imperial cult (Roman), 140, 148, 150, 152, 157n15; in landscape, 7, 8; in rites of passage, 127; and smell, 140, 248, 280, 289, 301; space, 70, 72, 75, 79, 81, 214, 287
rock art: at Chaco, 393; location of, 7, 40–43, 46; and sound, 8, 12, 36, 44

sacrifice, 137–157; Classical Greece and, 301; during *hajj,* 128; *hekatomb,* 141, 143, 152, 156; Kurban Bayram, 142; *Kourbánia,* 157n5; libation, 140, 275, 276, 292; *vicennalia,* 138–139, 152. *See also* offerings
scent. *See* smell
semiotics, 161, 311, 321, 326; architectural, 201; olfactory, 300
senses: five, 3, 4, 51, 162, 224, 248, 375, 384. *See also* hearing; taste; touch; sight; smell; sound; vision
sensorium, 11, 18, 21, 162, 280, 287, 288, 327; Christian, 161; Classical, 276; Mesoamerican, 302; Western, 3, 410, 411
sensotype, 327
Serres, Michel, 5, 50, 53, 59, 61, 63, 197, 411, 412, 413
shamanism, 43, 60, 129, 130
shell: abalone, 43; beads, 82, 393; conch trumpet, 117, 118, 132n1; mussels 84
sight, 4, 51, 55, 58, 59, 94, 130, 165, 248, 249, 267, 357, 360, 363; in museums, 284, 371, 373. *See also* vision
silence, 12, 55, 96, 196, 197, 198, 201, 208, 209, 210–214, 218
silver, 139, 163, 164, 166, 167, 354
skeuomorph, 296, 316
skill, 188; and craftsmanship, 292, 298, 314, 322, 336, 340, 343, 354, 355, 364, 365; oratorical, 95
skin, 4, 6, 97, 165, 178, 180, 181, 322, 411
smell, 3, 11, 14, 51, 97, 156, 287–288, 299, 384; bad smells and, 15, 16, 17, 20, 168, 252–253, 276, 277, 342; of blood, 144–146, 150, 152, 154, 301; of bodies, 52; of divinity, 168, 174n6, 301; and emotion, 248, 253, 289, 299, 302; of food, 69, 138, 235, 249, 256–257, 280, 299, 301; of herbs and spices, 256, 300, 375, 382; of icons, 413; and identity, 15, 246, 300; of incense, 140; and the Internet, 3, 21; in manufacturing, 342, 347, 355, 357; of manure, 146, 148, 153; and memory, 3, 14, 15, 55, 226, 244, 247, 258, 280, 302; in museums, 372, 375, 382, 384; of perfume manufacture, 244, 252, 254; pheromones and, 151; of slaughter, 144; symbol for, 304; in tombs, 277, 292, 302; virtual, 414; of wool, 149. *See also* olfactory system
smellscape, 15, 289, 345
sound, 11–12, 94, 101, 197, 411; of animals, 143, 215, 216, 217; of blood, 145, 152; in craft production, 322, 343, 355, 357, 359, 367n3; of cutlery, 215, 216; and flavor, 3; of jade, 96; and memory, 55, 178, 226, 344; in museums, 372, 375, 384; of organ, 211, 213; and power, 106–108; and ritual, 118, 138, 139–140, 149; of speech, 70, 165, 166; of vessels, 235, 236–237; of water, 36, 215. *See also* archaeoacoustics; auditory experiences; hearing
soundscape, 12, 118, 345
space syntax theory, 201
specialization: craft, 17, 92, 249, 328, 347, 353, 365; ritual, 127, 130, 132, 151, 153
spirituality, 8, 43, 45, 378, 379

synesthesia, 15, 51, 85, 162, 344; and experience, 410, 413; and material culture, 15, 292, 299, 302, 303

taboo, 13, 222
tactile: experience, 183, 372; and kinesthetic sense, 178, 184, 344; knowledge, 353, 359; materials, 169, 235, 293, 302, 311, 322, 328, 343; museum exhibits, 17, 372–374, 375, 378, 382, 383, 384, 385; vision, 10, 164–165, 173, 412, 413. *See also* haptics; touch
taskscape, 11, 178, 179, 180, 181, 182, 183, 189
taste, 13, 22n1, 50, 224–225, 237, 246, 288, 382, 411; of beverage, 299; elite, 314; and feasts, 85, 249; and memory, 14, 300; in museums, 371, 372, 382, 384; and ritual, 172, 173; and tastescape, 345; and *terroir*, 3; of soil, 113, 412; virtual, 414
temperature, 9, 152, 178, 355, 357, 411
temporality, 179, 183, 417; and color, 70; of sensorium, 327, 409; and smell, 301; of sound, 12, 216–217. *See also* time
textiles, 181, 197, 258, 289, 299, 300, 339; as clothing, 180, 184; haptic experience of, 181; manufacture at Pylos, 250, 254; perfumed, 255, 257
textual evidence, 9, 10, 15, 22n8, 94, 161, 163, 171, 199, 244, 251, 276, 355, 377
texture, 178, 322; of bread, 172; of ceramics, 286, 293; in craft, 355, 357, 363; of food, 227; of rock, 43; of soil, 412
Tilley, Christopher, 6, 18, 336, 345, 382
time, 6, 179, 326, 345, 355, 410; and color, 70, 72; *longue durée,* 50; and memory, 413. *See also* temporality
tomb. *See* burial
topography, 98, 184
touch, 10, 50, 147, 165, 178, 180, 411; in archaeology, 21; in craft production, 322, 343, 357; in museums, 17, 372, 373, 374, 379, 384; and touchscapes, 345; virtual, 17–18, 188, 189. *See also* haptics; tactile
Tringham, Ruth: "faceless blobs," 5, 20, 336, 346, 394

use-wear analysis, 180, 224, 227, 229, 234, 237, 339, 340

viewsheds, 9, 97
violence, 50, 61, 62; natural, 8, 53, 61, 62; and touch deprivation, 178
virtual reality, 3, 21, 189, 384, 414. *See also* digital technologies
visibility, 41, 55, 74, 121–122, 127
vision, 411; and affordance, 311; in archaeology, 6, 7, 21; control of, 79, 98, 106, 127; in craftsmanship, 322; field of, 124; hegemony of, 4, 94, 122, 224, 248, 276, 321, 374, 412; intellectualization of, 4; in perception, 8, 11; politics of, 415; as tactile, 164–165, 412

weapon, 139, 249, 250, 313, 316, 352
weather: climate change and, 53; and rock art, 40, 41, 42, 44; sensory experiences of, 182, 185, 187, 412; and smell, 152, 252; and sound, 217
wine, 140, 163, 166, 167, 172, 173, 251, 273, 298, 315; and press for, 197, 216
writing: in archaeology, 6, 7, 18–19, 21, 61, 223, 396–398, 417. *See also* narrative